WileyPLUS

Macomb Community College Student Registration

To register, you will need your class section URL.
Your class section URL is provided by your instructor. To help you identify your URL, here is the format we use: http://edugen.wileyplus.com/edugen/class/cls (followed by 6 numbers).
The last 6 numbers are unique to your class section.

Enter the section URL in your web browser and bookmark (add to favorites).

Confirm your section details, review the End User License Agreement, click the box next to "I agree to these terms", then click Continue.

Click on the plus sign ➕ **next to one of the 3 registration options:**

➕ I have a Registration Code. What's this?

If you have a registration code, enter your registration code exactly as it appears on your code card and click Continue. If you purchased a *new* textbook *from the MCC campus bookstore*, a code was included.

➕ I want to purchase instant access to WileyPLUS. What's this?

To purchase WileyPLUS with a credit card, (includes entire online version of your textbook), click on "Buy".

➕ I'm not ready to buy, I'd like to use the 14 day Grace Period. What's this?

If you do not have the funds to purchase your course materials yet, (i.e. you are waiting for your Financial Aid) use the Grace Period. You will receive 14 days of free access. Click on "Begin Grace Period".

Complete the steps and create your student account. NOTE: your email address will also be your WileyPLUS login username.

For all 3 options listed above, you will receive a confirmation that you registered successfully.

To immediately access your course materials, click "Access Course Now". For all future access, you can login at www.wileyplus.com

If you prefer to watch a registration video, visit **www.wileyplus.com/register**

If you experience any difficulties, **do not contact your instructor!**
Instead, contact WileyPLUS technical support at
www.wileyplus.com/support

Use the "Live Chat" tab for assistance

Nutrition 1400 Biology

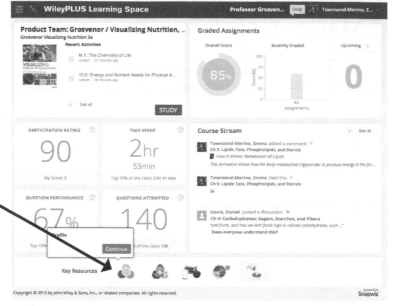

To access the online diet analysis software from your WileyPLUS Learning Space dashboard, click on the iProfile icon and then choose "Continue".

A new window will open to the iProfile home page.
To learn how to use iProfile or to answer any questions that come up during the semester, click on HELP.

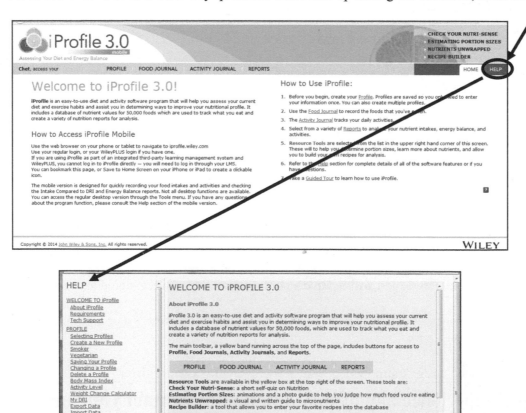

WileyPLUS with ORION

Nutrition: Everyday Choices by Grosvenor 3rd - Custom text for Macomb Community College

Top 7 reasons to use WileyPLUS Learning Space

1. WileyPLUS contains the **entire interactive e-book** – giving you **24/7** access to the text, iProfile, quizzes, and other resources.

2. WileyPLUS contains **iProfile** which will be used for a graded homework assignment.

3. Research shows that WileyPLUS improves student outcomes by as much as **one letter grade.**

4. **Save time and take control of your own learning with ORION.** Use the reports to help you know what to study before a test.

5. **Quiz** yourself with practice questions before exams.

6. Videos and animations are specific to the book – **don't waste your time** Googling topics – these are built right into the e-book and WileyPLUS.

7. ORION Is **FUN** and **EASY** to use!

"Excellent use of graphs to identify what I know and what I do not know. Excellent program!" - Dakota Jackson, Macomb Community College student

WileyPLUS with ORION

DO you want to be prepared for your quizzes, tests, and exams?

**ORION will help you figure out what you
know and what you don't know.
(yes, really!)**

Step 1 – Begin
Making it easy to figure out where to start!

First, ORION asks you to try a few questions so that you get an idea of where you stand.

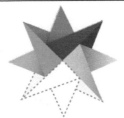

Step 2 – Practice
Making it easy to learn new things!

ORION recommends some options for you, and you pick where to go next.

Step 3 – Maintain
Making it easy to remember everything you learn!

ORION will remind you to go and check back on the things that you have already worked on.

Helping you learn by learning about you.™

Based on Cognitive Science, *WileyPLUS* with ORION provides students with a personal, adaptive learning experience so they can build their proficiency on topics and use their study time most effectively. ORION helps students learn by learning about them.

- Unique to ORION, students **BEGIN** by taking a quick diagnostic for any chapter. This will determine each student's baseline proficiency on each topic in the chapter.

- For each topic, students can either **STUDY** or **PRACTICE**. Study directs students to the specific topic they choose in *WileyPLUS*, where they can read from the e-textbook or use the variety of relevant resources available there. Students can also practice, using questions and feedback powered by ORION's adaptive learning engine. Based on the results of their diagnostic and ongoing practice, ORION presents students with questions appropriate for their current level of understanding and continuously adapts to each student.

- *WileyPLUS* with ORION includes a number of reports and ongoing recommendations for students to help them **MAINTAIN** their proficiency over time for each topic.

Students can easily access ORION from multiple places within *WileyPLUS*. This adaptive learning system does not require any additional registration, and there will not be an additional charge for students.

The questions used for the adaptive practice are numerous and are not found in the *WileyPLUS* assignment area.

I would use this even if my instructor didn't make it required. It would really help me feel more confident going into a test if I spent my time practicing where I was weakest.

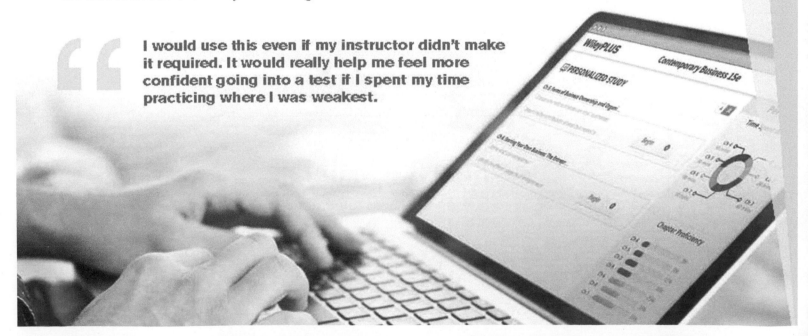

The Student Experience

If you need a boost for studying, need to prepare for a test, or even work ahead, ORION will work with you to help you use your study time quickly and effectively.

Step 1 - Begin

Making it easy to figure out where to start!

First, ORION asks you to try a few questions so that you get an idea of where you stand.

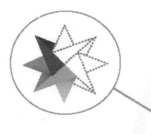

WileyPLUS
ORION Test Version   **Visualiz.**

↩ **Q9** (QId 238392): An order of french fries provides 380 calories ; provides 161 calories and 17 mg of vitamin C. these two foods?

- (A) The french fries are high in nutrient density.
- (B) The french fries are a good source of vitamin C.
- ✓ (C) The baked potato is high in nutrient density.
- (D) Potato products contain a high amount of calories.

Step 2 - Practice

Making it easy to learn new things!

ORION recommends some options for you, and you pick where to go next.

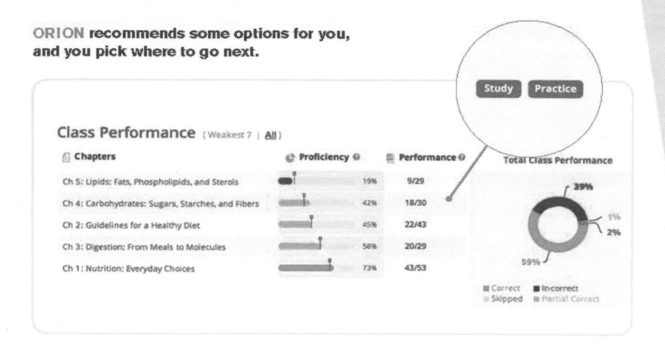

ORION will ask you questions and help you build your proficiency.

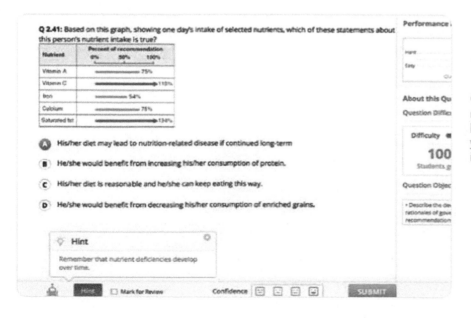

ORION will continuously make adjustments based on how you respond, helping you spend your time where it makes the most sense.

Step 3 - Maintain

Making it easy to remember everything you learn!

ORION will remind you to go and check back on the things that you have already worked on.

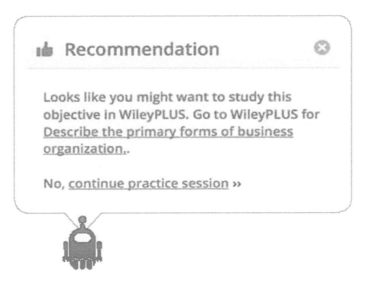

ORION will provide you with a number of views into your overall proficiency so you can quickly review the things you might have forgotten.

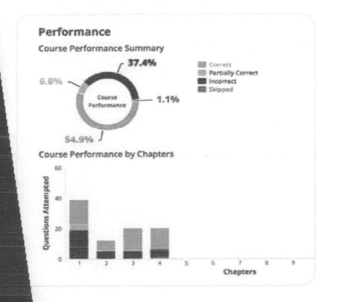

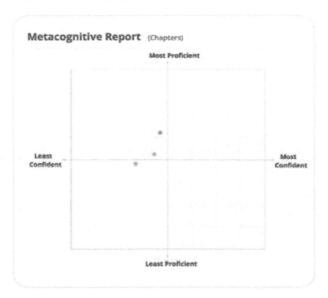

Visualizing Nutrition

Third Edition

MARY B. GROSVENOR • LORI A. SMOLIN

Macomb Community College

Wiley Custom Learning Solutions

Third Edition

VISUALIZING
NUTRITION
EVERYDAY CHOICES

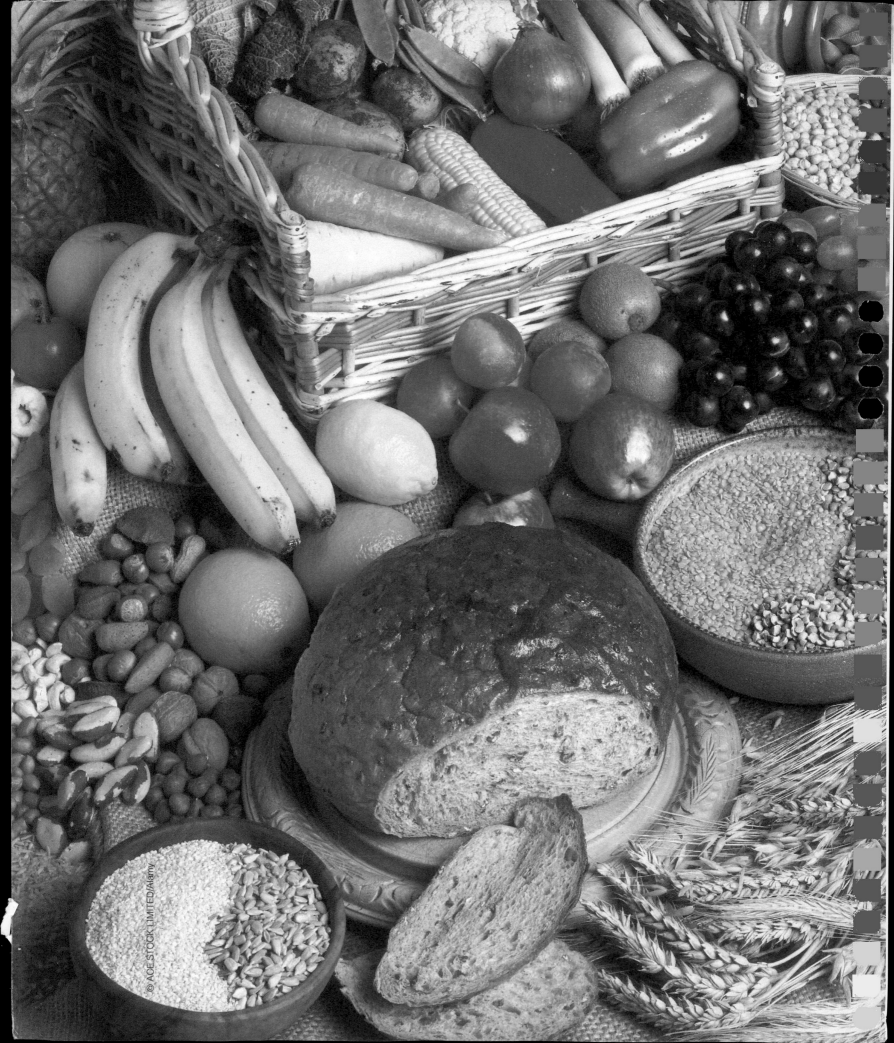

VISUALIZING
NUTRITION
EVERYDAY CHOICES

—————— **Third Edition** ——————

Mary B. Grosvenor, MS, RD

Lori A. Smolin, Ph.D.

University of Connecticut

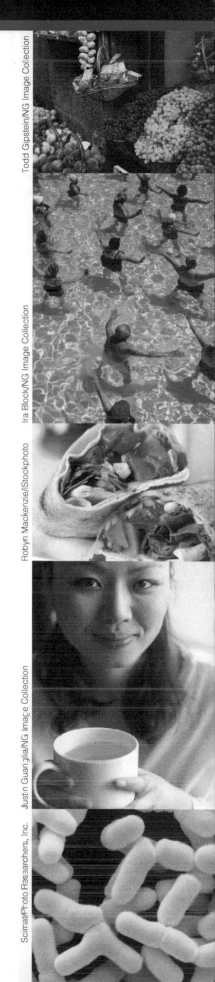

Todd Gipstein/NG Image Collection

Ira Block/NG Image Collection

Robyn Mackenzie/iStockphoto

Justin Guariglia/NG Image Collection

Scimat/Photo Researchers, Inc.

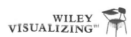

WILEY VISUALIZING™

WILEY

Wiley Visualizing is designed for engaging and effective learning

The visuals and text in *Visualizing Nutrition: Everyday Choices, 3e* are integrated to present complex processes in clear steps, organize information, and integrate related pieces of information with one another. This approach minimizes unproductive cognitive load and helps students engage with the content. When students are engaged, they are reading and learning; this leads to both greater acquisition of knowledge and academic success. Examples of this integration of textual concepts with visual elements include the following:

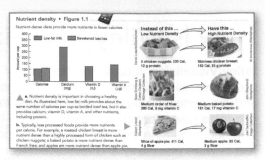

Figure 1: Nutrient density To augment the definition of nutrient density, which appears in the text, this 2-part figure integrates a graphical depiction of the concept of nutrient density with a photographic illustration. The arrows visually guide students to the more nutrient dense choice while captions add specific information about the nutrient density of each food.

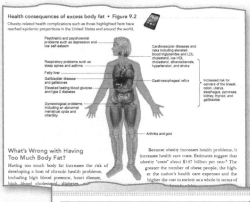

Figure 2: Health consequences of excess body fat This visual overview enhances learning by visually relating the health conditions associated with obesity to the area of the body affected. Organizing the list of health conditions and their effects reduces cognitive load.

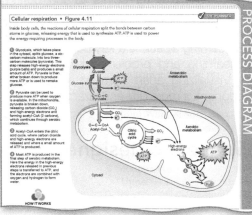

Figure 3: Cellular respiration (process diagram) Visually ordering the steps in this process diagram makes metabolism easier to understand. Analogous metabolism process illustrations appear throughout the book to review, reinforce, and build student's metabolism knowledge.

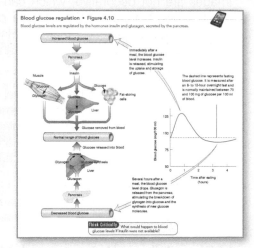

Figure 4: Blood glucose regulation Physically integrating textual elements with the visual elements, as shown here, eliminates split attention (when we must divide our attention between several sources of different information).

Research shows that well-designed visuals, integrated with comprehensive text, can improve the efficiency with which a learner processes information. In this regard, SEG Research, an independent research firm, conducted a national, multisite study evaluating the effectiveness of Wiley Visualizing. Its findings indicate that students using Wiley Visualizing products (both print and multimedia) were more engaged in the course, exhibited greater retention throughout the course, and made significantly greater gains in content area knowledge and skills, as compared to students in similar classes that did not use Wiley Visualizing.[3]

The use of *WileyPLUS Learning Space* can also increase learning. According to a white paper titled "Leveraging Blended Learning for More Effective Course Management and Enhanced Student Outcomes" by Peggy Wyllie of

Evince Market Research & Communications, studies show that effective use of online resources can increase learning outcomes. Pairing supportive online resources with face-to-face instruction can help students to learn and reflect on material, and deploying multimodal learning methods can help students to engage with the material and retain their acquired knowledge. *WileyPLUS Learning Space* provides students with an environment that stimulates active learning and enables them to optimize the time they spend on their coursework. Continual assessment/remediation is also key to helping students stay on track. The *WileyPLUS Learning Space* system facilitates instructors' course planning, organization, and delivery and provides a range of flexible tools for easy design and deployment of activities and tracking of student progress for each learning objective.

[3] SEG Research (2009). Improving Student-Learning with Graphically-Enhanced Textbooks: A Study of the Effectiveness of the Wiley Visualizing Series

New To This Edition

This third edition of *Visualizing Nutrition: Everyday Choices* includes the most recent nutrition information and recommendations along with improved illustrations and critical thinking pedagogy.

- **Metabolism: Energy for Life:** Metabolism topics have always been integrated through the *Visualizing Nutrition* texts. For those who require slightly more in-depth coverage of metabolism, want to cover it as a single topic, or who want help integrating the metabolic roles of macro- and micronutrients, a new separate chapter called *Metabolism: Energy for Life* is available online. This chapter consolidates material presented in the text and expands on topics such as oxidation-reduction reactions, the coenzyme roles of vitamins, and biochemical adaptations that occur between the fed and fasted states.

- **Food Label Legislation:** The Food Labeling Modernization Act of 2013 is currently before Congress. Coverage of this topic in Chapter 2 compares the current food label to the one proposed by this act. The relevance of these proposed changes are also addressed in all applicable subsequent chapters. Although these labels have not been adopted, they offer a launching pad for student discussion and critical thinking regarding the purpose of food labels, the effectiveness of current and proposed labels in providing consumer guidance, and how best to present nutrition information about individual foods to consumers.

- **Chapter introductions:** New chapter introductions have been written for the core chapters. These intriguing narratives, which are accompanied by vivid photographs, are designed to draw readers into the nutrition topics that will be addressed in the chapter. These capture student interest by relating nutrition concepts covered in the chapter to health, history, and culture.

- **New health management guidelines:** Recently published guidelines for the management of cardiovascular disease and overweight and obesity have been integrated into Chapters 5 and 9, respectively. New diagnostic criteria for eating disorders are included in Chapter 9. The World Health Organization's infant growth charts, which are now recommended for infants in the United States, are included in Chapter 11.

- **Choice (Exchange) Lists:** The Choice Lists, which update and replace the Exchange Lists, are discussed in Chapter 2 and provided in the online appendices.

- **Thinking it Through:** These critical thinking case study exercises have been redesigned and updated to more effectively promote critical thinking. The questions have been refined to make them more specific and to better emphasize current nutrition goals such as increasing consumption of whole grains and fresh fruits and vegetables and eating more whole foods and fewer processed foods.

- **Most current information:** The entire text has been updated and re-referenced to reflect the most current nutrition science and guidelines. For example, the Debate boxes have been updated and a new Debate, *Is Personalized Nutrition the Best Approach to Reducing Chronic Disease?*, has been included in Chapter 6 to reflect expanding study and interest in the topic of nutritional genomics. A new illustration and a more in-depth explanation of nutritional genomics have also been added to Chapter 1.

- **Improved art and labeling of illustrations:** Many illustrations have been replaced or revised to be more visually appealing or better illustrate concepts. For example, all digestion figures have been replaced with art that is more anatomically accurate. Figure layout, labels, arrow placement, color, and font size have been improved to make figures easier to understand and more informative. To help organize information and interconnect related pieces of information all multipart figures now include a unifying legend.

- **Online Features:** Critical and Creative Thinking Questions, gradable Self-Test questions, and links to Additional Resources for each chapter have been moved to an online format. This puts Additional Resources a click away and allows students to quickly check to see if they have answered all Self-Test questions correctly. Gradable Concept Check questions are also new online for this edition. Concept Questions apply to every learning objective and provide students with instant feedback on their understanding of the content.

How Does Wiley Visualizing Support Instructors?

Wiley Visualizing Site

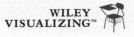

The Wiley Visualizing site hosts a wealth of information for instructors using Wiley Visualizing, including ways to maximize the visual approach in the classroom and a white paper titled "How Visuals Can Help Students Learn," by Matt Leavitt, instructional design consultant. Visit Wiley Visualizing at www.wiley.com/college/visualizing.

Wiley Custom Select

Wiley Custom Select gives you the freedom to build your course materials exactly the way you want them, offering your students a cost-efficient alternative to traditional texts. In a simple three-step process create a solution containing the content you want, in the sequence you want, delivered how you want. Visit Wiley Custom Select at http://customselect.wiley.com.

PowerPoint Presentations

(available in *WileyPLUS Learning Space* and on the book companion site)

A complete set of highly visual PowerPoint presentations—one per chapter—by Jennifer Zimmerman, Tallahassee Community College, is available online and in WileyPLUS *Learning Space* to enhance classroom presentations. Tailored to the text's topical coverage and learning objectives, these presentations are designed to convey key text concepts, illustrated by embedded text art.

Test Bank

(available in *WileyPLUS Learning Space* and on the book companion site)

The visuals from the textbook are also included in the Test Bank by Melanie Burns, Eastern Illinois University. The Test Bank has approximately 75 questions per chapter, many of which incorporate visuals from the book. The test items include multiple-choice and essay questions testing a variety of comprehension levels. The test bank is available online in MS Word files, as a Respondus Test Bank, and within *WileyPLUS Learning Space*. The easy-to-use test-generation program fully supports graphics, print tests, student answer sheets, and answer keys. The software's advanced features allow you to produce an exam to your exact specifications.

Instructor's Manual

(available in *WileyPLUS Learning Space* and on the book companion site)

The Instructor's Manual includes a lecture outline and chapter summary.

Nutrition Bytes Blog

The Nutrition Bytes Blog provides an ongoing dialogue of trending topics and controversies in nutrition that spark discussion, highlight the relevance of nutrition in our lives, and encourage critical thinking. Nutrition Bytes is accessible on mobile devices and available from both the student and instructor companion sites, as well as within *WileyPLUS Learning Space*. The blog is written by Katie Ferraro, University of California, San Francisco, and updated on a weekly basis, ensuring that discussions focus on the most current and relevant issues in nutrition. Blogs are searchable for topics of interest and students and instructors can join the discussion by posting their own comments. Users can subscribe to the newsfeed, which will automatically add it to their Favorites Center and be kept up to date.

Nutrition Visual Library

Visuals from the text are online and in *WileyPLUS Learning Space* and can be used as you wish in the classroom. These online electronic files allow you to easily incorporate images into your PowerPoint presentations as you choose, or to create your own handouts. Images are available labeled, with leader lines only, or unlabeled.

Book Companion Site

All instructor resources (the Test Bank, Instructor's Manual, PowerPoint presentations, and all textbook illustrations and photos in jpeg format) are housed on the book companion site (www.wiley.com/college/grosvenor). Student resources include self-quizzes and flashcards.

Wiley Faculty Network

The Wiley Faculty Network (WFN) is a global community of faculty, connected by a passion for teaching and a drive to learn, share, and collaborate. Their mission is to promote the effective use of technology and enrich the teaching experience. Connect with the Wiley Faculty Network to collaborate with your colleagues, find a mentor, attend virtual and live events, and view a wealth of resources all designed to help you grow as an educator. Visit the Wiley Faculty Network at www.wherefacultyconnect.com.

How Does *WileyPLUS Learning Space* Support Instructors and Students?

WileyPLUS Learning Space is designed for personalized, active learning. Several new resources are available for instructors and students within *WileyPLUS Learning Space*.

Hear This Illustration Audio Tutorials

Select figures in each chapter are accompanied by audio that narrates and discusses the important elements of that particular illustration. Figures with audio tutorials are indicated in the text with an audio player icon. All audio files are accompanied by downloadable scripts of the narration.

Nutrition Interactivities

The third edition of *Visualizing Nutrition* includes 15 new activities for student practice. Each activity is embedded within the e-book so that students can practice as they are learning the content. Activities include food source identification drag-n-drop exercises for the macro- and micro-nutrient chapters and calculating and critical thinking activities that ask students to compute caloric intake and percent RDA. These types of exercises include informative feedback about the health consequences of specific nutrient toxicities or deficiencies. New activities are available in most chapters, including the online chapter Metabolism: Energy for Life.

Create-a-Plate and Revise-a-Recipe Activities

New to this edition, each chapter includes an activity that asks students to create a balanced meal or snack to meet specific nutrient recommendations, incorporating MyPlate guidelines. Students can also practice altering meals by substituting foods with healthier choices.

Videos

New videos focus on topics that pique student interest. Videos address current topics and discussions in nutrition, such as gluten allergies and increasing portion sizes in the American diet. These videos can be used as part of lecture presentations, as discussion tools, or can be assigned through *WileyPLUS Learning Space* with gradable accompanying assessments. All videos have closed captioning for the hearing-impaired.

iProfile Mobile

The iProfile dietary analysis program now contains a database of over 50,000 foods and is available as a mobile-enabled website. Students can enter their food intakes and activities into their journal on the go via their smartphones and tablets. iProfile is also available, with additional functionality, fully integrated with *WileyPLUS Learning Space*. *WileyPLUS Learning Space* includes a few types of assessments around iProfile, including computer graded iProfile Dietary Analysis Exercises in Chapters 4 through 9, written by Lori A. Smolin and Mary B. Grosvenor. These exercises ask students to analyze and modify a diet in relation to the specific nutrients discussed in the chapter. iProfile Case Study Assignments are also available in every chapter, which have students focus on a specific nutritional concept related to that chapter's content. Students can analyze the impact of different food and activity choices using iProfile reports.

Personalized Practice

ORION adaptive practice exercises meet students at just above their level in order to keep them challenged, but not frustrated. ORION adaptive practice assesses student understanding at the objective level. All students begin with a unique, short diagnostic quiz that establishes a baseline from which each student develops his own unique path. Adaptive practice includes extensive actionable reports that focus student study in key areas individual to each learner. Our rich question database contains nearly 6000 questions at every level of difficulty and all Bloom's levels.

Mobile Enabled Assets

All of the key resources students need to succeed in their nutrition course are now accessible on mobile devices. These include the How It Works, Estimating Portion Sizes, and MyPlate animations. Also mobile are the new Nutrition Interactivities, Create-a-Plate and Revise-a-Recipe activities, and Interactive Process Diagrams.

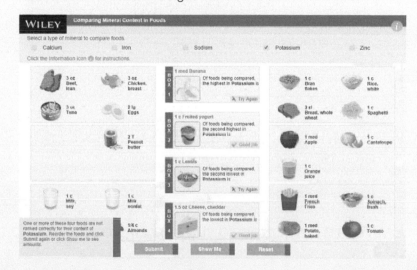

WileyPLUS Learning Space

An easy way to help your students learn, collaborate, and grow.

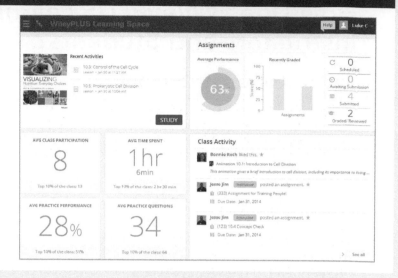

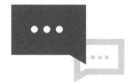

Personalized Experience

Students create their own study guide while they interact with course content and work on learning activities.

Flexible Course Design

Educators can quickly organize learning activities, manage student collaboration, and customize their course—giving them full control over content as well as the amount of interactivity between students.

Clear Path to Action

With visual reports, it's easy for both students and educators to gauge problem areas and act on what's most important.

Instructor Benefits

- Assign activities and add your own materials
- Guide students through what's important in the interactive e-textbook by easily assigning specific content
- Set up and monitor collaborative learning groups
- Assess learner engagement
- Gain immediate insights to help inform teaching

Student Benefits

- Instantly know what you need to work on
- Create a personal study plan
- Assess progress along the way
- Participate in class discussions
- Remember what you have learned because you have made deeper connections to the content

We are dedicated to supporting you from idea to outcome.

WILEY

How Has Wiley Visualizing Been Shaped by Contributors?

Instructor Contributions

Throughout the process of developing this edition, we benefited from the comments and constructive criticism provided by the instructors and colleagues listed below. We offer our sincere appreciation to these individuals for their helpful reviews, invaluable contributions to the online resources, and continued involvement with the Wiley nutrition program:

Katherine Alaimo, Michigan State University
Celine Santiago Bass, Kaplan University
William Banz, Southern Illinois University
Abbe Breiter-Fineberg, Kaplan University
Amy Allen-Chabot, Anne Arundel Community College
Elizabeth Chu, San Diego Mesa College
Kara Egan, Indiana University-Purdue University Indianapolis
Elizabeth Eilender, Montclair State University
Nicolle Fernandes, Ball State University
Katie Ferraro, University of California, San Francisco
Melany Gilbert, Ozarks Technical Community College
Mindy Haar, New York Institute of Technology
Donna Huisenga, Illinois Central College
Karen Friedman-Kester, Harrisburg Area Community College
Rose Martin, Iowa State University
Deborah Murray, Ohio University
Melissa Silva, Bryant University

Nutrition Advisory Board
Jeremy Akers, James Madison University
Jeanne Boone, Palm Beach State College

Nancy Berkoff, Los Angeles Trade Technical College
Jayne Byrne, College of St. Benedict
Linda Brown, Florida State University
Melanie Burns, Easting Illinois University
Laura Christoph, Holyoke Community College
James F. Collins, University of Florida
Sylvia Crixell, Texas State University
Barbara Goldman, Palm Beach State College
Timaree Hagenburger, Consumnes River College
Donna Handley, University of Rhode Island
Karen Israel, Anne Arundel Community College
Shanil Juma, Texas Women's University
Younghee Kim, Bowling Green State University
George Liepa, Eastern Michigan University
Owen Murphy, Central Oregon Community College
Judy Myhand, Louisiana State University
Cheryl Neudauer, Minneapolis Community and Technical College
Kristen Hilbert, SUNY Oneonta
Priya Venkatesan, Pasadena City College
Shahla Wunderlich, Montclair State University

Special Thanks

Special thanks to Peter Ambrose for providing a fresh eye by writing the chapter introductions for this project. We appreciate his "non-nutritionist" view of the science we know too well. His ability to help us organize and articulate our thoughts throughout the text is greatly appreciated.

Our sincere appreciation goes to Rose Martin, Iowa State University, for helping us develop the new nutrition interactivities for this edition. We are grateful for her vision and hands-on involvement throughout the development process.

We are extremely grateful to the many members of the editorial and production staff at John Wiley & Sons who guided us through the challenging steps of developing this book. Their tireless enthusiasm, professional assistance, and endless patience smoothed the path as we found our way. We thank in particular Associate Publisher, Kevin Witt, who continually works to provide support and guidance and develop new ways to ensure the book's success; and Trish McFadden, Senior Production Editor, who guided the production process. Our sincere thanks also go to Kaye Pace, Vice President and Executive Publisher, who oversaw the entire project; Clay Stone, Executive Marketing Manager, who adeptly represents the Visualizing imprint. We appreciate the expertise of Mary Ann Price, Senior Photo Editor, in managing and researching our photo program. We also wish to thank Media Specialist, Svetlana Barskaya, who worked on the wide assortment of media resources. We are grateful to Emma Townsend-Merino, Senior Editorial Assistant for helping to bring this project to fruition. And thanks to Senior Associate Editor, Lauren Elfers, for her support through developing and writing this text and its ancillary materials.

About the Authors

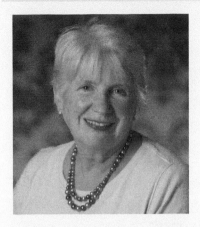

Mary B. Grosvenor holds a bachelor of arts in English and a master of science in Nutrition Science, affording her an ideal background for nutrition writing. She is a registered dietitian and has worked in clinical as well as research nutrition, in hospitals and communities large and small in the western United States. She teaches at the community college level and has published articles in peer-reviewed journals in nutritional assessment and nutrition and cancer. Her training and experience provide practical insights into the application and presentation of the science in this text.

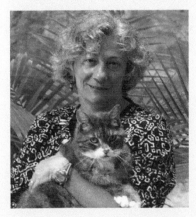

Lori A. Smolin received a bachelor of science degree from Cornell University, where she studied human nutrition and food science. She received a doctorate from the University of Wisconsin at Madison, where her doctoral research focused on B vitamins, homocysteine accumulation, and genetic defects in homocysteine metabolism. She completed postdoctoral training both at the Harbor–UCLA Medical Center, where she studied human obesity, and at the University of California—San Diego, where she studied genetic defects in amino acid metabolism. She has published articles in these areas in peer-reviewed journals. Dr. Smolin is currently at the University of Connecticut, where she has taught both in the Department of Nutritional Science and in the Department of Molecular and Cell Biology. Courses she has taught include introductory nutrition, life cycle nutrition, food preparation, nutritional biochemistry, general biochemistry, and introductory biology.

Dedication

To my sons, David and John, and my husband, Peter. In the beginning, their contribution was support and patience with my long hours but over the years it has grown to include editing and writing as well. Thanks for keeping my projects, and me, on track.

(from Mary Grosvenor)

To my sons, Zachary and Max, who have grown up along with my textbooks, helping me to keep a healthy perspective on the important things in life. To my husband, David, who has continuously provided his love and support and is always there to assist with the computer and technological issues that arise when writing in the electronic age.

(from Lori Smolin)

Contents in Brief

Todd Gipstein/NG Image Collection

Contents

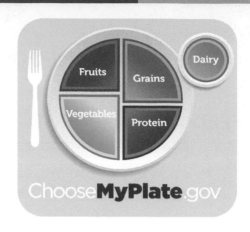

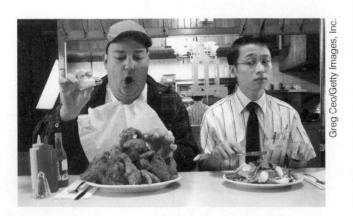

Greg Ceo/Getty Images, Inc.

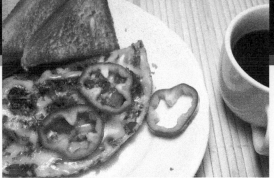
dirkr/iStockphoto

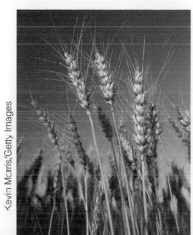
Kevin Morris/Getty Images

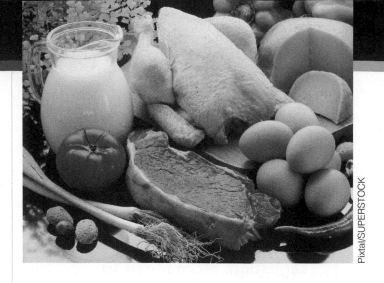

Pixtal/SUPERSTOCK

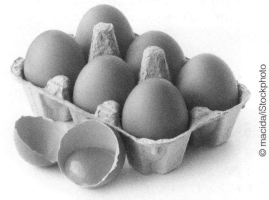

© macida/iStockphoto

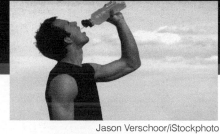
Jason Verschoor/iStockphoto

Abraham Newitz/NG Image Collection

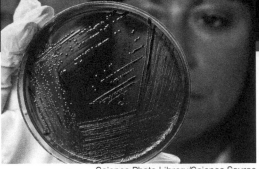

Science Photo Library/Science Source

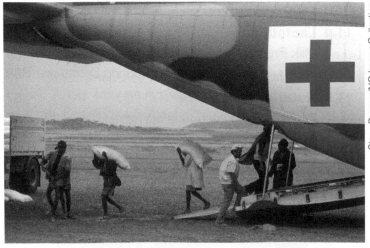

Steve Raymer/NG Image Collection

Third Edition

VISUALIZING
NUTRITION
EVERYDAY CHOICES

1 Nutrition: Everyday Choices

How do you choose what to eat? For most of the world's population, the answer is simple: You eat what you can grow, raise, catch, kill, or purchase. Fundamentally, subsistence is the principal motivator of food consumption: If you don't eat, you die. Historically, the game or crops people could kill or cultivate successfully became staples of their diet. As agriculture and food production became more sophisticated,

a greater array of food choices became available. Colonization and exploitation of native peoples introduced new foods to the colonizers: Corn became part of the diet of European settlers in North America, for instance, and the potato was brought to the Old World from the New. Today, in a cosmopolitan, global society, one may literally choose from the world's dinner table.

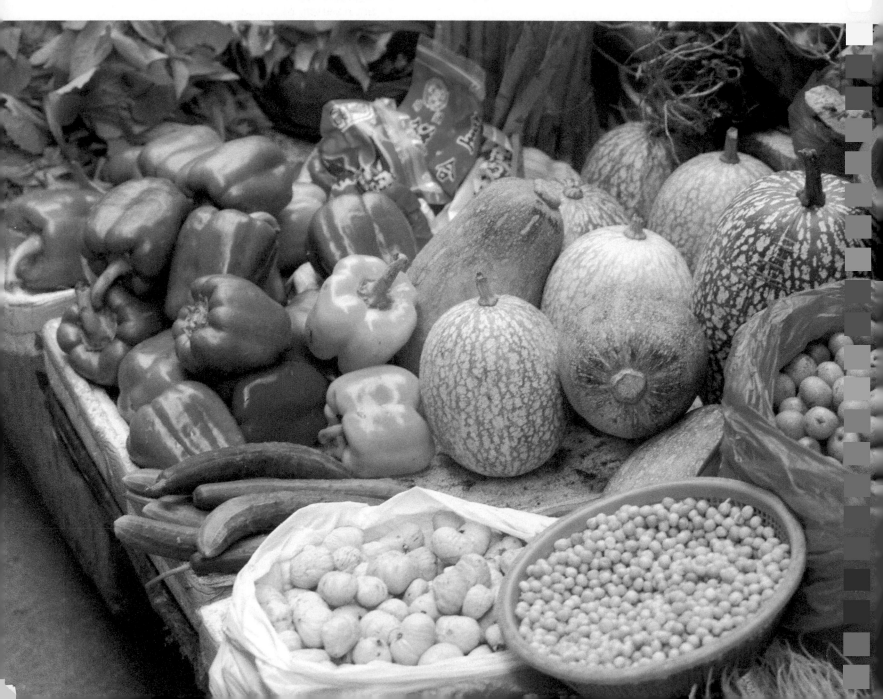

The implications of food choices are significant not only because what you eat affects your health but also because what you like affects what you choose to eat. Hundreds of millions of people enjoy eating insects, raw fish, horses, and even dogs, while hundreds of millions of others abhor pork, beef, shellfish, dairy products, and even chocolate! Most of us enjoy the sweet and avoid the bitter, yet some of us choose the zip of the bitter or the bite of the zesty.

Because the nutrients in the food we eat form and maintain the structure of our bodies, we really are what we eat. The challenge is to find a satisfying balance between what we like and what optimizes our health. The choice is ours.

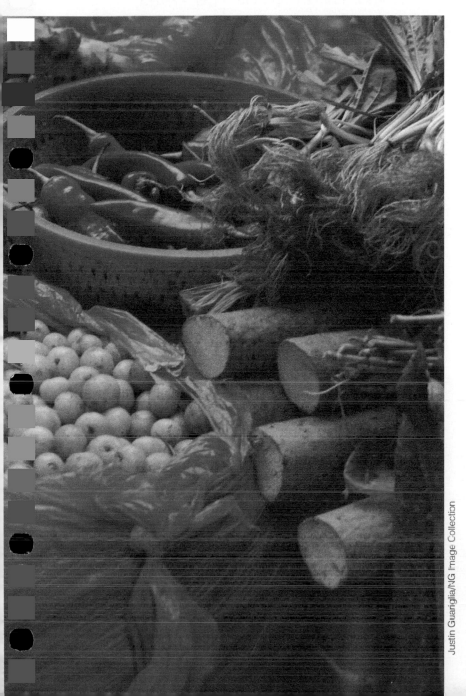

Justin Guariglia/NG Image Collection

CHAPTER OUTLINE

CHAPTER PLANNER ✓

☐ Stimulate your interest by reading the opening story and looking at the visual.

☐ Scan the Learning Objectives in each section:
   p. 4 ☐ p. 8 ☐ p. 12 ☐ p. 15 ☐ p. 18 ☐

☐ Read the text and study all figures and visuals. Answer any questions.

Analyze key features:

☐ Nutrition InSight, p. 6 ☐ p. 11 ☐

☐ Debate, p. 10 ☐

☐ Thinking It Through, p. 17 ☐

☐ Process Diagram, p. 18 ☐

☐ What a Scientist Sees, p. 21 ☐

☐ Stop: Answer the Concept Checks before you go on:
   p. 7 ☐ p. 12 ☐ p. 14 ☐ p. 17 ☐
   p. 24 ☐

End of chapter and online review:

☐ Review the Summary, Key Terms, and online links to Additional Resources.

☐ Answer the online Critical and Creative Thinking Questions.

☐ Answer What is happening in this picture?

☐ Complete the online Self-Test and check your answers.

1.1 Food Choices and Nutrient Intake

LEARNING OBJECTIVES

1. **Define** nutrient density.
2. **Compare** fortified foods and dietary supplements.
3. **Distinguish** essential nutrients from phytochemicals.
4. **Identify** factors that determine food choices.

What are you going to eat today? Will breakfast be a vegetable omelet or a bowl of sugar-coated cereal? How about lunch—a burger or a turkey sandwich? The foods we choose determine the **nutrients** we consume. To stay healthy, humans need more than 40 **essential nutrients**. Because the foods we eat vary from day to day, so do the amounts and types of nutrients and the number of **calories** we consume.

nutrient A substance in food that provides energy and structure to the body and regulates body processes.

nutrient-dense foods. Foods with a high **nutrient density** contain more nutrients per calorie than do foods with a lower nutrient density (**Figure 1.1**). If a large proportion of your diet consists of foods that are low in nutrient density, such as soft drinks, chips, and candy, you could have a hard time meeting your nutrient needs without exceeding your calorie needs. By choosing nutrient-dense foods, you can meet all your nutrient needs and have calories left over for occasional treats that are lower in nutrients and higher in calories.

essential nutrient A nutrient that must be consumed in the diet because it cannot be made by the body or cannot be made in sufficient quantities to maintain body functions.

calorie A unit of measure used to express the amount of energy provided by food.

nutrient density A measure of the nutrients provided by a food relative to its calorie content.

Nutrients from Foods, Fortified Foods, and Supplements

Any food you eat adds some nutrients to your diet, but to make your diet healthy, it is important to choose

Nutrient density • Figure 1.1

Nutrient-dense diets provide more nutrients in fewer calories.

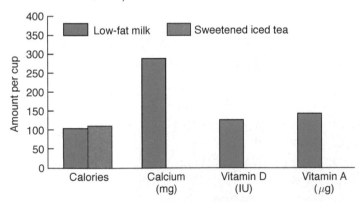

a. Nutrient density is important in choosing a healthy diet. As illustrated here, low-fat milk provides about the same number of calories per cup as bottled iced tea, but it also provides calcium, vitamin D, vitamin A, and other nutrients, including protein.

b. Typically, less processed foods provide more nutrients per calorie. For example, a roasted chicken breast is more nutrient dense than a highly processed form of chicken such as chicken nuggets; a baked potato is more nutrient dense than French fries; and apples are more nutrient dense than apple pie.

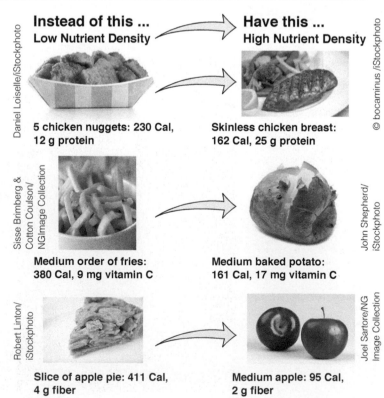

Instead of this ...
Low Nutrient Density

5 chicken nuggets: 230 Cal, 12 g protein

Medium order of fries: 380 Cal, 9 mg vitamin C

Slice of apple pie: 411 Cal, 4 g fiber

Have this ...
High Nutrient Density

Skinless chicken breast: 162 Cal, 25 g protein

Medium baked potato: 161 Cal, 17 mg vitamin C

Medium apple: 95 Cal, 2 g fiber

In addition to nutrients that occur naturally in foods, we obtain nutrients from fortified foods. The **fortification** of foods was begun to help eliminate nutrient deficiencies in the population, with the federal government mandating that certain nutrients be added to certain foods. Foods such as milk with added vitamin D and grain products with added B vitamins and iron are examples of this mandated fortification that have been part of the U.S. food supply for decades.

Recently, however, voluntary fortification of foods has become common practice. Vitamins and minerals are routinely added to breakfast cereals and a variety of snack foods. The amounts and types of nutrients added to these voluntarily fortified foods are at the discretion of the manufacturer. These added nutrients contribute to the diet but are not necessarily designed to address deficiencies and may increase the likelihood of consuming an excess of some nutrients.

fortification The addition of nutrients to foods.

dietary supplement A product sold to supplement the diet; may include nutrients (vitamins, minerals, amino acids, fatty acids), enzymes, herbs, or other substances.

phytochemical A substance found in plant foods that is not an essential nutrient but may have health-promoting properties.

Dietary supplements are another source of nutrients; about half of U.S. adults take some sort of daily dietary supplement. Supplements provide nutrients but do not offer all the benefits of food (see Chapters 2 and 7).[1]

Food Provides More Than Nutrients

In addition to nutrients, food contains substances that, though not essential to life, can be beneficial for health. In plants, these health-promoting substances are called **phytochemicals** (**Figure 1.2**). Although fewer such substances have been identified in animal foods, animal foods also contain substances with health-promoting properties. These are called **zoochemicals**.

Some foods, because of the complex mixtures of nutrients and other chemicals they contain, provide health benefits that extend beyond basic nutrition. Such foods

Foods that are high in phytochemicals • Figure 1.2

Fruits, vegetables, and whole grains provide a variety of phytochemicals, such as those highlighted here. Supplements of individual phytochemicals are available, but there is little evidence that they provide the health benefits obtained from foods that are high in phytochemicals.[1]

Know these ↙

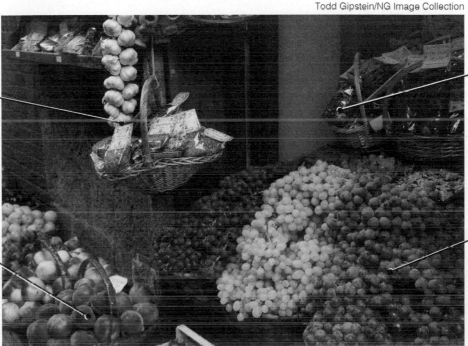

Todd Gipstein/NG Image Collection

Garlic, broccoli, and onions provide sulfur-containing phytochemicals that help protect us from some forms of cancer by inactivating carcinogens or stimulating the body's natural defenses.[4,5]

Soybeans are a source of phytoestrogens, hormone-like compounds found in plants that may affect the risk of certain types of cancer and delay the progression of heart disease.[6,7]

Yellow–orange fruits and vegetables, such as peaches, apricots, carrots, and cantaloupe, as well as leafy greens, are rich in carotenoids, which are phytochemicals that may prevent oxygen from damaging our cells.[8]

Purple grapes, berries, and onions provide red, purple, and pale yellow pigments called flavonoids, which prevent oxygen damage and may reduce the risk of cancer and heart disease.[9,10]

Know these

Functional foods provide benefits beyond their nutrients	Table 1.1
Food	**Potential health benefit**
Blueberries	May reduce the risk of heart disease and cancer.[10,11]
Breakfast cereal with added flaxseed	Helps reduce blood cholesterol levels and the overall risk of heart disease.[12]
Chocolate	May help reduce blood pressure and other risk factors for heart disease.[13]
Garlic	Helps reduce blood cholesterol levels and the overall risk of heart disease.[14]
Kale	May reduce the risk of age-related blindness (macular degeneration).[15]
Margarine with added plant sterols	Reduces blood cholesterol levels.[16]
Nuts	May reduce the risk of heart disease.[17]
Oatmeal	Helps reduce blood cholesterol.[18]
Orange juice with added calcium	Helps prevent osteoporosis.
Salmon	Reduces the risk of heart disease.[19]
Green tea	May reduce the risk of certain types of cancer.[20]
Whole-grain bread	Helps reduce the risk of cancer, heart disease, obesity, and diabetes.[21]

functional food A food that has health-promoting properties beyond basic nutritional functions.

have been termed **functional foods**. The simplest functional foods are unmodified whole foods, such as broccoli and fish, that naturally contain substances that promote health and protect against disease, but some foods fortified with nutrients or enhanced with phytochemicals or other substances are also classified as functional foods (**Table 1.1**).[22]

Nutrition InSight   Food choices • Figure 1.3

The food choices we make are influenced by society, culture, attitudes, and emotions as well as by food availability.

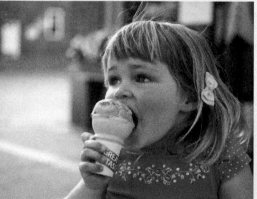

We use food as reward and punishment. A well-behaved child may be rewarded with an ice cream cone, while a child who misbehaves may be sent to bed without dessert. We also use food to commemorate milestones such as birthdays and anniversaries.

Tim Laman/NG Image Collection

Food can provide comfort and security. "Comfort foods" such as hot tea, chicken soup, and chocolate help us to feel better when we are sick, cold, tired, or lonely.

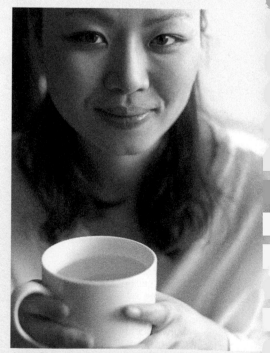

Justin Guariglia/NG Image Collection

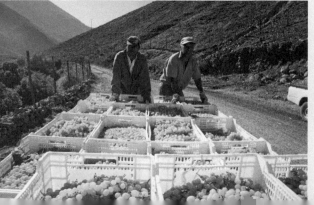

We can choose only from foods that are available to us. What is available is affected by season, geography, economics, health, and living conditions. In many parts of the world, food choices are limited to foods produced locally, but in more developed regions, many nonnative and seasonal foods, such as these grapes, are available year-round because they can be stored and shipped from distant locations.

Michael Hanson/NG Image Collection

These modified foods, such as water with added vitamins, oatmeal with added soy protein, and orange juice with added calcium, have also been called **designer foods.** The term **nutraceutical** refers to any food or supplement that delivers a health benefit. As food manufacturers fortify foods to cash in on the concept that "health sells," the line between what is a dietary supplement and what is a food has become blurred.

What Determines Food Choices?

Do you eat oranges to boost your vitamin C intake or ice cream to add a little calcium to your diet? Probably not. We need these nutrients to survive, but we generally choose foods for reasons other than the nutrients they contain. Sometimes we choose a food simply because it is put in front of us; often our choices also depend on what we have learned to eat, what is socially acceptable in our cultural heritage or religion, what we think is healthy, or what our personal convictions—such as environmental

consciousness or vegetarianism—demand. Tradition and values may dictate what foods we consider appropriate, but individual preferences for taste, smell, appearance, and texture affect which foods we actually consume. All these factors are involved in food choices because food does more than meet our physiological requirements. It also provides sensory pleasure and helps meet our social and emotional needs (**Figure 1.3**).

| CONCEPT CHECK | STOP |

1. **Which** has a higher nutrient density: a soda or a glass of milk?
2. **Why** are foods fortified?
3. **Why** is it better to meet your vitamin C needs by eating an orange than by taking a dietary supplement?
4. **What** factors determine the foods you eat at a family picnic?

✓ THE PLANNER

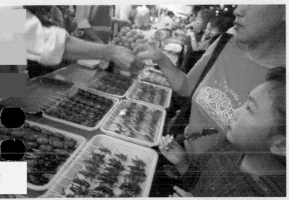

Food preferences and eating habits are learned as part of an individual's family, cultural, national, and social background. In many parts of the world, insects, such as these cicadas and grasshoppers, are considered a treat, but in U.S. culture, insects are considered food contaminants, and most people would refuse to eat them.

© Kevin Foy/Alamy

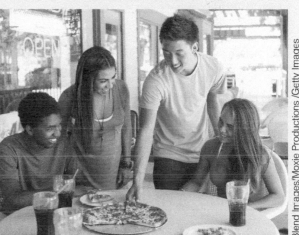

Blend Images/Moxie Productions /Getty Images

For an adolescent, stopping for pizza after school may be part of being accepted by his or her peers. Food is the centerpiece of everyday social interactions. We meet friends for dinner or a cup of coffee. The family dinner table is a focal point for communication, where experiences of the day are shared.

David Hoffman/Alamy

Often people's attitudes about what foods they think are good for them or are good for the environment affect what they choose. For example, you may choose green tea to increase your intake of cancer-fighting antioxidants or organic produce because you are concerned about the environmental impact of pesticides.

7

1.2 Nutrients and Their Functions

LEARNING OBJECTIVES

1. **List** the six classes of nutrients.
2. **Discuss** the three functions of nutrients in the body.

There are six classes of nutrients: carbohydrates, lipids, proteins, water, vitamins, and minerals. Carbohydrates, lipids, proteins, and water are considered **macronutrients** because they are needed in large amounts. Vitamins and minerals are referred to as **micronutrients** because they are needed in small amounts. Together, the macronutrients and micronutrients in our diet provide us with energy, contribute to the structure of our bodies, and regulate the biological processes that go on inside us. Each nutrient provides one or more of these functions, but all nutrients together are needed to provide for growth, maintain and repair the body, and support reproduction.

The Six Classes of Nutrients

Carbohydrates, lipids, and proteins are all **organic compounds** that provide energy to the body. Although we tend to think of each of them as a single nutrient, there are actually many different types of molecules in each of these classes. **Carbohydrates** include starches, sugars, and **fiber** (**Figure 1.4a**). Several types of **lipids** play important roles in nutrition (**Figure 1.4b**). The most recognizable of these are **cholesterol**, **saturated fats**, and **unsaturated fats**. There are thousands of different **proteins** in our bodies and our diets. All proteins are made up of units called **amino acids** that are linked together in different combinations to form different proteins (**Figure 1.4c**).

organic compound A substance that contains carbon bonded to hydrogen.

carbohydrates A class of nutrients that includes sugars, starches, and fibers. Chemically, they all contain carbon, along with hydrogen and oxygen, in the same proportions as in water (H_2O).

Water, unlike the other classes of nutrients, is only a single substance. Water makes up about 60% of an adult's body weight. Because we can't store water, the water the body loses must constantly be replaced by water obtained from the diet. In the body, water acts as a lubricant, a transport fluid, and a regulator of body temperature.

Vitamins are organic molecules that are needed in small amounts to maintain health. There are 13 vitamins, which perform a variety of unique functions in the body, such as regulating energy metabolism, maintaining vision, protecting cell membranes, and helping blood to clot. **Minerals** are **elements** that are essential nutrients needed in small amounts to provide a variety of diverse functions in the body. For example, iron is an element needed for the transport of oxygen in the blood, calcium is an element important in keeping bones strong. We consume vitamins and minerals in almost all the foods we eat. Some are natural sources: Oranges contain vitamin C, milk provides calcium, and carrots give us vitamin A. Other foods are fortified with vitamins and minerals; a serving of fortified breakfast cereal often has 100% of the recommended intake of many vitamins and minerals (see *Debate: Super-Fortified Foods: Are They a Healthy Addition to Your Diet?* on page 10). Dietary supplements are another source of vitamins and minerals for some people.

What Nutrients Do

Carbohydrates, lipids, and proteins are often referred to as **energy-yielding nutrients**; they provide energy that can be measured in calories. The calories people talk about and see listed on food labels are actually **kilocalories** (abbreviated kcalorie or kcal), units of 1000 calories. When spelled with a capital *C*, Calorie means kilocalorie. Carbohydrates provide 4 Calories/gram; they are the most immediate source of energy for the body. Lipids also help fuel our activities and are the major form of stored

fiber A type of carbohydrate that cannot be broken down by human digestive enzymes.

lipids A class of nutrients, commonly called fats, that includes saturated and unsaturated fats and cholesterol; most do not dissolve in water.

cholesterol A type of lipid that is found in the diet and in the body. High blood levels increase the risk of heart disease.

saturated fat A type of lipid that is most abundant in solid animal fats and is associated with an increased risk of heart disease.

unsaturated fat A type of lipid that is most abundant in plant oils and is associated with a reduced risk of heart disease.

protein A class of nutrients that includes molecules made up of one or more intertwining chains of amino acids.

Carbohydrates, lipids, and proteins • Figure 1.4

Varying combinations of carbohydrates, lipids, and proteins provide the energy in the foods we eat.

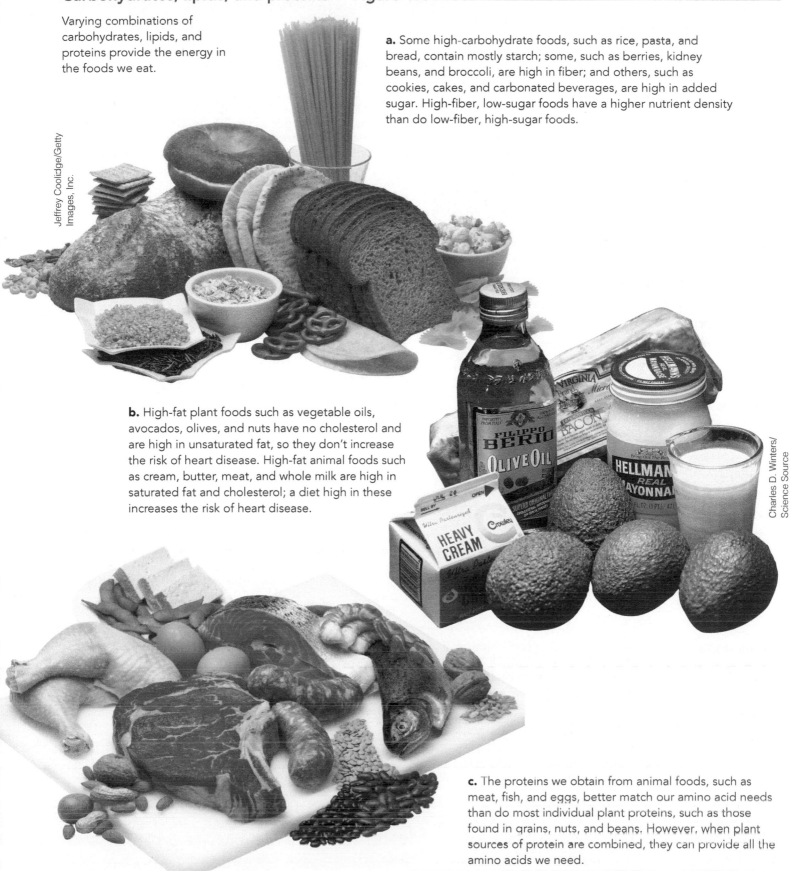

a. Some high-carbohydrate foods, such as rice, pasta, and bread, contain mostly starch; some, such as berries, kidney beans, and broccoli, are high in fiber; and others, such as cookies, cakes, and carbonated beverages, are high in added sugar. High-fiber, low-sugar foods have a higher nutrient density than do low-fiber, high-sugar foods.

b. High-fat plant foods such as vegetable oils, avocados, olives, and nuts have no cholesterol and are high in unsaturated fat, so they don't increase the risk of heart disease. High-fat animal foods such as cream, butter, meat, and whole milk are high in saturated fat and cholesterol; a diet high in these increases the risk of heart disease.

c. The proteins we obtain from animal foods, such as meat, fish, and eggs, better match our amino acid needs than do most individual plant proteins, such as those found in grains, nuts, and beans. However, when plant sources of protein are combined, they can provide all the amino acids we need.

Jeffrey Coolidge/Getty Images, Inc.

Charles D. Winters/Science Source

Jeffrey Coolidge/Getty Images, Inc.

Debate | Super-Fortified Foods: Are They a Healthy Addition to Your Diet?

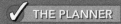 THE PLANNER

The Issue: Some foods, such as protein bars and energy drinks, are fortified with large amounts of nutrients. These super-fortified foods add nutrients to the diet, but if eaten in large quantities or in combination with other highly fortified foods, they may pose a risk of toxicity. Are they a safe, healthy addition to your diet?

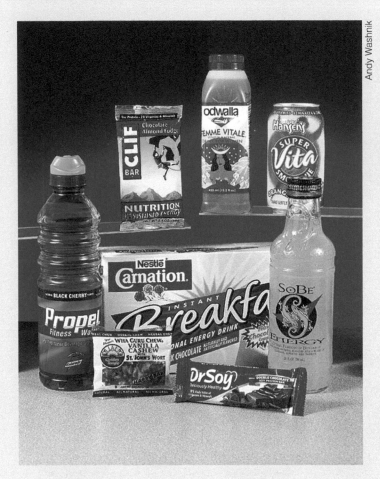

Andy Washnik

An orange, a tomato, a slice of whole-grain bread, and a piece of grilled salmon—these are foods that are part of a healthy diet. What about an energy drink with 23 added vitamins and minerals, a protein bar with 100% of your daily vitamin requirements, soft drinks with Echinacea and green tea extract, fruit juice with added phytochemicals, and bottled water fortified with vitamin C? Are these products foods, or are they supplements?

One could argue that fortified protein bars and juices are foods, not supplements, because they provide calories like traditional foods, and the substances added to them, such as vitamin C, fish oil, or phytochemicals, are also naturally found in food. On the other hand, by definition, a supplement is a product intended to add nutrients or other substances to the diet, which these products certainly do. Does it matter if these supplemental substances come in a food or in a pill? Opponents of these foods would argue that it does because our decisions about eating foods are different than our decisions about supplements. Typically, we consider the dose when taking a supplement pill. But we eat to satisfy our sensory desires, fill our stomachs, and quench our thirsts. We don't think about whether a food or beverage might provide toxic amounts of nutrients.

In general, traditional foods contain moderate amounts of a variety of nutrients, so the risk of consuming a toxic amount of any single nutrient is almost nonexistent. In contrast, it is not difficult to swallow a very high dose of one or more nutrients from an excess of supplement pills or excessive servings of super-fortified foods. For example, if you drank your recommended 2 to 3 liters of fluid as water fortified with vitamin C, niacin, vitamin E, and vitamins B_6 and B_{12}, you would exceed the recommended upper limit for these vitamins. Then if you also consumed 2 cups of fortified breakfast cereal and two protein bars during the day, your risk of toxicity would increase even more. The government labels these fortified products as foods, and we eat them like foods, but they may have the same toxicity risks as supplements.

Advocates of super-fortified foods point out that they add health-promoting substances to the diet. But do super-fortified foods provide the benefits that the original food would have? In some cases they do. For example, if you are getting your calcium from orange juice, studies show that you are absorbing just about as much calcium as you would from milk.[2] On the other hand, fish oil consumed in capsules does not have all the heart-health benefits of fish oil consumed in a piece of fish.[3]

So, are these products foods, or are they supplements? It is a fine line. Whether they are helpful or harmful depends on what is in them and how much you consume. Should the government get involved in regulating the amounts of nutrients that can be added to all foods? These answers depend on your view of the government's role in food regulation. Should we be gobbling them down without a thought? Probably not.

Think Critically: Should super-fortified foods carry a consumer warning to avoid overconsumption?

The nutrients we consume in our diet provide energy, form body structures, and regulate body processes.

Energy

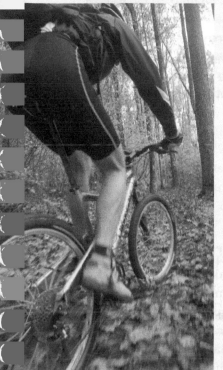

Whether riding a bike through the fall foliage, walking to the mailbox, or gardening, physical activity is fueled by the carbohydrate, fat, and protein in the food we eat.

Skip Brown/NG Image Collection

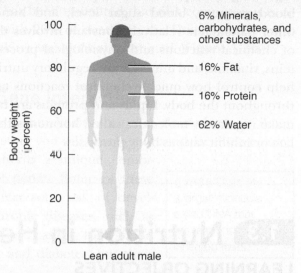

6% Minerals, carbohydrates, and other substances

16% Fat

16% Protein

62% Water

Body weight (percent)

Lean adult male

Structure

Proteins, lipids, carbohydrates, minerals, and water all contribute to the shape and structure of our bodies.

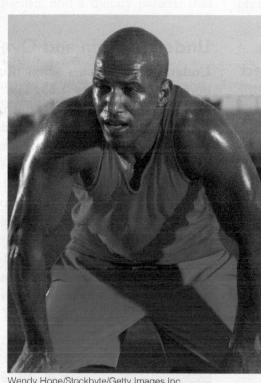

Wendy Hope/Stockbyte/Getty Images,Inc.

Regulation

Water helps regulate body temperature. When body temperature increases, sweat is produced, cooling the body as it evaporates from the skin.

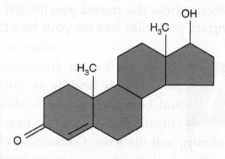

Regulation

Lipids, such as the hormone testosterone, illustrated here, help regulate body processes. Testosterone is made from cholesterol. In men, it stimulates sperm production and the development of secondary sex characteristics, such as body and facial hair, a deep voice, and increased muscle mass.

energy in the body. One gram of fat provides 9 Calories. Protein can supply 4 Calories/gram but is not the body's first choice for meeting energy needs because protein has other roles that take priority. Alcohol, though it is not a nutrient because it is not needed for life, provides about 7 Calories/gram. Water, vitamins, and minerals do not provide energy (calories) (**Figure 1.5**).

With the exception of vitamins, all the classes of nutrients are involved in forming and maintaining the body's structure. Fat deposited under the skin contributes to our body shape, for instance, and proteins form the ligaments and tendons that hold our bones together and attach our muscles to our bones. Minerals harden bone. Protein and water make up the structure of the muscles, which help define our body contours, and protein and carbohydrates form the cartilage that cushions our joints. On a smaller scale, lipids, proteins, and water form the structure of individual cells. Lipids and proteins make up the membranes that surround each cell, and water and dissolved substances fill the cells and the spaces around them.

Nutritional genomics • Figure 1.8

Both the genes you inherit and your dietary choices directly affect your health and disease risk. There is also interplay between these such that your genes, through nutrigenetics, influence how your diet affects your health and your diet, through nutrigenomics, affects how your genes impact your health.

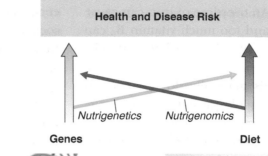

Health and Disease Risk

Nutrigenetics   *Nutrigenomics*

Genes   **Diet**

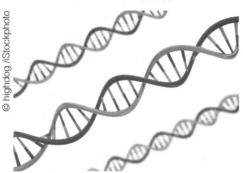

© highdog /iStockphoto

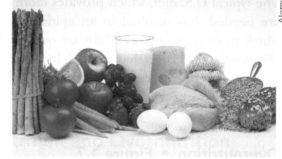

Alamy

Think Critically Can you become obese even if both of your parents are thin?

The genes you inherit affect your tendency to develop nutrition-related chronic diseases such as heart disease and diabetes.

The diet you consume affects your risk of developing nutrition-related chronic diseases.

---

impact is affected by what you eat. Your genetic makeup also determines the impact a certain nutrient will have on you. For example, some people inherit a combination of genes that results in a tendency to have high blood pressure. When these individuals consume even an average amount of sodium, their blood pressure increases (discussed further in Chapter 8). Others inherit genes that allow them to consume more sodium without much of a rise in blood pressure. Those whose genes dictate a significant rise in blood pressure with a high-sodium diet can reduce their blood pressure, and the complications associated with high blood pressure, by eating a diet that is low in sodium.

Our increasing understanding of human genetics has given rise to the discipline of **nutritional genomics**, which explores the interaction between human genes and nutrition and health.[27] It encompasses both the effect that the genes a person inherits have

nutritional genomics The study of how our genes affect the impact of nutrients or other food components on health (nutritgenetics) and how nutrients affect the activity of our genes (nutrigenomics).

on how their diet affects health (**nutrigenetics**) and the effect the nutrients and other food components they consume has on gene activity (**nutrigenomics**) **(Figure 1.8)**. Research in these areas has led to the development of the concept of "personalized nutrition." The goal of personalized nutrition is to prescribe a diet based on the genes an individual has inherited in order to prevent, moderate, or cure chronic disease (see Chapter 6 Debate). Although today we do not have the tools to take a sample of everyone's DNA and use it to tell them what to eat to optimize their health, we do know that certain dietary patterns can reduce the risk of many chronic diseases.

CONCEPT CHECK   **STOP**

1. **What** causes malnutrition?
2. **How** can your diet today affect your health 20 years from now?
3. **Why** might the diet that optimizes health be different for different people?

1.4 Choosing a Healthy Diet

LEARNING OBJECTIVES

1. **List** three reasons it is important to eat a variety of foods.
2. **Explain** why you can sometimes eat foods that are low in nutrient density and still have a healthy diet.
3. **Discuss** how dietary moderation can reduce the risk of chronic disease.

A healthy diet is one that provides the right number of calories to keep your weight in the desirable range; the proper balance of carbohydrate, protein, and fat; plenty of water; and sufficient but not excessive amounts of vitamins and minerals. This healthy diet is rich in whole grains, fruits, and vegetables; high in fiber; moderate in fat, sugar, and sodium; and low in unhealthy fats (saturated fat, cholesterol, and *trans* fat). In short, a healthy diet is based on variety, balance, and moderation (see *What Should I Eat?*).

Eat a Variety of Foods

In nutrition, choosing a variety of foods is important because no single food can provide all the nutrients the body needs for optimal health. *Variety* means choosing foods from different food groups—vegetables, grains, fruits, dairy products, and high-protein foods. Some of these foods are rich in vitamins and phytochemicals, others are rich in protein and minerals, and all are important.

Variety also means choosing diverse foods from within each food group. Different vegetables provide different nutrients. Potatoes, for example, are the only vegetable in many Americans' diets. Potatoes provide vitamin C but are low in vitamin A. If potatoes are your only vegetable, it is unlikely that you will meet your nutrient needs. If instead you have a salad, potatoes, and broccoli, you will be getting plenty of vitamins C and A, as well as many other vitamins and minerals. Making varied choices both from the different food groups and from within each food group is also important because nutrients and other food components interact. Such interactions may be positive, enhancing nutrient utilization, or negative, inhibiting nutrient availability. Variety averages out these interactions. Some foods may also contain toxic substances. Eating a variety of foods reduces the risk that you will consume enough of any one toxin to be harmful. For example, tuna may contain traces of mercury, but as long as you don't eat tuna too often, you are unlikely to consume a toxic amount.

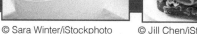

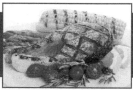

© Sara Winter/iStockphoto   © Jill Chen/iStockphoto   © Steve Mcsweeny/iStockphoto

WHAT SHOULD I EAT?

A Healthy Diet

Eat a variety of foods

- Mix up your snacks. Have salsa and chips one day and fruit, yogurt, or nuts another day.
- Add almonds and diced apples to your salad.
- Try a new vegetable or fruit each week. Tired of carrots? Try jicama.
- Vary your protein sources. Eat fish one day and beef the next—or skip the meat and have beans.

Balance your choices

- Going out to dinner? Have a salad for lunch.
- Add a vegetable instead of pepperoni to your pizza.
- When you have cookies for a snack, have fruit for dessert.
- Had soda with lunch? Have low-fat milk with dinner.

Practice moderation

- Push back from the table before you are stuffed and go for a walk.
- Reduce your portions by using a smaller bowl.
- Skip the seconds and split your restaurant meal with a friend.
- If you eat some extra fries, take some extra steps.

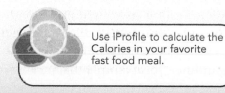

Use iProfile to calculate the Calories in your favorite fast food meal.

Balance calories in with calories out • Figure 1.9

To keep your weight stable, you need to burn the same number of calories as you consume. Extra calories consumed during the day can be balanced by increasing the calories you burn in physical activity.

Picturenet/Blend Images/GettyImages, Inc.

Andy Washnik

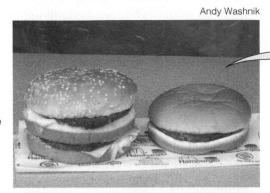

Choosing a Big Mac over a smaller burger means you will need to increase your energy expenditure by 300 Calories to maintain your weight.

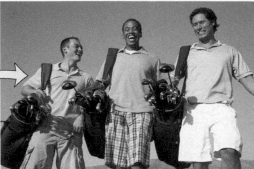

You could do this by playing golf for about an hour, carrying your own clubs.

Andy Washnik

Kate Thompson/NG Image Collection

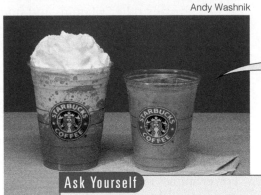

Choosing a grande Mocha Frappuccino over a regular iced coffee means you will need to increase your energy expenditure by 370 Calories to maintain your weight.

You could do this by jogging for about 30 minutes.

Ask Yourself

If you add a daily grande Mocha Frappuccino to your usual diet and do not increase your activity, what will happen to your weight?

Variety involves choosing different foods not only each day but also each week and throughout the year. If you had apples and grapes today, for example, have blueberries and cantaloupe tomorrow. If you can't find tasty tomatoes in December, replace them with a winter vegetable such as squash.

Balance Your Choices

Choosing a healthy diet is a balancing act. Healthy eating doesn't mean giving up your favorite foods. There is no such thing as a good food or a bad food—only healthy diets and unhealthy diets. Any food can be part of a healthy diet, as long as your diet throughout the day or week provides enough of all the nutrients you need without excesses of any. When you choose a food that is lacking in fiber, for example, balance it with one that provides lots of fiber. When you choose a food that is very high in fat, balance that choice with a low-fat one.

A balanced diet also balances the calories you take in with the calories you burn in your daily activities so that your body weight stays in the healthy range (**Figure 1.9**).

Practice Moderation

Moderation means not overdoing it—not having too many calories, too much fat, too much sugar, too much salt, or too much alcohol. Choosing moderately will help you maintain a healthy weight and prevent some of the chronic diseases, such as heart disease and cancer, that are on the rise in the U.S. population

The fact that more than 68% of adult Americans are overweight or obese demonstrates that we have not been practicing moderation when it comes to calorie intake.[23] One of the main culprits is likely the size of our food portions. The sandwiches, soft drinks, and French fry orders

A Case Study on Choosing a Healthy Diet

For many college students, their freshman year is the first time they are making all their own food choices, and they don't always make the best ones. Learning to apply the principles of variety, balance, and moderation can help improve these choices.

Helen doesn't really know how to choose a healthy diet so she picks what she knows. Every day she eats cereal for breakfast, a peanut butter sandwich for lunch, and chicken, broccoli, and rice for dinner.

 What's wrong with Helen's diet?

Your answer:

Amad's favorite breakfast is doughnuts and he always has fast food for lunch—usually a burger and fries. He knows these are not the most nutrient-dense choices, but he is always in a hurry rushing between school and work.

 Suggest some more nutrient-dense foods that would be just as easy to grab as Amad's current breakfast and lunch choices.

Answer: He could grab yogurt for breakfast just as easily as a doughnut. If he has a doughnut for breakfast, he could balance this with a sandwich on whole-grain bread with turkey, lettuce, tomatoes, and peppers for lunch. He can get this meal just as quickly and easily as a burger and fries.

 Suggest a nutrient-dense dinner that would help balance Amad's poor breakfast and lunch choices.

Your answer:

Sam has gained a few pounds and is worried that he will become a victim of the "freshman 15"—the 15 or so pounds gained by college students during the first year away from home. He thinks his weight gain is due to the dinner he eats on his all-you-can-eat college meal plan. He piles food on his plate thinking he will only eat what he likes best but then ends up eating it all while he sits and relaxes with his friends.

 Suggest two changes Sam could make to practice moderation with his dinner choices.

Your answer:

Marty knows that beans are a healthy choice, so she decides to try some Mexican food. She orders the beef and bean burrito platter shown here.

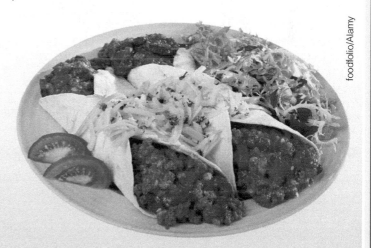

foodfolio/Alamy

How does Marty's meal stack up in terms of variety, balance, and moderation?

Your answer:

(Check your answers in online appendix L.)

served in fast-food restaurants today are two to five times larger than what they were 40 years ago. The sizes of the snacks and meals we eat at home have also increased. As these portion sizes have grown, so has the amount we eat—and so has our weight.[28] Moderation makes it easier to balance your diet and allows you to enjoy a greater variety of foods (see *Thinking It Through: A Case Study on Choosing a Healthy Diet*).

CONCEPT CHECK **STOP**

1. **Why** is variety in a diet important?
2. **What** could you have for lunch to balance a breakfast that provides no vitamin C or A?
3. **How** are obesity and dietary moderation related?

1.5 Evaluating Nutrition Information

LEARNING OBJECTIVES

1. **List** the steps of the scientific method and give an example of how it is used in nutrition.
2. **Discuss** three different types of experiments used to study nutrition.
3. **Describe** the components of a sound scientific experiment.
4. **Distinguish** between reliable and unreliable nutrition information.

We are bombarded with nutrition information almost every day. The evening news, the morning papers, and the World Wide Web continually offer us tantalizing tidbits of nutrition advice. Food and nutrition information that used to take professionals years to disseminate now travels with lightning speed, reaching millions of people within hours or days. Much of this information is reliable, but some can be misleading. In order to choose a healthy diet, we need to be able to sort out the useful material in this flood of information.

The Science Behind Nutrition

Like all other sciences, the science of nutrition is constantly evolving. As new discoveries provide clues to the right combination of nutrients needed for optimal health, new nutritional principles and recommendations are developed. Sometimes established beliefs and

PROCESS DIAGRAM

The scientific method • Figure 1.10

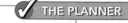 THE PLANNER

The scientific method is a process used to ask and answer scientific questions through observation and experimentation.

 The first step of the scientific method is to make an observation and ask questions about that observation.

Observation
More people get colon cancer in the United States than in Japan.

⬇

❷ The next step is to propose an explanation for this observation. This proposed explanation is called a hypothesis.

Hypothesis
The lower incidence of colon cancer in Japan than in the United States is due to differences in the diet.

⬇

❸ Once a hypothesis has been proposed, experiments like this one are designed to test it. To generate reliable theories, the experiments done to test hypotheses must produce consistent, quantifiable results and must be interpreted accurately.

Experiment
Compare the incidence of colon cancer of Japanese people who move to the United States and consume a typical U.S. diet with Caucasian Americans who eat the same diet. **Result:** The Japanese people who eat the U.S. diet have the same higher incidence of colon cancer as Caucasian Americans.

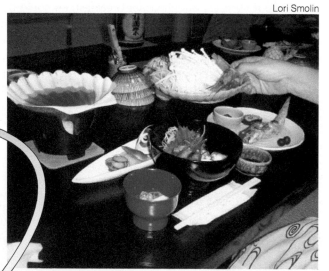
Lori Smolin

❺ If experimental results do not support the hypothesis, a new hypothesis can be formulated.

⬇

❹ If the results from repeated experiments support the hypothesis, a scientific theory can be developed. A single experiment is not enough to develop a theory; rather, repeated experiments showing the same conclusion are needed to develop a sound theory.

Theory
The U.S. diet contributes to the development of colon cancer.

 As new information becomes available, even a theory that has been accepted by the scientific community for years can be proved wrong.

Think Critically A scientist has hypothesized that the difference in the incidence of colon cancer in Japan and the United States is due to differences in the genetic makeup of the populations. Based on the results of the experiment described in this illustration, explain why this hypothesis is not supported.

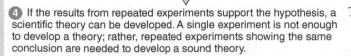

Types of nutrition studies • Figure 1.11

Scientists use a variety of methods to expand our understanding of nutrition.

a. Epidemiological studies Epidemiological studies of populations around the world explore the impact of nutrition on health. If you were to measure saturated fat intake and the incidence of heart attacks in different populations, you might get a graph that looks like this one. It indicates that diets with a high percentage of calories from saturated fat are associated with an increased incidence of heart attacks. However, epidemiology does not determine cause-and-effect relationships—it just identifies patterns. Therefore, it cannot determine whether the higher incidence of heart attacks is caused by the high intake of saturated fat.

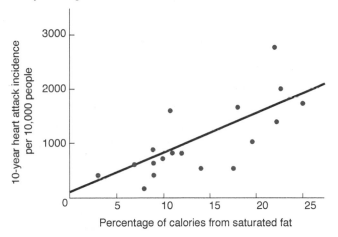

Percentage of calories from saturated fat

©kickers/iStockphoto

b. Clinical trials The observations and hypotheses that arise from epidemiology can be tested using clinical trials. In nutrition, clinical trials explore the health effects of altering people's diets—for instance, the possible effects of reducing saturated fat intake on blood cholesterol levels.

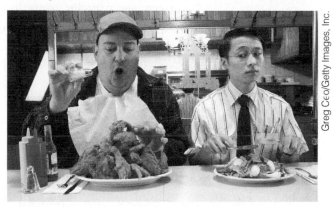

Greg Ceo/Getty Images, Inc.

d. Biochemistry and molecular biology Laboratory-based techniques can be used to study nutrient functions in the body. For example, biochemistry can be used to study the chemical reactions that provide energy or synthesize molecules, such as cholesterol, and molecular biology can be used to study how nutrients regulate our genes.

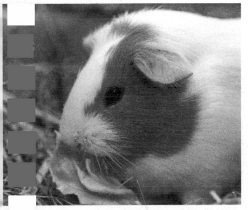

c. Animal studies Ideally, studies of human nutrition should be done with human subjects. However, because studying humans is costly, time consuming, inconvenient for the subjects, and in some cases impossible for ethical reasons, many studies are done using animals. Guinea pigs are a good model for studying heart disease, but even the best animal model is not the same as a human, and care must be taken when extrapolating animal results to humans.

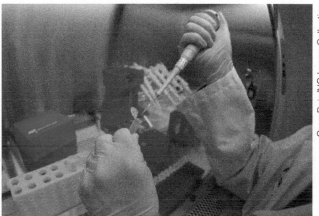

Greg Dale/NG Image Collection

---

concepts give way to new information. Understanding the process of science can help consumers understand the nutrition information they encounter.

The systematic, unbiased approach that allows any science to acquire new knowledge and correct and update previous knowledge is the **scientific method**. The scientific method involves making observations of natural events, formulating **hypotheses** to explain these events, designing and performing experiments to test these hypotheses, and developing **theories** that explain the observed phenomenon

> **hypothesis** A proposed explanation for an observation or a scientific problem that can be tested through experimentation.
>
> **theory** A formal explanation of an observed phenomenon made after a hypothesis has been tested and supported through extensive experimentation.

based on the results of many studies (**Figure 1.10**). In nutrition, the scientific method is used to develop nutrient recommendations, understand the functions of nutrients, and learn about the role of nutrition in promoting health and preventing disease.

How Scientists Study Nutrition

Many different types of experiments are used to expand our knowledge of nutrition (**Figure 1.11**). Some make observations about relationships between diet and health; these are based

epidemiology The branch of science that studies health and disease trends and patterns in populations.

on the science of **epidemiology**. Other types of experiments evaluate the affect of a particular dietary change on health. Some of these experiments study humans, others use animals; some look at whole populations, others study just a few individuals; and some use just cells or molecules.

A sound nutrition experiment studies the right experimental population, collects quantifiable data, includes proper experimental controls, and interprets the data accurately. The experimental population must be chosen to answer a specific question. For example, if a dietary supplement claims to increase bone strength in older women, a study to test this should use older women as subjects. For an experiment to determine whether a treatment does or does not have an effect, it must include enough subjects to demonstrate that the treatment causes the effect to occur more frequently than it would by chance. The number of subjects needed depends on how likely an effect is to occur without the treatment. For example, if weight training without a muscle-building supplement causes an increase in muscle mass, a large number of experimental subjects may be needed to demonstrate that there is a greater increase in muscle mass with the treatment, in this case the muscle-building supplement. Results from studies with only a few subjects may not be able to distinguish effects that occur due to chance and should therefore be interpreted with caution.

Data collected in experiments must be quantifiable, that is it must include parameters that can be measured reliably and repeatedly, such as body weight or blood pressure. Individual testimonies or opinions alone are not quantifiable, objective measures.

control group In a scientific experiment, the group of participants used as a basis of comparison. They are similar to the participants in the experimental group but do not receive the treatment being tested.

experimental group In a scientific experiment, the group of participants who undergo the treatment being tested.

In order to know whether what is being tested has an effect, one must compare it with something. A **control group** acts as a standard of comparison for the factor, or **variable**, being studied. A control group is treated in the same way as the **experimental group** except that the control group does not receive the treatment being tested. For example, in a study examining the effect of a dietary supplement on muscle strength, the control group would consist of individuals of similar age, gender, and ability, eating similar diets and following similar workout regimens as individuals in the experimental group. Instead of the supplement, the control subjects would consume a **placebo**, a fake product that is identical in appearance to the dietary supplement.

When an experiment has been completed, the results must be interpreted. Accurate interpretation is just as important as conducting a study carefully. If a study conducted on a large group of young women indicates that a change in diet reduces breast cancer risk later in life, the results of that study cannot be used to claim that the same effect will occur if older women make a similar dietary change. Likewise, if the study looks only at the connection between a change in diet and breast cancer, the findings can't be used to claim a reduced risk for other cancers.

One way to ensure that the results of experiments are interpreted correctly is to have them reviewed by experts in the field who did not take part in the study being evaluated. Such a **peer-review process** is used in determining whether experimental results should be published in scientific journals. The reviewing scientists must agree that the experiments were conducted properly and that the results were interpreted appropriately. Nutrition articles that have undergone peer review can be found in many journals, including *The American Journal of Clinical Nutrition, The Journal of Nutrition, The Journal of the Academy of Nutrition and Dietetics, The New England Journal of Medicine,* and *The International Journal of Sport Nutrition.* Newsletters from reputable institutions, such as the *Tufts Health and Nutrition Letter,* the *Harvard Health Letter,* and *Nutrition Action Healthletter* are also reliable sources of nutrition and health information. The information in these newsletters comes from peer-reviewed articles but is written for a consumer audience.

Recommendations and policies regarding nutrition and health care are made by compiling the evidence from the wealth of well-controlled, peer-reviewed studies that are available. This is referred to as **evidence-based practice**.

Judging for Yourself

Not everything you hear is accurate. Because much of the nutrition information we encounter is intended to sell products, that information may be embellished to make it more appealing. Understanding the principles scientists use to perform nutrition studies can help consumers judge the nutrition information they encounter in their daily lives (see *What a Scientist Sees*). Some things that may

WHAT A SCIENTIST SEES
Behind the Claims

This product must be amazing! It will increase your muscle strength, decrease your body fat, and boost your drive and motivation. This is what consumers see. The claims sound great, but a scientist looking at the same ad may have some concerns.

First of all, the claims about muscle strength and motivation are testimonials based on individuals' feelings and impressions, and these are not objective measures.

A scientist would also question whether the research evidence supports the claim that the product increases muscle mass and decreases body fat. The study measured the amount of lean tissue (muscle, bone, and other nonfat body tissues) and

fat tissue in weightlifters before and four weeks after they began consuming the POWER BOOST drink. The measures used provide quantifiable, repeatable data. The results report a gain of 5.2 lb of lean tissue and a loss of 4.5 lb of fat tissue in weightlifters taking POWER BOOST. This looks convincing, but the results for the control group are not reported in the ad. When the results for the experimental group are compared to those for the control group, a different picture emerges. This comparison (see graph) shows that the control group gained almost as much lean mass and lost slightly more fat mass than the group taking POWER BOOST.

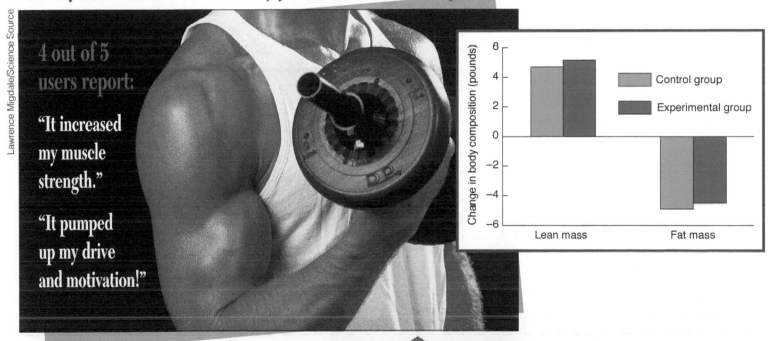

Lawrence Migdale/Science Source

POWER**BOOST**
BOOST your STRENGTH • POWER up your DRIVE • MAXIMIZE your MASS

4 out of 5 users report:

"It increased my muscle strength."

"It pumped up my drive and motivation!"

POWER BOOST
Years of research were needed to develop this special nutritional formulation. Just mix with water and drink one shake with every meal or snack.

In a university study, 25 experienced weightlifters consumed one POWER BOOST shake at meals and snacks, 5 times a day for 4 weeks.

Lean body mass and fat mass were measured by underwater weighing before the study began and after 4 weeks of training while taking POWER BOOST.

RESULTS
The weight lifters gained an average of 5.2 lb of lean muscle and lost 4.5 lb of unwanted fat.

Think Critically Based on the information in the graph, explain why you would or would not recommend this product.

tip you off to misinformation are claims that sound too good to be true, information from unreliable sources, information intended to sell a product, and information that is new or untested.

Let's now look at questions that can help you evaluate any piece of nutrition information you encounter.

Does it make sense? Some claims are too outrageous to be true. For example, if a product claims to increase your muscle size without any exercise or decrease your weight without a change in diet, common sense should tell you that the claim is too good to be true. In contrast, an article that tells you that adding exercise to your daily routine will help you lose weight and increase your stamina is not so outrageous.

What's the source? If a claim seems reasonable, find out where it came from. Personal testimonies are not a reliable source (**Figure 1.12**), but government recommendations regarding healthy dietary practices and information disseminated by universities generally are. Government recommendations are developed by committees of scientists who interpret the latest well-conducted research studies and use their conclusions to develop recommendations for the population as a whole. The information is designed to improve the health of the population. Information that comes from universities is supported by research studies that are well scrutinized and published in peer-reviewed journals. Many universities also provide information that targets the general public. Not-for-profit organizations such as the Academy of Nutrition and Dietetics and the American Medical Association are also reliable sources of nutrition information.

If you are looking at an article in print or posted on a Web site, checking the author's credentials can help you evaluate the credibility of the information. Where does the author work? Does this person have a degree in nutrition or medicine? Although "nutrition counselors" may provide accurate information, this term is not legally

Individual testimonies are not proof • Figure 1.12

Weight-loss product advertisements commonly show before-and-after photos of people who have successfully lost weight using the product. These individuals' success stories are not a guarantee that the product will produce the same results for you or anyone else. These individuals' results are not compared to those for a control group or subjected to scientific evaluation. Therefore, it cannot be assumed that similar results will occur in other people.

Ask Yourself

If an ad for a weight-loss product showed you these before-and-after photos with the quote saying, "In just 3 weeks I went from a size 14 to a size 8 and looked fabulous on my vacation," what questions should you ask to determine whether this is valid information?

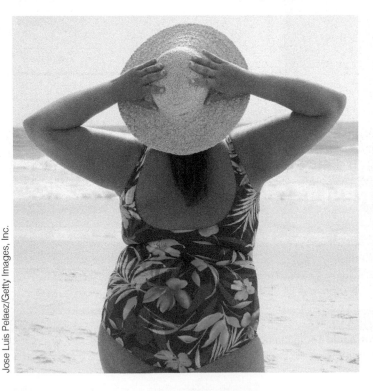

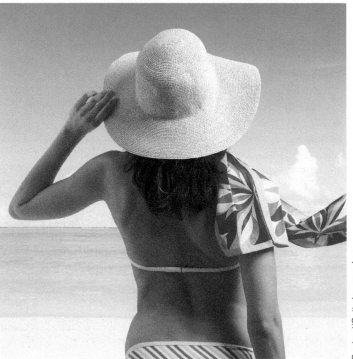

defined and can be used by individuals with no formal nutrition or medical training.

One reliable source of nutrition information is a registered dietitian or registered dietitian nutritionist (RD/RDN). RDs and RDNs are nutrition professionals who are certified to provide nutrition education and counseling. To obtain certification an RD/RDN must earn a four-year college degree that includes coursework approved by the Academy of Nutrition and Dietetics, complete a supervised internship, and pass a national exam.

Is it selling something? If a person or company will profit from the information presented, be wary. Advertisements are designed to increase product sales, and the company stands to profit if you believe the claims that are made. Information presented in newspapers and magazines and on television may also be biased or exaggerated because it is designed to help sell magazines or boost ratings, not necessarily to promote health and well-being. Even a well-designed, carefully executed study published in a peer-reviewed journal can be a source of misinformation if its results have been interpreted incorrectly or exaggerated (**Figure 1.13**).

Has it stood the test of time? Often the results of new scientific studies are on the news the same day they are presented at a meeting or published in a peer-reviewed journal. However, a single study cannot serve as a basis for a reliable theory. Results need to be reproduced and supported numerous times before they can be used as a foundation for nutrition recommendations.

Headlines based on a single study should therefore be viewed skeptically. The information may be accurate, but there is no way to know because there has not been enough time to repeat the work and reaffirm the conclusions. If, for example, someone has found the secret to easy weight loss, you will undoubtedly encounter this information again at some later time if the finding is valid. If the finding is not valid, it will fade away with all the other weight-loss concoctions that have come and gone.

CONCEPT CHECK STOP

1. **What** is the difference between a hypothesis and a theory?

2. **How** is an epidemiologic study different from a clinical trial?

3. **Why** are control groups important in any scientific experiment?

4. **Why** are personal testimonies not a source of reliable nutrition information?

Results may be misinterpreted in order to sell products • Figure 1.13

These rats, which were given large doses of vitamin E, lived longer than rats that consumed less vitamin E. Does this mean that dietary supplements of vitamin E will increase longevity in people? Not necessarily. The results of animal studies can't always be extrapolated to humans, but they are often the basis of claims in ads for dietary supplements.

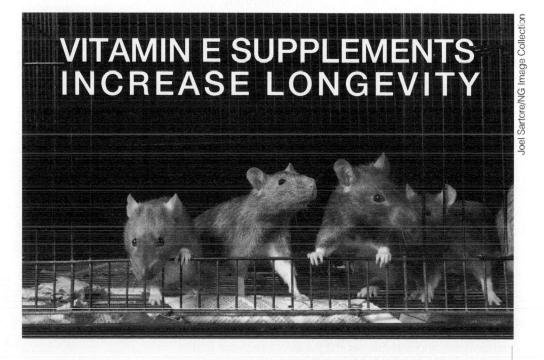

Joel Sartore/NG Image Collection

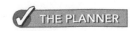

Summary

1 Food Choices and Nutrient Intake 4

- The foods you choose determine which **nutrients** you consume. Choosing foods that are high in **nutrient density** allows you to obtain more nutrients in fewer calories, as shown in this graph. Fortified foods and **dietary supplements** can also contribute nutrients to the diet.

Nutrient density • Figure 1.1a

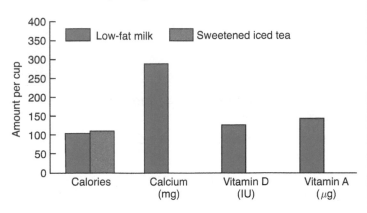

- Food contains not only nutrients but also nonnutritive substances, such as **phytochemicals**, that may provide additional health benefits. Foods that provide health benefits beyond basic nutrition are called **functional foods**. Some foods are naturally functional, and others are made functional through **fortification**.

- The food choices we make are affected by many factors other than nutrition, including food availability; what we learn to eat from family, culture, and traditions; personal tastes; and what we think we should eat to maintain health.

2 Nutrients and Their Functions 8

- Nutrients are grouped into six classes. **Carbohydrates, lipids, proteins**, and water are referred to as **macronutrients** because they are needed in large amounts. **Vitamins** and **minerals** are **micronutrients** because they are needed in small amounts to maintain health.

- Carbohydrates, lipids, and proteins are nutrients that provide energy, typically measured in **calories**. Lipids, proteins, carbohydrates, minerals, and water perform structural roles, as shown, forming and maintaining the structure of our bodies. All six classes of nutrients help regulate body processes. The

energy, structure, and regulation provided by nutrients are needed for growth, maintenance and repair of the body, and reproduction.

Nutrient functions • Figure 1.5b

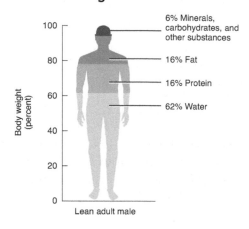

3 Nutrition in Health and Disease 12

- Your diet affects your health. The foods you choose contain the nutrients needed to keep you alive and healthy and prevent **malnutrition**. **Undernutrition** results from consuming too few calories and/or too few nutrients. **Overnutrition** can result from a toxic dose of a nutrient or from a chronic excess of nutrients or calories, which over time contributes to chronic diseases, such as those shown in this graph.

Overnutrition • Figure 1.7

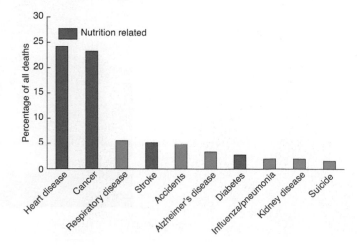

- Your genetic makeup and the diet you consume interact to affect your health risks. **Nutritional genomics** studies how the genes you inherit affect the impact of diet on health and how the diet you choose affects the activity of your genes.

4 Choosing a Healthy Diet 15

- A healthy diet includes a variety of nutrient-dense foods from the different food groups as well as a variety of foods from within each group. Variety is important because different foods provide different nutrients and health-promoting substances as well as a variety of tastes.

- Balance means mixing and matching foods and meals in order to obtain enough of the nutrients you need and not too much of the ones that can potentially harm your health. Extra calories you consume during the day can be balanced by increasing the calories you burn in physical activity, as shown.

- Moderation means not ingesting too many calories or too much fat, sugar, salt, or alcohol. Eating moderate portions helps you maintain a healthy weight and helps prevent chronic diseases such as heart disease and cancer.

Balance calories in with calories out • Figure 1.9

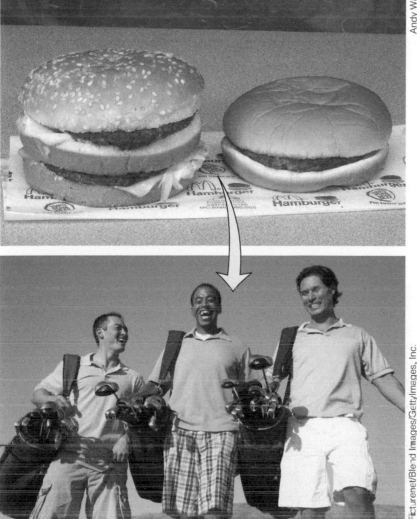

Andy Washnik

Picturenet/Blend Images/GettyImages, Inc.

5 Evaluating Nutrition Information 18

- Nutrition uses the **scientific method** to study the relationships among food, nutrients, and health. The scientific method, illustrated here, involves observing and questioning natural events, formulating **hypotheses** to explain these events, designing and performing experiments to test the hypotheses, and developing **theories** that explain the observed phenomena based on the experimental results.

- To be valid, a nutrition experiment must provide quantifiable measurements, study the right type and number of subjects, and use appropriate **control groups**. When a study has been completed, the results must be interpreted fairly and accurately. The **peer-review process** ensures that studies published in professional journals adhere to a high standard of experimental design and interpretation of results.

- Not all the nutrition information we encounter is accurate. The first step in deciding whether a nutritional claim is valid is to ask whether the claim makes sense. If it sounds too good to be true, it probably is. It is also important to determine whether the information came from a reliable source, whether it is trying to sell a product, and whether it has been confirmed by multiple studies.

The scientific method • Figure 1.10

 The first step of the scientific method is to make an observation and ask questions about that observation.

Observation
More people get colon cancer in the United States than in Japan.

 The next step is to propose an explanation for this observation. This proposed explanation is called a hypothesis.

Hypothesis
The lower incidence of colon cancer in Japan than in the United States is due to differences in the diet.

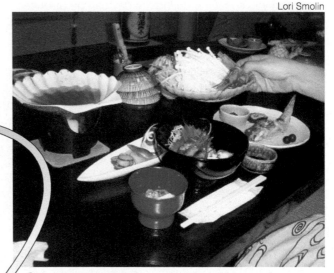

Lori Smolin

3 Once a hypothesis has been proposed, experiments like this one are designed to test it. To generate reliable theories, the experiments done to test hypotheses must produce consistent, quantifiable results and must be interpreted accurately.

Experiment
Compare the incidence of colon cancer of Japanese people who move to the United States and consume a typical U.S. diet with Caucasian Americans who eat the same diet. **Result:** The Japanese people who eat the U.S. diet have the same higher incidence of colon cancer as Caucasian Americans.

5 If experimental results do not support the hypothesis, a new hypothesis can be formulated.

4 If the results from repeated experiments support the hypothesis, a scientific theory can be developed. A single experiment is not enough to develop a theory; rather, repeated experiments showing the same conclusion are needed to develop a sound theory.

Theory
The U.S. diet contributes to the development of colon cancer.

6 As new information becomes available, even a theory that has been accepted by the scientific community for years can be proved wrong.

Key Terms

- amino acid 8
- calorie 4
- carbohydrates 8
- cholesterol 8
- control group 20
- designer food or nutraceutical 7
- dietary supplement 5
- element 8
- energy-yielding nutrient 8
- epidemiology 20
- essential nutrient 4
- evidence-based practice 20
- experimental group 20
- fiber 8
- fortification 5
- functional food 6
- genes 13
- hormone 12
- hypothesis 19
- kilocalorie 8
- lipids 8
- macronutrient 8
- malnutrition 12
- micronutrient 8
- mineral 8
- nutrient 4
- nutrient density 4
- nutrigenetics 14
- nutrigenomics 14
- nutritional genomics 14
- organic compound 8
- osteoporosis 12
- overnutrition 13
- peer-review process 20
- phytochemical 5
- placebo 20
- protein 8
- saturated fat 8
- scientific method 19
- theory 19
- undernutrition 12
- unsaturated fat 8
- variable 20
- vitamin 8
- zoochemical 5

What is happening in this picture?

Instead of playing basketball and hide-and-seek like American kids a generation ago, this boy is sitting in front of the television snacking and playing video games.

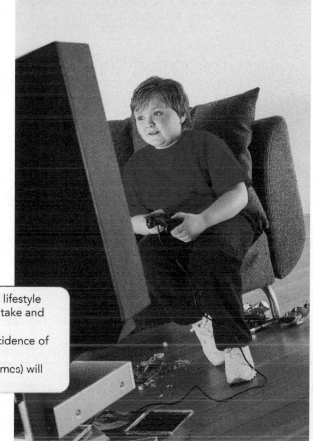

Digital Vision/Getty Images, Inc.

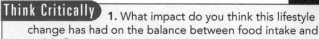

Think Critically

1. What impact do you think this lifestyle change has had on the balance between food intake and activity?
2. How do you think video games impacted the incidence of childhood obesity?
3. Do you think active video games (such as Wii games) will help American children increase their activity?

THE PLANNER ✓

Review your Chapter Planner on the chapter opener and check off your completed work.

Guidelines for a Healthy Diet

"What you don't know could kill you," may have been the first nutrition recommendation. To swallow the wrong berry or gulp down water from a suspect source could have been fatal to early humans. Such lessons served as anecdotal guideposts to survival. As societies developed, dietary cautions turned into taboos, sometimes laws, and ultimately, nutrition recommendations.

Governments have been providing what we would call modern nutrition information for the past 150 years. As the Industrial Revolution swept through Great Britain, urban populations—and poverty and hunger—swelled. To ensure a healthy workforce, the British government developed minimum dietary guidelines utilizing the cheapest foods. It wasn't until World War I that the

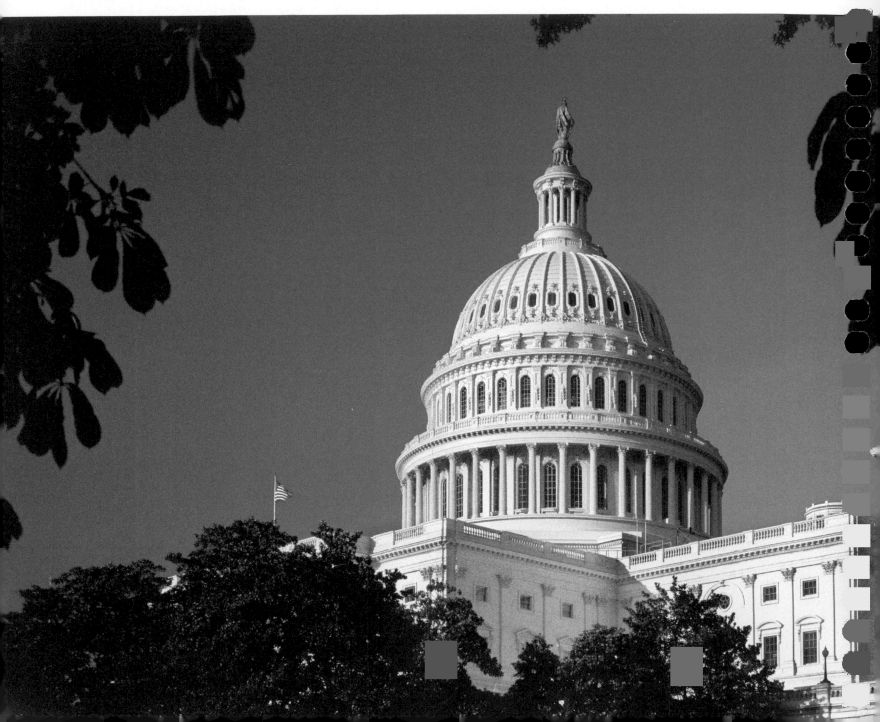

British Royal Society determined that a healthy workforce required a healthy diet—not necessarily the cheapest. So fruits, vegetables, and milk became elements of nutritional guidance. Since then, virtually every nation has sought to establish dietary standards for its citizens.

Today, modern public health agencies provide valuable information regarding healthy food choices. However, this information isn't always understood or used properly. As portion sizes grow, so do waistlines—and the attendant health concerns. "What you don't know could kill you," remains as vital an admonition today as it was 40,000 years ago.

Rex A. Stucky/NG Image Collection

CHAPTER OUTLINE

CHAPTER PLANNER ✓

- ❏ Stimulate your interest by reading the introduction and looking at the visual.
- ❏ Scan the Learning Objectives in each section:
  p. 30 ❏   p. 34 ❏   p. 37 ❏   p. 47 ❏
- ❏ Read the text and study all figures and visuals. Answer any questions.

Analyze key features:

- ❏ What a Scientist Sees, p. 31 ❏
- ❏ Process Diagram, p. 32 ❏
- ❏ Debate, p. 38 ❏
- ❏ Nutrition InSight, p. 40 ❏   p. 43 ❏   p. 48 ❏
- ❏ Thinking It Through, p. 50 ❏
- ❏ Stop: Answer the Concept Checks before you go on:
  p. 33 ❏   p. 36 ❏   p. 47 ❏   p. 54 ❏

End of chapter and online review:

- ❏ Review the Summary, Key Terms, and online links to Additional Resources.
- ❏ Answer the online Critical and Creative Thinking Questions.
- ❏ Answer What is happening in this picture?
- ❏ Complete the online Self-Test and check your answers.

2.1 Nutrition Recommendations

LEARNING OBJECTIVES

1. **Explain** the purpose of government nutrition recommendations.
2. **Discuss** how U.S. nutrition recommendations have changed over the past 100 years.
3. **Describe** how nutrition recommendations are used to evaluate nutritional status and set public health policy.

What should we be eating if we want to satisfy our nutrient needs? Our taste buds, food marketers and advertisers, and magazine and newspaper headlines all influence our choices. These choices may not always be healthy ones, however. Our taste buds respond to flavor and sensation, not necessarily to sensible nutrition; manufacturers want to sell products; and magazines want to sell subscriptions. Government recommendations, on the other hand, are designed with individual health as well as public health in mind. They can be used to plan diets and to evaluate what we are eating, both as individuals and as a nation.

Past and Present U.S. Recommendations

The federal government has been making nutritional recommendations for over 100 years. These recommendations have changed over time as our food intake patterns have changed and our knowledge of what constitutes a healthy diet has evolved.

The first dietary recommendations in the United States, published in 1894 by the U.S. Department of Agriculture (USDA), suggested amounts of protein, carbohydrate, fat, and "mineral matter" needed to keep Americans healthy.[1] At the time, specific vitamins and minerals essential for health had not been identified; nevertheless, this work set the stage for the development of the first **food guides**. Food guides are used to translate nutrient-intake recommendations into food choices (**Figure 2.1**). The food guide *How to Select Foods*, released in 1917, made recommendations based on five food groups: meat and milk, cereals, vegetables and fruit, fats and fatty foods, and sugars and sugary foods.

In the early 1940s, as the United States entered World War II, the Food and Nutrition Board was established to advise the Army and other federal agencies regarding problems related to food and the nutritional health of the armed forces and the general population. The Food and Nutrition Board developed the first set of recommendations for specific amounts of nutrients. These came to be

known as the Recommended Dietary Allowances (RDAs). The original RDAs made recommendations on amounts of energy and on specific nutrients that were most likely to be deficient in people's diets—protein, iron, calcium, vitamins A and D, thiamin, riboflavin, niacin, and vitamin C. Recommended intakes were based on amounts that would prevent nutrient deficiencies.

Over the years since those first standards were developed, dietary habits and disease patterns have changed, and dietary recommendations have had to change along with them. Overt nutrient deficiencies are now rare in the United States, but the incidence of nutrition-related chronic diseases, such as heart disease, diabetes, osteoporosis, and obesity, has increased. To combat these more recent health concerns, recommendations are now intended to promote health as well as prevent deficiencies. The original RDAs have been expanded into the Dietary Reference Intakes, which address problems of excess as well as deficiency. The *Dietary Guidelines for Americans*, introduced in 1980 to make diet and lifestyle recommendations that promote health and reduce the risks of obesity and chronic disease, have

Today's food guide • Figure 2.1 _____

How food guides present recommendations has changed over the years, but the basic message has stayed the same: Choose the right combinations of foods to promote health. MyPlate, shown here, is the latest food guide.

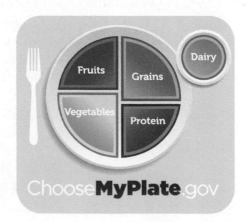

WHAT A SCIENTIST SEES

Trends in Milk Consumption

The graph below shows estimates of milk consumption in the United States from 1910 to 2005, based on the amount of milk available for human consumption during that period.[3,4] Anyone looking at the graph can tell that overall milk consumption and consumption of whole milk both declined, while consumption of lower-fat milks increased. A nutrition scientist looking at this graph, however, would see not just changes in the amounts and types of milk consumed but the nutritional and public health implications of these changes as well.

Because whole milk is high in saturated fat, replacing whole milk with lower-fat milk decreases saturated fat intake. This is good from the standpoint of heart health, but the decline in total milk consumption may be bad for bone health. Milk is one of the most important sources of calcium in the North American diet. The scientist will be alerted to the fact that calcium intake from milk has been declining. Unless more calcium from other sources is being consumed, this drop in milk consumption may indicate that the population is at risk for fragile bones and an increase in fractures.

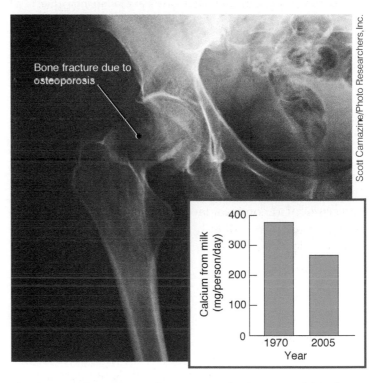

Bone fracture due to osteoporosis

Scott Camazine/Photo Researchers, Inc.

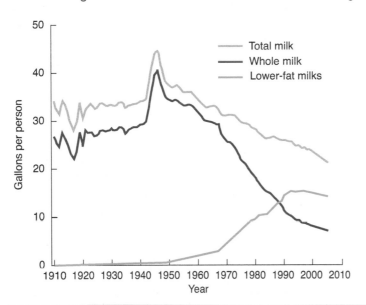

This bar graph compares the amount of calcium available from milk in 1970 and 2005. If the decrease is indicative of overall calcium intake, it could contribute to an increase in the risk of bone fractures such as the one shown here.

Think Critically Based on this analysis, what measures would you suggest to increase the population's calcium intake?

---

been revised every 5 years.[2] Early food guides have evolved into *MyPlate*, which suggests amounts and types of food from five food groups to meet the recommendations of the Dietary Guidelines (see Figure 2.1). In addition, standardized food labels have been developed to help consumers choose foods that meet these recommendations.

How We Use Nutrition Recommendations

Nutrition recommendations are developed to address the nutritional concerns of the population and help individuals meet their nutrient needs. These recommendations can also be used to evaluate the nutrient intake of populations and of individuals within populations. Determining what people eat and how their nutrient intake compares to nutrition recommendations is important for assessing their nutritional status.

When evaluating the nutritional status of a population, food intake can be assessed by having individuals record or recall their food intake or by using information about the amounts and types of food available to the population to identify trends in the diet (see *What a Scientist Sees*).

> **nutritional status**
> An individual's health, as it is influenced by the intake and utilization of nutrients.

PROCESS DIAGRAM

Assessing nutritional status • Figure 2.2

✓ THE PLANNER

A complete assessment of an individual's nutritional status includes a diet analysis, a physical exam, a medical history, and an evaluation of nutrient levels in the body. An interpretation of this information can determine whether an individual is well nourished, malnourished, or at risk of malnutrition.

1 Determine typical food intake. People's typical food intake can be evaluated by having them record their food as they consume it or recall what they have eaten during the past day or so. Because food intake varies from day to day, to obtain a realistic picture, an individual's intake should be monitored for more than one day. An accurate food record includes the amounts of all foods and beverages consumed, along with descriptions of cooking methods and brand names of products. It is often difficult to obtain an accurate record because people may change what they are eating rather than record it, or they may forget what they ate when trying to recall it.

2 Analyze nutrient intake. A quick diet analysis can be done by comparing an individual's food intake to the recommendations of MyPlate. A more thorough analysis can be done by using a computer program that compares nutrient intake to recommendations. In this example, which shows only a few nutrients, intake of vitamin A, iron, and calcium is below the recommended amounts, and intake of vitamin C and saturated fat is above the recommended amounts.

Nutrient	My DRI	My Intake	Percent of My DRI
Vitamin A (RAE)	700 µg	525	75%
Vitamin C	75 mg	86	115%
Iron	18 mg	9.7	54%
Calcium	1000 mg	750	75%
Saturated fat	< 23.8 g	31.9	Above recommended range

FOOD DIARY

Record all the food and beverages you eat. Include the food, how it was prepared, the amount you ate and the brand name. Don't forget to list all fats used in cooking and all spreads and sauces added.

Time	Food	Kind and how prepared	Amount
7:00 A.M.	Eggs	scrambled	2
	Butter	in eggs	1 tsp.
	toast	whole wheat	2 slices
	Butter	on toast	2 tsp.
	Milk	non-fat	8 oz.
	Orange juice	from frozen concentrate	8 oz.
12:00 P.M.	Big Mac	McDonald's	1

3 Evaluate physical health. A physical examination can detect signs of nutrient deficiencies or excesses. Measures of body dimensions such as height and weight can be monitored over time or compared with standards for a given population. Drastic changes in measurements or measurements that are significantly above or below the standards could indicate nutritional deficiency or excess.

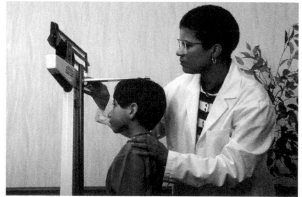

Blair Seitz/Photo Researchers

When food intake data are evaluated in conjunction with information about the health and nutritional status of individuals in the population (**Figure 2.2**), relationships between dietary intake and health and disease can be identified. This is important for developing public health policies and programs that address nutritional problems. For example, population surveys such as the National Health and Nutrition Examination Survey (NHANES), which collects diet and health information, have helped public health officials recognize that low iron levels are a problem for many people, including young women, preschool children, and elderly people. This information led to the fortification of grain products with iron beginning in the 1940s. Recent NHANES data have also shown that the number of calories Americans consume per day has increased over the past few decades and that the incidence of obesity has increased dramatically during the same period. This has led public health experts to develop programs to improve both the diet and the fitness of Americans.

The information obtained from population health and nutrition surveys is also used to determine whether

4 **Consider medical history and lifestyle.** Personal and family medical histories are important because genetic risk factors affect an individual's risk of developing a nutrition-related disease. For example, if you have high cholesterol and your father died of a heart attack at age 50, you have a higher-than-average risk of developing heart disease. Lifestyle factors such as physical activity level and eating habits can add to or reduce your inherited risk.

5 **Assess with laboratory tests.** Measures of nutrients, their by-products, or their functions in the blood, urine, or body cells can help detect nutrient deficiencies and excesses or the risk of nutrition-related chronic diseases (see online Appendix F). For instance, an individual's iron status can be assessed by drawing a blood sample, measuring hemoglobin (an iron-carrying protein) and hematocrit (the proportion of blood volume that is red blood cells), and then comparing the values to the healthy range.

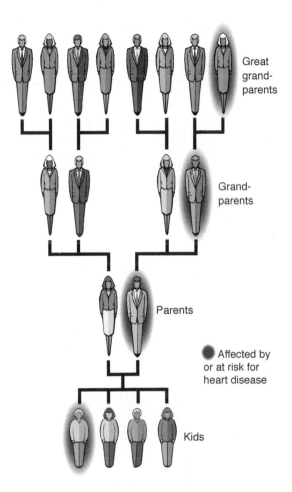

Great grand-parents

Grand-parents

Parents

● Affected by or at risk for heart disease

Kids

Patient: Jane Doe, female, age 20

Laboratory test	Laboratory Result	Healthy Range
Hemoglobin	14 g/100 ml	12-16 g/100 ml
Hematocrit	40 ml/100 ml	36-47 ml/100 ml

Think Critically If a medical history reveals that one of your parents has had a heart attack, what other components of nutrition assessment would help you to determine your overall risk for heart disease? Why?

the nation is meeting health and nutrition goals, such as those established by **Healthy People**. This set of health-promotion and disease-prevention objectives is revised every 10 years, with the goal of increasing the quality and length of healthy lives for the population as a whole and eliminating health disparities among different segments of the population. The latest version of these objectives has been released as *Healthy People 2020*. The long-term goal is to create a social climate in which everyone has a chance to live long, healthy lives (see online Appendix G).[5]

CONCEPT CHECK

1. **How** do nutrition recommendations benefit individual and public health?

2. **Why** do the current DRIs focus on preventing chronic disease?

3. **What** factors are considered in evaluating nutritional status?

LEARNING OBJECTIVES

1. **Summarize** the purpose of the DRIs.
2. **Describe** the four sets of DRI values used in recommending nutrient intake.
3. **List** the factors that are considered when estimating an individual's energy needs.
4. **Explain** the concept of the Acceptable Macronutrient Distribution Ranges (AMDRs).

The **Dietary Reference Intakes (DRIs)** are recommendations for the amounts of energy, nutrients, and other food components that healthy people should consume in order to stay healthy, reduce the risk of chronic disease, and prevent deficiencies.[6] The DRIs can be used to evaluate whether a person's diet provides all the essential nutrients in adequate amounts. They include several types of recommendations that address both nutrient intake and energy intake and include values that are appropriate for people of different genders and stages of life (**Figure 2.3**).

Recommendations for Nutrient Intake

The DRI recommendations for nutrient intake include four sets of values. The **Estimated Average Requirements (EARs)** are average amounts of nutrients or other dietary components required by healthy individuals in a population (**Figure 2.4**). They are used to assess the adequacy of a population's food supply or typical nutrient intake and are not appropriate for evaluating an individual's intake. The **Recommended Dietary Allowances (RDAs)** are set higher than the EARs and represent amounts of nutrients and other dietary components that will meet the needs of most healthy people (see Figure 2.4).

> **Estimated Average Requirements (EARs)** Nutrient intakes estimated to meet the needs of 50% of the healthy individuals in a given gender and life-stage group.
>
> **Recommended Dietary Allowances (RDAs)** Nutrient intakes that are sufficient to meet the needs of almost all healthy people in a specific gender and life-stage group.

DRIs for all population groups • Figure 2.3

The DRIs include four types of nutrient intake recommendations and two types of recommendations related to energy intake. Because gender and life stage affect nutrient needs, recommendations have been set for each gender and for various life-stage groups. These values take into account the physiological differences that affect the nutrient needs of men and women, infants, children, adolescents, adults, older adults, and pregnant and lactating women.

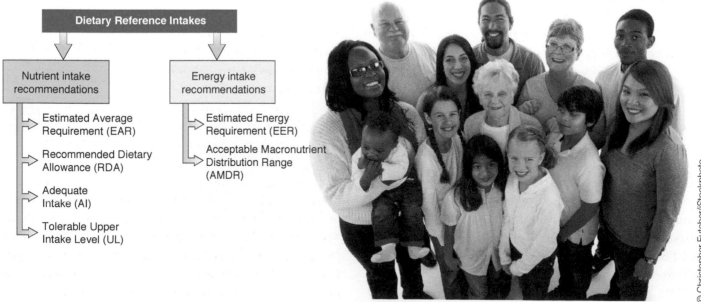

Dietary Reference Intakes

Nutrient intake recommendations
- Estimated Average Requirement (EAR)
- Recommended Dietary Allowance (RDA)
- Adequate Intake (AI)
- Tolerable Upper Intake Level (UL)

Energy intake recommendations
- Estimated Energy Requirement (EER)
- Acceptable Macronutrient Distribution Range (AMDR)

© Christopher Futcher/iStockphoto

The EAR and RDA for a nutrient are determined by measuring the amount of the nutrient required by different individuals in a population group and plotting all the values. The resulting plot is a bell-shaped curve; a few individuals in the group need only a small amount of the nutrient, a few need a large amount, and the majority need an amount that falls between the extremes.

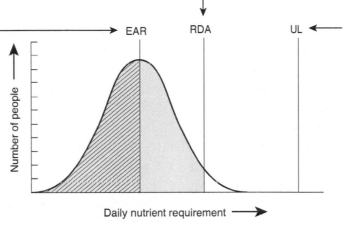

The RDA is set by adding a safety factor to the EAR. About 97% of the population meets its needs by consuming this amount (shown as yellow shading). If nutrient intake meets the RDA, the risk of deficiency is very low. As intake falls, the risk of a deficiency increases.

An EAR is the average amount of a nutrient required for good health. If everyone in the population consumed this amount, only 50% would obtain enough of the nutrient to meet their requirements (shown as diagonal lines).

The UL is set well above the needs of everyone in the population and represents the highest amount of the nutrient that will not cause toxicity symptoms in the majority of healthy people. As intake rises above the UL, the likelihood of toxicity increases.

EAR   RDA   UL

Number of people

Daily nutrient requirement

Ask Yourself

1. Which DRI value(s) is/are set at a level that will meet the needs of most healthy people in the population?
2. Which DRI value represents the amount above which toxicity becomes more likely?

When there aren't enough data about nutrient requirements to establish RDAs, **Adequate Intakes (AIs)** are set, based on what healthy people typically eat. RDA or AI values can be used as goals for individual intake and to plan and evaluate individual diets (see Appendix A and the inside covers). They are meant to represent the amounts that most healthy people should consume, on average, over several days or even weeks, not each and every day.

Because they are set high enough to meet the needs of almost all healthy people, intake below the RDA or AI does not necessarily mean that an individual is deficient, but the risk of deficiency is greater than if the individual consumed the recommended amount.

> **Adequate Intakes (AIs)** Nutrient intakes that should be used as a goal when no RDA exists. AI values are an approximation of the nutrient intake that sustains health.

The fourth set of values, **Tolerable Upper Intake Levels (ULs)**, specifies the maximum amount of a nutrient that most people can consume on a daily basis without some adverse effect (see Figure 2.4). For most nutrients, it is difficult to exceed the UL by consuming food. Most foods do not contain enough of any one nutrient to cause toxicity; however, some dietary supplements and fortified foods may. For some nutrients, the UL is set for total intake from all sources, including food, fortified foods, and dietary supplements. For other nutrients, the UL refers to intake from supplements alone or from supplements and fortified foods. For many nutrients, there is no UL because not enough information is available to determine it.

> **Tolerable Upper Intake Levels (ULs)** Maximum daily intake levels that are unlikely to pose risks of adverse health effects to almost all individuals in a given gender and life-stage group.

Meeting energy needs • Figure 2.5

Think Critically If this 19-year-old gains 20 pounds, how will it affect her EER?

The DRIs recommend amounts of energy (calories) and proportions of carbohydrate, fat, and protein that provide a healthy diet.

a. The EER represents the amount of energy required to maintain weight. Based on the EER calculation, a 19-year-old girl who is 5'4" tall, weighs 127 pounds, and gets no exercise needs about 1940 Calories a day. If she adds an hour of moderate activity to her daily routine, her EER will increase by 460 Calories; she would need to eat an additional 460 Calories more per day to maintain her current weight.[6]

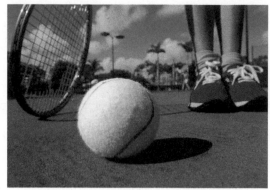

b. The AMDRs are a guide for selecting healthy proportions of carbohydrate, protein, and fat. As shown by these two meals, many different food combinations can provide a healthy diet. Although only the meal on the left provides proportions of carbohydrate, protein, and fat that fall within the AMDRs, the meal on the right can still be part of a healthy diet if other meals that day are lower in protein and fat and higher in carbohydrate.

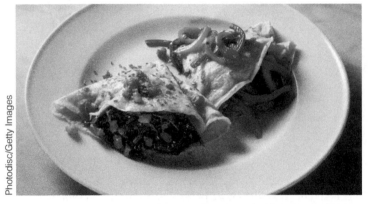

This meal contains approximately 480 Calories, of which about 55% is from carbohydrate, 20% is from protein, and 25% is from fat.

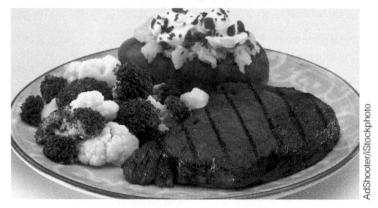

This meal contains approximately 740 Calories, of which about 30% is from carbohydrate, 35% is from protein, and 35% is from fat.

Recommendations for Energy Intake

The DRIs make two types of recommendations about energy intake. The first, called **Estimated Energy Requirements (EERs)**, provides an estimate of how many calories are needed to keep body weight stable. EER calculations take into account a person's age, gender, weight, height, and level of physical activity (see Appendix A). A change in any of these variables changes the person's energy needs (**Figure 2.5a**).

The second type of energy recommendation, called **Acceptable Macronutrient Distribution Ranges (AMDRs)**, makes recommendations about the proportions of calories that should come from carbohydrate, fat, and protein in a healthy diet. AMDRs are ranges—10 to 35% of calories from protein, 45 to 65% of calories from carbohydrate, and 20 to 35% of calories from fat—not exact values. This is because a wide range of macronutrient distributions is associated with health. AMDRs are intended to promote diets that minimize disease risk and allow flexibility in food intake patterns (**Figure 2.5b**).

> **Estimated Energy Requirements (EERs)** Energy intakes that are predicted to maintain body weight in healthy individuals
>
> **Acceptable Macronutrient Distribution Ranges (AMDRs)** Healthy ranges of intake for carbohydrate, fat, and protein, expressed as percentages of total energy intake.

CONCEPT CHECK STOP

1. **What** are RDAs and AIs used for?
2. **How** might you use ULs?
3. **What** are five variables that affect your energy needs?
4. **Why** are AMDR values given as ranges rather than as single numbers?

2.3 Tools for Diet Planning

LEARNING OBJECTIVES

1. **Discuss** how following the recommendations of the Dietary Guidelines can help prevent chronic disease.
2. **Explain** the purpose of MyPlate.
3. **Plan** a diet that meets your daily food plan.
4. **Identify** foods that are high in empty calories.

The DRIs tell you how much of each nutrient you need, but they do not help you choose foods that will meet these needs. To help consumers choose diets that will meet their needs, the U.S. government has developed the *Dietary Guidelines for Americans* and **MyPlate**. The Dietary Guidelines are a set of diet and lifestyle recommendations designed to promote health and reduce the risk of overweight, obesity, and chronic diseases in the U.S. population.[2] MyPlate is the USDA's most recent food guide. It divides foods into groups, based on the nutrients they supply most abundantly, and illustrates the appropriate proportions of foods from each food group that make up a healthy diet.

Recommendations of the *Dietary Guidelines for Americans*

The 2010 *Dietary Guidelines for Americans* provide evidence-based nutritional guidance to promote health and reduce the prevalence of overweight and obesity and the risk of chronic disease. The recommendations of this 7th edition of the *Dietary Guidelines for Americans* focus on balancing calorie intake with physical activity and consuming nutrient dense foods and beverages (**Table 2.1**).

Key Recommendation of the 2010 Dietary Guidelines[2]   Table 2.1

Balancing calories to manage weight
- Prevent and/or reduce overweight and obesity through improved eating and physical activity behaviors.
- Control total calorie intake to manage body weight. For people who are overweight or obese, this means consuming fewer calories from foods and beverages.
- Increase physical activity and reduce time spent in sedentary behaviors.
- Maintain appropriate caloric balance during each stage of life—childhood, adolescence, adulthood, pregnancy and breastfeeding, and older age.

Foods and nutrients to increase. Individuals should meet the following recommendations as part of a healthy eating pattern while staying within their calorie needs:
- Increase vegetable and fruit intake.
- Eat a variety of vegetables, especially dark-green and red and orange vegetables and beans and peas.
- Consume at least half of all grains as whole grains. Increase whole-grain intake by replacing refined grains with whole grains.
- Increase intake of fat-free or low-fat milk and milk products, such as milk, yogurt, cheese, or fortified soy beverages.
- Choose a variety of protein foods, including seafood, lean meat and poultry, eggs, beans and peas, soy products, and unsalted nuts and seeds.
- Increase the amount and variety of seafood consumed by choosing seafood in place of some meat and poultry.
- Replace protein foods that are higher in solid fats with choices that are lower in solid fats and calories and/or are sources of oils.
- Use oils to replace solid fats where possible.
- Choose foods that provide more potassium, dietary fiber, calcium, and vitamin D, which are nutrients of concern in U.S. diets. These foods include vegetables, fruits, whole grains, and milk and milk products.

Foods and food components to reduce
- Reduce daily sodium intake to less than 2300 milligrams (mg) and further reduce intake to 1500 mg among persons who are 51 and older and those of any age who are African American or have hypertension, diabetes, or chronic kidney disease. The 1500 mg recommendation applies to about half of the U.S. population, including children, and the majority of adults.
- Consume less than 10% of calories from saturated fatty acids by replacing them with monounsaturated and polyunsaturated fatty acids.
- Consume less than 300 mg per day of dietary cholesterol.
- Keep *trans* fatty acid consumption as low as possible by limiting foods that contain synthetic sources of *trans* fats, such as partially hydrogenated oils, and by limiting other solid fats.
- Reduce intake of calories from solid fats and added sugars.
- Limit consumption of foods that contain refined grains, especially refined grain foods that contain solid fats, added sugars, and sodium.
- If alcohol is consumed, consume it in moderation—up to one drink per day for women and two drinks per day for men—and only by adults of legal drinking age.

Building healthy eating patterns
- Select an eating pattern that meets nutrient needs over time at an appropriate calorie level.
- Account for all foods and beverages consumed and assess how they fit within a total healthy eating pattern.
- Follow food safety recommendations when preparing and eating foods to reduce the risk of food-borne illnesses.

The Issue: Poor dietary habits in the United States have resulted in a largely unfit, unhealthy nation. Should the government intervene to change the types of food we can purchase?

The typical U.S. diet is not as healthy as it could be. Our lack of dietary discretion has contributed to our high rates of obesity, diabetes, high blood pressure, and heart disease.[2] This is not only the concern of the individuals whose lives are affected by these conditions but also the government. The dollar cost to our health care system is huge; half of the $147 billion per year the United States spends on obesity comes from government-funded Medicare and Medicaid.[7] Government concern is not just financial. The fact that almost one in four applicants to the military is rejected for being overweight is suggested to be a threat to national security and military readiness.[8]

So, who is responsible for our unhealthy diet, and who should be responsible for changing what we eat? Proponents of more government involvement in our food choices suggest that our food environment is the cause of our unhealthy eating habits. Obesity expert Kelly Brownell believes that environment plays a more powerful role in determining food choices than does personal irresponsibility.[9] Brownell and other proponents of government intervention argue that the government should treat our noxious food environment like any other public health threat and develop programs to keep us safe and healthy. Just as government regulations help to ensure that our food is not contaminated with harmful bacteria, laws could ensure that what you order at a restaurant will not contribute to heart disease or cancer. Unfortunately, unlike bacteria, individual foods are difficult to classify as healthy or unhealthy. Almost all food has some nutritional benefits, and the arguments as to what is a "junk food" and what we should add or subtract from our diets are ongoing. However, many people believe there are things that could be done to ensure healthier choices.

One option to encourage healthier choices suggested by proponents of government intervention is to tax junk food, making it more expensive, and to increase subsidies for fruits and vegetables, making them less expensive. Other suggestions include zoning restrictions to keep fast-food restaurants away from schools and child-care facilities and limitations on the types of foods that can be advertised on children's television. All these ideas have pros and cons, and none will absolve individuals of the responsibility for getting more exercise and making healthier food choices.

Opponents of government involvement believe it is an infringement on personal freedom and suggest that individuals need to take responsibility for their actions. They propose that the food industry work with the public to make healthier food more available and affordable. Many food companies have already responded to the need for a better diet; General Mills and Kellogg's offer whole-grain cereals. And the giant food retailer Wal-Mart is working with suppliers to reduce the amount of sodium and added sugar and eliminate *trans* fat from packaged foods.

Our current food environment makes unhealthy eating easy. Fatty, salty, and sugary foods are available 24/7, and the portions offered are often massive. To preserve our public health, the United States needs to change the way it eats. This change could be driven by government regulations and taxes, it could come from changes in the food industry, or it could come from individuals taking more responsibility for their choices and their health. A synergy of policy intervention, industry cooperation, and personal efforts is likely needed to solve the crisis.

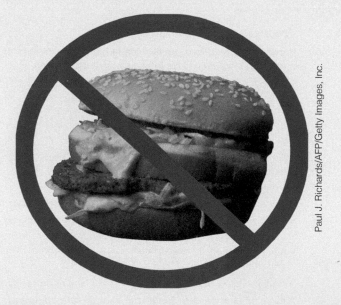

Paul J. Richards/AFP/Getty Images, Inc.

Americans want the personal freedom to choose what they eat, but that has not stopped people from blaming fast food for their health problems.

Think Critically: If someone eats fast food daily and becomes obese, is that person to blame for eating the food, or is the restaurant to blame for not informing the person of the health risks?

These recommendations are designed for Americans 2 years of age and older. Additional recommendations target specific subpopulations (see online Appendix G). Adopting the recommendations of the Dietary Guidelines will help Americans live healthier lives, which will lower health-care costs and help to strengthen America's long-term economic competitiveness and overall productivity. (see *Debate: How Involved Should the Government be in Your Food Choices?*).

Balancing calories to manage weight About two-thirds of adults and a third of children in the United

States weigh more than they should.[10] This is not only a cosmetic problem but increases the risk of diabetes, heart disease, and a variety of other ailments. To address this problem, the 2010 Dietary Guidelines emphasize balancing the calories consumed in food and beverages with the calories expended through physical activity in order to achieve and maintain a healthy weight. Weight maintenance requires consuming the same number of calories as you burn; this means that if you eat more, you need to exercise more (see Chapter 9). Losing weight requires consuming fewer calories than you burn. This weight loss can be accomplished by reducing energy intake and increasing energy expenditure through exercise (**Figure 2.6**). The Dietary Guidelines recommend enjoying your food but eating less of it.

Foods and nutrients to increase The Dietary Guidelines recommend that we increase our vegetable and fruit intake to at least 2½ cups per day and improve our choices by selecting more fruits than fruit juices and eating a variety of vegetables, especially dark-green and red and orange vegetables and beans and peas. The Dietary Guidelines suggest that we replace refined grains with whole grains so that at least half of our grain servings are whole grains. They also suggest that Americans increase their intake of fat-free or low-fat milk and milk products, while limiting consumption of high-fat dairy products such as cheese. This pattern of fruit, vegetable, grain, and dairy consumption will increase our intake of potassium, dietary fiber, calcium, vitamin A, vitamin C, and vitamin D, which are nutrients of concern in American diets. Protein choices should include a variety of protein foods, such as lean meat, poultry, seafood, eggs, beans and peas, soy products, and unsalted nuts and seeds. We should increase the variety and amount of seafood by choosing it in place of meat

Healthy weight and exercise recommendations • Figure 2.6

The Dietary Guidelines suggest that most Americans consume more calories than they expend. To achieve calorie balance, adults should decrease calorie intake and increase physical activity gradually over time to achieve a healthy weight.

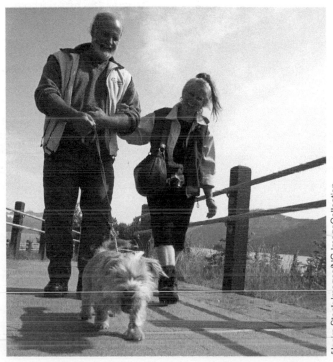

b. To promote health and reduce disease risk, a minimum of 150 minutes of moderate-intensity aerobic exercise is recommended each week. Some adults will need a higher level of physical activity than others (the equivalent of more than 300 minutes of moderate-intensity activity per week) to achieve and maintain a healthy body weight.

a. Limiting portion sizes and reducing consumption of added sugars, solid fats, and alcohol, which provide calories but few essential nutrients, can help promote a healthy weight. There is no optimal proportion of macronutrients that can facilitate weight management; the critical issue is the right number of calories needed to maintain or lose weight over time.

Jose Luis Pelaez/Getty Images, Inc.

Alaska Stock Images/NG ImageCollection

Healthy eating patterns are high in fruits and vegetables and whole grains, and include low-fat dairy products, fish, legumes, nuts, seeds, and healthy oils. They are low in solid fats, sodium, and added sugar.

a. The current U.S. dietary pattern is not as healthy as it could be. The graph shown here illustrates the usual U.S. intake of selected foods and nutrients as a percentage of the recommended goal or limit. ▼

[Bar graph: "Percentage of goal or limit" on x-axis (0 to 300)]

Goal
- Whole grains
- Vegetables
- Fruits
- Dairy
- Seafood
- Oils

Limit
- *SoFAS
- Calories
- Sodium
- Saturated fat

*Calories from solid fats and added sugars

b. The *Dietary Guidelines for Americans* suggest that there are many ways to choose a healthy diet, including the USDA Food Patterns (see Appendix B), the DASH Eating Plan, and Mediterranean-style eating patterns. These patterns all focus on similar types of foods. ▶

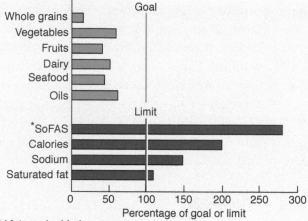

Keen Press/NG Image Collection

c. It is important to consider ◀ beverages as part of any healthy dietary pattern. Currently, American adults ages 19 years and older consume an average of about 400 Calories per day from beverages. Many of the most commonly consumed beverages, including sugar-sweetened sodas, fruit drinks, and alcoholic beverages, contain calories but provide few essential nutrients. The Dietary Guidelines recommend replacing sugary drinks with water.

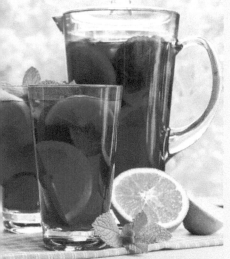

Elena Elisseeva/iStockphoto

Courtesy Jonathan Liss, MD

and poultry. The Dietary Guidelines also recommend that we use oils in place of solid fats when possible.

Foods and food components to reduce The Dietary Guidelines recommend reducing intake of saturated fat, *trans* fat, and cholesterol—the types of lipids that increase the risk of heart disease (see Chapter 5).

In order to prevent high blood pressure, the Dietary Guidelines recommend limiting sodium intake to less than 2300 mg/day. Those who are 51 and older, and those of any age who are African American or have hypertension, diabetes, or chronic kidney disease should limit sodium to less than 1500 mg/day. They also recommend that Americans reduce their intake of added

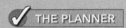
Joe Petersburger/NG
Image Collection

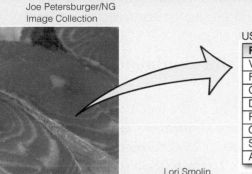

USDA Food Patterns

Food group	Amount/day
Vegetables	2.5 cups
Fruit and juices	2.0 cups
Grains	6.0 ounces
Dairy products	3.0 cups
Protein foods	5.5 ounces
Oils	27 grams
Solid fats	16 grams
Added sugars	32 grams

Lori Smolin

The USDA Food Patterns suggest amounts of foods from different food groups and subgroups for different calorie levels (2000 Calories shown here). The USDA Food Patterns and their vegetarian variations (see Appendix B and Chapter 6) were developed to help individuals follow the Dietary Guidelines recommendations and are the basis for the MyPlate recommendations.

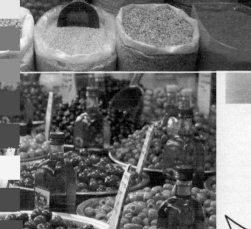

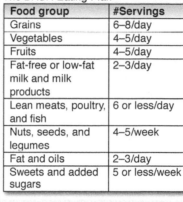

The DASH Eating Plan

Food group	#Servings
Grains	6–8/day
Vegetables	4–5/day
Fruits	4–5/day
Fat-free or low-fat milk and milk products	2–3/day
Lean meats, poultry, and fish	6 or less/day
Nuts, seeds, and legumes	4–5/week
Fat and oils	2–3/day
Sweets and added sugars	5 or less/week

The DASH Eating Plan focuses on increasing foods rich in potassium, calcium, magnesium, and fiber. It is plentiful in fruits and vegetables, whole grains, low-fat dairy, fish, poultry, beans, nuts, and seeds. It was first developed for lowering blood pressure and is discussed further in Chapter 8.

Masterfile

Mediterranean Eating Pattern

Foods	How often
Fruits, vegetables, grains (mostly whole), olive oil, nuts, legumes and seeds, herbs and spices	Every meal
Fish and seafood	At least twice a week
Cheese and yogurt	Moderate portions daily or weekly
Poultry and eggs	Moderate portions every 2 days or weekly
Meats and sweets	Less often

Traditional Mediterranean eating patterns are based on fruits, vegetables, grains, olive oil, legumes, nuts, and seeds. They include moderate portions of cheese and yogurt. Fish and seafood are consumed at least twice a week; poultry and eggs every few days; and red meat and sweets less often. The incidence of chronic diseases such as heart disease is low in populations consuming this diet (see Chapter 5).

Courtesy Jonathan Liss, MD

sugars and refined grains and consume alcohol only in moderation.

Building healthy eating patterns There is no single diet that defines healthy. Rather, there are a variety of healthy eating patterns that can accommodate differences in cultural, ethnic, traditional, and personal preferences and differences in food cost and availability (**Figure 2.7**).[11] All these patterns are abundant in nutrient-dense foods, including vegetables, fruits, and whole grains; include moderate amounts of a variety of high-protein foods; and are low in full-fat dairy products. Healthy eating patterns include more oils than solid fats and limit added sugars and sodium. The *Dietary Guidelines for Americans* discuss three healthy eating patterns. There are also other dietary patterns that promote health. The Healthy Eating Plate in **Figure 2.8** is a healthy dietary pattern developed by the Harvard School of Public Health.

A fundamental premise of the Dietary Guidelines is that nutrients should come primarily from foods; supplements and fortified foods may be advantageous in specific situations to increase intake of a specific vitamin or mineral. Fortification can provide a food-based means for increasing the intake of particular nutrients.

Paying attention to food safety is also part of healthful eating. Currently, food-borne illness affects about 48 million individuals in the United States every year and leads to 128,000 hospitalizations and 3000 deaths (see Chapter 13).[12] Consumers can prevent food-borne illness at home by washing hands, rinsing vegetables and fruits, preventing cross-contamination, cooking foods to safe internal temperatures, and storing foods safely.

MyPlate: Putting the Guidelines into Practice

MyPlate can be used to plan a diet based on the recommendations of the Dietary Guidelines. The plate icon illustrates the proportions of food recommended from each of five food groups: Fruits, vegetables, grains, protein foods, and dairy. Half of your plate should be fruits and vegetables, about a quarter grains, and about a quarter protein foods. Dairy should accompany meals as shown by the small circle to the side (**Figure 2.9a**)

The Healthy Eating Plate • Figure 2.8

The Healthy Eating Plate emphasizes that a healthy diet is based on whole grains, fruits, vegetables, healthy protein sources, and oils. This dietary pattern recommends limiting red meat, refined grains, and dairy and avoiding sugary soft drinks, *trans* fat, and processed meats.

Think Critically How does the Healthy Eating Plate differ from MyPlate? Which of these tools will better help Americans improve their diets? Why?

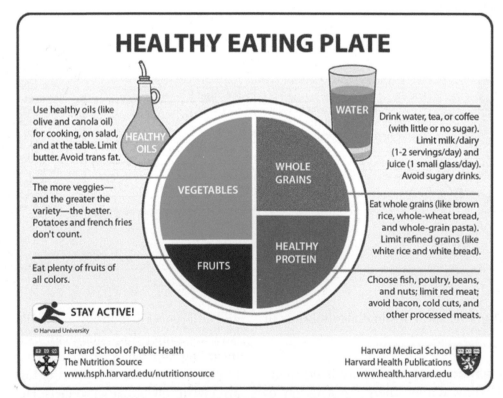

Copyright © 2011 Harvard University. For more information about The Healthy Eating Plate, please see The Nutrition Source, Department of Nutrition, Harvard School of Public Health, http://www.thenutritionsource.org.

MyPlate recommends proportions of foods that make up a healthy diet and offers personalized food plans to determine the amounts from each food group that are appropriate for you.

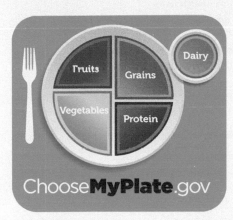

Balancing Calories

- Enjoy your food, but eat less.
- Avoid oversized portions.

Foods to Increase

- Make half your plate fruits and vegetables.
- Make at least half your grains whole grains.
- Switch to fat-free or low-fat (1%) milk.

Foods to Reduce

- Compare sodium in foods such as soup, breads, and frozen meals—and choose the foods with lower numbers.
- Drink water instead of sugary drinks.

a. The MyPlate icon shows what a balanced meal should look like. It is based on the recommendations of the Dietary Guidelines. Shown here are some key messages to help consumers balance calories and increase the nutrient density of their diet.

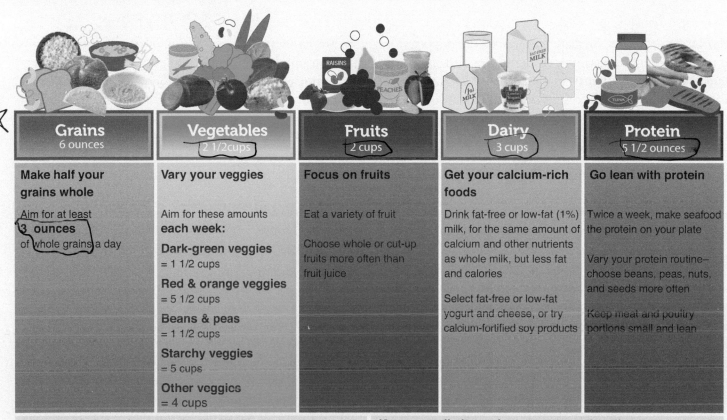

Grains 6 ounces	Vegetables 2 1/2 cups	Fruits 2 cups	Dairy 3 cups	Protein 5 1/2 ounces
Make half your grains whole Aim for at least 3 ounces of whole grains a day	**Vary your veggies** Aim for these amounts **each week:** **Dark-green veggies** = 1 1/2 cups **Red & orange veggies** = 5 1/2 cups **Beans & peas** = 1 1/2 cups **Starchy veggies** = 5 cups **Other veggies** = 4 cups	**Focus on fruits** Eat a variety of fruit Choose whole or cut-up fruits more often than fruit juice	**Get your calcium-rich foods** Drink fat-free or low-fat (1%) milk, for the same amount of calcium and other nutrients as whole milk, but less fat and calories Select fat-free or low-fat yogurt and cheese, or try calcium-fortified soy products	**Go lean with protein** Twice a week, make seafood the protein on your plate Vary your protein routine—choose beans, peas, nuts, and seeds more often Keep meat and poultry portions small and lean

Find your balance between food and physical activity

Be physically active for at least **150 minutes** each week.

Know your limits on fats, sugars, and sodium

Your allowance for oils is **6 teaspoons** a day. Limit calories from solid fats and added sugars to **260 Calories** a day. Reduce sodium intake to less than **2300 mg a day.**

b. The MyPlate Daily Food Plan shown here is for a person who needs 2000 Calories per day. You can obtain your personalized food plan by looking up the USDA Food Plan that meets your calorie needs in Appendix B or by going to the Web site www.ChooseMyPlate.gov, clicking on "Supertracker and Other Tools," and selecting "Daily Food Plans."

WHAT SHOULD I EAT?

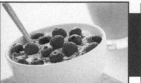
© Sara Winter/iStockphoto

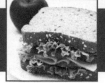
© Jill Chen/iStockphoto

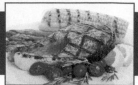
© Steve Mcsweeny/iStockphoto

To Fill My Plate

Balance calories to manage weight
- Choose low-calorie snacks such as vegetables and fruits.
- Walk an extra 1000 steps; the more you exercise, the easier it is to keep your weight at a healthy level.
- Ride your bike to work or when running errands.
- Watch your portions. When you eat out, split an entrée with a friend.

Increase foods that promote health
- Have strawberries rather than strawberry shortcake for dessert.
- Make sure your breakfast cereal is a whole-grain cereal.
- Be colorful by adding some red and orange vegetables to your salad.
- Toss some salmon on the grill to increase your seafood intake.

Limit nutrients that increase health risks
- Choose lean meat, fish, and low-fat dairy products in order to limit saturated fat.
- Have water and skip sugary soft drinks.
- Pass on the salt; instead, try lemon juice or some basil and oregano.
- If you drink alcohol, stop after one drink.

Use iProfile to look up the saturated fat and sugar content of your breakfast cereal.

MyPlate messages MyPlate emphasizes the importance of proportionality, variety, moderation, and nutrient density in a healthy diet (see *What Should I Eat?*). Proportionality means eating more of some types of foods than others. The MyPlate icon shows how much of your plate should be filled with foods from various food groups.

Variety is important for a healthy diet because no one food or food group provides all the nutrients and food components the body needs. A variety of foods should also be selected from within each food group. The vegetables food group includes choices from five subgroups: dark-green vegetables such as broccoli, collard greens, and kale; red and orange vegetables such as carrots, sweet potatoes, and red peppers; starchy vegetables such as corn, green peas, and potatoes; other vegetables such as cabbage, asparagus, and artichokes; and beans and peas such as lentils, chickpeas, and black beans. Beans and peas are good sources of the nutrients found in both vegetables and protein foods, so they can be counted in either food group. Protein foods include meat, poultry, seafood, beans and peas, eggs, processed soy products, nuts, and seeds. Grains include whole grains such as whole-wheat bread, oatmeal, and brown rice as well as refined grains such as white bread, white rice, and white pasta (see Chapter 4). Fruits include fresh, canned, or dried fruit and 100% fruit juice. Dairy includes all fluid milk products and many foods made from milk such as cheese, yogurt, and pudding, as well as calcium-fortified soy products.

Moderation involves limiting portion sizes and choosing nutrient-dense foods to balance calories consumed with calories expended. Tips such as "make half your grains whole," "choose whole or cut-up fruits more often than juice," "select fat-free or low-fat dairy products," "keep meat and poultry portions small and lean," and many more found on the MyPlate website, are designed to help consumers make wise choices.

A Daily Food Plan Your Daily Food Plan tells you how much food to eat from each food group (**Figure 2.9b**). The amounts from the grains group are expressed in ounces. An ounce of grains is 1 cup of cold cereal, 1/2 cup of cooked cereal or grains, or a slice of bread. So if you have 2 cups of cereal and 2 slices of toast at breakfast, you have already consumed 4 ounces of grains for the day (two-thirds of the total for a 2000-Calorie diet). The amounts recommended for protein foods are also expressed in ounces. One ounce is equivalent to an ounce of cooked meat, poultry, or fish; one egg; 1 tablespoon of peanut butter; 1/4 cup of cooked dry beans; or 1/4 cup of nuts or seeds. The amounts recommended for fruits, vegetables, and dairy are given in cups.

It is easy to see where some foods in your diet fit on MyPlate. For example, a chicken breast is 3 ounces from the protein group; a scoop of rice is 2 ounces from the grains group. It is more difficult to see how much mixed foods such as pizza, stews, and casseroles contribute to each food group. To fit these on your plate, individual ingredients must be considered. For example, a slice of pizza provides 1 ounce of grains, 1/8 cup of vegetables, and 1/2 cup of dairy. Having meat on your pizza adds about 1/4 ounce from the protein group (**Figure 2.10**).

How meals fit • Figure 2.10

The lunch that is part of this 2000-Calorie menu includes about a third of the amounts of grains, protein foods, and dairy recommended for the day, a quarter of the recommended fruit, and half the recommended oils, but only a small proportion of the vegetables recommended. The lettuce and celery fit into to the "other vegetables" category, so choices at other meals should come from dark green, red and orange, and starchy vegetables as well as beans and peas. To find out what counts as an ounce or a cup, go to each food group at www.ChooseMyPlate.gov.

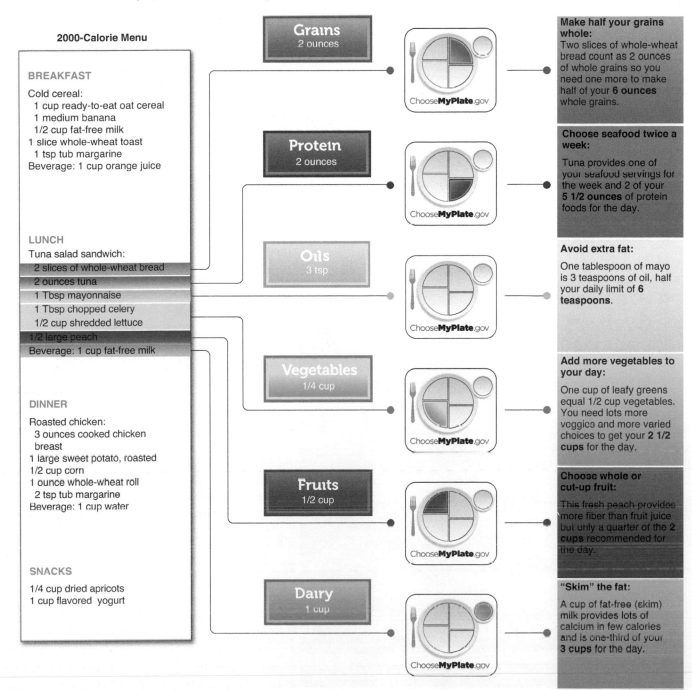

A Daily Food Plan also includes recommendations about the amounts of oils (in teaspoons) that should be included in your diet (see Figure 2.9b and Figure 2.10). Oils are fats that are liquid at room temperature; they come from plants and fish. They are rich in unsaturated fats, which help protect against heart disease. Solid fats are fats that are solid at room temperature, such as butter, lard, and shortening. They provide saturated and *trans* fat and should be limited in the diet.

A MyPlate Daily Food Plan recommends at least 150 minutes of activity each week to help balance food and physical activity and includes a calorie limit for **empty calories** from solid fats and added sugars. It is important to limit empty calories because consuming too many means you can't meet your nutrient needs without exceeding your calorie needs. (**Figure 2.11**).

One way to see how your daily intake matches the MyPlate recommendations is to use the interactive tools (such as Supertracker) on the MyPlate website to help track your progress toward choosing a healthy diet.

> **empty calories**
> Calories from solid fats and/or added sugars, which add calories to the food but few nutrients.

Empty calorie allowance • Figure 2.11

Many of the foods we choose are high in empty calories. In order to meet your nutrient needs without exceeding your calorie needs, you can include only small amounts of these foods.

a. Some empty calories come from foods that belong to a food group but contain added sugars and solid fats. These donuts, for example, are in the grains group, but about half of their calories are empty calories from solid fat and added sugars. Some foods, such as butter, table sugar, soft drinks, and candy, don't belong in any food group, because all their calories are empty. Oils are healthy fats, so they are not considered empty calories. ▼

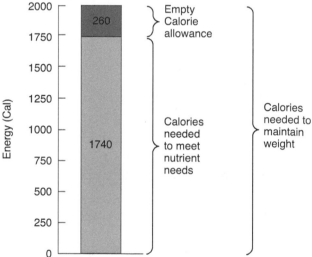

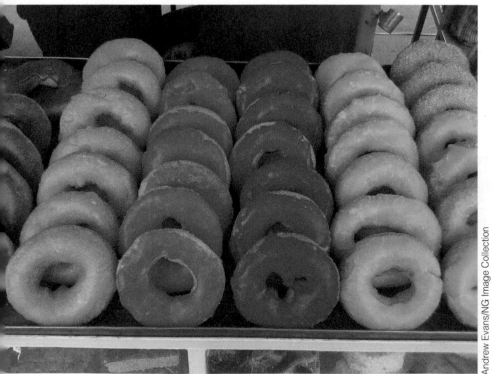

▲ **b.** If you are at a healthy weight and you choose nutrient-dense foods, you can satisfy all your nutrient needs with fewer calories than you need to maintain your weight. The "extra" calories needed to maintain your weight can come from additional nutrient-dense choices or from foods such as candy, soda, or butter that are high in added sugar or solid fats.

Andrew Evans/NG Image Collection

Choice (Exchange) Lists

The Exchange Lists are a set of food-group recommendations developed in the 1950s to plan diets for people with diabetes. Since then, their use has been expanded to planning diets for anyone who has to monitor calorie intake. The most recent version, published as *Choose Your Foods: Food Lists for Diabetes*, has replaced the term "exchange" with "choice." The Choice Lists group foods based their calorie and macronutrient composition. Foods in the same list contain approximately the same amounts of energy, carbohydrate, protein, and fat. The food groupings of the Choice Lists differ from the MyPlate food groups because the lists are designed to meet energy and macronutrient criteria, whereas the MyPlate groups are designed to be good sources of nutrients regardless of their energy content. For example, the Choice Lists include a potato in the starch list because it contains about the same amount of energy, carbohydrate, protein, and fat as breads and grains, but in MyPlate a potato is in the vegetable group because it is a good source of vitamins, minerals, and fiber. The Choice Lists provide a useful tool whether you are controlling calorie intake for purposes of weight loss or carbohydrate intake for purposes of diabetes management (see online Appendix H).

CONCEPT CHECK — STOP

1. **How** can the recommendations of the Dietary Guidelines help Americans manage body weight?
2. **What** does the MyPlate graphic tell you about a healthy diet?
3. **How** many ounces from the grains group does your Daily Food Plan recommend?
4. **Which** contains more empty calories—a bowl of oatmeal or a bowl of Froot Loops?

2.4 Food and Supplement Labels

LEARNING OBJECTIVES

1. **Discuss** how the information on food labels can help you choose a healthy diet.
2. **Determine** whether a food is high or low in fiber, sodium, or saturated fat.
3. **Explain** how the order of ingredients on a food label is determined.
4. **Explain** the types of claims that are common on food and dietary supplement labels.

The Dietary Guidelines and MyPlate recommend appropriate amounts of nutritious foods, but sometimes it is difficult to tell how nutritious a particular food is. How do you know whether your frozen entrée is a good source of iron, how much fiber your breakfast cereal provides, or how much calcium is in your daily vitamin/mineral supplement? You can find this information on food and supplement labels.

Food Labels

Standardized food labels are designed to help consumers make informed food choices by providing information about the nutrient composition of a food and how that food fits into the overall diet.[13] They are required on all packaged foods, except those produced by small businesses and those in packages too small to accommodate the information. Raw fruits, vegetables, and seafood are not required to carry individual food labels. However, grocery stores are asked to provide nutrition information voluntarily for the raw fruits, vegetables, and seafood most frequently purchased in the United States. The information can appear on large placards or in consumer pamphlets or brochures. Food served in restaurants, delicatessens, and bakeries is not required to carry labels unless the food is from an establishment that has 20 or more locations. These food chains must list calorie content information for standard menu items and provide other nutrient information upon request.[14]

Knowing how to interpret the information on food labels can help you choose a healthy diet.

a. The current Nutrition Facts panel can help you evaluate the nutritional contribution a food makes to your diet.

Standard serving sizes are required to allow consumers to compare products. For example, the number of calories in one serving of this product can be compared to the number of calories in a similar product because the values for both are for a standard 2/3rd-cup serving.

Food labels must list the "% Daily Value" for total fat, saturated fat, cholesterol, sodium, total carbohydrate, and dietary fiber, as well as for vitamins A and C, calcium, and iron. A % Daily Value of 5% or less is considered low, and a value of 20% or more is considered high.

The label provides information about the amounts of nutrients whose intake should be limited—total fat, saturated fat, *trans* fat, cholesterol, and sodium.

The label provides information about the amounts of nutrients that tend to be low in the American diet—fiber, vitamins A and C, calcium, and iron.

The footnote gives the Daily Values for 2000 and 2500 Calorie diets to illustrate that for some nutrients the Daily Value increases with increasing caloric intake.

Nutrition Facts

Serving Size 2/3 cup (55g)
Servings Per Container About 8

Amount Per Serving

Calories 230   **Calories from Fat** 40

	% Daily Value*
Total Fat 8g	12%
Saturated Fat 1g	5%
Trans Fat 0g	
Cholesterol 0mg	0%
Sodium 160mg	7%
Total Carbohydrate 37g	12%
Dietary Fiber 4g	16%
Sugars 1g	
Protein 3g	

Vitamin A	10%
Vitamin C	8%
Calcium	20%
Iron	45%

* Percent Daily Values are based on a 2,000 calorie diet. Your daily value may be higher or lower depending on your calorie needs.

	Calories:	2,000	2,500
Total Fat	Less than	65g	80g
Sat Fat	Less than	20g	25g
Cholesterol	Less than	300mg	300mg
Sodium	Less than	2,400mg	2,400mg
Total Carbohydrate		300g	375g
Dietary Fiber		25g	30g

Interpret the Data

How much sodium would you consume if you ate 2 cups of this product? What percentage of the Daily Value would that represent?

Since 1990, food labels have included a **Nutrition Facts** panel and an ingredient list. The only major change that has been made to this standard format since 1990 is the addition of *trans* fat to the label in 2006. In 2013, the Food Labeling Modernization Act was introduced in Congress, proposing changes in the food labels based on current understanding of nutrition science with the goal of providing consumers with more accessible information.[15] If passed, manufacturers will have 2 years to make required changes to their food labels (**Figure 2.12**).

b. This revised Nutrition Facts panel illustrates the changes proposed to help consumers make informed food choices and follow guidelines for a healthy diet.

Nutrition Facts

8 servings per Container

Serving size   2/3 cup (55g)

Amount Per 2/3 cup

Calories   **230**

12%	**Total Fat** 8g
5%	Saturated Fat 1g
	Trans Fat 0g
0%	**Cholesterol** 0mg
7%	**Sodium** 160mg
12%	**Total Carbs** 37g
16%	Dietary Fiber 4g
	Sugars 1g
	Added Sugars 0mg
	Protein 3g
10%	**Vitamin D** 2mcg
20%	**Calcium** 200mg
45%	**Iron** 8 mg
5%	**Potassium** 235mg

* Footnote on Daily Values (DV) and calories reference to be inserted here.

Standard serving sizes will be updated based on what people actually eat, not on what they should eat. The information on servings per container will also be in a larger, bolder font.

The Calories per serving will be more prominent to highlight this information, which is important to address current public health concerns such as obesity, diabetes, and heart disease.

The % Daily Values will be listed in front of the nutrients and the Daily Values used to calculate the % Daily Value will be updated.

Information about amounts of nutrients that should be limited will include added sugars.

The information on nutrients that tend to be low in the diet will include potassium and vitamin D along with iron and calcium. Vitamins A and C will not be required. Actual amounts of these nutrients as well as % Daily Values will be included.

A new footnote will more clearly explain the meaning of % Daily Values

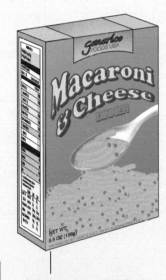

c. The ingredient list shows the exact contents of a food. This information can be useful for those who must avoid certain ingredients because of allergies, have other dietary restrictions, or are just curious about what is in the food they eat.

The ingredients are listed in descending order by weight, from the most abundant to the least abundant. The wheat flour in the macaroni is the most abundant ingredient in this product.

Ingredients:
Enriched macaroni product (wheat flour, niacin, ferrous sulfate [iron], thiamine mononitrate, riboflavin, folic acid); cheese sauce mix (whey, modified food starch, milk fat, salt, milk protein concentrate, contains less tha 2% of sodium tripolyphosphate, cellulose gel, cellulose gum, citric acid, sodium phosphate, lactic acid, calcium phosphate, milk, yellow 5, yellow 6, enzymes, cheese culture)

Labels must contain basic product information, such as the name of the product, the weight or volume of the contents, and the name and place of business of the manufacturer, packager, or distributor.

Nutrition Facts All food labels must contain a Nutrition Facts panel that lists the serving size and the number of Calories and the amounts of specific nutrients in that standard serving (see Figures 2.12a and b).[13,16] If a person eats twice the standard serving, he or she is consuming twice the number of Calories and other nutrients listed (*See Thinking it Through: A Case Study on Using Tools for Diet Planning*).

For most nutrients, the Nutrition Facts panel also lists the amounts contained in a serving as a percentage of the

A Case Study on Using Tools for Diet Planning

Frieda is trying to improve her diet. She decides to start with the Dietary Guidelines recommendation to increase her intake of fruits and vegetables. Frieda needs to eat about 2000 Calories/day to maintain her weight.

 1 Based on the MyPlate recommendations in Figure 2.9, how many cups of fruit and how many of vegetables should she eat each day?

Your answer:

Frieda likes fruits and vegetables but they always seem to go bad in her refrigerator before she eats them. While shopping she notices vegetable chips. The bag says she will get a serving (1/2 cup) of vegetables in every ounce.

Vegetable Chips

Nutrition Facts
Serving Size 1 oz (28g/about 14 chips)
Servings Per Container about 7

Amount Per Serving		
Calories		150
Calories from Fat		80
		% Daily Value**
Total Fat 9g		14%
Saturated Fat 1g		5%
Trans Fat 0g		
Cholesterol 0mg		0%
Sodium 50mg		2%
Total Carbohydrate 16g		5%
Dietary Fiber 3g		12%
Sugars 3g		
Protein 1g		

 2 If Frieda ate all of her vegetable servings as vegetable chips, what percentage of her calorie needs would this provide?

Your answer:

Another easy choice for Frieda would be a fruit and vegetable juice blend. The package says that it provides 1/2 cup of fruit and 1/2 cup of vegetables in 8 ounces.

 3 If Frieda wants to get all her fruits and vegetables from the juice, how much would she have to drink? Based on the label shown here, how many Calories would this provide?

Juice Blend

Nutrition Facts
Serving Size 8 fl oz (240 mL)
Servings Per Container 1

Amount Per Serving		
Calories 110		
Calories from Fat 0		
		% Daily Value*
Total Fat 0g		0%
Saturated Fat 0g		0%
Trans Fat 0g		
Cholesterol 0mg		0%
Sodium 70mg		3%
Total Carbohydrate 28g		9%
Dietary Fiber 0g		0%
Sugars 24g		
Protein 1g		

Your answer:

Although the vegetable chips and juice are convenient, Frieda wonders if she could meet her needs with fewer calories if she ate whole foods. She decides to take the juice with her lunch but have whole fruits and vegetables for dinner. Use the Food-A-Pedia feature of SuperTracker at ChooseMyPlate.gov to look up the nutrient information for the 1 cup of cooked broccoli and 1 cup of raw strawberries she plans to have for dinner.

 4 Which provides more Calories, 16 ounces of juice blend (see label) or the broccoli and strawberries? Which provides more fiber?

Your answer:

Which choice do you think will be more filling?

Your answer:

 5 What are the advantages and disadvantages of the juice versus whole fruits and vegetables?

Your answer:

(Check your answers in online Appendix L.)

Daily Value A reference value for the intake of nutrients used on food labels to help consumers see how a given food fits into their overall diet.

Daily Value. The % Daily Value is the amount of a nutrient in a food as a percentage of the amount recommended for a 2000-Calorie diet. For example, if a food provides 10% of the Daily Value for calcium, it provides 10% of the recommended daily intake for calcium in a 2000-Calorie diet (see Appendix C). These percentages help consumers see how a given food fits into their overall diet. Because a Daily Value is a single standard for all consumers, it may overestimate the amount of a nutrient needed for some population groups, but it does not underestimate the requirement for any group except pregnant and lactating women.

Ingredient List Do you want to know exactly what goes into your food? The ingredient list is the place to look (see Figure 2.12c). The ingredient list presents the contents of the product in order of their prominence by weight. An ingredient list is required on all products containing more than one ingredient and optional on products that contain a single ingredient. Food additives, including food colors and flavorings, must be listed among the ingredients.

Nutrient content and health claims Looking for low-fat or high-fiber foods? You may not even need to look at the Nutrition Facts panel. Food labels often contain **nutrient content claims**. These are statements that highlight specific characteristics of a product that might be of interest to consumers, such as "fat free" or "low sodium." Standard definitions for these descriptors have been established by the Food and Drug Administration (FDA) (**Table 2.2** and online Appendix I). These definitions also apply to food sold in restaurants.

Nutrient content claims[16]   Table 2.2   *Not needed to know*

Claim	Description
Free	Used on products that contain no amount of or only a trivial amount of fat, saturated fat, cholesterol, sodium, sugars, or calories. For example, "sugar free" and "fat free" both mean < 0.5 g per serving. Synonyms for *free* include *without*, *no*, and *zero*.
Low	Used for foods that can be eaten frequently without exceeding the Daily Value for fat, saturated fat, cholesterol, sodium, or calories. Specific definitions have been established for each of these nutrients. For example, *low-fat* means that the food contains ≤ 3 g of fat per serving, and *low cholesterol* means that the food contains ≤ 20 mg of cholesterol per serving. Synonyms for *low* include *little*, *few*, and *low source of*.
Lean and extra lean	Used to describe the fat content of meat, poultry, seafood, and game meats. *Lean* means that the food contains < 10 g fat, ≤ 4.5 g saturated fat, and < 95 mg of cholesterol per serving and per 100 g. *Extra lean* is defined as containing < 5 g fat, < 2 g saturated fat, and < 95 mg of cholesterol per serving and per 100 g.
High	Used for foods that contain 20% or more of the Daily Value for a particular nutrient. Synonyms for *high* include *rich in* and *excellent source of*.
Good source	Used for foods that contain 10 to 19% of the Daily Value for a particular nutrient per serving.
Reduced	Used on nutritionally altered products that contain 25% less of a nutrient or energy than the regular or reference product.
Less	Used on foods, whether altered or not, that contain 25% less of a nutrient or energy than the reference food. For example, pretzels may claim to have "less fat" than potato chips. *Fewer* may be used as a synonym for *less*.
Light	Used in different ways. First, it can be used on a nutritionally altered product that contains one-third fewer calories or half the fat of a reference food. Second, it can be used when the sodium content of a low-calorie, low-fat food has been reduced by 50%. The term *light* can be used to describe properties such as texture and color, as long as the label explains the intent—for example, "light and fluffy."
More	Used when a serving of food, whether altered or not, contains a nutrient in an amount that is at least 10% of the Daily Value more than the reference food. Synonyms for *more* are *fortified*, *enriched*, and *added*.
Healthy	Used to describe foods that are low in fat and saturated fat, contain limited amounts of sodium and cholesterol, and provide at least 10% of the Daily Value for vitamins A or C, or iron, calcium, protein, or fiber.
Fresh	Used on foods that are raw and have never been frozen or heated and contain no preservatives.

When a claim is made about a menu item's nutritional content or health benefits, such as "low-fat" or "heart healthy," nutrition information must be available upon request.[17]

Because of the importance of certain types of foods and dietary components in disease prevention, food labels are permitted to include a number of **health claims**. Health claims refer to a relationship between a nutrient, food, food component, or dietary supplement and reduced risk of a disease or health-related condition. All health claims are reviewed by the FDA. To carry a health claim, a food must be a naturally good source of one of six nutrients (vitamin A, vitamin C, protein, calcium, iron, or fiber) and must not contain more than 20% of the Daily Value for fat, saturated fat, cholesterol, or sodium. Authorized health claims are supported by strong scientific evidence (**Figure 2.13** and online Appendix I). Health claims for which there is emerging but not well-established evidence are called **qualified health claims**; such a claim must be accompanied by an explanatory statement to avoid misleading consumers.

Dietary Supplement Labels

Products ranging from multivitamin pills to protein powders and herbal elixirs can all be defined as **dietary supplements**. These products are considered foods, not drugs, and therefore are regulated by the laws that govern food safety and labeling. To help consumers understand what they are choosing when they purchase these products, dietary supplements are required to carry a **Supplement Facts** panel similar to the Nutrition Facts panel found on food labels (**Figure 2.14**).[18] Along with changes in the Nutrition Facts label the FDA is proposing changes to the current Supplement Facts label that will update the Daily Values and units of measure.

Labels on dietary supplements may also include nutrient content claims and FDA-approved health claims similar to those on food labels. For example, a product can claim to be an excellent source of a particular

> **dietary supplement** A product sold to supplement the diet; may include nutrients, enzymes, herbs, or other substances.

Health claims • Figure 2.13

Oatmeal contains enough soluble fiber to be permitted to include this health claim about the relationship between soluble fiber and the risk of heart disease. Other health claims you may see on food labels are listed below and included in online Appendix I.[16]

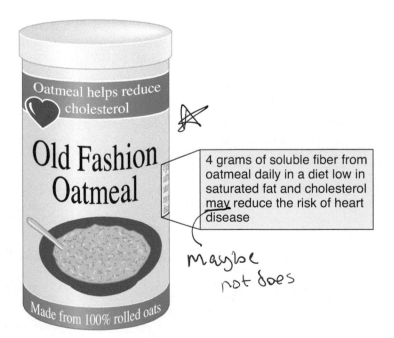

4 grams of soluble fiber from oatmeal daily in a diet low in saturated fat and cholesterol may reduce the risk of heart disease

- Calcium intake and calcium and vitamin D intake and the risk of osteoporosis
- Sodium intake and the risk of high blood pressure
- Saturated fat and cholesterol intake and the risk of heart disease
- Fiber-containing fruit, vegetable, and grain intake and the risk of heart disease and cancer
- Fruit and vegetable intake and the risk of cancer
- Dietary fat and the risk of cancer
- Whole-grain foods and the risk of heart disease and certain cancers

Dietary supplement label • Figure 2.14

Unlike food labels, dietary supplement labels must include directions for use and must provide information about ingredients that are not nutrients and for which Daily Values have not been established. For such ingredients, it is difficult to tell from the label whether the amount included in a serving is helpful, is harmful, or has no effect at all.

Think Critically What classes of nutrients might you miss out on if you chose to take this supplement instead of eating a piece of salmon to get your omega-3s?

The serving size tells you the recommended dose.

SUGGESTED USE : Take 3 capsules daily with meals.

Supplement Facts

Serving Size 3 Capsules   Servings Per Container 33

	Amount Per Serving	% Daily Value*
Calories	20	
Calories from Fat	20	
Total Fat	2 g	3%
Total Omega-3 Fatty Acids	1100 mg	
EPA (Eicosapentaenoic Acid)	450 mg	†
DHA (Docosahexaenoic Acid)	500 mg	†
DPA (Docosapentaenoic Acid)	60 mg	†
Stearidonic, Eicosatrienoic, Eicosatetraenoic, Heneicosapentaenoic, and Alpha-Linolenic Acids	90 mg	†

* Percent Daily Values are based on 2,000 calorie diet
† Daily Value not established

INGREDIENTS: Salmon Oil, UHPO3 Omega-3 Fatty Acid Concentrate (Sardines, Tuna, Anchovies), Gelatin, Glycerin and Water.

Each serving of Fish Oil Omega A–C provides the complete spectrum of healthful Omega-3 fatty acids equivalent to approximately one serving of fresh salmon.

*Research shows Omega-3 fatty acids play a role in the health and function of the cardiovascular system, central nervous system, vision, connective tissue, and the inflammatory response.

*These statements have not been evaluated by the Food and Drug Administration. This product is not intended to diagnose, treat, cure or prevent any disease.

The name, quantity per serving, and % Daily Values for nutrients are listed. You can use this information to assess how that amount compares to the recommended intake and UL for each nutrient. Nutrients with Daily Values are listed first, followed by ingredients without Daily Values.

All ingredients must be listed on the label either in the Supplement Facts panel or in the ingredient list below the panel. Ingredients are listed in descending order of prominence by weight.

FISH OIL OMEGA A-C

DIETARY SUPPLEMENT
100 soft gel caps

All these products must include the words *dietary supplement* on the label.

Because structure/function claims are based on the manufacturer's interpretation and are not approved by the FDA, products with these claims must include this disclaimer.

nutrient. To make this claim, one serving of the product must contain at least 20% of the Daily Value for that nutrient. A label may say "high potency" if one serving provides 100% or more of the Daily Value for the nutrient it contains. For multinutrient products, "high potency" means that a serving provides more than 100% of the Daily Value for two-thirds of the vitamins and minerals present.

Dietary supplement labels may also carry **structure/function claims**, which describe the role of a dietary ingredient in maintaining normal structure, function, or general well-being. For example, a structure/function claim about calcium may state that "calcium builds strong bones"; one about fiber may say "fiber maintains

bowel regularity." These statements can be misleading. For example, the health claim "lowers cholesterol" requires FDA approval, but the structure/function claim "helps maintain normal cholesterol levels" does not. It would not be unreasonable for consumers with high cholesterol to conclude that a product that "helps maintain normal cholesterol levels" would help lower their elevated blood cholesterol level to within the normal range.

Manufacturers must notify the FDA when including a structure/function claim on a dietary supplement label and are responsible for ensuring the accuracy and truthfulness of these claims. Structure/function claims are not approved by the FDA. For this reason, the law says that if a dietary supplement label includes such a claim, it must state in a disclaimer that the FDA has not evaluated the claim. The disclaimer must also state that the dietary supplement product is not intended to "diagnose, treat, cure, or prevent any disease" because only a drug can legally make such a claim (see Figure 2.14). Structure/function claims may also appear on food labels, but the FDA does not require conventional food manufacturers to notify the FDA about their structure/function claims, and disclaimers are not required.

CONCEPT CHECK

1. **Why** are serving sizes standardized on food labels?

2. **What** food label information helps you find foods that are low in saturated fat and cholesterol?

3. **Where** should you look to see if a food contains nuts?

4. **How** do structure/function claims differ from health claims?

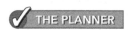

Summary

1 Nutrition Recommendations 30

- Nutrition recommendations are designed to encourage consumption of a diet that promotes health and prevents disease. Some of the earliest nutrition recommendations in the United States were in the form of **food guides**, which translate nutrient intake recommendations into food intake recommendations. The first set of Recommended Dietary Allowances, developed during World War II, focused on energy and the nutrients most likely to be deficient in a typical diet. Current recommendations focus on promoting health and preventing chronic disease as well as nutrient deficiencies.

- Dietary recommendations can be used as a standard for assessing the **nutritional status** of individuals and of populations. Records of dietary intake, such as the one shown here, along with information obtained from a physical examination, a medical history, and laboratory tests, can be used to assess an individual's nutritional status. Collecting information about the food intake and health of individuals in the population or surveying the foods available can help identify potential and actual nutrient deficiencies and excesses within a population and help policymakers improve nutrition recommendations.

Dietary Diet looks like

Assessing nutritional status • Figure 2.2

FOOD DIARY

Record all the food and beverages you eat. Include the food, how it was prepared, the amount you ate and the brand name. Don't forget to list all fats used in cooking and all spreads and sauces added.

Time	Food	Kind and how prepared	Amount
7:00 A.M.	Eggs	scrambled	2
	Butter	in eggs	1 tsp.
	toast	whole wheat	2 slices
	Butter	on toast	2 tsp.
	Milk	non-fat	8 oz.
	Orange juice	from frozen concentrate	8 oz.
12:00 P.M.	Big Mac	McDonald's	1

2 Dietary Reference Intakes (DRIs) 34

- **Dietary Reference Intakes (DRIs)** are recommendations for the amounts of energy, nutrients, and other food components that should be consumed by healthy people to promote health, reduce the incidence of chronic disease, and prevent deficiencies. **Estimated Average Requirements (EARs)** are average requirements, as seen in the illustration, and can be used to evaluate the adequacy of a population's nutrient intake. **Recommended Dietary Allowances (RDAs)** and **Adequate Intakes (AIs)** can be used by individuals as goals for nutrient intake, and **Tolerable Upper Intake Levels (ULs)** indicate safe upper intake limits.

Understanding EARs, RDAs, and ULs • Figure 2.4

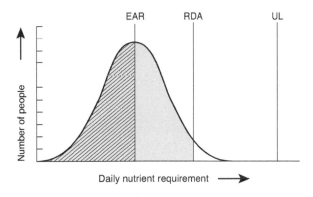

- The DRIs make two types of energy-intake recommendations. **Estimated Energy Requirements (EERs)** provide an estimate of how many calories are needed to maintain body weight. **Acceptable Macronutrient Distribution Ranges (AMDRs)** make recommendations about the proportion of energy that should come from carbohydrate, fat, and protein in a healthy diet.

3 Tools for Diet Planning 37

- The **Dietary Guidelines for Americans** are a set of diet and lifestyle recommendations designed to promote health and reduce the risk of overweight and obesity and chronic disease in the U.S. population. They emphasize balancing the calories consumed in food and beverages with the calories expended through physical activity in order to achieve and maintain a healthy weight. To accomplish this, they recommend that Americans increase their activity level and choose a healthy eating pattern. Healthy eating patterns are higher in fruits, vegetables, whole grains, low-fat dairy products, and seafood than current American diets, and they are lower in saturated fat, *trans* fat, cholesterol, salt, and added sugar.

- **MyPlate**, shown here, is the USDA's current food guide. It shows the proportions of foods from five food groups that make up a healthy diet and recommends amounts of food from each group based on individual energy needs. It also makes recommendations about the amounts of oils and the number of **empty calories** that can be included in an individual's diet. MyPlate stresses using variety, proportionality, and moderation in choosing a healthy diet and promotes the physical activity recommendations included in the Dietary Guidelines.

MyPlate recommendations • Figure 2.9

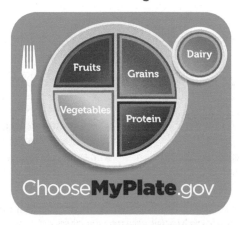

- Choice (Exchange) Lists are a food group system used to plan individual diets that provide specific amounts of energy, carbohydrate, protein, and fat.

- Standardized food labels are designed to help consumers make healthy food choices by providing information about the nutrient composition of foods and about how a food fits into the overall diet. The **Nutrition Facts** panel, as illustrated to the right, presents information about the amounts of various nutrients in a standard serving. For most nutrients, the amount is also given as a percentage of the **Daily Value**. A food label's ingredient list states the contents of the product, in order of prominence by weight. Food labels often include FDA-defined **nutrient content claims**, such as "low fat" or "high fiber," and **health claims**, which refer to a relationship between a nutrient, food, food component, or dietary supplement and the risk of a particular disease or health-related condition. All health claims are reviewed by the FDA and permitted only when they are supported by scientific evidence, but the level of scientific support for such claims varies

- A **Supplement Facts** panel appears on the label of every dietary supplement. Because **structure/function claims** are not FDA approved, when they appear on supplement labels, they must be accompanied by a disclaimer.

Food labels • Figure 2.12

Nutrition Facts		
Serving Size 2/3 cup (55g)		
Servings Per Container 8		
Amount Per Serving		
Calories 230	**Calories from Fat** 40	
		% Daily Value*
Total Fat 8g		12%
Saturated Fat 1g		5%
Trans Fat 0g		
Cholesterol 0mg		0%
Sodium 160mg		7%
Total Carbohydrate 37g		12%
Dietary Fiber 4g		16%
Sugars 1g		
Protein 3g		
Vitamin A		10%
Vitamin C		8%
Calcium		20%
Iron		45%

Key Terms

- Acceptable Macronutrient Distribution Ranges (AMDRs) 36
- Adequate Intakes (AIs) 35
- Daily Value 51
- dietary supplement 52
- *Dietary Guidelines for Americans* 37

- Dietary Reference Intakes (DRIs) 34
- empty calories 46
- Estimated Average Requirements (EARs) 34
- Estimated Energy Requirements (EERs) 36
- food guide 30

- health claim 52
- *Healthy People* 33
- MyPlate 37
- nutrient content claim 51
- Nutrition Facts 48
- nutritional status 31
- qualified health claim 52

- Recommended Dietary Allowances (RDAs) 34
- structure/function claim 53
- Supplement Facts 52
- Tolerable Upper Intake Levels (ULs) 35

What is happening in this picture?

In September of 2013 New York City's Board of Health attempted to enact legislation that would prohibit restaurants, sports stadiums, movie theaters, and food carts from selling sugar-sweetened drinks in cups larger than 16 ounces. This photo compares the amount of sugar in 32- and 64-ounces of soda.

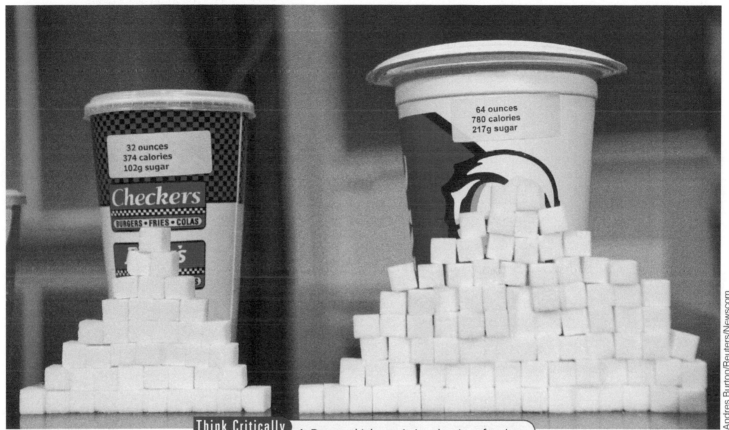

32 ounces
374 calories
102g sugar

Checkers
BURGERS • FRIES • COLAS

64 ounces
780 calories
217g sugar

Andres Burton/Reuters/Newscom

Think Critically

1. Do you think restricting the size of sodas sold will help curb obesity? Why or why not?
2. Should government organizations be able to control what Americans eat and drink?

THE PLANNER ✓

Review your Chapter Planner on the chapter opener and check off your completed work.

Digestion: From Meals to Molecules

The human body has been compared to a car: We fill the tank of our car with gasoline to get down the highway; we fill our body with food to get on with life. In both "machines," combustion with oxygen releases energy.

Our bodies are machine-like in another way as well: They are virtually identical to one another. Like cars, we look different on the outside but are basically the same on the inside. The processes that drive us—like the internal combustion engine, no matter where it's manufac-

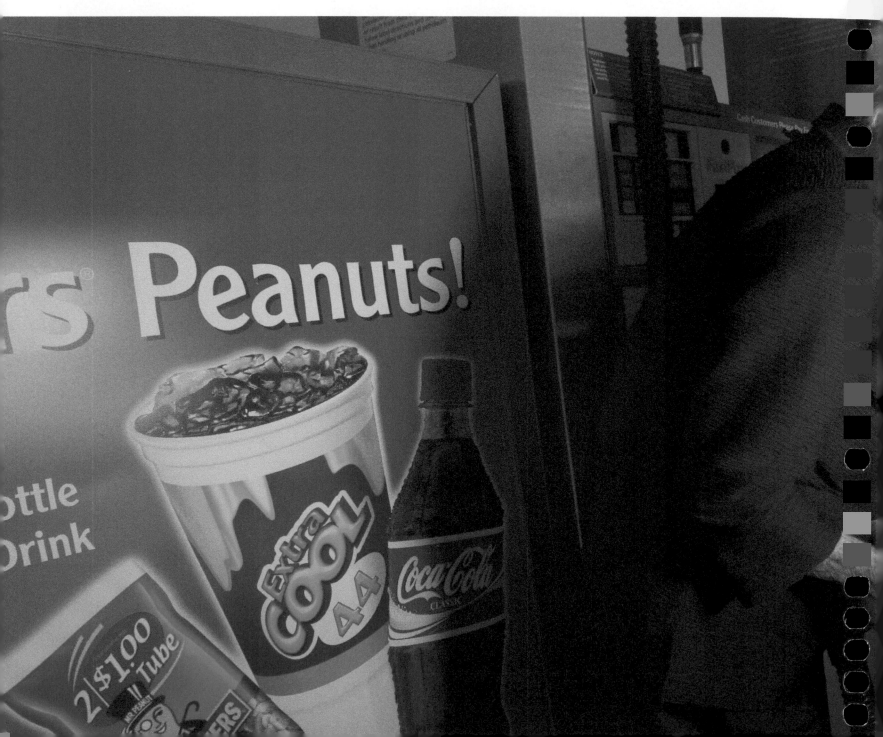

tured—are more similar than different because they are based on the same fundamental chemical reactions.

Despite the similarities, there are differences between human bodies and machines. An automobile cannot use gasoline to heal itself or to grow, as we do with nutrients. Although a gas tank and a stomach both store fuel, gasoline travels unchanged through the fuel line to the engine, whereas in humans the digestive system must break down the fuel into smaller units *before* it can be used by the body. Gas-powered cars are fueled only by gasoline, but the human digestive system must process fuel from many sources for use by the "high-performance machine" that is the human body.

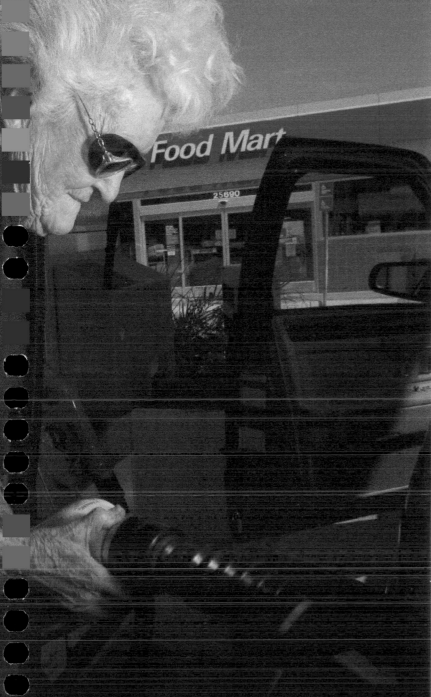

David McLan/Aurora Photos

CHAPTER PLANNER ✓

- ☐ Stimulate your interest by reading the opening story and looking at the visual.
- ☐ Scan the Learning Objectives in each section:
  p. 60 ☐   p. 64 ☐   p. 66 ☐   p. 75 ☐   p. 81 ☐   p. 86 ☐
- ☐ Read the text and study all figures and visuals. Answer any questions.

Analyze key features:

- ☐ Process Diagram, p. 60 ☐   p. 70 ☐   p. 72 ☐   p. 82 ☐   p. 86 ☐
- ☐ Nutrition InSight, p. 71 ☐   p. 79 ☐
- ☐ What a Scientist Sees, p. 74 ☐
- ☐ Debate, p. 77 ☐
- ☐ Thinking It Through, p. 80 ☐
- ☐ Stop: Answer the Concept Checks before you go on:
  p. 63 ☐   p. 66 ☐   p. 75 ☐   p. 81 ☐   p. 85 ☐   p. 87 ☐

End of chapter and online review:

- ☐ Review the Summary, Key Terms, and online links to Additional Resources.
- ☐ Answer the online Critical and Creative Thinking Questions.
- ☐ Answer What is happening in this picture?
- ☐ Complete the online Self-Test and check your answers.

3.1 The Organization of Life

LEARNING OBJECTIVES

1. **Describe** the organization of living things, from atoms to organisms.

2. **Name** the organ systems that work with the digestive system to deliver nutrients and eliminate wastes.

Matter, be it a meal you are about to eat or the plate you are about to eat it from, is made up of **atoms** (**Figure 3.1**). Atoms combine to form **molecules**, which can have different properties from those of the atoms they contain. In any living system, the molecules are organized into **cells**, the smallest units of life. Cells that are similar in structure and function form **tissues**. The human body contains four types of tissue: muscle, nerve, epithelial, and connective. These tissues are organized in varying combinations to form

> **atom** The smallest unit of an element that retains the properties of the element.
>
> **molecule** A group of two or more atoms of the same or different elements bonded together.
>
> **cell** The basic structural and functional unit of living things.

PROCESS DIAGRAM

From atoms to organisms • Figure 3.1

The organization of life begins with atoms that form molecules, which are then organized into cells to form tissues, organs, and whole organisms.

1 Atoms linked by chemical bonds form molecules.

2 Molecules form the structures that make up cells. Each cell is bounded by a membrane. In multicellular organisms, cells are usually specialized to perform specific functions.

3 Groups of similar cells form tissues, such as the muscle shown here.

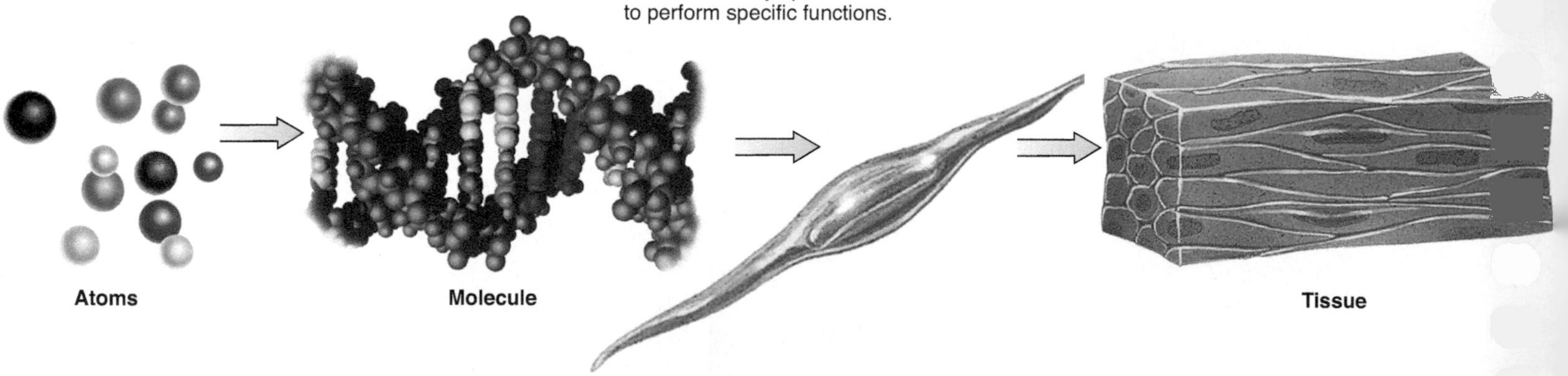

Atoms　　　　　**Molecule**　　　　　　　　　　　　　　　　　**Tissue**

organ A discrete structure composed of more than one tissue that performs a specialized function.

organs. In most cases, an organ does not function alone but is part of an **organ system.** Moreover, an organ may be part of more than one organ system. For example, the pancreas is part of the endocrine system and also part of the digestive system.

The body's 11 organ systems interact to perform all the functions necessary for life (**Table 3.1**). For example, the digestive system, which is the primary organ system responsible for moving nutrients into the body, is assisted by the endocrine system, which secretes **hormones** that help regulate how much we eat and how quickly food and nutrients travel through the digestive system. The digestive system is also aided by the nervous system, which sends nerve signals that help control the passage of food through the digestive tract; by the cardiovascular system, which transports nutrients to individual cells in the body; and by the urinary, respiratory, and integumentary systems, which eliminate wastes generated in the body.

hormone A chemical messenger that is produced in one location in the body, is released into the blood and travels to other locations, where it elicits responses.

✔ THE PLANNER

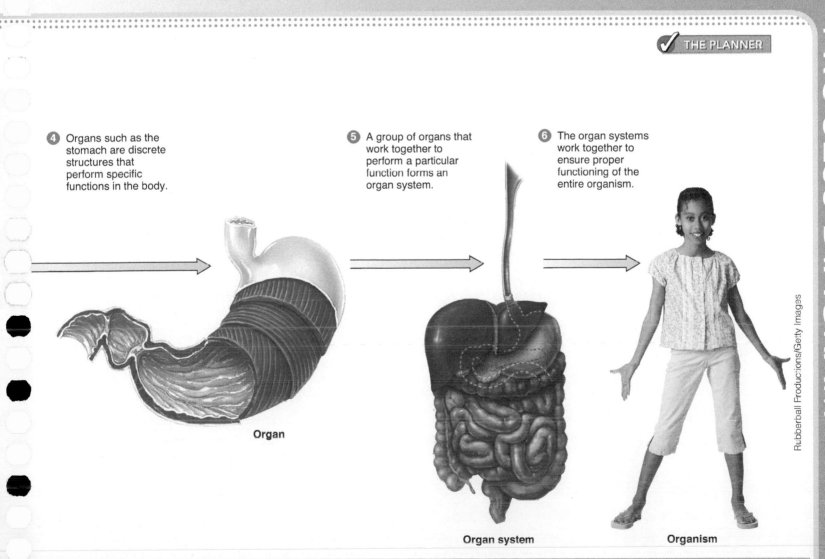

4 Organs such as the stomach are discrete structures that perform specific functions in the body.

5 A group of organs that work together to perform a particular function forms an organ system.

6 The organ systems work together to ensure proper functioning of the entire organism.

Organ

Organ system

Organism

Rubberball Productions/Getty Images

The major organ systems of the human body   Table 3.1

Organ system	What it includes	What it does
Nervous	Nerves, sense organs, brain, and spinal cord	Responds to stimuli from external and internal environments; conducts impulses to activate muscles and glands; integrates activities of other systems.
Respiratory	Lungs, trachea, and air passageways	Supplies the blood with oxygen and removes carbon dioxide.
Urinary	Kidneys, bladder, and associated structures	Eliminates wastes and regulates the balance of water, electrolytes, and acid in the blood.
Reproductive	Testes, ovaries, and associated structures	Produces offspring.
Cardiovascular/circulatory	Heart and blood vessels	Transports blood, which carries oxygen, nutrients, and wastes.
Lymphatic/immune	Lymph and lymph structures, white blood cells	Defends against foreign invaders; picks up fluid leaked from blood vessels; transports fat-soluble nutrients.

Organ system		What it includes	What it does
Muscular		Skeletal muscles	Provides movement and structure.
Skeletal		Bones and joints	Protects and supports the body, provides a framework for the muscles to use for movement.
Endocrine		Pituitary, adrenal, thyroid, pancreas, and other ductless glands	Secretes hormones that regulate processes such as growth, reproduction, and nutrient use.
Integumentary		Skin, hair, nails, and sweat glands	Covers and protects the body; helps control body temperature.
Digestive		Mouth, esophagus, stomach, intestines, pancreas, liver, and gallbladder	Ingests and digests food; absorbs nutrients into the blood; eliminates nonabsorbed food wastes.

CONCEPT CHECK   STOP

1. **How** are atoms, molecules, and cells related to one another?

2. **How** do the endocrine and nervous systems interact with the digestive system?

3.2 The Digestive System

LEARNING OBJECTIVES

1. **Define** digestion and absorption.
2. **List** the organs that make up the digestive system.
3. **Describe** the tissue layers that make up the wall of the gastrointestinal tract.
4. **Explain** the roles of mucus, enzymes, nerves, and hormones in digestion.

The digestive system is the organ system that is primarily responsible for **digestion** and for the **absorption** of nutrients into the body. When you eat a taco, for example, the tortilla, meat, cheese, lettuce, and tomato are broken apart, releasing the nutrients and other food components they contain. Water, vitamins, and minerals are taken into the body without being broken into smaller units, but proteins, carbohydrates, and fats must be digested further. Proteins are broken down into amino acids, most of the carbohydrate is broken down into sugars, and most fats are digested to produce molecules with long carbon chains called **fatty acids**. The sugars, amino acids, and fatty acids can then be absorbed into the body. The fiber in whole grains, fruits, and vegetables cannot be digested and therefore is not absorbed into the body. It and other unabsorbed substances pass through the digestive tract and are eliminated in **feces**.

> **digestion** The process by which food is broken down into components small enough to be absorbed into the body.
>
> **absorption** The process of taking substances from the gastrointestinal tract into the interior of the body.
>
> **feces** Body waste, including unabsorbed food residue, bacteria, mucus, and dead cells, which is eliminated from the gastrointestinal tract by way of the anus.

is not technically inside the body because it has not been absorbed. When you swallow something that cannot be digested, such as a whole sesame seed or an unpopped kernel of popcorn, it passes through your digestive tract and exits in the feces, without ever entering your blood or cells. Only after substances have been absorbed into the cells that line the intestine can they be said to be inside the body.

The lumen is lined with a layer of **mucosal cells** called the **mucosa** (see Figure 3.2b). Because mucosal cells are in direct contact with churning food and harsh digestive secretions, they live only about two to five days. The dead cells are sloughed off into the lumen, where some components are digested and absorbed and the rest are eliminated in feces. New mucosal cells are formed continuously to replace those that die. To allow for this rapid replacement, the mucosa has high nutrient requirements and is one of the first parts of the body to be affected by nutrient deficiencies.

The time it takes food to travel the length of the GI tract from mouth to anus is called the **transit time**. The shorter the transit time, the more rapidly material is passing through the digestive tract. In a healthy adult, transit time is 24 to 72 hours, depending on the composition of the individual's diet and his or her level of physical activity, emotional state, health status, and use of medications.

Organs of the Digestive System

The digestive system is composed of the **gastrointestinal tract** and accessory organs (**Figure 3.2a**). The gastrointestinal tract is a hollow tube, about 30 feet long, that runs from the mouth to the anus. It is also called the gut, GI tract, alimentary canal, or digestive tract. The inside of the tube is the **lumen** (**Figure 3.2b**). Food in the lumen

Digestive System Secretions

Digestion is aided by substances secreted into the digestive tract from cells in the mucosa and from a number of accessory organs. One of these substances is **mucus**, which moistens, lubricates,

> **mucus** A viscous fluid secreted by glands in the digestive tract and other parts of the body. It lubricates, moistens, and protects cells from harsh environments.

Structure of the digestive system • Figure 3.2

This overview of the digestive system illustrates its structure and summarizes the functions of specific organs.

a. The digestive system consists of the organs of the digestive tract—mouth, pharynx, esophagus, stomach, small intestine, and large intestine—plus four accessory organs—salivary glands, liver, gallbladder, and pancreas.

Ask Yourself

Bile is made in the _____ and stored in the _____. It is released into the _____, where it is important for the digestion and absorption of _____.

Organs of the gastrointestinal tract

Mouth: Chews food and mixes it with saliva

Pharynx: Swallows chewed food mixed with saliva

Esophagus: Moves food to the stomach

Stomach: Churns and mixes food; secretes acid and a protein-digesting enzyme

Small intestine: Completes digestion; absorbs nutrients into blood or lymph

Large intestine: Absorbs water and some vitamins and minerals; home to intestinal bacteria; passes waste material

{ Colon

{ Rectum

Anus: Opens to allow waste to leave the body

Accessory organs

Salivary glands: Produce saliva, which contains a starch-digesting enzyme

Liver: Makes bile, which aids in digestion and absorption of fat

Pancreas: Releases bicarbonate to neutralize intestinal contents; produces enzymes that digest carbohydrate, protein, and fat

Gallbladder: Stores bile and releases it into the small intestine when needed

Layers of smooth muscle

External layer of connective tissue

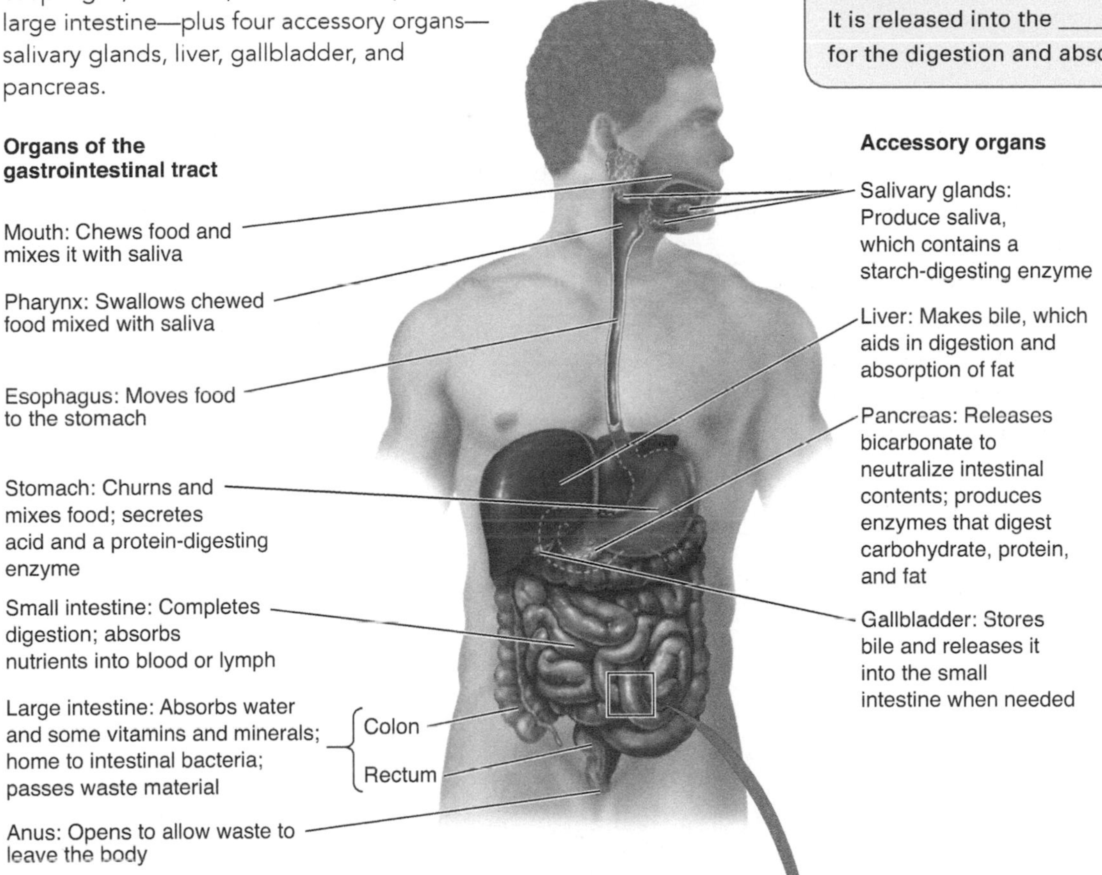

b. This cross section through the wall of the small intestine reveals the lumen and the four tissue layers that make up the wall of the gastrointestinal tract.

Lumen

Connective tissue

Mucosa

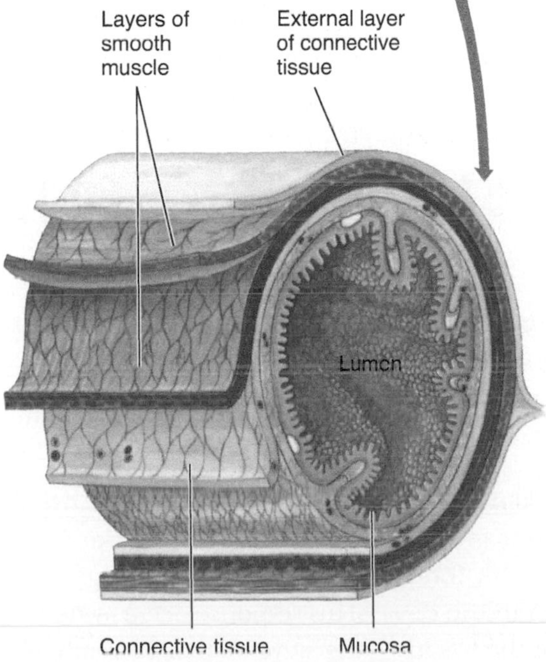

Think Critically Why is food in the lumen still outside the body?

The Digestive System 65

Enzyme activity • Figure 3.3

Enzymes are needed to break down different food components. The enzyme shown here, called an *amylase*, breaks large carbohydrate molecules, such as those in bread, into smaller ones. Amylases have no effect on fat, whereas enzymes called *lipases* digest fat and have no effect on carbohydrate.

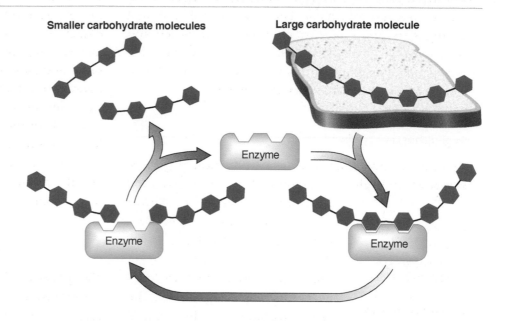

Smaller carbohydrate molecules

Large carbohydrate molecule

Enzyme

Enzyme

Enzyme

> **enzyme** A protein molecule that accelerates the rate of a chemical reaction without itself being changed.

and protects the digestive tract. **Enzymes** are also present in digestive system secretions. They accelerate the chemical reactions that break down food into units small enough to be absorbed (**Figure 3.3**).

The gastrointestinal tract is part of the endocrine system as well as the digestive system. It releases hormones that help prepare different parts of the gut for the arrival of food and thus regulate digestion and the rate at which food moves through the digestive system. Some hormonal signals slow digestion, whereas others facilitate it. For

example, when the nutrients from your lunch reach your small intestine, they trigger the release of hormones that signal the pancreas and gallbladder to secrete digestive substances into the small intestine.

CONCEPT CHECK STOP

1. **What** happens during digestion and absorption?
2. **Which** organs make up the gastrointestinal tract?
3. **What** are mucosal cells?
4. **How** are enzymes important for digestion and absorption?

3.3 Digestion and Absorption of Nutrients

LEARNING OBJECTIVES

1. **Describe** what happens in each of the organs of the gastrointestinal tract.

2. **Discuss** factors that influence how quickly food moves through the GI tract.

3. **Explain** how the structure of the small intestine aids in its function.

4. **Distinguish** passive diffusion from active transport.

Imagine warm slices of freshly baked bread smeared with melting butter. Is your mouth watering? You don't even need to put food in your mouth for activity to begin in the digestive tract. Sensory input alone—the sight of the bread

being lifted out of the oven, the smell of the bread, the clatter of the butter knife—may make your mouth water and your stomach begin to secrete digestive substances. This response occurs when the nervous system signals the digestive system to ready itself for a meal. In order for food to be used by the body, however, you need to do more than smell your meal. The food must be ingested and digested, and the nutrients must be absorbed and transported to the body's cells. This involves the combined functions of all the organs of the digestive system, as well as the help of some other organ systems.

The Mouth

Digestion involves chemical and mechanical processes, both of which begin in the mouth. The presence of food in the mouth stimulates the flow of saliva from the salivary glands. Saliva moistens the food and carries dissolved food molecules to the taste buds, most of which are located on the tongue. Signals from the taste buds, along with the aroma of food, allow us to enjoy the taste of the food we eat. Saliva contains the enzyme **salivary amylase**, which begins the chemical digestion of food by breaking starch molecules into shorter sugar chains (see Figure 3.3). Saliva also helps protect against tooth decay because it washes away food particles and contains substances that inhibit the growth of bacteria that cause tooth decay.

> **saliva** A watery fluid that is produced and secreted into the mouth by the salivary glands. It contains lubricants, enzymes, and other substances.

Chewing food begins the mechanical aspect of digestion. Adult humans have 32 teeth, which are specialized for biting, tearing, grinding, and crushing foods. Chewing breaks food into small pieces. This makes the food easier to swallow and increases the surface area in contact with digestive juices. The tongue helps mix food with saliva and aids chewing by constantly repositioning food between the teeth. Chewing also breaks up fiber, which traps nutrients. If the fiber is not broken up, some of the nutrients in the food cannot be absorbed. For example, if the fibrous skin of a raisin is not broken open by the teeth, the nutrients inside the raisin remain inaccessible, and the raisin travels, undigested, through the intestines for elimination in the feces.

The Pharynx

The **pharynx**, the part of the gastrointestinal tract that is responsible for swallowing, is also part of the respiratory tract. Food passes through the pharynx on its way to the stomach, and air passes through the pharynx on its way to and from the lungs. As we prepare to swallow, the tongue moves the bolus of chewed food mixed with saliva to the back of the mouth. During swallowing, the air passages are blocked by a valvelike flap of tissue called the **epiglottis** so that food goes to the esophagus and not to the lungs (**Figure 3.4a**).

> **epiglottis** A piece of elastic connective tissue that covers the opening to the lungs during swallowing.

The role of the epiglottis • Figure 3.4

The epiglottis reduces the risk of food entering the airway, and the Heimlich maneuver can expel food if it becomes lodged there.

a. When a bolus of food is swallowed, it normally pushes the epiglottis down over the opening to the passageway that leads to the lungs.

b. If food becomes lodged in the passageway leading to the lungs, it can block the flow of air. The Heimlich maneuver, which involves a series of thrusts directed upward from under the diaphragm (the muscle separating the chest and abdominal cavities), forces air out of the lungs, blowing the lodged food out of the air passageway.

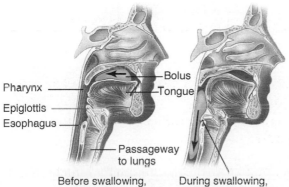

Pharynx
Bolus
Tongue
Epiglottis
Esophagus
Passageway to lungs

Before swallowing, the passageway to the lungs is open.

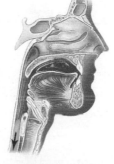

During swallowing, the bolus forces the epiglottis down to cover the passageway to the lungs.

After swallowing, the epiglottis returns to its original position, reopening the airway to the lungs.

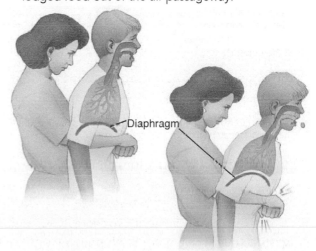

Diaphragm

Sometimes eating too quickly or talking while eating interferes with the movement of the epiglottis, and food passes into an upper air passageway. This food can usually be dislodged with a cough, but if it becomes stuck and causes choking, it may need to be forced out by means of the Heimlich maneuver (**Figure 3.4b**).

The Esophagus

The esophagus connects the pharynx with the stomach. In the esophagus, the bolus of food is moved along by rhythmic contractions of the smooth muscles, an action called peristalsis (**Figure 3.5**). The contractions of peristalsis are strong enough so that even if you ate while standing on your head, food would reach your stomach. This contractile movement, which is controlled automatically by the nervous system, occurs throughout the gastrointestinal tract,

> **peristalsis**
> Coordinated muscular contractions that move material through the GI tract.

pushing the bolus along from the pharynx through the large intestine.

To leave the esophagus and enter the stomach, food must pass through a **sphincter**, a muscle that encircles the tube of the digestive tract and acts as a valve. When the sphincter contracts, the valve is closed; when it relaxes, the valve is open, allowing food to pass (see Figure 3.5). The sphincter, located between the esophagus and the stomach, prevents food from moving from the stomach back into the esophagus, but occasionally stomach contents do move in this direction. This is what occurs with heartburn (as discussed later in this chapter): Some of the acidic stomach contents leak up through this sphincter into the esophagus, causing a burning sensation.

Food also moves from the stomach into the esophagus during vomiting. Vomiting is initiated by a complex series of signals from the brain that cause the sphincter to relax and the muscles to contract, forcing the stomach contents upward, out of the stomach and toward the mouth.

Moving food through the GI tract • Figure 3.5

The food we swallow doesn't just fall down the esophagus and into the stomach. It is pushed along by muscular contractions and enters the stomach in response to the opening and closing of the sphincter, located where the esophagus meets the stomach.

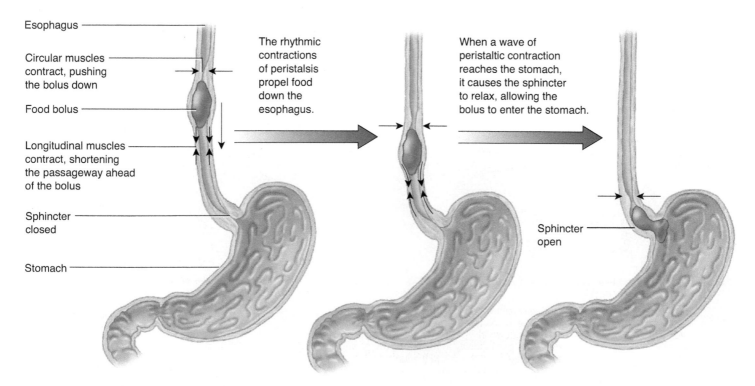

Esophagus

Circular muscles contract, pushing the bolus down

Food bolus

The rhythmic contractions of peristalsis propel food down the esophagus.

Longitudinal muscles contract, shortening the passageway ahead of the bolus

Sphincter closed

Stomach

When a wave of peristaltic contraction reaches the stomach, it causes the sphincter to relax, allowing the bolus to enter the stomach.

Sphincter open

The Stomach

The stomach is an expanded portion of the gastrointestinal tract that serves as a temporary storage place for food. Here the bolus is mashed and mixed with highly acidic stomach secretions to form a semiliquid food mass called **chyme**. The mixing of food in the stomach is aided by an extra layer of smooth muscle in the stomach wall (**Figure 3.6a**). Some digestion takes place in the stomach, but, with the exception of some water, alcohol, and a few drugs, such as aspirin and acetaminophen (Tylenol), very little absorption occurs here.

Gastric juice Gastric juice, which is produced by gastric glands in pits that dot the stomach lining, promotes chemical digestion in the stomach (**Figure 3.6b**). Gastric juice is a mixture of water, mucus, hydrochloric acid, and an inactive form of the protein-digesting enzyme **pepsin**. This enzyme is secreted in an inactive form so that it will not damage the gastric glands that produce it. The hydrochloric acid in gastric juice kills most of the bacteria present in food. It also stops the activity of the carbohydrate-digesting enzyme salivary amylase and helps begin the digestion of protein by activating pepsin and unfolding proteins. A thick layer of mucus prevents the protein that makes up the stomach wall from being damaged by the hydrochloric acid and pepsin in gastric juice.

Regulation of stomach activity How much your stomach churns and how much gastric juice is released are regulated by signals from both nerves and hormones.

Stomach structure and function • Figure 3.6

The stomach contributes to both the mechanical and chemical breakdown of food.

a. Most of the gastrointestinal tract is surrounded by two layers of smooth muscle, one that is longitudinal and one that is circular, but the stomach contains a third smooth muscle layer running diagonally. The presence of this diagonal layer allows for the powerful contractions that churn and mix the stomach contents. The sphincter at the bottom of the stomach controls the flow of chyme into the small intestine.

b. The lining of the stomach is covered with gastric pits. Inside these pits are the gastric glands, made up of different types of cells that produce the mucus, hydrochloric acid, and the inactive form of pepsin contained in gastric juice.

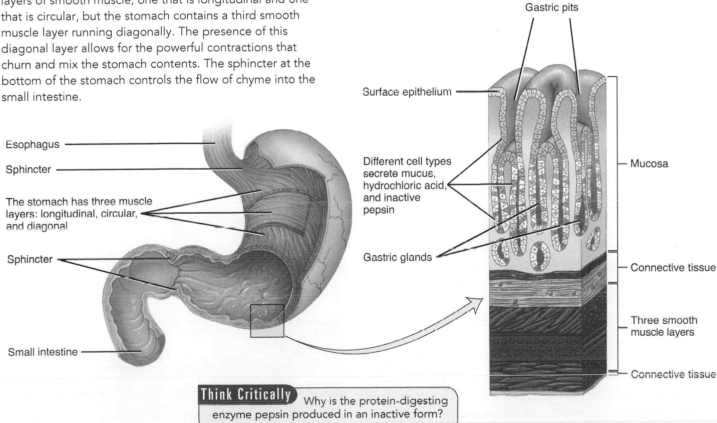

Esophagus

Sphincter

The stomach has three muscle layers: longitudinal, circular, and diagonal

Sphincter

Small intestine

Gastric pits

Surface epithelium

Different cell types secrete mucus, hydrochloric acid, and inactive pepsin

Gastric glands

Mucosa

Connective tissue

Three smooth muscle layers

Connective tissue

Think Critically Why is the protein-digesting enzyme pepsin produced in an inactive form?

The regulation of stomach motility and secretion • Figure 3.7

Stomach activity is affected by food that has not yet reached the stomach, by food that is in the stomach, and by food that has left the stomach.

HOW IT WORKS

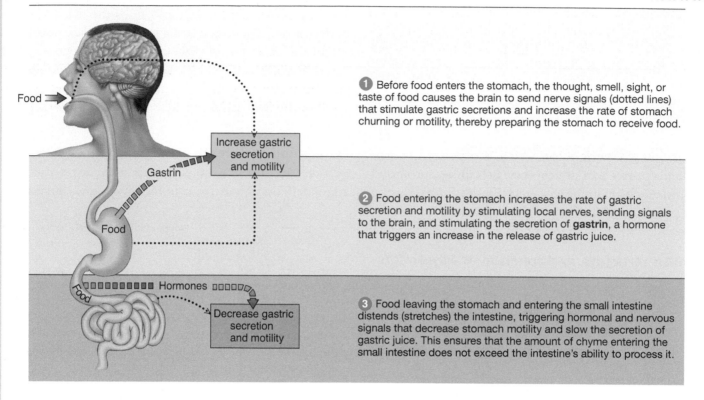

Food

Gastrin

Increase gastric secretion and motility

Food

Food

Hormones

Decrease gastric secretion and motility

1 Before food enters the stomach, the thought, smell, sight, or taste of food causes the brain to send nerve signals (dotted lines) that stimulate gastric secretions and increase the rate of stomach churning or motility, thereby preparing the stomach to receive food.

2 Food entering the stomach increases the rate of gastric secretion and motility by stimulating local nerves, sending signals to the brain, and stimulating the secretion of **gastrin**, a hormone that triggers an increase in the release of gastric juice.

3 Food leaving the stomach and entering the small intestine distends (stretches) the intestine, triggering hormonal and nervous signals that decrease stomach motility and slow the secretion of gastric juice. This ensures that the amount of chyme entering the small intestine does not exceed the intestine's ability to process it.

These signals originate from three sites—the brain, the stomach, and the small intestine (**Figure 3.7**).

As chyme moves out of the stomach, signals sent by the small intestine help regulate the rate at which the stomach empties. The small intestine stretches as it fills with chyme; this distension inhibits the stomach from emptying. Chyme normally empties from the stomach within two to six hours, but this rate varies with the size and composition of the meal that has been consumed. A large meal takes longer to leave the stomach than does a small meal. Liquids empty quickly, but solids linger until they are well mixed with gastric juice and are liquefied; hence, solids leave the stomach more slowly than liquids.

The nutritional composition of a meal also affects how long it stays in the stomach. A meal that consists primarily of starch or sugar leaves quickly, but a meal that is high in fiber or protein takes longer to leave the stomach. A high-fat meal stays in the stomach the longest. Because the nutrient composition of a meal affects how quickly it leaves your stomach, it affects how soon after eating you will feel hungry again (**Figure 3.8**).

Hunger and meal composition • Figure 3.8

What you choose for breakfast can affect how soon you become hungry for lunch. A small, carbohydrate-rich meal of dry toast and coffee will leave your stomach far more quickly than a larger meal containing more protein, fiber, and fat, such as a vegetable-and-cheese omelet with whole-wheat toast and butter.

dirkr/iStockphoto

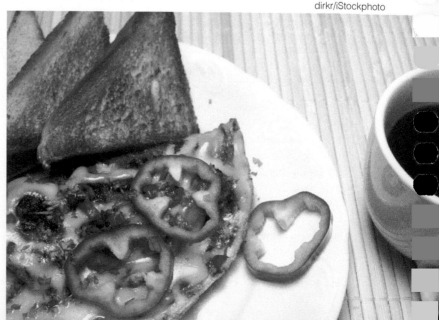

The Small Intestine

The small intestine is a narrow tube about 20 feet long. Here the chyme is propelled along by peristalsis and mixed by rhythmic constrictions called **segmentation** that slosh the material back and forth. The small intestine is the main site for the chemical digestion of food, completing the process that the mouth and stomach have started. It is also the primary site for the absorption of water, vitamins, minerals, and the products of carbohydrate, fat, and protein digestion.

The small intestine has a number of unique structural features that contribute to its digestive function and enhance the amount of surface area available for absorption (**Figure 3.9**). Together these features provide a surface area that is about the size of a tennis court (about 2700 ft²).

Secretions that aid digestion In the small intestine, secretions from the pancreas, the gallbladder, and the small intestine itself aid digestion. The pancreas secretes **pancreatic juice**, which contains **bicarbonate**, and

Nutrition InSight   The structure of the small intestine • Figure 3.9

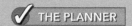

The structure of the small intestine helps to maximize its absorptive function.

Ask Yourself
What are the three structural features of the small intestine that increase its surface area?

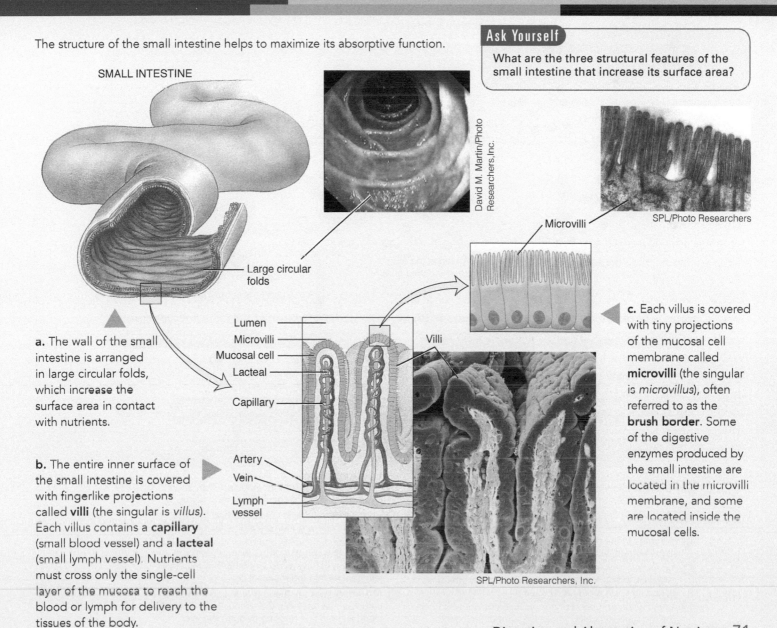

SMALL INTESTINE

David M. Martin/Photo Researchers, Inc.

Microvilli

SPL/Photo Researchers

Large circular folds

Lumen
Microvilli
Mucosal cell
Lacteal
Capillary

Villi

Artery
Vein
Lymph vessel

SPL/Photo Researchers, Inc.

a. The wall of the small intestine is arranged in large circular folds, which increase the surface area in contact with nutrients.

b. The entire inner surface of the small intestine is covered with fingerlike projections called **villi** (the singular is *villus*). Each villus contains a **capillary** (small blood vessel) and a **lacteal** (small lymph vessel). Nutrients must cross only the single-cell layer of the mucosa to reach the blood or lymph for delivery to the tissues of the body.

c. Each villus is covered with tiny projections of the mucosal cell membrane called **microvilli** (the singular is *microvillus*), often referred to as the **brush border**. Some of the digestive enzymes produced by the small intestine are located in the microvilli membrane, and some are located inside the mucosal cells.

Digestion and Absorption of Nutrients 71

digestive enzymes. Bicarbonate, which is a base, neutralizes the acid in the chyme, making the environment in the small intestine neutral or slightly basic rather than acidic, as in the stomach. This neutrality allows enzymes from the pancreas and small intestine to function.

Pancreatic amylase is an enzyme that continues the job of breaking down starches into sugars that was started in the mouth by salivary amylase. Pancreatic **proteases** (protein-digesting enzymes), such as trypsin and chymotrypsin, break protein into shorter and shorter chains of amino acids, and fat-digesting enzymes called **lipases**

break down fats into fatty acids. The pancreatic proteases, like the pepsin produced by the stomach, are released in an inactive form so that they will not digest the glands that produce them. Intestinal digestive enzymes, found in the cell membranes or inside the mucosal cells lining the small intestine, aid the digestion of double sugars (those that contain two sugar units) into single sugar units and the digestion of short amino acid chains into single amino acids. The sugars from carbohydrate digestion and the amino acids from protein digestion pass into the blood and are delivered to the liver (**Figure 3.10**).

PROCESS DIAGRAM

Digestion and absorption in the small intestine • Figure 3.10

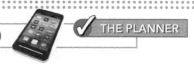 THE PLANNER

Most digestion and absorption occurs in the small intestine.

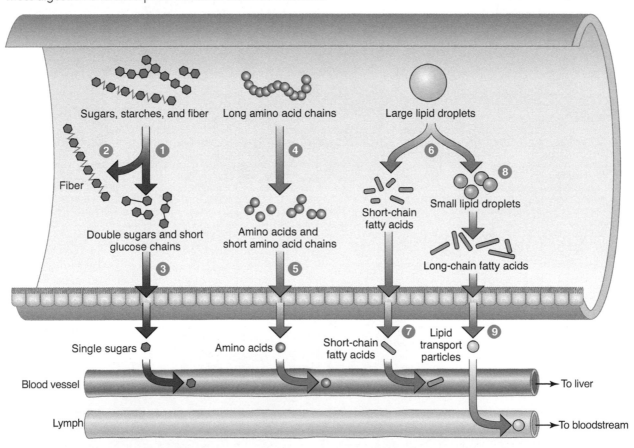

1️⃣ Pancreatic amylase digests starch to double sugars and short glucose chains.

2️⃣ Fiber, which cannot be digested by human enzymes, passes to the large intestine.

3️⃣ Enzymes in the microvilli digest double sugars into single sugars, which are absorbed into the blood.

4️⃣ Pancreatic proteases, along with proteases in the microvilli, digest long amino acid chains into amino acids and short amino acid chains.

5️⃣ Amino acids and short amino acid chains are absorbed into the mucosal cells, where they are digested into single amino acids, which pass into the blood.

6️⃣ Bile helps divide large fat globules. Pancreatic lipases digest fat molecules into fatty acids.

7️⃣ Short-chain fatty acids are absorbed into the mucosal cells and then pass directly into the blood.

8️⃣ Long-chain fatty acids and other lipids combine with bile to form small droplets that aid the absorption of fatty acids and other fat-soluble substances into the mucosal cell.

9️⃣ Absorbed lipids are incorporated into transport particles that pass into the lymph. They enter the blood without first passing through the liver.

The gallbladder stores and secretes **bile**, a fluid containing bile acids and cholesterol, which is produced in the liver and is necessary for the digestion and absorption of fat. Bile that is secreted into the small intestine mixes with fat. Bile acids help divide the large lipid droplets into small globules, allowing lipases to access and digest the fat molecules more efficiently. The bile acids and digested fats then form small droplets that facilitate the absorption of fat into the mucosal cells. Once inside the mucosal cells, the products of fat digestion are incorporated into transport particles. These are absorbed into the lymph before passing into the blood (see Figure 3.10).

> **bile** A digestive fluid made in the liver and stored in the gallbladder that is released into the small intestine, where it aids in fat digestion and absorption.

Absorption The small intestine is the main site for the absorption of nutrients. To be absorbed, nutrients must pass from the lumen of the GI tract into the mucosal cells lining the tract and then into either the blood or the lymph. Several different mechanisms are involved (**Figure 3.11**). Some rely on **diffusion**, which is the net movement of substances from an area of higher concentration to an area of lower concentration. **Simple diffusion**, in which material moves freely across a cell membrane; **osmosis**, which is the diffusion of water; and **facilitated diffusion**, in which a carrier molecule is needed for the substance to cross a cell membrane, depend on diffusion and are passive, requiring no energy. **Active transport** requires energy and a carrier molecule. This process can transport material from an area of lower concentration to one of higher concentration.

> **simple diffusion** The unassisted diffusion of a substance across a cell membrane.
>
> **osmosis** The unassisted diffusion of water across a cell membrane.
>
> **facilitated diffusion** Assisted diffusion of a substance across a cell membrane.
>
> **active transport** The transport of substances across a cell membrane with the aid of a carrier molecule and the expenditure of energy.

Absorption mechanisms • Figure 3.11

A variety of mechanisms are involved in transporting nutrients from the lumen of the small intestine into the mucosal cells.

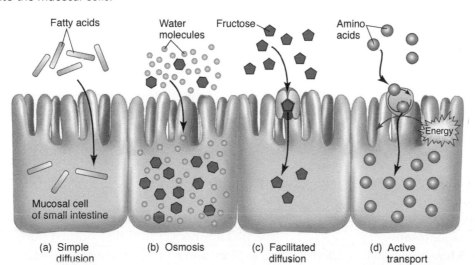

(a) Simple diffusion   (b) Osmosis   (c) Facilitated diffusion   (d) Active transport

Ask Yourself

1. Which absorption mechanism(s) can only move nutrients from an area with a higher concentration of that nutrient to an area with a lower concentration?
2. Which absorption mechanism(s) require(s) a carrier molecule?
3. Which absorption mechanism(s) require(s) energy?

a. In simple diffusion, substances such as the fatty acids shown here pass freely across a cell membrane from an area of higher concentration to an area of lower concentration, and no energy is required.

b. Osmosis is the passage of water molecules from an area with a lower concentration of dissolved substances, such as the glucose shown here (red hexagons), to an area with a higher concentration of dissolved substances. Water can move both into and out of the lumen of the GI tract by osmosis.

c. Facilitated diffusion is a type of passive diffusion that requires a carrier molecule. Here fructose molecules move from an area of higher concentration to an area of lower concentration, with the help of a carrier molecule.

d. Active transport requires energy and a carrier molecule and can transport substances from an area of lower concentration to an area of higher concentration. Active transport allows nutrients, such as the amino acids shown here, to be absorbed even when they are present in higher concentrations in the mucosal cell than in the lumen.

WHAT A SCIENTIST SEES
Bacteria on the Menu

Ads claim that eating specialized yogurts such as those shown in the photo will help regulate the digestive system. Consumers see these products as a tasty way to help regulate digestion. Scientists recognize that these products as well as most other yogurts contain active cultures of beneficial bacteria, including *Lactobacillus* and *Bifidobacterium*. The human gut is home to 15,000 to 36,000 species of bacteria.[1] The right mix of bacteria is important for immune function, proper growth and development of colon cells, and optimal intestinal motility and transit time.[2] Having healthy microflora can inhibit the growth of harmful bacteria and has been shown to prevent the diarrhea associated with antibiotic use and to reduce the duration of diarrhea resulting from intestinal infections and other causes.[3] There is also evidence that having healthy microflora may relieve constipation, reduce allergy symptoms, and modify the risk of inflammatory bowel disease, colon cancer, obesity, diabetes, and heart disease.[4–7] Consuming these beneficial bacteria, called **probiotics**, is one way of promoting healthy microflora (see illustration).[8] Another way is to consume **prebiotics**, substances that serve as a food supply for beneficial bacteria.

Think Critically Why might consuming a prebiotic increase the number of beneficial bacteria in the gut?

● Beneficial bacteria ● Harmful bacteria

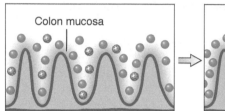
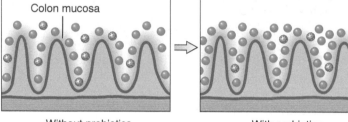

Colon mucosa

Without probiotics   With probiotics

When beneficial bacteria are consumed in sufficient amounts, they live temporarily in the colon, where they inhibit the growth of harmful bacteria (as shown on the right) and confer other health benefits on the host. However, the bacteria must be consumed frequently because they are flushed out in the feces.

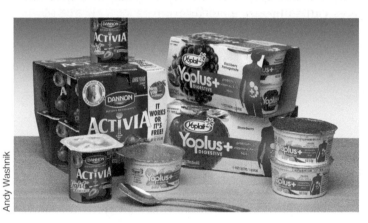
Andy Washnik

The Large Intestine

Materials not absorbed in the small intestine pass through a sphincter between the small intestine and the large intestine. This sphincter prevents material from the large intestine from reentering the small intestine.

The large intestine is about 5 feet long and is divided into the colon, which makes up the majority of the large intestine, and the rectum, the last 8 inches. The large intestine opens to the exterior of the body at the anus. Although most nutrient absorption occurs in the small intestine, water and some vitamins and minerals are also absorbed in the colon.

Peristalsis occurs more slowly in the large intestine than in the small intestine. Water, nutrients, and fecal matter may spend 24 hours in the large intestine, in contrast to the 3 to 5 hours it takes these materials to move through the small intestine. This slow movement favors the growth of bacteria. These bacteria, called the **intestinal microflora**, are permanent, beneficial residents of this part of the gastrointestinal tract (see *What a Scientist Sees*). They break down unabsorbed portions of food, such as fiber, and synthesize nutrients that can be used by the microflora or, in some cases, absorbed into the body. For example, the microflora synthesize small amounts of certain B vitamins and vitamin K, some of which can be absorbed. As the microflora break down material in the colon, they produce gas, which causes flatulence. In a healthy adult, between 200 and 2000 ml of gas is produced in the intestine each day.

Material that is not absorbed in the colon passes into the rectum, where it is stored temporarily and then evacuated through the anus as feces. The feces are a mixture of undigested, unabsorbed matter, dead cells, secretions from the GI tract, water, and bacteria. The amount of bacteria varies but can make up more than half the weight of the feces. The amount of water in the feces is affected by fiber and fluid intake. Because fiber retains water, when adequate fiber and fluids are consumed, feces have a higher water content and are more easily passed.

CONCEPT CHECK **STOP**

1. **What** are the functions of the stomach?
2. **How** does food move through the GI tract?
3. **How** do the villi and microvilli aid absorption?
4. **Why** must some nutrients be absorbed by active transport rather than passive diffusion?

3.4 Digestion in Health and Disease

LEARNING OBJECTIVES

1. **Explain** how the gastrointestinal tract protects against infection.
2. **Describe** how a food allergy is triggered.
3. **Discuss** the causes and consequences of ulcers, heartburn, and GERD.
4. **Explain** how dental problems and gallstones might affect food intake.

T he health of the GI tract is essential to our overall health. The gut acts as a defense against invasion by disease-causing organisms and other contaminants and allows us to obtain nutrients efficiently. Food allergies, which can be life-threatening, have their origins in the GI tract, but most common gastrointestinal problems are minor and do not affect long-term health.

The Digestive System and Disease Prevention

Food almost always contains bacteria and other contaminants, but it rarely makes us sick. This is because the mucosa of the GI tract contains tissue that is part of the immune system (**Figure 3.12a**). This tissue prevents disease-causing bacteria and toxins from damaging the GI tract and invading the body.

Immune function in the small intestine • Figure 3.12

The intestinal lining and the blood contain cells that participate in the immune system's efforts to prevent harmful organisms or materials that enter the GI tract from making us ill.

a. The darkly stained areas shown here are called Peyer's patches. They are made up of immune system tissue and are embedded throughout the mucosa of the small intestine.

b. The cells shown here in pink are a type of white blood cell called *phagocytes*, that can engulf and destroy invading substances. The cells shown in green are *lymphocytes*, which are specific with regard to which invaders they can attack. Some lymphocytes directly kill invaders, while others secrete antibodies that help destroy antigens.

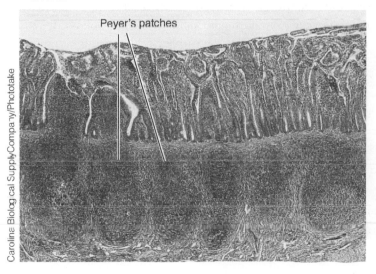

Peyer's patches

Caroline Biological Supply Company/Phototake

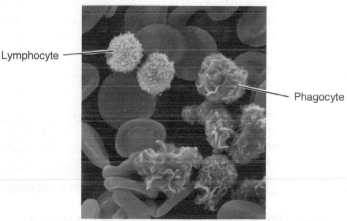

Lymphocyte

Phagocyte

Dennis Kunkel Microscopy, Inc./Phototake

cause abdominal pain, diarrhea, and fatigue. Eventually this damage can lead to malnutrition, weight loss, anemia, osteoporosis, intestinal cancer, and other chronic illnesses.[11,12] Celiac disease, also called gluten intolerance, celiac sprue, nontropical sprue, and gluten-sensitive enteropathy, is an inherited condition that affects an estimated 1 in 133 people in the population. Although gluten-free diets are a current trend, gluten intolerance can be diagnosed only by a blood test or an intestinal biopsy. For people with celiac disease, consuming a diet that eliminates gluten provides relief from symptoms. This means eliminating products containing wheat, barley, or rye, including most breads, crackers, pastas, cereals, cakes, and cookies. It also requires eliminating foods ranging from packaged gravies to soy sauce that are processed with these grains.

Digestive System Problems and Discomforts

Almost everyone experiences digestive system problems from time to time. These problems often cause discomfort and frequently limit the types of foods a person can consume (**Figure 3.14a**). They also can interfere with nutrient digestion and absorption. Problems may occur anywhere in the digestive tract, from the mouth to the anus, and can affect the accessory organs that provide the secretions that are essential for proper GI function.

Heartburn and GERD Heartburn occurs when the acidic contents of the stomach leak back into the esophagus (**Figure 3.14b**). The medical term for the leakage of stomach contents into the esophagus is *gastroesophageal reflux.*

> **heartburn** A burning sensation in the chest or throat caused when acidic stomach contents leak back into the esophagus.
>
> **gastroesophageal reflux disease (GERD)** A chronic condition in which acidic stomach contents leak into the esophagus, causing pain and damaging the esophagus.

Occasional heartburn is common, but if it occurs more than twice a week, it may indicate a condition called **gastroesophageal reflux disease (GERD)**. If left untreated, GERD can eventually lead to more serious health problems, such as esophageal bleeding, ulcers, and cancer.

The discomforts of heartburn and GERD can be reduced by limiting the amounts and types of foods consumed. Eating small meals and consuming beverages between rather than with meals prevents heartburn by reducing the volume of material in the stomach. Avoiding fatty and fried foods, chocolate, peppermint, and caffeinated beverages, which increase stomach acidity or slow stomach emptying, can help minimize symptoms. Remaining upright after eating, wearing loose clothing, avoiding smoking and alcohol, and losing weight may also help prevent heartburn. For many people, medications that neutralize acid or reduce acid secretion are needed to manage symptoms.

Peptic ulcers Peptic ulcers occur when the mucus barrier protecting the stomach, esophagus, or upper small intestine is penetrated and the acid and pepsin in digestive secretions damage the gastrointestinal lining (**Figure 3.14c**). Mild ulcers cause abdominal pain; more severe ulcers can cause life-threatening bleeding.

> **peptic ulcer** An open sore in the lining of the stomach, esophagus, or upper small intestine.

Peptic ulcers can result from GERD or from misuse of medications such as aspirin or nonsteroidal anti-inflammatory drugs (such as Motrin and Aleve) but are more often caused by infection with the bacterium *Helicobacter pylori* (*H. pylori*). These bacteria burrow into the mucus and destroy the protective mucosal layer.[13] Over half of the world's population is infected with *H. pylori*, but not everyone who is infected develops ulcers.[14] *H. pylori* infection can be treated using antibiotics.

Gallstones Clumps of solid material that accumulate in either the gallbladder or the bile duct are referred to as **gallstones** (**Figure 3.14d**). They can cause pain when the gallbladder contracts in response to fat in the intestine. Gallstones can interfere with bile secretion and reduce fat absorption. They are usually treated by removing the gallbladder. After the gallbladder has been removed, bile, which is produced in the liver, drips directly into the intestine as it is produced rather than being stored and squeezed out in larger amounts when fat enters the intestine.

Diarrhea and constipation Diarrhea and constipation are common discomforts that are related to problems in the intestines. **Diarrhea** refers to frequent, watery stools. It occurs when material moves through the colon too quickly for sufficient water to be absorbed or when water is drawn into the lumen from cells lining the intestinal tract.

Diarrhea can be caused by bacterial or viral infections, irritants that inflame the lining of the GI tract, the

Abnormalities in any of the organs of the digestive system can affect nutritional status and overall health.

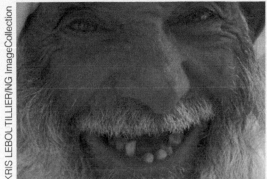

KRIS LEBOL TILLIER/NG ImageCollection

a. Tooth loss and dental pain can make chewing difficult. This may limit the intake of certain foods and reduce nutrient absorption because poorly chewed food may not be completely digested. Tooth decay and gum disease are more likely when saliva production is reduced. Reduced saliva production, which is a side effect of many medications, can also cause changes in taste and difficulty swallowing.

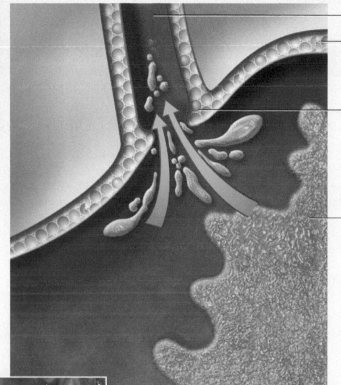

Esophagus

Stomach wall

Sphincter

Acidic stomach contents

b. Heartburn and GERD occur when stomach acid leaks back through the sphincter and irritates the lining of the esophagus. Stomach contents also pass through this sphincter during vomiting. Vomiting may be caused by an illness, a food allergy, medication, or pregnancy.

CNRI/SPL/Photo Researchers

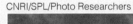

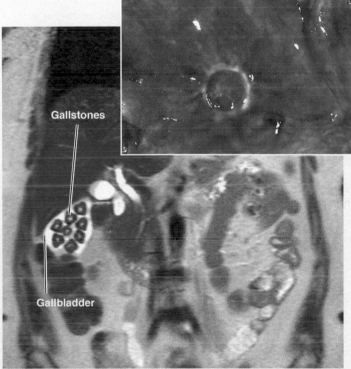

Gallstones

Gallbladder

Simon Fraser/Photo Researchers, Inc.

c. Peptic ulcers occur when the mucosa is destroyed, exposing underlying tissues to gastric juices. Damage that reaches the nerve layer causes pain, and bleeding can occur if blood vessels are damaged. An ulcer that perforates the wall of the stomach or esophagus can be life-threatening.

e. Constipation increases pressure in the colon and can lead to outpouches in the colon wall, shown here, called diverticula (discussed further in Chapter 4).

Colon wall

Dr. Larpent/CNRI/Photo Researchers, Inc.

Diverticula

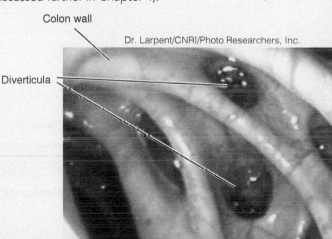

d. Gallstones, visible in this image of the abdomen, are deposits of cholesterol, bile pigments, and calcium that can be in the gallbladder or the bile duct. They can block bile from entering the small intestine, cause pain when the gallbladder contracts, and reduce fat digestion and absorption.

passage of undigested food into the large intestine, medications, and chronic intestinal diseases. Diarrhea causes loss of fluids and minerals. Severe diarrhea lasting more than a day or two can be life-threatening.

Constipation refers to hard, dry stools that are difficult to pass (**Figure 3.14e**). Constipation can be caused by a diet containing insufficient fluid or fiber, lack of exercise, a weakening of the muscles of the large intestine, and a variety of medications. It can be prevented by drinking plenty of liquids consuming a high-fiber diet, and getting enough exercise (see *Thinking It Through* and *What Should I Eat?*).

A Case Study on How Changes in the Digestive System Affect Nutrition

Changes in the digestive system affect how our bodies process the food we eat. For each patient described here, think about how digestion and absorption are affected and the consequences for the patient's nutritional health.

A 50-year-old man is taking medication that reduces the amount of saliva he produces.

 What effect might this have on his nutrition and dental health?

Your answer:

An 80-year-old woman wearing dentures that don't fit well likes raw carrots and still eats them but can't chew them thoroughly.

 How might this affect the digestion and absorption of nutrients contained in the carrots?

Your answer:

A 47-year-old woman undergoes treatment for colon cancer, which requires that most of her large intestine be surgically removed.

 How does this change affect the amount of fluid she needs to consume?

Your answer:

A 56-year-old man has gallstones, which cause pain when his gallbladder contracts.

 What types of food should he avoid and why?

Your answer:

A 50-year-old man has a deficiency of pancreatic enzymes.

 How would this affect nutrient digestion?

Your answer:

A 40-year-old woman weighing 300 pounds has undergone a surgical procedure called gastric banding to help her lose weight. The diagram shows how her stomach was altered.

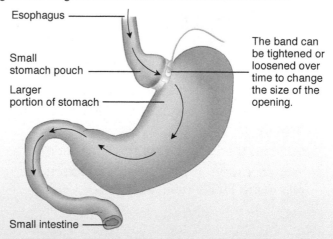

Esophagus

Small stomach pouch

Larger portion of stomach

The band can be tightened or loosened over time to change the size of the opening.

Small intestine

 Why can't she eat as much food as before? Will the procedure affect nutrient absorption? Why or why not?

Your answer:

(Check your answers in online Appendix L.)

WHAT SHOULD I EAT?

For Digestive Health

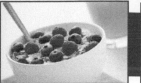
© Sara Winter/iStockphoto

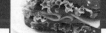
© Jill Chen/iStockphoto

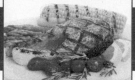
© Steve Mcsweeny/iStockphoto

Reduce your risk of adverse reactions
- Avoid foods that you are allergic to by reading food labels carefully.
- Chew each bite thoroughly to maximize digestion and avoid choking.
- Don't talk with food in your mouth.
- Learn the Heimlich maneuver: You could save a life.

Reduce your chances of heartburn
- Eat enough to satisfy your hunger but not so much that you are stuffed.
- Wait 10 minutes between your first and second courses to see how full you feel.
- Stay upright after you eat; don't flop on the couch in front of the television.

Avoid constipation by consuming enough fiber and fluid
- Choose whole-grain cereals and breads.
- Double your servings of vegetables at dinner.
- Eat two pieces of fruit with your lunch.
- Add beans to your salad.
- Have one or two beverages with or before each meal.

Use iProfile to find the fiber content of your favorite fruits and vegetables.

CONCEPT CHECK 🛑 STOP

1. **Why** is the immune function of the GI tract so important?
2. **How** can food allergy symptoms be prevented?
3. **When** can antibiotics be used to treat ulcers?
4. **What** foods should be avoided by people with gallstones?

3.5 Delivering Nutrients and Eliminating Wastes

LEARNING OBJECTIVES

1. **Trace** the path of blood circulation.
2. **Discuss** how blood flow is affected by eating and by activity.
3. **Explain** the functions of the lymphatic system.
4. **List** four ways in which waste products are eliminated from the body.

fter food has been digested and the nutrients have been absorbed, the nutrients must be delivered to the cells. This delivery is handled by the **cardiovascular system**, which consists of the heart and blood vessels. Amino acids from protein, single sugars from carbohydrate, and the water-soluble products of fat digestion are absorbed into **capillaries** in the villi of the small intestine

> **capillary** A small, thin-walled blood vessel through which blood and the body's cells exchange gases and nutrients.

and transported via the blood to the liver (see Figure 3.9b). The products of digestion that are not water soluble, such as cholesterol and large fatty acids, are absorbed into **lacteals**, which are part of the **lymphatic system**, before entering the blood.

> **lacteal** A lymph vessel in the villi of the small intestine that picks up particles containing the products of fat digestion.

The Cardiovascular System

The cardiovascular system circulates blood throughout the body. Blood carries nutrients and oxygen to the cells of all the organs and tissues of the body and removes carbon dioxide and other waste products from these cells. Blood also carries other substances, such as hormones, from one part of the body to another.

Delivering Nutrients and Eliminating Wastes 81

Blood circulation • Figure 3.15

Blood pumped to the lungs picks up oxygen and delivers nutrients. Blood pumped to the rest of the body delivers oxygen and nutrients.

1 Oxygen-poor blood that reaches the heart from the rest of the body is pumped through the arteries to the capillaries of the lungs.

2 In the capillaries of the lungs, oxygen from inhaled air is picked up by the blood, and carbon dioxide is released into the lungs and exhaled.

3 Oxygen-rich blood returns to the heart from the lungs via veins.

4 Oxygen-rich blood is pumped out of the heart into the arteries that lead to the rest of the body.

5 In the capillaries of the body, nutrients and oxygen move from the blood to the body's tissues, and carbon dioxide and other waste products move from the tissues to the blood, to be carried away.

6 Oxygen-poor blood returns to the heart via veins.

Think Critically Why is the cardiovascular system important in nutrition?

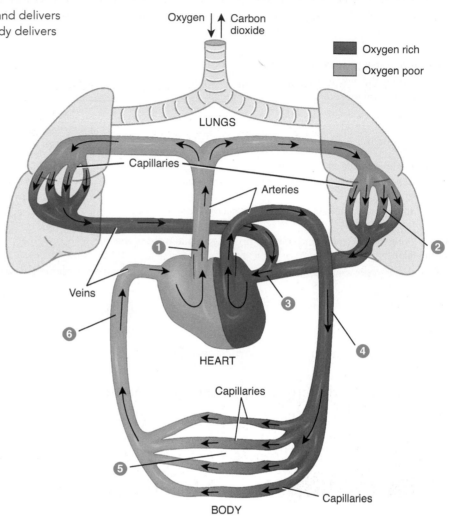

The exchange of nutrients and gases occurs across the thin walls of the capillaries. In most body tissues, oxygen and nutrients carried by the blood pass from the capillaries into the cells, and carbon dioxide and other waste products pass from the cells into the capillaries. In the capillaries of the lungs, blood releases carbon dioxide to be exhaled and picks up oxygen to be delivered to the cells. In the capillaries of the GI tract, blood delivers oxygen and picks up water-soluble nutrients absorbed from the diet.

The amount of blood, and hence the amounts of nutrients and oxygen, delivered to a specific organ or tissue depends on the need. When you are resting, about 25% of your blood goes to your digestive system, about 20% to your skeletal muscles, and the rest to your heart, kidneys, brain, skin, and other organs.[15] This distribution changes

The heart and blood vessels The heart is the workhorse of the cardiovascular system. It is a muscular pump with two circulatory loops—one that carries blood to and from the lungs and one that carries blood to and from the rest of the body (**Figure 3.15**).

The blood vessels that transport blood and dissolved substances toward the heart are called **veins**, and those that transport blood and dissolved substances away from the heart are called **arteries**. As arteries carry blood away from the heart, they branch many times to form smaller and smaller blood vessels. The smallest arteries are called **arterioles**. Arterioles branch to form capillaries. Blood from capillaries then flows into the smallest veins, the **venules**, which converge to form larger and larger veins for returning blood to the heart.

when you eat or exercise. When you have eaten a large meal, a greater proportion of your blood goes to your digestive system to provide the oxygen and nutrients needed by the GI muscles and glands for digestion of the meal and absorption of nutrients. When you are exercising strenuously, about 70% of your blood is directed to your skeletal muscles to deliver nutrients and oxygen and remove carbon dioxide and other waste products (**Figure 3.16**).

Blood flow at rest and during exercise • Figure 3.16

Blood flow changes depending on the needs of various organs and tissues.

a. At rest between meals, the amount of blood directed to the abdomen, which includes the organs, muscles, and glands of the digestive system, is similar to the amount that goes to the skeletal muscles.[15]

b. During exercise, blood flow increases to the muscles so that more oxygen and nutrients can be delivered. As a result, only a small proportion of the blood is directed to the abdomen.[15] You may get cramps if you exercise right after eating a big meal because your body cannot direct enough blood to the intestines and the muscles at the same time. The muscles win out, and food remains in your intestines, often causing cramps.

ALASKA STOCK IMAGES/NGImage Collection

TAYLOR S. KENNEDY/NG ImageCollection

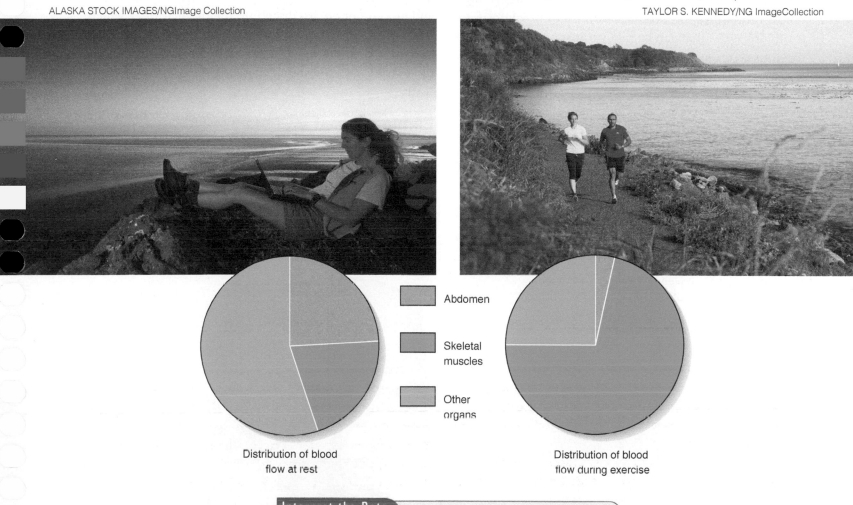

Abdomen

Skeletal muscles

Other organs

Distribution of blood flow at rest

Distribution of blood flow during exercise

Interpret the Data

Based on these charts, which area receives the least blood flow during exercise?
a. skeletal muscle
b. abdomen
c. other organs
d. Blood flow is equal to all areas.

Delivering nutrients to the liver Water-soluble molecules in the small intestine, including amino acids, sugars, water-soluble vitamins, and the water-soluble products of fat digestion, cross the mucosal cells of the villi and enter the capillaries (see Figures 3.9 and 3.10). Once in the capillaries, these molecules are carried to the liver via the **hepatic portal vein** (**Figure 3.17**).

The liver acts as a gatekeeper between the body and substances absorbed from the intestine. Some nutrients are stored in the liver, some are changed into different forms, and others are allowed to pass through unchanged. The liver determines whether individual nutrients are stored or delivered immediately to the cells, depending on the body's needs. The liver is also important in the synthesis and breakdown of amino acids, proteins, and lipids. It modifies the products of protein breakdown to form molecules that can be safely transported to the kidney for excretion. The liver also contains enzyme systems that protect the body from toxins absorbed by the gastrointestinal tract.

The Lymphatic System

The lymphatic system consists of a network of tubules (lymph vessels) and lymph organs that contain infection-fighting cells. Fluid that collects in tissues and between cells drains into the lymphatic system. This prevents the fluid from accumulating and causing swelling.

The lymphatic system is an important part of the immune system. Fluid that drains into lymph vessels is filtered past a collection of infection-fighting cells before being returned to the blood. If the fluid contains antigen, an immune response is triggered. White blood cells and antibodies produced by this response enter the blood and help destroy the foreign substance.

In the small intestine, the lymph vessels aid in the absorption and transport of fat-soluble substances such as cholesterol, fatty acids, and fat-soluble vitamins. These nutrients pass from the intestinal mucosa into the lacteals located in the villi (see Figure 3.9b). The lacteals drain into larger lymph vessels. Lymph vessels from the intestine and most other organs drain into the thoracic duct, which empties into the blood near the neck. Therefore, substances absorbed into the lymphatic system do not pass through the liver before entering the general blood circulation.

Elimination of Wastes

Material that is not absorbed from the gut into the body is eliminated from the gastrointestinal tract in the feces. Wastes that originate in the body, such as carbon dioxide, minerals, and nitrogen-containing wastes, must also

Hepatic portal circulation • Figure 3.17 _____

The hepatic portal circulation delivers nutrients to the liver. Water-soluble substances absorbed into the capillaries of the villi move into venules, which merge to form larger veins that eventually form the hepatic portal vein.

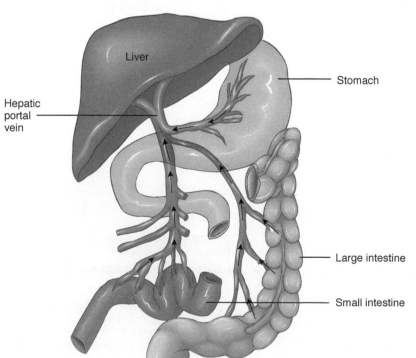

Liver

Stomach

Hepatic portal vein

Large intestine

Small intestine

Organ systems involved in elimination of wastes • Figure 3.18

Substances in food that cannot be absorbed are eliminated in the feces. Nutrients that are absorbed from the digestive system and the oxygen taken in by the respiratory system are distributed to all the cells in the body by the cardiovascular system. Wastes generated from nutrient metabolism, called metabolic wastes, are eliminated from the body through the skin and the urinary and respiratory systems.

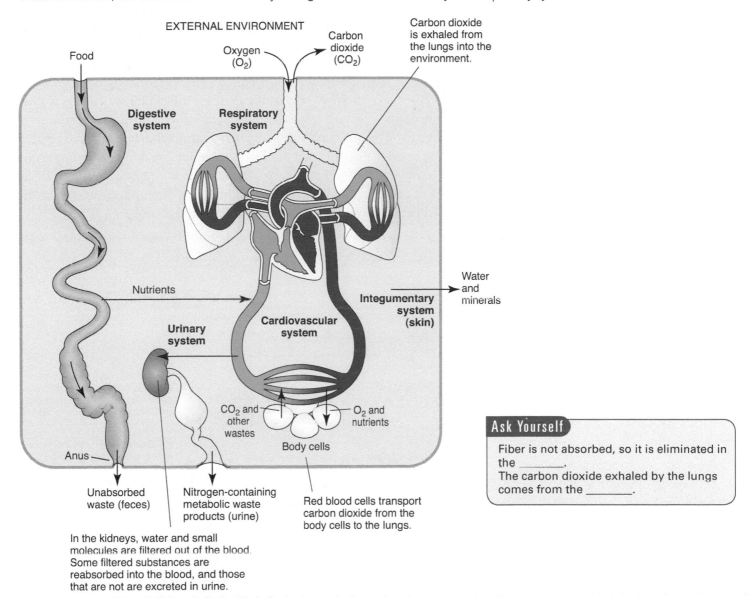

EXTERNAL ENVIRONMENT

Food

Oxygen (O_2)

Carbon dioxide (CO_2)

Carbon dioxide is exhaled from the lungs into the environment.

Digestive system

Respiratory system

Nutrients

Integumentary system (skin)

Water and minerals

Urinary system

Cardiovascular system

CO_2 and other wastes

O_2 and nutrients

Body cells

Anus

Unabsorbed waste (feces)

Nitrogen-containing metabolic waste products (urine)

Red blood cells transport carbon dioxide from the body cells to the lungs.

In the kidneys, water and small molecules are filtered out of the blood. Some filtered substances are reabsorbed into the blood, and those that are not are excreted in urine.

Ask Yourself

Fiber is not absorbed, so it is eliminated in the _____.
The carbon dioxide exhaled by the lungs comes from the _____.

be eliminated. The same highway of blood vessels that picks up absorbed nutrients and oxygen helps remove wastes from the body (**Figure 3.18**). Carbon dioxide and some water are lost via the lungs, and some water, minerals, and nitrogen-containing wastes are lost through the skin, but the kidney is the primary site for the excretion of metabolic wastes. Water, minerals, and the nitrogen-containing by-products of protein breakdown are filtered out of the blood by the kidneys and excreted in the urine.

CONCEPT CHECK STOP

1. **Where** does blood go after it leaves the lungs?
2. **Why** is it not a good idea to exercise after eating a large meal?
3. **What** is the role of the lymphatic system in nutrient absorption?
4. **What** wastes are excreted by the kidneys? by the lungs?

3.6 An Overview of Metabolism

LEARNING OBJECTIVES

1. **Discuss** the two general ways in which nutrients can be used after they have been absorbed.

2. **Describe** what happens in cellular respiration.

3. **List** the types of molecules that can be made from glucose, from fatty acids, and from amino acids.

Once they are inside the body's cells, nutrients are used either for energy or to synthesize all the structural and regulatory molecules needed for growth and maintenance. Together, the chemical reactions that break down molecules to provide energy and those that synthesize larger molecules are referred to as **metabolism**. Many of the reactions of metabolism occur in series known as **metabolic pathways**. Molecules that enter these pathways are modified at each step, with the help of enzymes. Some of the pathways use energy to build body structures, and others break large molecules into smaller ones, releasing energy. Reactions that synthesize molecules occur in different cellular compartments from those that break down molecules for energy. For example, ribosomes are cellular structures that specialize in the synthesis of proteins, and **mitochondria** are cellular organs that are responsible for breaking down molecules to release energy. Metabolism is discussed in more detail in appropriate individual chapters and expanded in the online minichapter: *Metabolism: Energy for Life.*

PROCESS DIAGRAM

Producing ATP • Figure 3.19

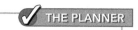 THE PLANNER

Cellular respiration uses oxygen to convert glucose, fatty acids, and amino acids into carbon dioxide, water, and energy, in the form of ATP.

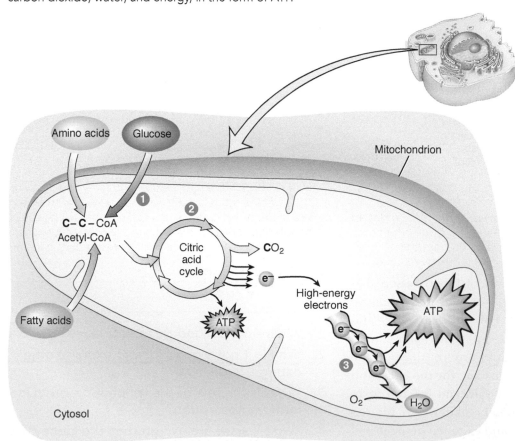

❶ In the presence of oxygen, glucose, fatty acids, and amino acids can be metabolized to produce a two-carbon molecule (acetyl-CoA).

❷ Each acetyl-CoA molecule enters a circular pathway, called the citric acid cycle, that produces two molecules of carbon dioxide (CO_2).

❸ In the final step of this metabolic pathway, most of the energy released from the glucose, fatty acid, or amino acid molecules is used to produce ATP, and oxygen combines with hydrogen to form water.

HOW IT WORKS

Releasing Energy

In the mitochondria, glucose, fatty acids, and amino acids derived from carbohydrates, fats, and proteins, respectively, are broken down in the presence of oxygen to produce carbon dioxide and water and release energy. This process, called **cellular respiration**, is like cell breathing: Oxygen goes into the cell, and carbon dioxide comes out. The energy released by cellular respiration is used to make a molecule called **adenosine triphosphate (ATP)** (**Figure 3.19**). ATP can be thought of as the cell's energy currency. The chemical bonds of ATP are very high in energy, and when they break, the energy is released and can be used either to power body processes, such as muscle contraction or the transport of molecules across membranes, or to synthesize new molecules needed to maintain and repair body tissues.

> **adenosine triphosphate (ATP)** A high-energy molecule that the body uses to power activities that require energy.

Synthesizing New Molecules

Glucose, fatty acids, and amino acids that are not broken down for energy are used, with the input of energy from ATP, to synthesize structural, regulatory, or storage molecules. Glucose molecules are used to synthesize the glucose-storage molecule glycogen and, in some cases, fatty acids. Fatty acids are used to make body fat, cell membranes, and regulatory molecules. Amino acids are used to synthesize various proteins and non-protein molecules that the body needs and, when necessary, to make glucose. Excess amino acids can also be converted into fatty acids.

CONCEPT CHECK STOP

1. **What** are absorbed nutrients used for?
2. **Why** can cellular respiration be thought of as cell breathing?
3. **What** types of molecules can be made from amino acids?

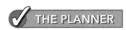 THE PLANNER

Summary

1 The Organization of Life 60

- Our bodies and the foods we eat are all made from the same building blocks—**atoms**. Atoms are linked together by chemical bonds to form **molecules**. Molecules can form **cells**, and cells with similar structures and functions are organized into **tissues**. Tissues are organized into **organs**, such as the stomach shown here, and the **organ systems** that make up an organism. The body organ systems work together; for example, the passage of food through the digestive system and the secretion of digestive substances are regulated by the nervous and endocrine systems.

From atoms to organisms • Figure 3.1

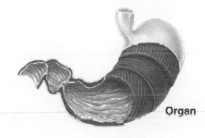

Organ

2 The Digestive System 64

- The digestive system has two major functions: **digestion** and **absorption**. Digestion breaks down food and nutrients into units that are small enough to be absorbed. Absorption transports nutrients into the body. The main component of the digestive system, illustrated here, is the **gastrointestinal tract**, which consists of a hollow tube that begins at the mouth and continues through the pharynx, esophagus, stomach, small intestine, and large intestine, ending at the anus.

Structure of the digestive system • Figure 3.2a

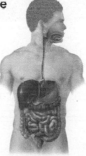

- The digestion of food and absorption of nutrients are aided by the secretion of **mucus** and **enzymes**.

Digestion and Absorption of Nutrients 66

- The processes involved in digestion begin in response to the smell or sight of food and continue as food enters the digestive tract at the mouth, where it is broken down into smaller pieces by the teeth and mixed with **saliva** to form a bolus. Carbohydrate digestion is begun in the mouth by **salivary amylase**. From the mouth, the bolus passes through the **pharynx** and into the esophagus. The rhythmic contractions of **peristalsis** propel it down the esophagus to the stomach.

- The stomach is a temporary storage site for food. The muscles of the stomach mix the food into a semiliquid mass called **chyme**, and **gastric juice**, which contains hydrochloric acid and **pepsin**, begins the digestion of protein. The rate at which the stomach empties varies with the amount and composition of food consumed and is regulated by nervous and hormonal signals.

- The small intestine is the primary site for nutrient digestion and absorption. The circular folds, **villi**, shown here, and microvilli of the small intestine, ensure a large absorptive surface area. In the small intestine, **bicarbonate** from the pancreas neutralizes stomach acid, and pancreatic and intestinal enzymes digest carbohydrate, fat, and protein. The digestion and absorption of fat in the small intestine are aided by **bile** from the gallbladder.

The structure of the small intestine • Figure 3.9b

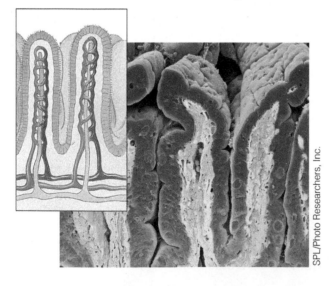

SPL/Photo Researchers, Inc.

- The absorption of nutrients across the intestinal **mucosa** occurs by means of several different transport mechanisms. **Simple diffusion**, **osmosis**, and **facilitated diffusion** do not require energy, but **active transport** does.

- Components of **chyme** that are not absorbed in the small intestine pass on to the large intestine, where some water and other nutrients are absorbed. The large intestine is populated by **intestinal microflora** that digest some of the unabsorbed materials, such as fiber, producing small amounts of nutrients and gas. The remaining unabsorbed materials are eliminated in the **feces**.

Digestion in Health and Disease 75

- Immune system cells and tissues located in the gastrointestinal tract help prevent disease-causing organisms or chemicals from entering the body. An **antigen** entering the digestive tract is attacked first by **phagocytes**. If it is not eliminated by the phagocytes, **lymphocytes** respond specifically to the antigen by producing **antibodies**. The immune system protects us from disease but can also cause **food allergies**.

- Diseases or discomforts that affect any part of the digestive system can interfere with food intake, digestion, or nutrient absorption. Common difficulties include dental problems, reduced saliva production, **heartburn**, **GERD**, **peptic ulcers** (such as the one shown here), **gallstones**, vomiting, **diarrhea**, and **constipation**.

Digestive disorders • Figure 3.14c

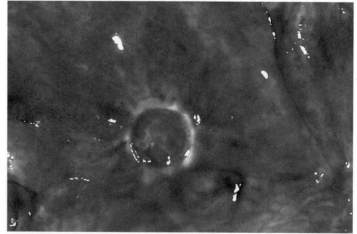

CNRI/SPL/Photo Researchers

5 Delivering Nutrients and Eliminating Wastes 81

- Absorbed nutrients are delivered to the cells by the **cardiovascular system**. The heart pumps blood to the lungs to pick up oxygen and release carbon dioxide. From the lungs, blood returns to the heart and is then pumped to the rest of the body to deliver oxygen and nutrients and remove carbon dioxide and other wastes before returning to the heart. Exchange of nutrients and gases occurs at the **capillaries**.

- The products of carbohydrate and protein digestion and the water-soluble products of fat digestion enter capillaries in the intestinal villi and are transported to the liver via the **hepatic portal vein**, as illustrated here. The liver removes the absorbed substances for storage, converts them into other forms, or allows them to pass unaltered. The liver also protects the body from toxic substances that may have been absorbed.

Hepatic portal circulation • Figure 3.17

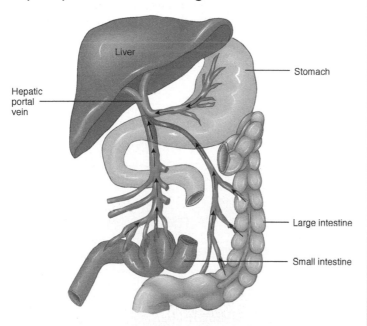

- The fat-soluble products of digestion enter **lacteals** in the intestinal villi. Lacteals join larger lymph vessels. The nutrients absorbed via the **lymphatic system** enter the blood without first passing through the liver.

- Unabsorbed materials are eliminated in the feces. The waste products of metabolism are excreted by the lungs, skin, and kidneys.

6 An Overview of Metabolism 86

- In the cells, glucose, **fatty acids**, and amino acids absorbed from the diet can be broken down by means of **cellular respiration**, as shown here, to provide energy in the form of **ATP**.

Producing ATP • Figure 3.19

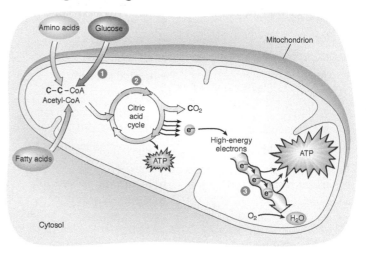

- In the presence of ATP, glucose, fatty acids, and amino acids can be used either to synthesize structural or regulatory molecules or to synthesize energy-storage molecules.

Key Terms

- absorption 64
- active transport 73
- adenosine triphosphate (ATP) 87
- allergen 76
- antibody 76
- antigen 76
- arteriole 82
- artery 82
- atom 60
- bicarbonate 71
- bile 73
- brush border 71
- capillary 81
- cardiovascular system 81
- celiac disease 76
- cell 60
- cellular respiration 87
- chyme 69

- constipation 80
- diarrhea 78
- diffusion 73
- digestion 64
- enzyme 66
- epiglottis 67
- facilitated diffusion 73
- fatty acid 64
- feces 64
- food allergy 76
- gallstone 78
- gastric juice 69
- gastrin 70
- gastroesophageal reflux disease (GERD) 78
- gastrointestinal tract 64
- heartburn 78
- hepatic portal vein 84
- hormone 61

- intestinal microflora 74
- lacteal 81
- lipase 72
- lumen 64
- lymphatic system 81
- lymphocyte 76
- metabolic pathway 86
- metabolism 86
- microvilli 71
- mitochondrion 86
- molecule 60
- mucosa 64
- mucosal cells 64
- mucus 64
- organ 61
- organ system 61
- osmosis 73
- pancreatic amylase 72
- pancreatic juice 71

- pepsin 69
- peptic ulcer 78
- peristalsis 68
- phagocyte 76
- pharynx 67
- prebiotic 74
- probiotic 74
- protease 72
- saliva 67
- salivary amylase 67
- segmentation 71
- simple diffusion 73
- sphincter 68
- tissue 60
- transit time 64
- vein 82
- venule 82
- villi 71

What is happening in this picture?

This patient has Crohn's disease, an inflammatory disease of the intestine that is interfering with his ability to absorb nutrients. Doctors are ensuring that he is being nourished by infusing a nutrient solution into his blood through a process called total parenteral nutrition (TPN).

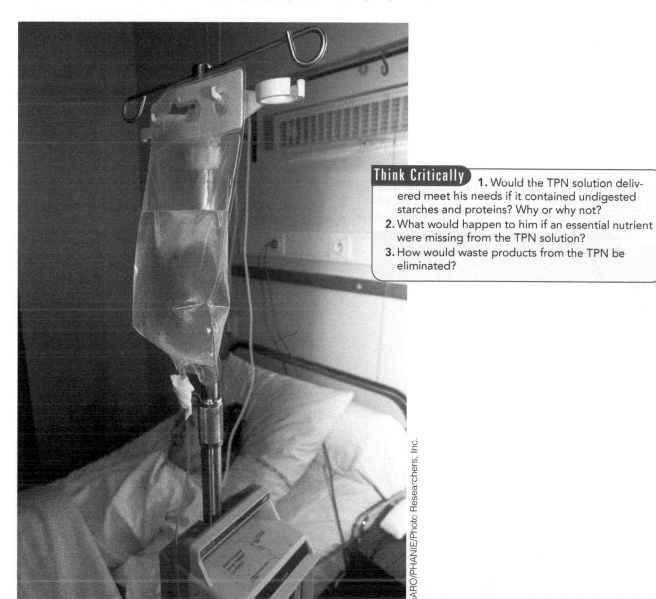

GARO/PHANIE/Photo Researchers, Inc.

Think Critically

1. Would the TPN solution delivered meet his needs if it contained undigested starches and proteins? Why or why not?
2. What would happen to him if an essential nutrient were missing from the TPN solution?
3. How would waste products from the TPN be eliminated?

THE PLANNER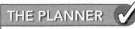

Review your Chapter Planner on the chapter opener and check off your completed work.

4.1 Carbohydrates in Our Food

LEARNING OBJECTIVES

1. **Distinguish** refined carbohydrates from unrefined carbohydrates.

2. **Compare** the nutrients in whole grains to those in enriched grains.

3. **Discuss** how added refined sugars and naturally occurring sugars differ from each other.

Our hunter-gatherer ancestors ate very differently from the way we eat. Their diet consisted almost entirely of **unrefined foods**—foods eaten either just as they are found in nature or with only minimal processing, such as cooking. Today we still consume some unrefined sources of carbohydrate, but many of the foods we consume are made with **refined** grains and contain added refined sugar (**Figure 4.1**).

The increased consumption of refined carbohydrates that has occurred around the world over the past few decades has been implicated as one of the causes of the current obesity epidemic and the rising incidence of chronic diseases. Recommendations for a healthy diet suggest that we select more unrefined sources of carbohydrates, including whole grains, vegetables, and fruits, and that

> **refined** Refers to foods that have undergone processing that changes or removes various components of the original food.
>
> **enrichment** The addition to food of specific amounts of nutrients to replace those lost during processing.

we limit foods high in refined carbohydrates, such as candies, cookies, and sweetened beverages.

What Is a Whole Grain?

When you eat a bowl of oatmeal or a slice of whole-wheat toast, you are consuming a **whole-grain product**. Whole-grain products include the entire kernel of the grain: the **germ**, the **bran**, and the **endosperm** (**Figure 4.2a**). Refined grain products, such as white bread, include just the endosperm. The bran and germ are discarded during refining, and along with them the fiber and some vitamins and minerals are lost. To make up some of these losses, refined grains sold in the United States are required to be enriched. **Enrichment**, adds back some, but not all, of the nutrients lost in processing (**Figure 4.2b**). For example, the thiamin, niacin, riboflavin, and iron that are lost when grains are milled are later added back to levels that are equal to or higher than originally present. Since 1998, folic acid has also been added to enriched grains. Other nutrients, including vitamin E and vitamin B_6 are also removed by milling, but they are not added back. Therefore, foods made with refined grains contain more of some nutrients and less of others than foods made from whole grains.

Unrefined and refined foods • Figure 4.1

Corn is an unrefined source of carbohydrate, but it can be refined through grinding, cooking, extruding, and drying to eventually end up as cornflakes in your cereal bowl. The sugar you sprinkle on cornflakes is also a refined carbohydrate; it has been refined from sugar cane or sugar beets.

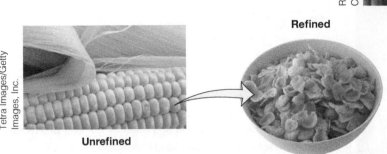

Raul Touzon/NG Image Collection

Unrefined

Refined

Image Source/Getty Images, Inc

Refined

Tetra Images/Getty Images, Inc.

Unrefined

Carlos Alvarez/iStockphoto

Ask Yourself

Which is less refined: canned peaches or fresh peaches? Whole-wheat bread or white bread? Granola cereal or oatmeal?

Whole grains • Figure 4.2

Whole-grain products provide greater amounts of many nutrients than refined grains, but lesser amounts of a few nutrients that are added in the enrichment process.

a. A kernel of grain is made up of three parts that together provide all of the nutrients present in whole grain.

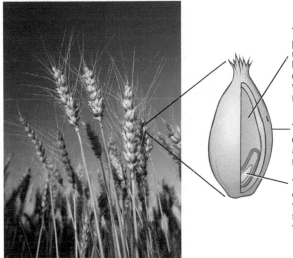

Kevin Morris/Getty Images

The **endosperm** is the largest part of the kernel. It is made up of primarily starch, but it also contains most of the kernel's protein, along with some vitamins and minerals.

The outermost **bran** layers contain most of the fiber and are a good source of many vitamins and minerals.

The **germ**, located at the base of the kernel, is the embryo where sprouting occurs. It is a source of oil and is rich in vitamin E.

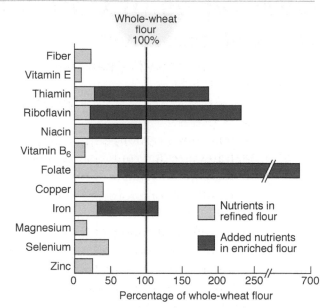

Whole-wheat flour 100%

Fiber
Vitamin E
Thiamin
Riboflavin
Niacin
Vitamin B$_6$
Folate
Copper
Iron
Magnesium
Selenium
Zinc

□ Nutrients in refined flour
■ Added nutrients in enriched flour

0   50   100   150   200   250   700
Percentage of whole-wheat flour

b. The amounts of many nutrients in refined flour (yellow bars) are much lower than the amounts originally present in the whole grain (100% line). In enriched flour, thiamin, riboflavin, niacin, iron, and folate have been added back in amounts that equal or exceed the original levels (red bars).

What Is Added Refined Sugar?

Refined sugars added to food during processing or at the table account for almost 15% of the calories consumed in the typical American diet.[1] Refined sugars are nutritionally and chemically identical to sugars that occur naturally in foods. When separated from their plant sources, however, refined sugars no longer contain the fiber, vitamins, minerals, and other substances found in the original plant. Therefore, added refined sugars contribute empty calories to the diet. Foods that naturally contain sugars, such as fruits and milk, provide vitamins, minerals, and phytochemicals, along with the calories from the sugar, making them higher in nutrient density (**Figure 4.3**). To help consumers identify packaged foods that are high in added sugars, one of the changes proposed to food labels is to list the amount of added sugars on the Nutrition Facts panel.

CONCEPT CHECK 🛑 STOP

1. **What** is the difference between a whole-grain product and a product made with a refined grain?

2. **Why** is there more vitamin B$_6$ and less thiamin in a slice of whole-wheat bread than in a slice of white bread?

3. **Why** are foods high in added refined sugars said to contribute empty calories?

Added versus naturally occurring sugar • Figure 4.3

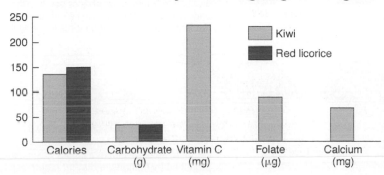

250
200
150
100
50
0

□ Kiwi
■ Red licorice

Calories   Carbohydrate Vitamin C   Folate   Calcium
            (g)   (mg)   (µg)   (mg)

Choosing three kiwis rather than four pieces of red licorice is a more nutrient-dense choice. The kiwis are an unrefined source of sugar that also provides fiber and vitamin C, folate, and calcium. Most of the calories in the licorice are from added sugar; it is lower in nutrient density because it provides almost no other nutrients.

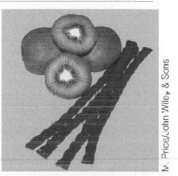

M. Price/John Wiley & Sons

4.2 Types of Carbohydrates

LEARNING OBJECTIVES

1. **Name** the basic unit of carbohydrate.
2. **Classify** carbohydrates as simple or complex.
3. **Describe** the types of complex carbohydrates.
4. **Distinguish** soluble fiber from insoluble fiber.

Chemically, carbohydrates are a group of compounds made up of one or more sugar units that contain carbon (*carbo*) as well as hydrogen and oxygen in the same two-to-one proportion found in water (*hydrate*, H_2O). Carbohydrates made up of only one sugar unit are called **monosaccharides**, those made up of two sugar units are called **disaccharides**, and those made up of more than two sugar units are called **polysaccharides**.

> **sugar unit** A sugar molecule that cannot be broken down to yield other sugars.
>
> **monosaccharide** A carbohydrate made up of a single sugar unit.

> **disaccharide** A carbohydrate made up of two sugar units.
>
> **polysaccharide** A carbohydrate made up of many sugar units linked together.

Nutrition InSight — Carbohydrate structures and sources • Figure 4.4

Simple carbohydrates include monosaccharides and disaccharides. Complex carbohydrates include glycogen, starches, and fiber.

a. Glucose, fructose, and galactose are monosaccharides that have the same chemical formulas, but the atoms are arranged differently.

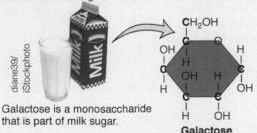

Glucose is a monosaccharide that circulates in the blood. It is rarely found alone in food, but is a component of sucrose and starch.

Glucose

Fructose is a monosaccharide found in fruits and vegetables. It makes up about half the sugar in honey and in the high-fructose corn syrup used to sweeten many foods and beverages.

Fructose

Galactose is a monosaccharide that is part of milk sugar.

Galactose

b. Maltose, sucrose, and lactose are disaccharides made up of different pairs of monosaccharides.

Maltose (Glucose + Glucose)

Maltose, made of two glucose units, is formed when starch is digested. When you chew bread and then hold it in your mouth, the slightly sweet taste you experience is due to the maltose formed as the enzyme salivary amylase digests the starch present in the bread.

Sucrose (Glucose + Fructose)

Sucrose, the disaccharide made by linking glucose to fructose, is table sugar. It is the only sweetener that can be called "sugar" in the ingredient list on food labels in the United States.

Lactose (Galactose + Glucose)

Lactose, made of glucose linked to galactose, is produced by humans and other mammals. It is often called milk sugar because it is found in milk, as well as ice cream, and other dairy products.

Simple Carbohydrates

Monosaccharides and disaccharides are classified as **simple carbohydrates** and are what we commonly refer to as *sugars*. The three most common monosaccharides in the diet are **glucose**, **fructose**, and **galactose**. Each contains 6 carbon, 12 hydrogen, and 6 oxygen atoms ($C_6H_{12}O_6$), but these three sugars differ in the arrangement of these atoms (**Figure 4.4a**). Glucose, often called *blood sugar*, is the most important carbohydrate fuel for the human body.

The most common disaccharides in our diet are **maltose, sucrose,** and **lactose** (**Figure 4.4b**).

glucose A 6-carbon monosaccharide that is the primary form of carbohydrate used to provide energy in the body.

glycogen The storage form of carbohydrate in animals, made up of many glucose molecules linked together in a highly branched structure.

starch A carbohydrate found in plants, made up of many glucose molecules linked in straight or branched chains.

Complex Carbohydrates

Complex carbohydrates are polysaccharides; they are generally not sweet tasting the way simple carbohydrates are. They include **glycogen** in animals and starches and fibers in plants (**Figure 4.4c**). Glycogen is the storage form of glucose in humans and other animals. It is found in the liver and muscles, but we don't consume it in our diet because the glycogen in animal muscles is broken down soon after the animal is slaughtered.

Starch is made up of glucose molecules linked together in either straight or branched chains (see Figure 4.4c). It is the storage form of carbohydrate in plants and provides energy

✓ THE PLANNER

c. Glycogen, starches, and the fiber cellulose are polysaccharides made up of straight or branching chains of glucose.

Think Critically How do the bonds that link the glucose units in a molecule of starch differ from those in a molecule of cellulose fiber?

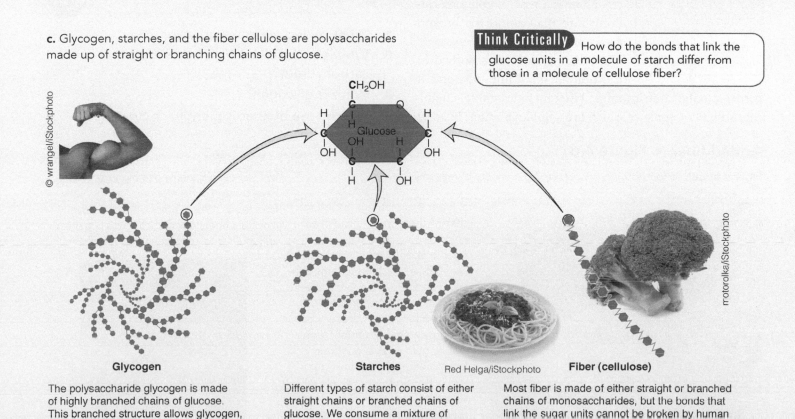

Glycogen

The polysaccharide glycogen is made of highly branched chains of glucose. This branched structure allows glycogen, which is found in muscle and liver, to be broken down quickly when the body needs glucose.

Starches   Red Helga/iStockphoto

Different types of starch consist of either straight chains or branched chains of glucose. We consume a mixture of starches in grain products, legumes, and other starchy vegetables.

Fiber (cellulose)

Most fiber is made of either straight or branched chains of monosaccharides, but the bonds that link the sugar units cannot be broken by human digestive enzymes. For example, cellulose, shown here, is a fiber made up of straight chains of glucose molecules. Sources include wheat bran and broccoli.

Photosynthesis • Figure 4.5

Glucose is produced in plants through the process of **photosynthesis**, which uses energy from the sun to convert carbon dioxide and water to glucose. Plants most often convert glucose to starch. When a human eats plants, digestion converts the starch back to glucose.

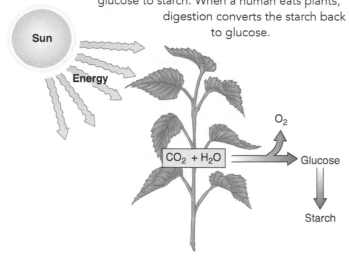

Sun

Energy

O_2

$CO_2 + H_2O$ → Glucose

Starch

---

soluble fiber Fiber that dissolves in water or absorbs water and is readily broken down by intestinal microflora. It includes pectins, gums, and some hemicelluloses.

for plant growth and reproduction. When we eat plants, we consume the energy stored in the starch (**Figure 4.5**).

Fiber is a type of complex carbohydrate that cannot be broken down by human digestive enzymes. Thus fiber cannot be absorbed in the human small intestine, and it passes into the large intestine. Fiber includes several chemical substances, some of which are soluble in water. Soluble

fiber, found around and inside plant cells, dissolves in water to form viscous solutions. Although human enzymes can't digest soluble fiber, bacteria in the large intestine can break it down. Beans contain soluble fiber and small polysaccharides, called **oligosaccharides**, that cannot be broken down by human digestive enzymes. Both of these pass into the large intestine, where they are digested by bacteria creating gas and other by-products. Other foods that contain soluble fiber include oats, apples, and seaweed (**Figure 4.6a**).

Fiber that does not dissolve in water is called **insoluble fiber**. Insoluble fiber comes primarily from the structural parts of plants, such as cell walls. This type of fiber adds bulk to fecal matter because it passes, relatively unchanged, through the gastrointestinal tract. Food sources of insoluble fiber include wheat and rye bran, broccoli, and celery (**Figure 4.6b**).

---

oligosaccharide A carbohydrate made up of 3 to 10 sugar units.

insoluble fiber Fiber that does not dissolve in water and is less readily broken down by bacteria in the large intestine. It includes cellulose, some hemicelluloses, and lignin.

CONCEPT CHECK   STOP

1. **What** molecules make up starch?
2. **Why** is sucrose classified as a simple carbohydrate?
3. **What** is glycogen?
4. **Which** type of fiber is plentiful in beans?

Added fiber • Figure 4.6

Fiber is added to food during processing for a variety of reasons.

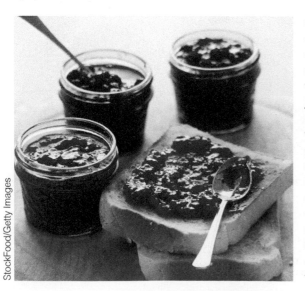

a. Fiber is sometimes added to change the physical properties of foods. Pectin, which is a soluble fiber found in fruits and vegetables, is added to jams and jellies as a thickener. Gums are also used as thickeners because they combine with water to keep solutions from separating; gum arabic, gum karaya, guar gum, locust bean gum, xanthan gum, and gum tragacanth, which are extracted from shrubs, trees, and seedpods, and agar, carrageenan, and alginates, which are gums derived from seaweed, are frequently added to foods.

b. The health benefits of a high-fiber diet have created consumer demand for high-fiber foods. Wheat bran, which provides insoluble fiber, is added to foods like breads and muffins to increase their fiber content.

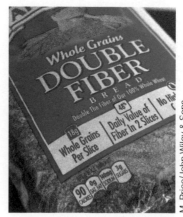

StockFood/Getty Images

M. Price/John Wiley & Sons

LEARNING OBJECTIVES

1. **Describe** the steps of carbohydrate digestion.
2. **Explain** what is meant by lactose intolerance.
3. **Discuss** how indigestible carbohydrates affect the colon and feces.
4. **Draw** a graph that compares blood glucose levels after drinking soda and after eating beans.

D isaccharides and complex carbohydrates must be digested to monosaccharides before they can be absorbed into the body. Carbohydrates that cannot be completely digested cannot be absorbed but still have an impact on the gastrointestinal tract and overall health. Once absorbed, carbohydrates travel in the blood to the liver.

Carbohydrate Digestion

Carbohydrate digestion begins in the mouth, but most starch digestion and the breakdown of disaccharides occur in the small intestine (**Figure 4.7**). Carbohydrate that cannot be digested passes into the colon. Some of this is broken down by bacteria. Material that cannot be absorbed is excreted in the feces.

Carbohydrate digestion • Figure 4.7

THE PLANNER

During digestion, enzymes break starches and sugars into monosaccharides, which are absorbed. Most of the fiber and other indigestible carbohydrates are excreted in the feces.

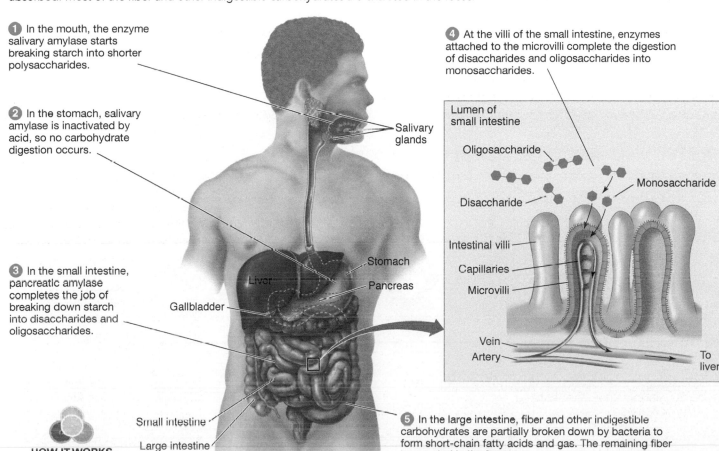

1 In the mouth, the enzyme salivary amylase starts breaking starch into shorter polysaccharides.

2 In the stomach, salivary amylase is inactivated by acid, so no carbohydrate digestion occurs.

3 In the small intestine, pancreatic amylase completes the job of breaking down starch into disaccharides and oligosaccharides.

4 At the villi of the small intestine, enzymes attached to the microvilli complete the digestion of disaccharides and oligosaccharides into monosaccharides.

Lumen of small intestine

Oligosaccharide

Monosaccharide

Disaccharide

Intestinal villi

Capillaries

Microvilli

Vein

Artery

To liver

Salivary glands

Stomach

Liver

Pancreas

Gallbladder

Small intestine

Large intestine

HOW IT WORKS

5 In the large intestine, fiber and other indigestible carbohydrates are partially broken down by bacteria to form short-chain fatty acids and gas. The remaining fiber is excreted in the feces.

PROCESS DIAGRAM

Lactose intolerance The disaccharide lactose is broken down by the enzyme lactase in the small intestine. We are all born with adequate levels of lactase, but in many people, levels decline so much with age that lactose cannot be completely digested, a condition called **lactose intolerance**. When these individuals consume milk and other dairy products, the lactose passes into the large intestine, where it draws in water and is metabolized by bacteria, producing gas and causing abdominal distension, cramping, and diarrhea. The incidence of lactose intolerance varies among populations (**Figure 4.8**).

Because milk is the primary source of calcium in the U.S. diet, lactose-intolerant individuals may have difficulty meeting calcium needs. Many people who are lactose intolerant can handle small amounts of lactose and therefore can meet their calcium needs by consuming small portions of milk throughout the day and eating cheese and yogurt, which contain less lactose than milk. Those who cannot tolerate any lactose can get their calcium from nondairy sources, such as tofu, legumes, dark-green vegetables, and canned salmon and sardines, which are consumed with the bones, as well as from calcium-fortified foods, calcium supplements, and lactase-treated milk (such as Lactaid). Another option is to take lactase tablets with or before consuming milk products

> **lactose intolerance** The inability to completely digest lactose due to a reduction in the levels of the enzyme lactase.
>
> **resistant starch** Starch that escapes digestion in the small intestine of healthy people.

to digest the lactose before it passes into the large intestine.

Indigestible carbohydrates Some carbohydrates are not digested and therefore are not readily absorbed. Fiber and some oligosaccharides are not digested because they cannot be broken down by human enzymes. **Resistant starch** is not digested either because the natural structure of the grain protects the starch molecules or because cooking and processing alter their digestibility. Legumes, unripe bananas, and cold cooked potatoes, rice, and pasta are high in resistant starch.

As indigestible carbohydrates pass through the gastrointestinal tract, they slow the rate at which nutrients, such as glucose, are absorbed (**Figure 4.9a**). Fiber can also bind to certain minerals, preventing their absorption. For instance, wheat bran fiber binds zinc, calcium, magnesium, and iron. Indigestible carbohydrates also speed transit through the intestine by increasing the amount of water and the volume of material in the intestine (**Figure 4.9b**). This stimulates peristalsis, causing the muscles of the large intestine to work more and function better, helping to prevent constipation.

Some carbohydrates that are not digested by human enzymes are digested by intestinal bacteria when they

Lactose intolerance • Figure 4.8

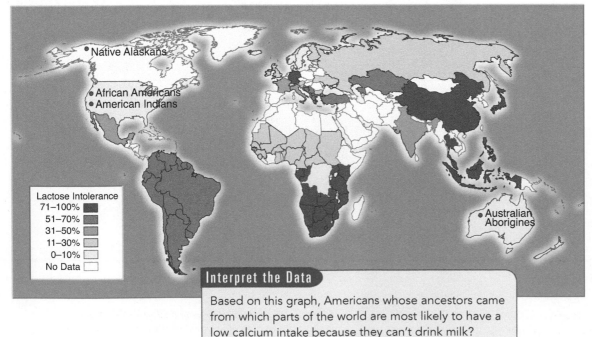

This map illustrates the dramatic variation in the incidence of lactose intolerance around the world. In the United States, between 30 and 50 million people are lactose intolerant; it is more common in some ethnic and racial populations than in others. Up to 80% of African Americans, 80 to 100% of Native Americans, and 90 to 100% of Asian Americans are lactose intolerant, but only about 15% of Caucasian Americans are.[2]

Interpret the Data

Based on this graph, Americans whose ancestors came from which parts of the world are most likely to have a low calcium intake because they can't drink milk?

Lactose Intolerance
71–100%
51–70%
31–50%
11–30%
0–10%
No Data

Fiber promotes health by slowing digestion and absorption, reducing transit time, increasing stool weight, and promoting the growth of healthy microflora.

a. As shown on the left, the bulk and volume of a high-fiber meal dilute the gastrointestinal contents. This dilution slows the digestion of food and absorption of nutrients (shown as green dots moving slowly out of the intestine), causing a delay and a blunting of the rise in blood glucose that occurs after a meal (see graph). With a low-fiber meal, as shown on the right, nutrients are more concentrated; digestion and absorption occur more rapidly (shown as green dots moving quickly out of the intestine), causing a quicker, sharper rise in blood glucose (see graph).

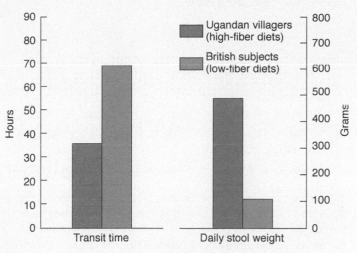

b. This study done in the 1970s compares Ugandan villagers, who consume a diet high in fiber, with British subjects living in Uganda, who consume a more refined, low-fiber diet. Stool weights are greater and transit times shorter for Ugandan villagers than for British subjects.[4]

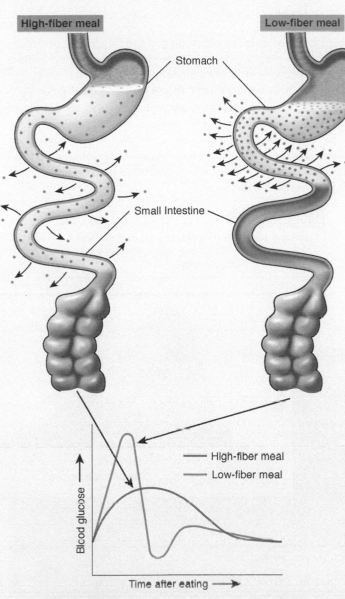

High-fiber meal   Low-fiber meal

Stomach

Small Intestine

High-fiber meal
Low-fiber meal

Blood glucose

Time after eating →

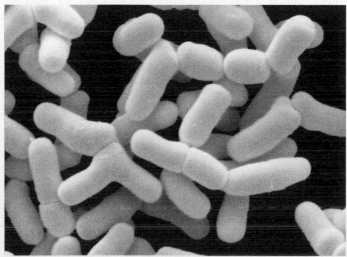

Scimat/Photo Researchers, Inc.

c. Indigestible carbohydrates are a food source for the bacteria in the colon. When bacteria break down these carbohydrates, short-chain fatty acids are formed. The acidic conditions that result inhibit the growth of undesirable bacteria and favor the growth of healthy ones, such as the *Bifidobacteria* shown here. Imbalances in these gut bacteria are related to numerous disorders, including colon cancer, inflammatory bowel disease, allergy, and diabetes.[5]

Ask Yourself

Why does blood glucose rise more slowly after a high-fiber meal than after a low-fiber meal?

reach the large intestine, producing short-chain fatty acids and gas. The fatty acids can be used as a fuel source for cells in the colon and other body tissues; they may play a role in regulating cellular processes and preventing disease (**Figure 4.9c**).[3]

Carbohydrate Absorption

After a meal, the monosaccharides from carbohydrate digestion enter the portal circulation and travel to the liver. Glucose can be used to provide energy, stored as

WHAT A SCIENTIST SEES
Glycemic Index

Potatoes and beans are both sources of unrefined carbohydrate, but scientists know that the effect potatoes have on blood glucose is very different from the effect beans have. Beans are much higher in fiber and protein, both of which slow digestion and absorption and therefore reduce the glycemic response.

The glycemic response of potatoes versus kidney beans is shown here graphically, but it can also be expressed using the **glycemic index**, which is a ranking of how a food affects blood glucose relative to the effect of an equivalent amount of carbohydrate from a reference food, such as white bread or pure glucose. For example, on a glycemic index scale on which white bread is 100, potatoes are 90 and kidney beans are about 25. This means that blood glucose levels do not increase as much after eating kidney beans as they do after eating white bread or potatoes.

A shortcoming of the glycemic index is that it is measured using a set amount of carbohydrate in a food (usually 50 grams), not the typical serving of food that we eat. For example, it takes over

4 cups of strawberries to supply 50 g of carbohydrate, but people typically eat only about 1 cup. **Glycemic load** compares the effect of typical portions of food on blood glucose, so it is a more practical way to assess the effect of a food on blood glucose levels.

A shortcoming of both the glycemic index and glycemic load is that they are determined for individual foods rather than for meals, which contain mixtures of foods. We typically eat meals, so knowing the glycemic index or glycemic load of a single food doesn't tell us much about the rise in blood glucose that will occur after eating a meal.

Think Critically How would the graph of blood glucose levels after eating a meal of meat and potatoes differ from the graph that would result after eating potatoes alone?

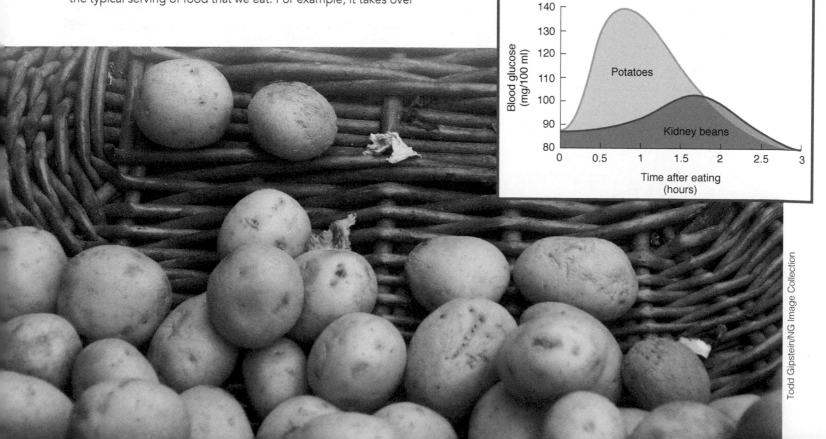

Todd Gipstein/NG Image Collection

glycemic response The rate, magnitude, and duration of the rise in blood glucose that occurs after food is consumed.

liver glycogen, or delivered via the general blood circulation to other body tissues, causing blood glucose levels to rise. **Glycemic response** is a measure of the impact a food has on blood glucose levels. How quickly and how high blood glucose levels rise are affected by how long it takes a food to leave the stomach and by how fast the food is digested and the glucose absorbed.

Refined sugars and starches generally cause a greater glycemic response than unrefined carbohydrates because sugars and starches consumed alone leave the stomach quickly and are rapidly digested and absorbed. For example, when you drink a bottle of sugary soda, your blood glucose increases within minutes. Because fiber takes longer to leave the stomach and slows absorption in the small intestine, a fiber-containing food such as oatmeal would take longer to leave your stomach and therefore cause a lower glycemic response (see *What a Scientist Sees*). When carbohydrate, fat, and protein are consumed together, stomach emptying is slowed, delaying both digestion and absorption of carbohydrate, so blood glucose rises more slowly than when carbohydrate is consumed alone. For instance, after a meal of chicken, brown rice, and green beans, which contains carbohydrate, fat, protein, and fiber, blood glucose doesn't begin to rise for 30 to 60 minutes.

CONCEPT CHECK STOP

1. **What** steps are involved in starch digestion?
2. **How** does lactose in the colon cause gas and diarrhea?
3. **Why** do indigestible carbohydrates affect the type of bacteria in the colon?
4. **How** does fiber affect the rate at which blood glucose rises after a meal?

4.4 Carbohydrate Functions

LEARNING OBJECTIVES

1. **Name** the main function of carbohydrate in the body.
2. **Contrast** the roles of insulin and glucagon in blood glucose regulation.
3. **Compare** anaerobic and aerobic metabolism.
4. **Discuss** what happens to protein and fat metabolism when dietary carbohydrate is insufficient.

The main function of carbohydrates is to provide energy, but carbohydrates also play other roles in the body. For example, nerve tissue needs the sugar galactose, and in breast-feeding women, galactose combines with glucose to produce the milk sugar lactose. The monosaccharides ribose and deoxyribose play nonenergy roles as components of RNA and DNA, respectively, the two molecules that contain a cell's genetic information. Ribose is also a component of the B vitamin riboflavin. Oligosaccharides are associated with cell membranes, where they help signal information about cells, and large polysaccharides found in connective tissue provide cushioning and lubrication.

Getting Enough Glucose to Cells

Glucose is an important fuel for body cells. Many body cells can use energy sources other than glucose, but brain cells, red blood cells, and a few others must have glucose to stay alive. In order to provide a steady supply of glucose, the concentration of glucose in the blood is regulated by the liver and by hormones secreted by the pancreas. The rise in blood glucose levels after eating stimulates the pancreas to secrete the hormone **insulin**, which allows glucose to enter muscle and fat cells, thereby lowering the level of glucose in the blood. In muscle insulin stimulates the synthesis of glycogen from glucose. In fat-storing cells, it promotes fat synthesis. In the liver,

insulin A hormone made in the pancreas that allows glucose to enter cells and stimulates the synthesis of protein, fat, and liver and muscle glycogen.

insulin promotes the storage of glucose as glycogen and, to a lesser extent, fat. Insulin also stimulates protein synthesis. The overall effect of insulin is to remove glucose from the blood and promote energy storage (**Figure 4.10**).

A few hours after eating, blood glucose levels—and consequently the amount of glucose available to the cells—have decreased enough

> **glucagon** A hormone made in the pancreas that raises blood glucose levels by stimulating the breakdown of liver glycogen and the synthesis of glucose.

to trigger the pancreas to secrete the hormone **glucagon** (see Figure 4.10). Glucagon raises blood glucose by signaling liver cells to break down glycogen into glucose, which is released into the blood. At the same time, glucagon signals the liver to synthesize new glucose molecules, which are also released into the blood, bringing blood glucose levels back to normal.

Blood glucose regulation • Figure 4.10

Blood glucose levels are regulated by the hormones insulin and glucagon, secreted by the pancreas.

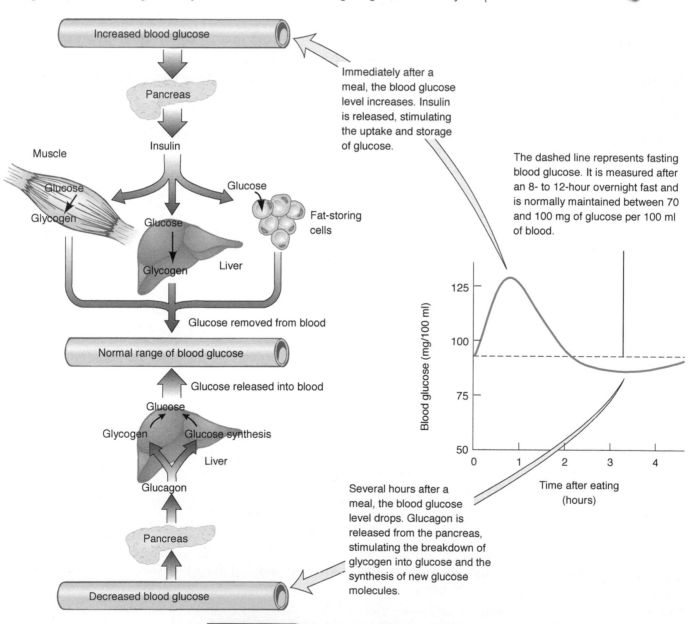

Increased blood glucose

Pancreas

Insulin

Muscle

Glucose

Glycogen

Glucose

Glucose

Fat-storing cells

Glucose

Glycogen   Liver

Glucose removed from blood

Normal range of blood glucose

Glucose released into blood

Glucose

Glycogen   Glucose synthesis

Liver

Glucagon

Pancreas

Decreased blood glucose

Immediately after a meal, the blood glucose level increases. Insulin is released, stimulating the uptake and storage of glucose.

The dashed line represents fasting blood glucose. It is measured after an 8- to 12-hour overnight fast and is normally maintained between 70 and 100 mg of glucose per 100 ml of blood.

Blood glucose (mg/100 ml)

125

100

75

50

0   1   2   3   4

Time after eating (hours)

Several hours after a meal, the blood glucose level drops. Glucagon is released from the pancreas, stimulating the breakdown of glycogen into glucose and the synthesis of new glucose molecules.

Think Critically What would happen to blood glucose levels if insulin were not available?

Cellular respiration • Figure 4.11

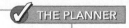

Inside body cells, the reactions of cellular respiration split the bonds between carbon atoms in glucose, releasing energy that is used to synthesize ATP. ATP is used to power the energy-requiring processes in the body.

1 Glycolysis, which takes place in the cytosol, splits glucose, a six-carbon molecule, into two three-carbon molecules (pyruvate). This step releases high-energy electrons (purple balls) and produces a small amount of ATP. Pyruvate is then either broken down to produce more ATP or is used to remake glucose.

2 Pyruvate can be used to produce more ATP when oxygen is available. In the mitochondria, pyruvate is broken down, releasing carbon dioxide (CO_2) and high-energy electrons and forming acetyl-CoA (2 carbons), which continues through aerobic metabolism.

3 Acetyl-CoA enters the citric acid cycle, where carbon dioxide and high-energy electrons are released and where a small amount of ATP is produced.

4 Most ATP is produced in the final step of aerobic metabolism. Here the energy in the high-energy electrons released in previous steps is transferred to ATP, and the electrons are combined with oxygen and hydrogen to form water.

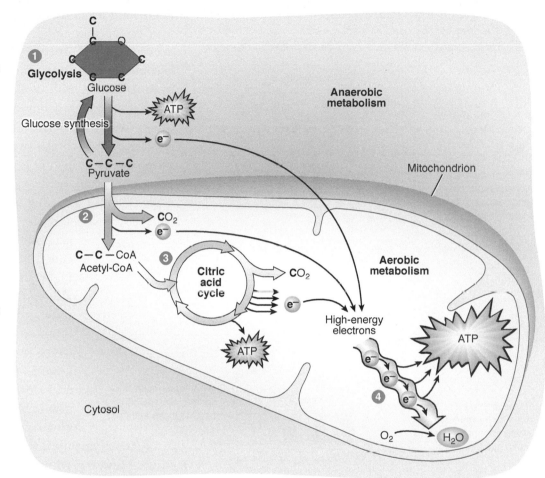

HOW IT WORKS

Glucose as a Source of Energy

Cells use glucose to provide energy via cellular respiration (see Chapter 3). Cellular respiration uses oxygen to convert glucose to carbon dioxide and water and provide energy in the form of ATP (**Figure 4.11**).

The first step in cellular respiration is **glycolysis** (*glyco* = "glucose," *lysis* = "to break down"). Glycolysis can rapidly produce two molecules of ATP from each glucose molecule. Because oxygen is not needed for this step, glycolysis is sometimes called anaerobic glycolysis, or **anaerobic metabolism**. When oxygen is available, the complete breakdown of glucose can proceed. This **aerobic metabolism** produces about 36 molecules of ATP for each glucose molecule, 18 times more ATP than is generated by anaerobic glycolysis.

glycolysis An anaerobic metabolic pathway that splits glucose into two three-carbon pyruvate molecules; the energy released from one glucose molecule is used to make two molecules of ATP.

anaerobic metabolism Metabolism in the absence of oxygen.

aerobic metabolism Metabolism in the presence of oxygen. It can completely break down glucose to yield carbon dioxide, water, and energy in the form of ATP.

What happens when carbohydrate is limited? • Figure 4.12

The availability of carbohydrate affects the metabolism of both protein and fat. When carbohydrate is limited, protein is broken down to supply amino acids that can be used to make glucose. Because the complete breakdown of fat requires some carbohydrate, when carbohydrate is limited, ketones are formed. Ketones can be used as a source of energy, but high levels can accumulate in the blood and be excreted in the urine.

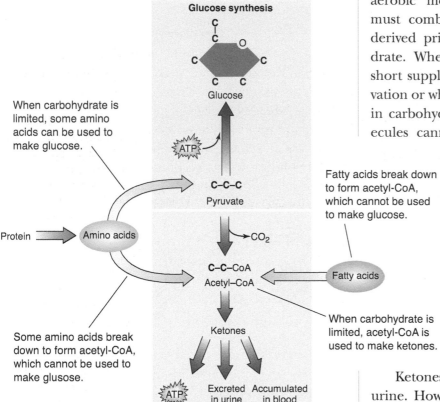

Limited carbohydrate increases protein breakdown

Glucose is an essential fuel for brain cells and red blood cells. If adequate amounts of glucose are not available, it can be synthesized from three-carbon pyruvate molecules (see Figure 4.11, step 1 on previous page). Fatty acids cannot be used to synthesize glucose because the reactions that break them down produce two-carbon, rather than three-carbon, molecules. Some of the amino acids from protein breakdown can supply the three-carbon molecules needed for glucose synthesis (**Figure 4.12**). However, this use of amino acids takes them away from body proteins. Body proteins that are broken down to make glucose are no longer available to do their job, whether that job is to speed up a chemical reaction or

contract a muscle. Sufficient dietary carbohydrate ensures that protein is not utilized in this way; carbohydrate is therefore said to *spare* protein.

Limited carbohydrate interferes with fat breakdown Most of the energy stored in the body is stored as fat. Fatty acids are broken down into two-carbon units that form acetyl-CoA. To proceed through aerobic metabolism, acetyl-CoA must combine with a molecule derived primarily from carbohydrate. When carbohydrate is in short supply, such as during starvation or when the diet is very low in carbohydrate, acetyl-CoA molecules cannot proceed through aerobic metabolism and instead react with each other to form molecules called **ketones** or **ketone bodies** (see Figure 4.12). The heart, muscle, and kidney can use ketones for energy. After about three days of fasting, even the brain adapts and can obtain about half of its energy from ketones. The use of ketones for energy helps spare glucose and decreases the amount of protein that must be broken down to synthesize glucose.

> **ketone** or **ketone body** An acidic molecule formed when there is not sufficient carbohydrate to break down acetyl-CoA.
>
> **ketosis** High levels of ketones in the blood.

Ketones not used for energy can be excreted in the urine. However, when ketone production is high, they build up in the blood, a condition known as **ketosis**. Mild ketosis can occur during starvation or when consuming a low-carbohydrate weight-loss diet and can cause symptoms such as reduced appetite, headaches, dry mouth, and odd-smelling breath. Severe ketosis can occur with untreated diabetes and can increase the blood's acidity so much that normal body processes are disrupted, resulting in coma and even death.

CONCEPT CHECK ⬛ STOP

1. **Why** is it important to keep blood glucose levels in the normal range?

2. **How** does insulin affect blood glucose levels?

3. **What** process breaks down glucose in the presence of oxygen to yield ATP?

4. **Why** is carbohydrate said to spare protein?

4.5 Carbohydrates in Health and Disease

LEARNING OBJECTIVES

1. **Define** diabetes and explain its health consequences.
2. **Describe** how carbohydrates contribute to the development of dental caries.
3. **Discuss** the role of carbohydrates in weight control.
4. **Explain** how fiber may help promote health.

A re carbohydrates good for you or bad for you? On the one hand, they have been blamed for everything from diabetes to obesity. On the other hand, U.S. guidelines for a healthy diet recommend that people base their diet on carbohydrate-rich foods in order to reduce disease risk. This incongruity relates to the health effects of different types of dietary carbohydrates: Diets high in unrefined carbohydrates from whole grains, fruits, and vegetables are associated with a lower incidence of a variety of chronic diseases, whereas diets high in refined carbohydrates, such as refined grains and foods high in added sugars, increase chronic disease risk.[6]

Diabetes

Diabetes mellitus, commonly referred to simply as diabetes, is a disease characterized by high blood glucose levels (**Figure 4.13**). Uncontrolled diabetes damages the heart, blood vessels, kidneys, eyes, and nerves. It is the leading cause of adult blindness and accounts for over 44% of new cases of kidney failure and more than 60% of nontraumatic lower-limb amputations. In the United States, over 29 million people have diabetes, and 8.1 million of these people have not been diagnosed.[7]

Types of diabetes Type 1 diabetes is an **autoimmune disease** in which the insulin-secreting pancreatic cells are destroyed by the body's immune system. This form of diabetes accounts for only 5 to 10% of diagnosed cases and usually develops before age 30. Because no insulin is produced, people with type 1 diabetes must inject insulin in order to keep blood glucose levels in the normal range. When insulin levels are low, the lack of glucose inside cells leads to

> **diabetes mellitus** A disease characterized by elevated blood glucose due to either insufficient production of insulin or decreased sensitivity of cells to insulin.
>
> **type 1 diabetes** The form of diabetes caused by autoimmune destruction of insulin-producing cells in the pancreas, usually leading to absolute insulin deficiency.
>
> **autoimmune disease** A disease that results from immune reactions that destroy normal body cells.

Blood glucose levels in diabetes • Figure 4.13

Normal blood glucose is less than 100 mg/100 ml blood after an 8 hour fast; a fasting blood level from 100 to 125 mg/100 ml is defined as prediabetes; a fasting level of 126 mg/100 ml or above is defined as diabetes. Two hours after consuming 75 g of glucose, normal blood levels are less than 140 mg/100 ml; prediabetes levels are from 140 to 199 mg/100 ml; diabetes levels are 200 mg/100 ml or greater.

Managing diabetes • Figure 4.16

To manage diabetes, blood glucose levels must be monitored and controlled with diet and exercise, and in some cases medication.

Diet

To avoid a rapid or prolonged rise in blood glucose, the diet needs to be carefully planned.

© Juanmonino/iStockphoto

© FreezeFrameStudio/iStockphoto

Medication

Exercise

© Ana Abejon/iStockphoto

Regular exercise helps control blood glucose. A change in the amount of exercise may change the amount of food and medication required to keep blood glucose in the normal range.

Blood glucose should be monitored regularly. It can be measured using a tiny drop of blood.

© Richard Cano/iStockphoto

Insulin is required to treat type 1 diabetes. Blood glucose levels in type 2 diabetes can be managed with a variety of oral medications as well as insulin.

exercise but may also require oral medications and/or insulin injections (**Figure 4.16**).

Carbohydrate intake and the risk of diabetes

Evidence is accumulating that the types of carbohydrate consumed may play a role in the development of type 2 diabetes in susceptible individuals.[9,10] In populations in which the diet is high in whole grains, the risk of developing type 2 diabetes is lower than in populations in which the diet is high in refined starches and added sugars.[11,12] Consuming foods high in refined carbohydrate causes a greater rise in blood glucose and hence a greater insulin demand than consuming foods high in whole grains. Epidemiological studies have shown that as sweetened beverage consumption increases, so does the risk of diabetes.[13] Regardless of whether or not sugar intake contributes to the development of diabetes, diets high in sugar are high in empty calories, which can contribute to weight gain, which does increase the risk of diabetes.

Hypoglycemia

Another condition that involves abnormal blood glucose levels is hypoglycemia.

hypoglycemia Abnormally low blood glucose levels.

Symptoms of hypoglycemia include low blood sugar (below 70 mg glucose/100 ml blood), irritability, sweating, shakiness, anxiety, rapid heartbeat, headache, hunger, weakness, and sometimes seizures and coma. Hypoglycemia occurs most frequently in people who have diabetes as a result of overmedication. It can also occur in people without diabetes; it is caused by abnormalities in insulin production or by abnormalities in the way the body responds to insulin or to other hormones.

Fasting hypoglycemia, which occurs when an individual has not eaten, is often related to some underlying condition, such as excess alcohol consumption, hormonal deficiencies, or tumors. Treatment involves identifying and treating the underlying disease. **Reactive hypoglycemia** occurs in response to the consumption of high-carbohydrate foods. The rise in blood glucose from the carbohydrate stimulates insulin release. However, too much insulin is secreted, resulting in a rapid fall in blood glucose to abnormally low levels. To prevent the rapid changes in blood glucose that occur with reactive hypoglycemia, the diet should consist of small, frequent meals that contain protein and fiber and are low in simple carbohydrates.

Dental Caries

Dental caries, or cavities, are the best-documented health problem associated with carbohydrate intake. Eighty-five percent of people 18 years and older have had caries. They occur when bacteria that live in the mouth form colonies, known as plaque, on the tooth surface. If the plaque is not brushed, flossed, or scraped away the bacteria metabolize carbohydrate from the food we eat, producing acids. These acids can dissolve tooth enamel and the underlying tooth structure, forming dental caries.

Although all carbohydrates can contribute to dental caries, sucrose is the most cariogenic because it is easily metabolized to acid by bacteria and it is needed for the synthesis of materials that help bacteria stick to the teeth and form plaque.[14] The longer teeth are exposed to carbohydrates—for example, through frequent snacking, consuming foods that stick to the teeth, sucking hard candy, and slowly sipping soda—the greater the risk of caries. Limiting intake of sweet or sticky foods and proper dental hygiene can help prevent dental caries.

Weight Management

As low-carbohydrate diets have gained popularity, carbohydrates have gotten a reputation for being fattening. In reality, carbohydrates are no more fattening than other nutrients, and there is no evidence that the proportion of total carbohydrate in the diet affects energy intake or body weight.[15] Weight gain is caused by excess intake of calories, no matter whether the excess is from carbohydrate, fat, or protein. Carbohydrates provide only 4 Calories/gram, less than half the 9 Calories/gram provided by fat.

Carbohydrates and weight loss The type of carbohydrates you consume can affect how hungry you feel and whether you lose or gain weight (**Figure 4.17**). A diet high in unrefined carbohydrates is high in fiber, which increases the sense of fullness by adding bulk and slowing digestion, allowing you to feel satisfied with less food. This can help promote weight loss.[16] However, diets high in fiber may be problematic for children, who have a small stomach capacity, because they may become satiated before meeting their nutrient requirements.

Foods high in refined carbohydrates cause a rapid rise in blood glucose and therefore stimulate release of insulin. Insulin promotes fat storage. Therefore, a diet high in refined carbohydrate, which causes more insulin release, may shift metabolism toward fat storage (see *Debate: Should You Avoid High-Fructose Corn Syrup?*).[17] In contrast, a low-carbohydrate diet causes less insulin release and hence does not promote fat storage. Low-carbohydrate diets lead to weight loss because they reduce insulin levels and raise blood ketone levels, both of which suppress appetite. In addition, these diets limit food choices to such an extent that the monotony of the diet may cause the dieter to eat less. The weight loss

Beverages and energy intake • Figure 4.17

A diet high in sugar-sweetened beverages may increase caloric intake because beverages do not induce satiety to the same extent as solid foods. Increases in the consumption of sugar-sweetened soft drinks are associated with weight gain.[18]

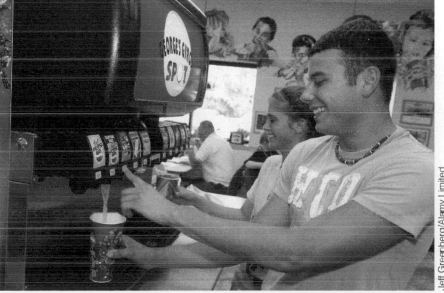

Jeff Greenberg/Alamy Limited

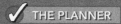
✓ THE PLANNER

The Issue: High-fructose corn syrup (HFCS) is the most common added sweetener in the American diet. The ubiquitous use of this sweetener has created concern about the effect it has on our health. Increased consumption of HFCS has been implicated in the development of obesity, heart disease, and diabetes, among other disorders.[19] Is HFCS just a convenient way to sweeten our food, or is it a threat to our health?

HFCS is a syrup made by extracting starch from corn and treating it to break the bonds between the glucose molecules. The resulting corn syrup is then treated to convert about half the glucose to fructose (hence "high-fructose" corn syrup). Manufacturers prefer HFCS as an added sweetener because it is cheaper and more stable during storage than other sweeteners. In 1970, the most common sweetener in the American diet was sucrose (see graph). Today HFCS has almost completely replaced sucrose in soft drinks and is found in many other foods, ranging from breakfast cereals to canned soups and salad dressings (see photo).

HFCS has been implicated in the growing obesity crisis because the increase in its use parallels the increase in obesity (see graph). Obesity in turn increases the risk of diabetes and heart disease. There is a physiological basis for a relationship between fructose and obesity. When excess energy is consumed, fructose is converted to fat more readily than glucose. In addition, fructose is not as effective as glucose at stimulating the release of hormones that suppress appetite or at inhibiting the release of hormones that stimulate appetite.[20] So, when compared to glucose, fructose consumption contributes more to fat synthesis and less to appetite suppression, potentially leading to overeating and weight gain. A study in humans found a greater amount of abdominal fat in subjects consuming diets high in fructose compared to glucose.[21]

There are a number of counterarguments to the contention that HFCS contributes to obesity more than other sweeteners. First, obesity has increased dramatically in countries that do not use HFCS, and in the United States obesity rates continued to increase even after HFCS consumption leveled off.[22] The most compelling argument as to why HFCS is not to blame for obesity is that it is really no different than sucrose. Sucrose is 50% fructose, while the HFCS used in soft drinks is about 55% fructose. There is no metabolic reason why the fructose in HFCS is more damaging than the fructose in sucrose, unless the slight difference in the amount of fructose in these two sweeteners is metabolically significant.

In an animal study, rats fed a diet supplemented with water sweetened with HFCS gained more weight and more fat than the rats supplemented with sucrose-sweetened water, despite actually consuming fewer calories.[23] However, studies in humans have found responses to consumption of HFCS and sucrose to be the same with regard to its biologic actions and effect on food intake.[22] In a study of weight-loss diets containing 20% of calories from HFCS or sucrose, similar weight changes were seen.[24]

Is HFCS worse than other sweeteners? We gain excess body weight by consuming more energy than we expend. Calories from beverages, whether sweetened with sucrose or HFCS, are a particular concern because the added calories are not compensated for by reductions in solid food intake.[25] Numerous studies have shown a positive association between sweetened beverage consumption and the risk of obesity in adults.[25] When consumed in large amounts, HFCS has the potential to both increase energy intake and promote the deposition of body fat. But will eliminating HFCS from our food supply necessarily make our diets healthier? Will replacing HFCS with sucrose help reduce obesity?

Think Critically: Compare the relationship between the percentage of adults who are obese and the intake of HFCS from 1970 to 2000 and from 2000 to 2005. Do they correlate with each other over both of these time periods? What do these relationships tell you about the role of HFCS in obesity?

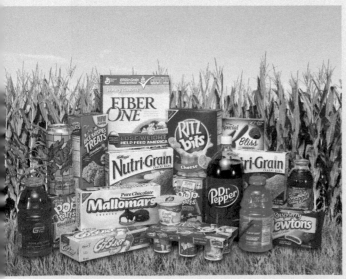

Since 1970, HFCS intake has increased dramatically, while sucrose use has declined. Over this same time period, the incidence of obesity has more than doubled.

◄ A large range of processed foods, from carbonated beverages and fruit drinks to cereals, crackers, barbeque sauce, and salad dressings, contain high-fructose corn syrup.

Andy Washnik

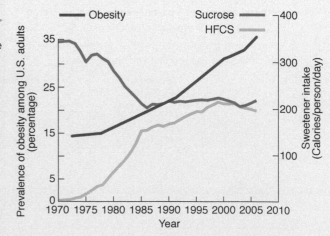

that is achieved with these diets is therefore caused by consuming fewer calories.

Pros and cons of nonnutritive sweeteners One way to reduce the amount of refined sugar in the diet is to replace sugar with **nonnutritive sweeteners** (also called **artificial sweeteners**). The FDA has approved saccharin, aspartame, sucralose, acesulfame K, neotame, and stevia as nonnutritive sweeteners and defined **acceptable daily intakes (ADIs)**—levels that can be consumed daily over a lifetime without appreciable health risk (**Table 4.1**).[26]

Nonnutritive sweeteners   Table 4.1

Sweetener	Brand names	What is it?	ADI
Saccharin	Sweet'N Low, SugarTwin Andy Washnik	The oldest of the nonnutritive sweeteners, developed in 1879. It was once considered a carcinogen but was taken off the government's list of cancer-causing substances in 2000. It is 300 times sweeter than sucrose and has a bitter aftertaste.	5 mg/kg of body weight/day; one packet contains 20 mg of saccharin. Beverages are limited to < 12 mg/fluid ounce. A 154-lb (70-kg) person would exceed the ADI by consuming 18 packets.
Aspartame	Equal, NutraSweet Andy Washnik	Made of two amino acids (phenylalanine and aspartic acid; see *What a Scientist Sees: Phenylketonuria*, in Chapter 6). Because it breaks down when heated, it is typically used in cold products or added after cooking. It is 200 times sweeter than sucrose.	50 mg/kg of body weight/day; one packet contains 37 mg of aspartame. To exceed the ADI, a 154-lb (70-kg) person would have to consume 95 packets or 16 12-oz aspartame-sweetened beverages. It must be limited in the diets of people with phenylketonuria (see Chapter 6).
Acesulfame K	Sunett, Sweet One ©Sara Wight	A heat-stable sweetener that is often used in combination with other sweeteners. It is 200 times sweeter than sucrose.	15 mg/kg of body weight/day; a 154-lb (70-kg) person could consume 2 gallons of beverages containing acesulfame K without exceeding the ADI.
Neotame	Neotame is not sold as a tabletop sweetener.	Made from the same two amino acids as aspartame, but because the bond between them is harder to break than the bond in aspartame, it is heat stable and can be used in baking. It is used in soft drinks, dairy products, and gum but is not sold as a tabletop sweetener. It is 8000 times sweeter than sucrose.	18 mg/kg of body weight/day.
Sucralose	Splenda Andy Washnik	Made from sucrose molecules that have been modified so that they cannot be digested or absorbed. It is heat stable so it can be used in cooking. It is 600 times sweeter than sucrose.	5 mg/kg of body weight/day; one packet contains about 12 mg of sucralose. A 154-lb (70-kg) person could consume 29 packets without exceeding the ADI.
Stevia	Truvia, Pure Via ©Sara Wight	A natural sweetener made from the leaf of the stevia plant.[22] It is the newest sweetener on the market and is about 250 times sweeter than sucrose.	4 mg/kg of body weight/day; to exceed the ADI, a 154-lb (70-kg) person would have to consume more than 10 packets of a stevia sweetener or drink about six 12-oz cans of a stevia-sweetened soda.

When nonnutritive sweeteners are used to replace added sugars in the diet, they can help reduce the incidence of dental caries and manage blood sugar levels. Whether use of these products promotes weight loss, however, depends on whether the calories they spare are added back from other food sources. Studies on the effects of nonnutritive sweeteners on body weight have had mixed results. The majority of studies suggest that obesity rates are lower when artificially sweetened beverages replace sugar-sweetened beverages and there is no evidence that the use of artificial sweeteners causes higher body weight in adults.[27,28] Animal studies suggest that artificial sweeteners may stimulate appetite, leading to weight gain, but this hypothesis has not been supported by studies done in humans.[29] Weight gain seen in some studies of artificial sweetener users is more likely to be due to the fact that individuals at higher risk of obesity are more likely to use artificial sweeteners to try to control weight.[27]

If you think switching to nonnutritive sweeteners will make your diet healthier, think again. Foods that are high in added sugar tend to be nutrient poor. Replacing them with artificially sweetened alternatives does not necessarily increase the nutrient density of the diet or improve overall diet quality.

Heart Disease

The effect of carbohydrate intake on heart disease risk depends on the type of carbohydrate. There is evidence that diets high in sugar can raise blood lipid levels and thereby increase the risk of heart disease,[30] whereas dietary patterns that are high in fiber from grains, vegetables, and fruits reduce the risk of heart disease.[16, 31, 32]

Dietary patterns high in fiber lower heart disease risk by helping to lower blood cholesterol, reduce blood pressure, normalize blood glucose levels, and prevent obesity, as well as by affecting a number of other parameters that impact heart disease risk.[31] Soluble fiber from foods such as legumes, oats, flaxseed, and brown rice lower blood cholesterol levels in several ways. In the digestive tract, soluble fiber helps eliminate cholesterol from the body by binding dietary cholesterol and bile acids, which are made from cholesterol, preventing them from being absorbed (**Figure 4.18**).[33,34] Soluble fiber may also help lower blood cholesterol because it lowers insulin levels and is broken down by bacteria in the colon. The lower insulin levels and the by-products of bacterial breakdown are hypothesized to inhibit cholesterol synthesis in the liver.[33] Insoluble fibers, such as wheat

Cholesterol and soluble fiber • Figure 4.18

Soluble fiber helps lower blood cholesterol by increasing excretion of bile acids and cholesterol.

a. In the absence of soluble fiber, dietary cholesterol and bile, which contains cholesterol and bile acids made from cholesterol, are absorbed into the blood and transported to the liver for use in the body.

b. When soluble fiber is present in the digestive tract, the fiber binds cholesterol and bile acids so that they are excreted rather than absorbed. This helps reduce the amount of cholesterol in the body.

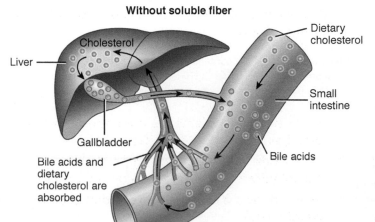

Without soluble fiber

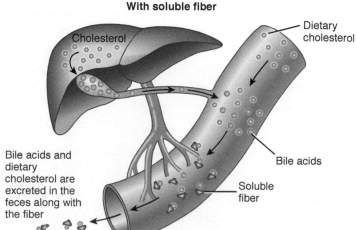

With soluble fiber

Diverticulosis • Figure 4.19

Diverticulosis is a condition in which outpouches form in the wall of the colon. These diverticula form at weak points due to pressure exerted when the colon contracts.

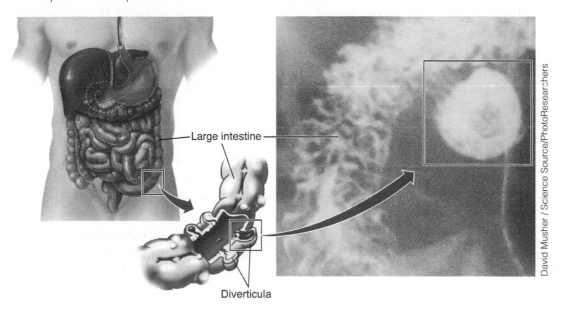

Large intestine

Diverticula

David Musher / Science Source/PhotoResearchers

bran and **cellulose**, are also beneficial for heart health but have less of an effect on blood cholesterol.

Bowel Health

Fiber and other indigestible carbohydrates add bulk and absorb water in the gastrointestinal tract, making the feces larger and softer and reducing the pressure needed for defecation. This helps reduce the incidence of constipation and **hemorrhoids**, the swelling of veins in the rectal or anal area. It also reduces the risk of developing outpouches in the wall of the colon called **diverticula** (the singular is *diverticulum*) (**Figure 4.19**). Fecal matter can accumulate in these pouches, causing irritation, pain, and inflammation—a condition known as **diverticulitis**. Diverticulitis may lead to infection. Treatment usually includes antibiotics to eliminate the infection and a low-fiber diet to prevent irritation of inflamed tissues. Once the inflammation is resolved, a high-fiber diet is recommended to ease stool elimination and reduce future attacks of diverticulitis.

Although fiber speeds movement of the intestinal contents, when the diet is low in fluid, fiber can contribute to constipation. The more fiber in the diet, the more water is needed to keep the stool soft. When too little fluid is consumed, the stool becomes hard and difficult to eliminate. In severe cases of excessive fiber intake and low fluid intake, intestinal blockage can occur.

A diet high in fiber, particularly from whole grains, may reduce the risk of colon cancer, although not all studies support this finding.[3,35,36] Fiber reduces contact between the cells lining the colon and potentially cancer-causing substances in the feces. Fiber in the colon also affects the intestinal microflora and their by-products. These by-products may directly affect colon cells or may change the environment of the colon in a way that can affect the development of colon cancer. Some of the protective effect may also be due to antioxidant vitamins and phytochemicals present in fiber-rich whole grains.

CONCEPT CHECK STOP

1. **What** health problems are common in people who have uncontrolled diabetes?
2. **Why** does frequent snacking on high-carbohydrate foods promote dental caries?
3. **When** does a low-carbohydrate diet promote weight loss?
4. **How** does fiber benefit colon health?

4.6 Meeting Carbohydrate Needs

LEARNING OBJECTIVES

1. **Discuss** how the carbohydrate intake of Americans compares with recommendations.

2. **Calculate** the percentage of calories from carbohydrate in a food or in a diet.

3. **Use** food labels to identify foods that are high in fiber and low in added sugar.

Recommendations for carbohydrate intake focus on two main points: getting enough carbohydrate to meet the need for glucose and choosing the types that promote health and prevent disease.

Carbohydrate Recommendations

The RDA for carbohydrate is 130 g/day, based on the average minimum amount of glucose used by the brain.[37] In a diet that meets energy needs, this amount provides adequate glucose and prevents ketosis. Additional carbohydrate provides an important source of energy in the diet, and carbohydrate-containing foods can add vitamins, minerals, fiber, and phytochemicals. Therefore, the Acceptable Macronutrient Distribution Range for carbohydrate is 45 to 65% of total calorie intake. A diet within this range meets energy needs without excessive amounts of protein or fat (**Figure 4.20**).

The typical U.S. diet meets the recommendation for the amount of carbohydrate, but most of this comes from refined sources, making the diet lower in fiber and higher in added sugar than recommended (see *Thinking It Through*). The Adequate Intake for fiber is 38 g/day for men and 25 g/day for women; the typical intake is only about 15 g/day.

American adults currently consume 14.6% of their calories as added sugars.[26] Although there is no RDA or Daily Value for added sugars, the 2010 Dietary Guidelines recommend that Americans reduce their consumption of added sugars and the American Heart Association recommends limiting the amount of added sugars to no more than half of one's empty calorie allowance.[38, 39] For most American women, that's no more than 100 Calories per day, or about 6 teaspoons of sugar. For men, it's no more than 150 Calories per day, or about 9 teaspoons.

Because no specific toxicity is associated with high intake of any type of carbohydrate, no UL has been established for total carbohydrate intake, for fiber intake, or for added sugar intake.

How much carbohydrate do you eat? • Figure 4.20

To calculate the percentage of calories from carbohydrate in a diet, first determine the number of grams of carbohydrate and multiply this value by 4 Calories/gram. For example, the vegetarian food shown here, which represents a day's intake, provides about 300 g of carbohydrate:

300 g × 4 Calories/g = 1200 Calories from carbohydrate

Next divide the number of Calories from carbohydrate by the total number of Calories in the diet and multiply by 100 to convert it to a percentage. In this example, the diet contains 2000 total Calories, and so it provides:

(1200 Calories from carbohydrate/2000 Calories total) × 100 = 60% of Calories from carbohydrate

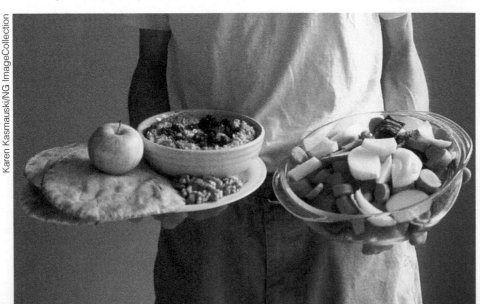

Karen Kasmauski/NG ImageCollection

Ask Yourself

What is the percentage of Calories from carbohydrate in a diet that provides 240 g of carbohydrate and 2400 Calories?

a. 10	**c.** 50
b. 40	**d.** 60

A Case Study on Healthy Carbohydrates

Trina is busy and tends to grab whatever is quick and easy to eat. She just read an article that says Americans make unhealthy carbohydrate choices. To evaluate her carbohydrate intake, Trina analyzes a typical day's diet using iProfile. For breakfast she has a bowl of presweetened cereal and a piece of fruit, lunch is chips and a soda, and dinner is a burrito. She always drinks milk with dinner. She has another soda at night while studying. Her iProfile analysis shows that she eats 2199 Calories, 70 g protein, 71 g fat, 320 g carbohydrate, and 12 g fiber per day.

 1 How does her intake compare with the recommended amounts of carbohydrate and fiber?

Answer: Trina calculates the percentage of calories from carbohydrate (320 g carbohydrate × 4 Calories/gram ÷ 2199 Calories × 100 = 58%), and is surprised to see that despite her poor choices, her carbohydrate intake is in the recommended range of 45 to 65% of calories. However, she consumes only 12 g of fiber, 13 g less than the 25 g recommended for women her age.

Based on her MyPlate Daily Food Plan, Trina is not consuming enough fruits, vegetables, or whole grains. Boosting her intake of these will help increase her fiber intake.

 2 Use iProfile to look up the fiber content of the fruits and vegetables listed below and choose a combination of these that will add at least 13 g of fiber to Trina's diet.

Vegetables	Fruits
Black beans, 1/2 cup	Pear, 1 medium
Green beans, 1/2 cup	Kiwi, 2 small
Iceberg lettuce, 1 cup	Apple, 1 medium
Broccoli, 1/2 cup	Banana, 1 medium
Asparagus, 1/2 cup	Watermelon, 1 cup
Raw spinach, 1 cup	Orange, 1 medium

Your answer:

Looking at her typical choices, Trina can see that much of her carbohydrate intake is from added sugars in her beverages and breakfast cereal.

 3 If Trina replaces the two 20-oz sodas she drinks per day with water, how many Calories and how much sugar will this eliminate from her diet?

Your answer:

To reduce the sugar and increase the fiber in her breakfast, Trina plans to choose between these two healthy-sounding breakfast cereals.

Raisin and Bran Cereal

Nutrition Facts
Serving Size 1 Cup (59g/2.1 oz.)
Servings Per Container about 8

Amount Per Serving	Cereal	Cereal with ½ cup Vitamins A&D Fat Free Milk
Calories	190	230
Calories from Fat	10	10
	% Daily Value**	
Total Fat 1g*	2%	2%
Saturated Fat 0g	0%	0%
Trans Fat 0g		
Cholesterol 0mg	0%	0%
Sodium 250mg	10%	13%
Potassium 320mg	9%	15%
Total Carbohydrate 46g	15%	17%
Dietary Fiber 5g	20%	20%
Sugars 17g		
Other Carbohydrate 24g		
Protein 5g		

INGREDIENTS: WHOLE GRAIN WHEAT, RAISINS, WHEAT BRAN, SUGAR, HIGH FRUCTOSE CORN SYRUP, CONTAINS 2% OR LESS OF SALT, MALT FLAVORING, INVERT SUGAR...

Multigrain Cereal

Nutrition Facts
Serving Size 1 cup (29g)
Servings Per Container about 8

Amount Per Serving	MultiGrain Cheerios	with ½ cup skim milk
Calories	110	150
Calories from Fat	10	10
	% Daily Value**	
Total Fat 1g*	2%	2%
Saturated Fat 0g	0%	3%
Trans Fat 0g		
Cholesterol 0mg	0%	1%
Sodium 160mg	7%	9%
Potassium 85mg	2%	8%
Total Carbohydrate 23g	8%	10%
Dietary Fiber 4g	16%	16%
Sugars 6g		
Other Carbohydrate 13g		
Protein 2g		

INGREDIENTS: WHOLE GRAIN CORN, WHOLE GRAIN OATS, SUGAR, WHOLE GRAIN BARLEY, WHOLE GRAIN WHEAT, WHOLE GRAIN RICE, CORN STARCH, BROWN SUGAR SYRUP, CORN BRAN, SALT...

 4 Use the ingredient list to identify the sources of whole grains and added sugars in these two products.

Your answer:

5 Which cereal would you recommend to Trina? Why?

Your answer:

(Check your answers in online Appendix L.)

Healthy MyPlate carbohydrate choices • Figure 4.21

The healthiest carbohydrate choices are whole grains, legumes, and fresh fruits and vegetables, which are low in added sugar and often are good sources of fiber. Foods containing refined carbohydrates should be limited because they are typically low in fiber and contain added sugars, which add empty calories.

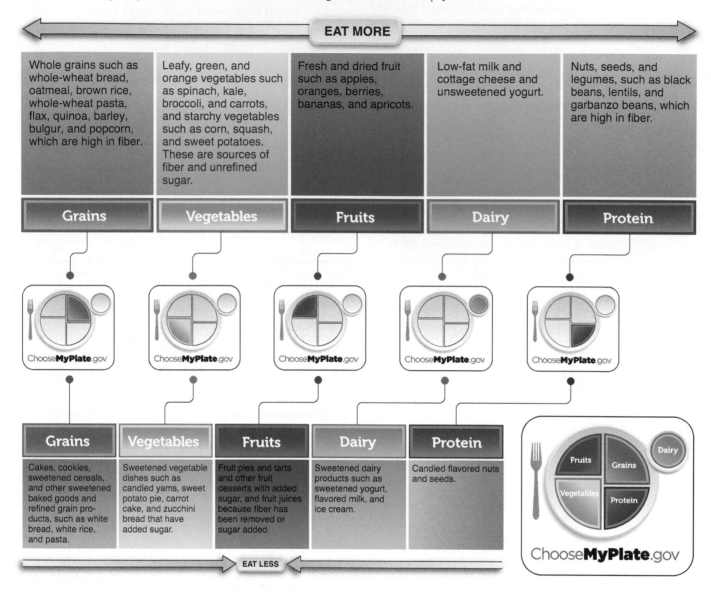

Choosing Carbohydrates Wisely

To promote a healthy, balanced diet, the 2010 Dietary Guidelines and MyPlate recommend increasing consumption of whole grains, fruits and vegetables, and low-fat dairy products while limiting foods high in refined grains and added sugars, such as soft drinks and other sweetened beverages, sweet bakery products, and candy. Because the majority of the added sugars Americans consume come from beverages, the Dietary Guidelines specifically recommend reducing intake of sugar-sweetened beverages such as soda, energy drinks, sports drinks, and sugar-sweetened fruit drinks.

Using MyPlate to make healthy choices For a 2000-Calorie diet, MyPlate recommends 6 oz of grains (half of which should be whole grains), 2 cups of fruit, and 2½ cups of vegetables. As **Figure 4.21** suggests, refined carbohydrates can be replaced with unrefined ones to make the diet healthier. For example, an apple provides about 80 Calories and 3.7 g of fiber, making it a better choice than 1 cup of apple juice, which has the same amount of energy but almost no fiber (0.2 g).

Interpreting food labels Food labels can help in choosing the right mix of carbohydrates (**Figure 4.22**).

Choosing carbohydrates from the label • Figure 4.22

Food labels provide information about the types and amounts of carbohydrates in packaged foods.

Whole Wheat Bread

Nutrition Facts	Amount/Serving	%DV*	Amount/Serving	%DV*
Serving Size 1 Slice (27g)	Total Fat 1g	2%	Total Carb. 12g	4%
Servings Per Container 17	Sat. Fat 0g	0%	Dietary Fiber 2g	8%
Calories 70	Trans Fat 0g	0%	Sugars 2g	
Calories from Fat 10	Cholesterol 0mg	0%	Protein 2g	
	Sodium 10mg	0%		

Vitamin A 0% • Vitamin C 0% • Calcium 4% • Iron 4%
Thiamin 4% • Riboflavin 2% • Niacin 4%

*Percent Daily Values (DV) are based on a 2,000-calorie diet. Your daily values may be higher or lower depending on your calorie needs:

		Calories:	2,000	2,500
Total Fat	Less than		65g	80g
Sat Fat	Less than		20g	25g
Cholesterol	Less than		300mg	300mg
Sodium	Less than		2,400mg	2,400mg
Total Carbohydrate			300g	375g
Dietary Fiber			25g	30g

NUTR SODIUM FREE FOOD

INGREDIENTS: WHOLE WHEAT FLOUR, WATER, SWEETENERS (HIGH FRUCTOSE CORN SYRUP, MOLASSES), WHEAT GLUTEN, SOYBEAN CONTAINS 2% OR LESS OF THE FOLLOWING: YEAST, DOUGH CONDITIONERS (MONO DIGLYCERIDES, ETHOXYLATED MONO & GLYCERIDES, CALCIUM STEAROYL-2-LACTYLATE), YEAST NUTRIENTS (CALCIUM SULFATE, MONO- CALCIUM PHOSPHA CALCIUM PROPIONATE (A PRESERVATIVE).

The Nutrition Facts panel of a food label lists the number of grams of total carbohydrate and fiber and gives these amounts as a percentage of the Daily Value.

The Daily Value for total carbohydrate is 60% of the diet's energy content, or 300 g for a 2000-Calorie diet. The Daily Value for fiber in a 2000-Calorie diet is 25 g.

To identify products made mostly from *whole* grains, look for the word "whole" before the name of the grain. If this is the first ingredient listed, the product is made from mostly whole grain. "Wheat flour" simply means it was made with wheat, not whole wheat. Note that foods labeled with the words "multigrain," "stone-ground," "100% wheat," "cracked wheat," "seven-grain," or "bran" are not necessarily 100% whole-grain products and may not contain any whole grains.

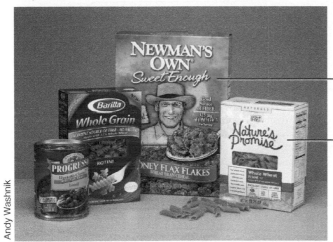

Foods labeled "high fiber" contain 20% or more of the Daily Value per serving.

Foods labeled "good source of fiber" contain between 10 and 19% of the Daily Value per serving.

Ask Yourself

Is a product that lists wheat flour as the first ingredient and whole-wheat flour as the second made mostly from whole grains? Why or why not?

Products labeled "reduced sugar" contain 25% less sugar than the regular, or reference, product.

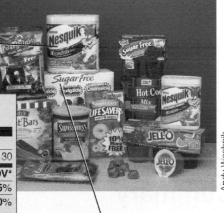

The ingredient list helps identify added sugars. Many products have more than one added sweetener. The closer the name of each sweetener appears to the beginning of the list, the more of it has been added.

INGREDIENTS: CULTURED PASTEURIZED GRADE A REDUCED FAT MILK, SUGAR, NONFAT MILK, HIGH FRUCTOSE CORN SYRUP, STRAWBERRY PUREE, MODIFIED CORN STARCH, KOSHER GELATIN, TRICALCIUM PHOSPHATE, NATURAL FLAVOR, COLORED WITH CARMINE, VITAMIN A ACETATE, VITAMIN D₃

On the ingredient list, all these are added sugar: Brown sugar, corn sweetener, corn syrup, dextrose, fructose, fruit juice, glucose, high fructose corn syrup, honey, invert sugar, lactose, maltose, malt syrup, molasses, raw sugar, sucrose, and sugar syrup concentrates.

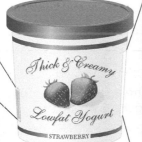

Nutrition Facts
Serving Size 1 Container

Amount Per Serving	
Calories 190 Calories from Fat 30	

Amount/Serving	% DV*
Total Fat 3.5g	5%
Saturated Fat 2g	10%
Trans Fat 0g	
Cholesterol 15mg	4%
Sodium 100mg	4%
Potassium 310g	9%
Total Carbohydrate 32g	11%
Dietary Fiber 0g	0%
Sugars 28g	
Protein 7g	14%

Vitamin A 15%   •   Calcium 30%

*Percent Daily Values (DV) are based on a 2,000 calorie diet.

Foods labeled "sugar free" contain less than 0.5 g of sugar per serving.

The number of grams of sugars listed includes the total amounts of mono- and disaccharides but does not distinguish between added sugar and the sugar that occurs naturally in the food. Proposed changes to the Nutrition Facts include putting grams of added sugars as a separate line below Sugars.

WHAT SHOULD I EAT?

Carbohydrates

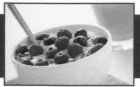
© Sara Winter/iStockphoto

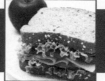
© Jill Chen/iStockphoto

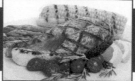
© Steve Mcsweeny/iStockphoto

Make half your grains whole
- Have your sandwich on whole-wheat, oat bran, rye, or pumpernickel bread.
- Switch to whole-wheat pasta and brown rice.
- Fill your cereal bowl with plain oatmeal and add a few raisins for sweetness.
- Check the ingredient list for the words *whole* or *whole grain* before the grain ingredient's name.

Increase your fruits and veggies
- Don't forget beans. Kidney beans, chickpeas, black beans, and others have more fiber and resistant starch than any other vegetables.
- Add berries and bananas to your cereal or dessert.
- Pile the veggies on your sandwich.
- Have more than one vegetable at dinner.

Limit added sugars
- Switch to a 12-oz can instead of a 20-oz bottle when you grab a soft drink or, better yet, have a glass of water or low-fat milk.
- Use one-quarter less sugar in your recipe next time you bake.
- Snack on a piece of fruit instead of a candy bar.
- Swap your sugary breakfast cereal for an unsweetened whole-grain variety.

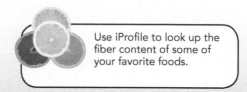
Use iProfile to look up the fiber content of some of your favorite foods.

The Nutrition Facts panel helps consumers find foods that are good sources of fiber and low in sugars. The ingredient list helps identify whole-grain products and the sources of added sugars. Nutrient content claims such as "high in fiber" or "no sugar added" and health claims such as those highlighting the relationship between fiber intake and the risk of heart disease and cancer help identify foods that meet the recommendations for fiber and added sugar intake (see *What Should I Eat?*).

CONCEPT CHECK — STOP

1. **How** does the U.S. diet compare with recommendations for fiber and added sugar?
2. **What** is the percentage of calories from carbohydrate in your breakfast cereal?
3. **Where** on the current food label can you find information about added sugars?

✓ THE PLANNER

Summary

1 Carbohydrates in Our Food 94

- Unrefined whole grains, fruits, and vegetables are good sources of fiber and micronutrients. When these foods are **refined**, nutrients and fiber are lost. Whole grains contain the entire kernel, as shown here, which includes the **endosperm, bran,** and **germ**; refined grains include only the endosperm. Refined grains are enriched with some of the B vitamins and iron, but not all the nutrients lost in refining are added back.

Whole grains • Figure 4.2

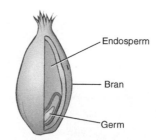
- Endosperm
- Bran
- Germ

- Refined sugars contain calories but few nutrients; for this reason, foods high in added refined sugar are low in nutrient density.

2 Types of Carbohydrates 96

- Carbohydrates contain carbon as well as hydrogen and oxygen, in the same proportion as water. **Simple carbohydrates** include **monosaccharides** and **disaccharides** and are found in foods such as table sugar, honey, milk, and fruit. **Complex carbohydrates** are **polysaccharides**; they include **glycogen** in animals and **starches**, illustrated here, and **fiber** in plants.

Carbohydrate structures and sources • Figure 4.4c

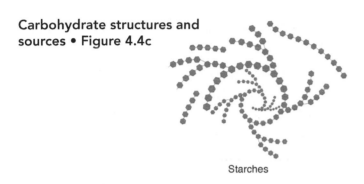

Starches

- Fiber cannot be digested in the stomach or small intestine and therefore is not absorbed into the body. **Soluble fiber** dissolves in water to form a viscous solution and is digested by bacteria in the colon; **insoluble fiber** is not readily digested by bacteria and adds bulk to fecal matter.

3 Carbohydrate Digestion and Absorption 99

- Disaccharides and starches must be digested to monosaccharides, as shown here, before they can be absorbed. In individuals with **lactose intolerance**, lactose passes into the colon undigested, causing cramps, gas, and diarrhea. Indigestible complex carbohydrates, including fiber, some **oligosaccharides**, and **resistant starch**, can increase intestinal gas, but they benefit health by increasing bulk in the stool, promoting growth of healthy microflora, and slowing nutrient absorption.

Carbohydrate digestion • Figure 4.7

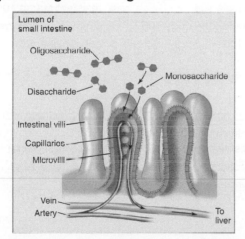

- After a meal, blood **glucose** levels rise. The rate, magnitude, and duration of this rise are referred to as the **glycemic response**. Glycemic response is affected by the amount and type of carbohydrate consumed and by other nutrients ingested with the carbohydrate.

4 Carbohydrate Functions 103

- Carbohydrate, primarily as glucose, provides energy to the body. Blood glucose levels are maintained by the hormones **insulin** and **glucagon**. As depicted here, when blood glucose levels rise insulin from the pancreas allows muscle and fat-storing cells to take up glucose from the blood and promotes the synthesis of glycogen, fat, and protein. When blood glucose levels fall, glucagon increases them by causing glycogen breakdown and glucose synthesis.

Blood glucose regulation • Figure 4.10

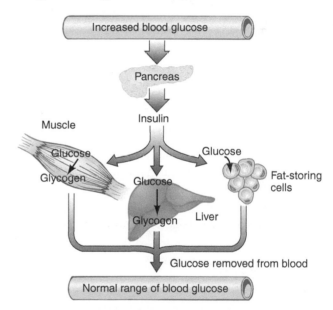

- Glucose is metabolized through cellular respiration. It begins with **glycolysis**, which breaks each six-carbon glucose molecule into two three-carbon pyruvate molecules, producing ATP even when oxygen is unavailable. The complete breakdown of glucose through **aerobic metabolism** requires oxygen and produces carbon dioxide, water, and more ATP than glycolysis.

- When carbohydrate intake is limited, amino acids from the breakdown of body proteins can be used to synthesize glucose. Therefore, an adequate carbohydrate intake is said to spare protein. Limited carbohydrate intake also results in the formation of **ketones** (**ketone bodies**) by the liver. These can be used as an energy source by other tissues. Ketones that accumulate in the blood can cause symptoms that range from headache and lack of appetite to coma and even death if levels are extremely high.

5 Carbohydrates in Health and Disease 107

- As shown in the graph, **diabetes mellitus** is characterized by high blood glucose levels, that occur either because insufficient insulin is produced or because of a decrease in the body's sensitivity to insulin. Over time, high blood glucose levels damage tissues and contribute to the development of heart disease, kidney failure, blindness, and infections that may lead to amputations. Treatment includes diet, exercise, and medication to keep glucose levels in the normal range.

Blood glucose levels in diabetes • Figure 4.13

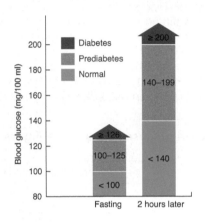

- **Hypoglycemia**, or low blood glucose, causes symptoms such as sweating, headaches, and rapid heartbeat.

- Diets high in carbohydrate, particularly sucrose, increase the risk of dental caries. Sucrose helps bacteria to stick to the teeth, and they then use sucrose and other carbohydrates as a food supply, producing acids that damage the teeth.

- Gram for gram, carbohydrates provide less energy than fat. High-fiber diets can prevent weight gain by making you feel full longer so that you eat less. Low-carbohydrate diets promote weight loss by causing a spontaneous reduction in food intake. **Nonnutritive sweeteners** aid weight loss if the sugar calories they replace are not added back from other food sources.

- Diets high in unrefined carbohydrates from whole grains, vegetables, fruits, and legumes may reduce the risk of heart disease, bowel disorders, and colon cancer. Soluble fiber helps prevent heart disease because it can lower blood cholesterol.

6 Meeting Carbohydrate Needs 116

- Guidelines for a healthy diet recommend 45 to 65% of energy from carbohydrates. Most of this should come from whole grains, legumes, fruits, and vegetables, such as those in this photo. Foods high in added sugar should be consumed in moderation.

How much carbohydrate do you eat? • Figure 4.20

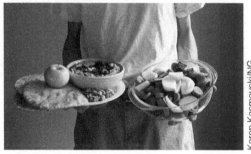

Karen Kasmauski/NG ImageCollection

- The recommendations of MyPlate and the information on food labels can be used to select healthy amounts and sources of carbohydrate.

Key Terms

- acceptable daily intake (ADI) 113
- aerobic metabolism 105
- anaerobic metabolism 105
- autoimmune disease 107
- bran 94
- cellulose 115
- complex carbohydrate 97
- diabetes mellitus 107
- disaccharide 96
- diverticula 115
- diverticulitis 115
- diverticulosis 115
- endosperm 94

- enrichment 94
- fasting hypoglycemia 110
- fiber 98
- fructose 97
- galactose 97
- germ 94
- gestational diabetes 108
- glucagon 104
- glucose 97
- glycemic index 102
- glycemic load 102
- glycemic response 103
- glycogen 97
- glycolysis 105
- hemorrhoid 115

- hypoglycemia 110
- insoluble fiber 98
- insulin 103
- insulin resistance 108
- ketoacidosis 108
- ketone or ketone body 106
- ketosis 106
- lactose 97
- lactose intolerance 100
- maltose 97
- monosaccharide 96
- nonnutritive sweetener or artificial sweetener 113
- oligosaccharide 98
- photosynthesis 98

- polysaccharide 96
- prediabetes 108
- reactive hypoglycemia 110
- refined 94
- resistant starch 100
- simple carbohydrate 97
- soluble fiber 98
- starch 97
- sucrose 97
- sugar unit 96
- type 1 diabetes 107
- type 2 diabetes 108
- unrefined food 94
- whole-grain product 94

What is happening in this picture?

These students may choose fruit drinks, and iced tea because they believe these beverages are healthier choices than soda.

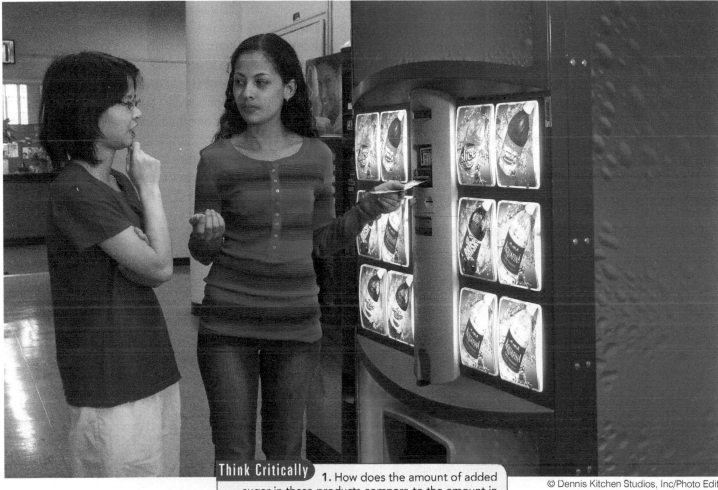

© Dennis Kitchen Studios, Inc/Photo Edit

Think Critically

1. How does the amount of added sugar in these products compare to the amount in soft drinks?
2. Do these beverages provide significant amounts of any essential nutrients?
3. Suggest beverage alternatives that would be lower in added sugar.

THE PLANNER ✓

Review your Chapter Planner on the chapter opener and check off your completed work.

5.1 Fats in Our Food

LEARNING OBJECTIVES

1. **Describe** the roles of fat in our food.
2. **Identify** sources of hidden fat in the diet.
3. **Discuss** how fat intake in the United States has changed since the 1970s.

The fats in our foods contribute to their texture, flavor, and aroma. It is the fat that gives ice cream its smooth texture and rich taste. Olive oil imparts a unique flavor to salads and many traditional Italian and Greek dishes. Sesame oil gives egg rolls and other Chinese foods their distinctive aroma. But while the fats in our foods contribute to their appeal, they also add more calories than other nutrients (9 Calories/gram compared to 4 Calories/gram for carbohydrate and protein), so consuming too much can contribute to weight gain. The types of fats we eat also can affect our health; too much of the wrong types can increase the risk of heart disease and cancer.

Sources of Fat in Our Food

Sometimes the fat in our food is obvious. You can see the stripes of fat in a slice of bacon sizzling in a frying pan, for example, or the layer of fat around the outside of your steak. Other visible sources of fat in our diets are the fats we add to foods at the table—the pat of butter melting on your steaming baked potato and the dressing you pour over your salad. When you choose these items, you know you are eating a high-fat food.

Not all sources of dietary fat are obvious. Cheese, ice cream, and whole milk are high in fat, and foods that we think of as sources of carbohydrate, such as crackers, doughnuts, cookies, and muffins, may also be quite high in fat (**Figure 5.1**). We also add invisible fat when we fry foods: French fries start as potatoes, which are low in fat, but when they are immersed in hot oil for frying, they soak up fat, increasing their calorie content.

America's Changing Fat Intake

Eating patterns in the United States have changed significantly over the past 40 years, even though total fat intake hasn't changed much. Beginning in the 1950s,

Americans were told that too much fat made them fat, increased their risk of heart disease, and maybe even increased their risk of cancer. In response to these messages, many Americans switched from whole milk to low-fat, chose chicken in place of beef, consumed fewer eggs, and used less butter and high-fat salad dressing. But in addition to these changes, they consumed more hidden fats from foods such as pizza, pasta dishes, snack foods, and fried potatoes.[1,2] Thus, even though the sources of fat in the U.S. diet have changed since 1970, the number of grams of fat Americans consume daily has changed little. What has changed in the past 40 years is our energy intake: It has increased. So although our fat intake (in grams) has not changed, the percentage of calories from fat has declined from 37% to 33% (**Figure 5.2**).[3,4]

Efforts to reduce the risk of chronic disease by cutting fat from our diets have failed not just because we haven't really cut our fat intake but also because fat does not deserve its bad reputation. Today we understand that the types of fat in the diet as well as the overall dietary pattern have a greater impact on chronic disease risk than

Visible and hidden fats • Figure 5.1

The amount of fat in a food is not always obvious. The two strips of bacon in this breakfast provide a total of 8 grams of fat, and the muffin provides 16 grams.

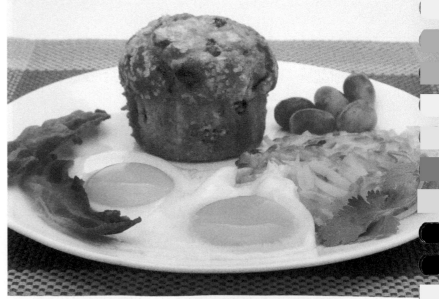

Donald Erickson/iStockphoto

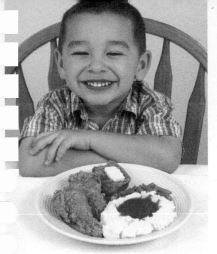

David Hernandez/iStockphoto

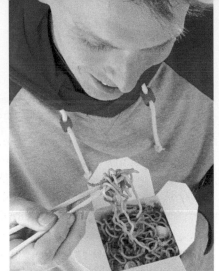

© Twin Designs/Shutterstock

a. In the 1970s, a typical dinner included high-fat meat, bread with butter, and mashed potatoes with lots of gravy, and it was usually served with a glass of whole milk.

b. Today we drink low-fat milk and eat leaner meats, but we eat more fat from takeout Chinese and Mexican foods and fast-food pizza, French fries, hamburgers, and cheeseburgers than we did in the 1970s.[1]

Interpret the Data

If the number of grams of fat in the U.S. diet has not changed, why has the percentage of fat in the diet gone down?

U.S. food intake in the 1970s and today • Figure 5.2

Changing food intake patterns over the past 50 years have resulted in changes in the sources of fat in our diet and an increase in the number of calories we eat.

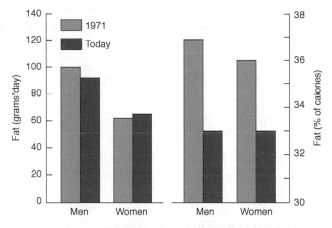

c. In 1971, U.S. men consumed an average of 2450 Calories/day and women 1540 Calories/day.[5] Today, men consume about 2500 Calories/day and women about 1780 Calories/day.[3] Because of this increase in energy intake, the percentage of calories from fat has decreased, but we don't consume any less total fat today than we did in the 1970s.

total fat intake. High intakes of **saturated fat** from meat and dairy products, and *trans* fat used in shortening and margarine and added to processed foods are associated with a higher incidence of heart disease and certain types of cancer. Diets high in **unsaturated fats** from fish, nuts, and vegetable oils seem to protect against chronic disease. A healthy diet includes the right kinds of fats along with plenty of whole grains, fruits, and vegetables.

CONCEPT CHECK STOP

1. **How** does adding fat affect the calorie content of a food?

2. **What** are some invisible sources of fat in the diet?

3. **How** have the sources of fat in the U.S. diet changed since the 1970s?

5.2 Types of Lipids

LEARNING OBJECTIVES

1. **Explain** the relationship between triglycerides and fatty acids.

2. **Compare** the structures of saturated, monounsaturated, polyunsaturated, omega-6, omega-3, and *trans* fatty acids.

3. **Describe** how phospholipids and cholesterol are used in the body.

4. **Name** foods that are sources of cholesterol and saturated, monounsaturated, polyunsaturated, omega-6, omega-3, and *trans* fatty acids.

Lipids are substances that do not dissolve in water. We tend to use the term *fat* to refer to lipids, but we are usually referring to types of lipids called **triglycerides**. Triglycerides make up most of the lipids in our food and in our bodies. The structure of triglycerides includes lipid molecules called **fatty acids**. Two other types of

triglyceride The major type of lipid in food and the body, consisting of three fatty acids attached to a glycerol molecule.

fatty acid A molecule made up of a chain of carbons linked to hydrogens, with an acid group at one end of the chain.

lipids that are important in nutrition but are present in the body in smaller amounts are **phospholipids** and **sterols**.

Triglycerides and Fatty Acids

A triglyceride consists of the three-carbon molecule glycerol with three fatty acids attached to it (**Figure 5.3**). A fatty acid is a chain of carbon atoms with an acid group at one end of the chain. Fatty acids vary in the length of their carbon chains and the types and locations of carbon–carbon bonds within the chain. Triglycerides may contain any combination of fatty acids. The fatty acids in a triglyceride determine its function in the body and the properties it gives to food. It is the fatty acids in triglycerides that we are really

phospholipid A type of lipid whose structure includes a phosphorus atom.

sterol A type of lipid with a structure composed of multiple chemical rings.

Triglycerides • Figure 5.3

A triglyceride contains glycerol and three fatty acids. The carbon chains of the fatty acids vary in length from short-chain fatty acids (4 to 7 carbons) to medium-chain (8 to 12 carbons) and long-chain fatty acids (more than 12 carbons). Most fatty acids in plants and animals contain between 14 and 22 carbons.

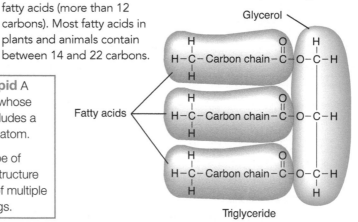

Nutrition InSight Fatty acids • Figure 5.4

The number and location of single (saturated) and double (unsaturated) carbon–carbon bonds in a fatty acid affect its physical properties. The types of fatty acids in a triglyceride determine its texture, taste, and physical characteristics.

a. Saturated Fatty Acids

Each carbon atom in the carbon chain of a fatty acid is attached to up to four other atoms. At the omega or methyl (CH_3) end of the carbon chain, three hydrogen atoms are attached to the carbon. At the other end of the chain, an acid group (COOH) is attached to the carbon. Each of the carbon atoms in between is attached to two carbon atoms and up to two hydrogen atoms. In saturated fatty acids, each carbon is attached to two hydrogen atoms so there are only single bonds between carbon atoms. Red meat, butter, cheese, and whole milk are high in saturated fatty acids, such as palmitic acid.

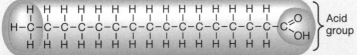

Palmitic acid

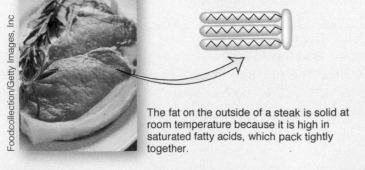

The fat on the outside of a steak is solid at room temperature because it is high in saturated fatty acids, which pack tightly together.

b. Unsaturated Fatty Acids

When the adjacent carbons in the carbon chain of a fatty acid have only one hydrogen atom attached, a double bond forms between the carbons. These are called unsaturated because not all the carbon atoms are saturated with hydrogen atoms; unsaturated fatty acids may have one or more carbon–carbon double bonds. Unsaturated fatty acids include monounsaturated fatty acids and polyunsaturated fatty acids.

Monounsaturated Fatty Acids

Monounsaturated fatty acids contain one carbon–carbon double bond. Canola, olive, and peanut oils, as well as nuts and avocados, are high in monounsaturated fatty acids, such as oleic acid.

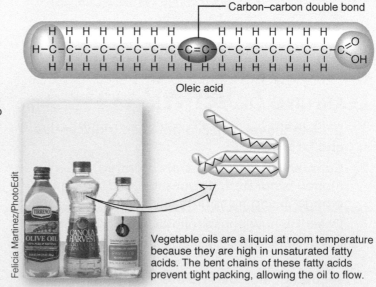

Oleic acid

Vegetable oils are a liquid at room temperature because they are high in unsaturated fatty acids. The bent chains of these fatty acids prevent tight packing, allowing the oil to flow.

talking about when we refer to *trans* fat or saturated fat—these terms really mean ***trans* fatty acids** and **saturated fatty acids**, respectively.

Saturated and unsaturated fatty acids

Fatty acids are classified as saturated fatty acids or **unsaturated fatty acids**, depending on whether they contain carbon–carbon double bonds (**Figure 5.4a and b**). The number and location of these double bonds affect the characteristics that fatty acids give to food and the health effects they have in the body. Saturated fatty acids have straight carbon chains that pack tightly together. Therefore, triglycerides that are high in saturated fatty acids, such as those found in beef, butter, and lard, tend to

saturated fatty acid A fatty acid in which the carbon atoms are bonded to as many hydrogen atoms as possible; it therefore contains no carbon–carbon double bonds.

unsaturated fatty acid A fatty acid that contains one or more carbon–carbon double bonds; may be either monounsaturated or polyunsaturated.

be solid at room temperature. Diets high in saturated fatty acids have been shown to increase the risk of heart disease. Unsaturated fatty acids have bent chains. This makes triglycerides that are higher in unsaturated fatty acids, such as those found in corn, safflower, and sunflower oils, liquid at room temperature. Unsaturated fats are susceptible to spoilage or *rancidity*, because the unsaturated bonds in fatty acids are easily damaged by oxygen. When fats go rancid, they give food an "off" flavor. Diets high in unsaturated fatty acids are associated with a lower risk of heart disease.

The body is capable of synthesizing most of the fatty acids it needs from glucose or other sources of carbon, hydrogen, and oxygen, but

Polyunsaturated Fatty Acids

Polyunsaturated fatty acids contain more than one carbon–carbon double bond.

Omega-6 Polyunsaturated Fatty Acids: When the first double bond occurs between the sixth and seventh carbon atoms (from the omega end), the fatty acid is called an **omega-6 fatty acid**. Corn oil, safflower oil, soybean oil, and nuts are sources of the omega-6 polyunsaturated fatty acid linoleic acid.

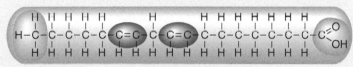

Linoleic acid

Omega-3 Polyunsaturated Fatty Acids: If the first double bond occurs between the third and fourth carbon atoms (from the omega end), the fatty acid is an **omega-3 fatty acid**. Flaxseed, canola oil, and nuts are sources of the omega-3 polyunsaturated fatty acid alpha-linolenic acid, and fish oils are high in longer-chain omega-3 fatty acids.

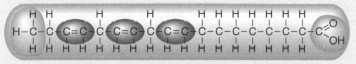

Alpha-linolenic acid

c. The fats and oils in our diets contain combinations of saturated, monounsaturated, and polyunsaturated fatty acids.

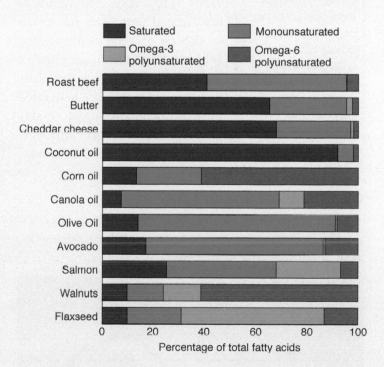

Percentage of total fatty acids

Interpret the Data

Based on the information in the graph:
1. Which two foods are highest in omega-3 fatty acids?
2. Which two foods are highest in saturated fatty acids?

Types of Lipids 129

the body cannot make some of the fatty acids it needs. These must be consumed in the diet and are referred to as **essential fatty acids**.

Saturated fatty acids are more plentiful in animal foods, such as meat and dairy products, than in plant foods. Plant oils are generally low in saturated fatty acids (**Figure 5.4c**). An exception to this are the **tropical oils**, which include palm oil, palm kernel oil, and coconut oil. These saturated plant oils are called tropical oils because they are found in plants that are common in tropical climates. Saturated oils are useful in food processing because they are less susceptible to spoilage than are more unsaturated oils. Even though tropical oils are high in saturated fats, the types of saturated fats they contain do not increase the risk of heart disease and may have some health benefits (**Figure 5.5**).[6,7]

essential fatty acid A fatty acid that must be consumed in the diet because it cannot be made by the body or cannot be made in sufficient quantities to meet the body's needs.

hydrogenation A process used to make partially hydrogenated oils in which hydrogen atoms are added to the carbon–carbon double bonds of unsaturated fatty acids, making them more saturated. *Trans* fatty acids are formed during the process.

Trans fatty acids The bonds in unsaturated fatty acids can occur in the *cis* or *trans* configuration (**Figure 5.6**). Small amounts of *trans* fatty acids occur naturally, and larger amounts are generated by **hydrogenation**, which makes unsaturated oils more saturated. Hydrogenation is used to solidify vegetable oils into hard margarine and shortening. Food manufacturers add hydrogenated oils to foods because they are more solid at room temperature and can be stored longer without becoming rancid. A disadvantage of hydrogenation is that in addition to converting some double bonds into saturated bonds, it transforms some double bonds from the *cis* to the *trans* configuration. Because the consumption of these synthetic *trans* fats increases the risk of developing heart disease, the use of **partially hydrogenated oils** in the food industry has been declining. The FDA has issued a preliminary determination that partially hydrogenated oils are not generally recognized as safe for use in our food. If the FDA finalizes this determination, it could lead to the elimination of synthetic *trans* fat from our food supply.[8]

Phospholipids

Phospholipids, though present in small amounts, are important in food and in the body because they allow water and fat to mix. They can do this because one side of the

Coconut oil • Figure 5.5

The triglycerides in coconut oil contain an unusual blend of short- and medium-chain fatty acids, primarily lauric and myristic acids, which may benefit heart health.

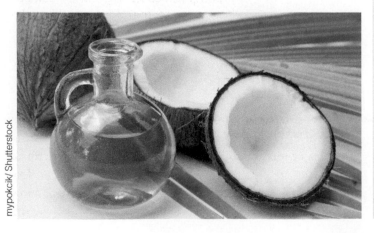

Cis and *trans* fatty acids • Figure 5.6

The orientation of hydrogen atoms around the carbon–carbon double bond distinguishes *cis* fatty acids from *trans* fatty acids. Most unsaturated fatty acids found in nature have double bonds in the *cis* configuration.

In *trans* fatty acids, the hydrogens are on opposite sides of the double bond, making the carbon chain straighter, similar to the shape of a saturated fatty acid.

In *cis* fatty acids, the hydrogens are on the same side of the double bond and cause a bend in the carbon chain.

The bond angles in saturated fatty acids allow the carbon chain to be straight.

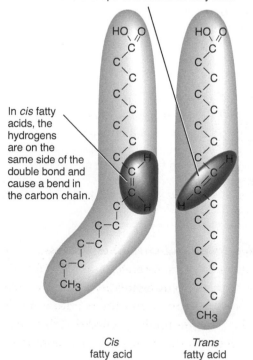

Cis fatty acid

Trans fatty acid

Saturated fatty acid

Phospholipid structure supports its function because it allows one end of the molecule to be soluble in fat, while the other end is soluble in water.

a. Like a triglyceride, a phospholipid, such as the lecithin molecule shown here, has a backbone of glycerol, but it contains two fatty acids rather than three. Instead of the third fatty acid, a phospholipid has a chemical group containing phosphorus, called a **phosphate group**. The fatty acids (the tails) at one end of a phospholipid molecule are soluble in fat, while the phosphate-containing region at the other end (the head) is soluble in water.

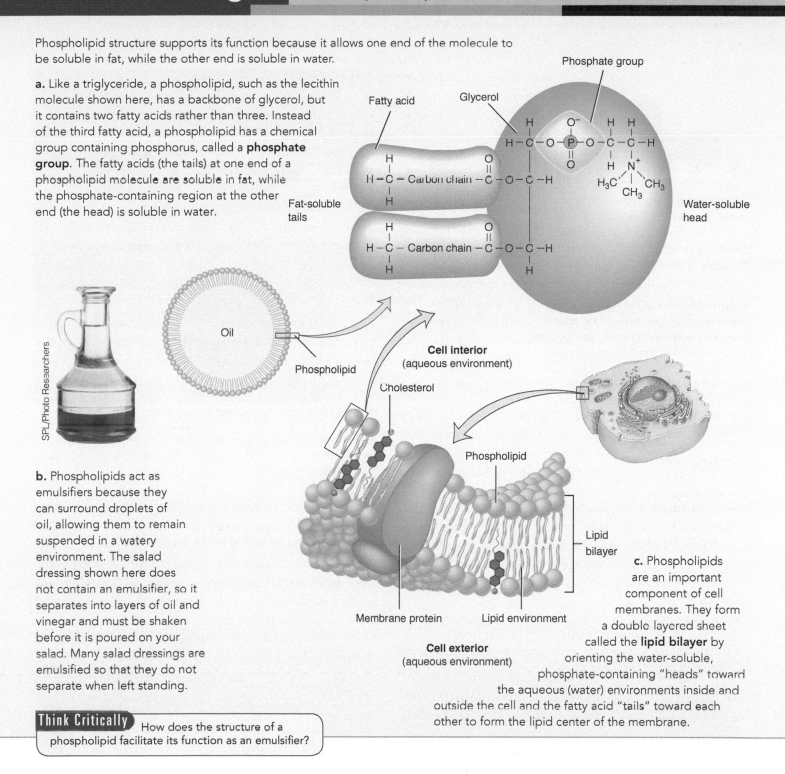

b. Phospholipids act as emulsifiers because they can surround droplets of oil, allowing them to remain suspended in a watery environment. The salad dressing shown here does not contain an emulsifier, so it separates into layers of oil and vinegar and must be shaken before it is poured on your salad. Many salad dressings are emulsified so that they do not separate when left standing.

c. Phospholipids are an important component of cell membranes. They form a double layered sheet called the **lipid bilayer** by orienting the water-soluble, phosphate-containing "heads" toward the aqueous (water) environments inside and outside the cell and the fatty acid "tails" toward each other to form the lipid center of the membrane.

Think Critically How does the structure of a phospholipid facilitate its function as an emulsifier?

molecule dissolves in water, and the other side dissolves in fat (**Figure 5.7a**). In foods, substances that allow fat and water to mix are referred to as **emulsifiers**. For example, the phospholipids in egg yolks allow the oil and water in cake batter to mix; phospholipids in salad dressings prevent the oil and vinegar in the dressing from separating.

One of the best-known phospholipids is **lecithin** (shown in Figure 5.7a). Eggs and soybeans are natural sources of lecithin. The food industry uses lecithin as an emulsifier in margarine, salad dressings, chocolate, frozen desserts, and baked goods to prevent oil from separating from the other ingredients (**Figure 5.7b**). In the

Cholesterol is a sterol that is only found in animal products.

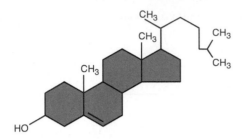

a. The cholesterol structure shown here illustrates the four interconnected rings of carbon atoms that form the backbone structure that is common to all sterols.

b. Egg yolks and organ meats such as liver and kidney are high in cholesterol. Lean red meats and skinless chicken are low in total fat but still contain some cholesterol. Cholesterol is not found in plant cell membranes, so even high-fat plant foods, such as nuts, peanut butter, and vegetable oils, do not contain cholesterol.

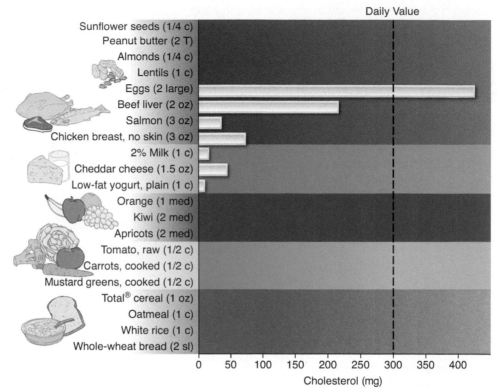

body, lecithin is a major constituent of cell membranes (**Figure 5.7c**). It is also used to synthesize the neurotransmitter acetylcholine, which activates muscles and plays an important role in memory.

Sterols

The best-known sterol is cholesterol (**Figure 5.8**). It is needed in the body, but because the liver manufactures it, it is not essential in the diet. More than 90% of the cholesterol in the body is found in cell membranes (see Figure 5.7c). It is also part of myelin, the insulating coating on many nerve cells. Cholesterol is needed to synthesize other sterols, including vitamin D; bile acids, which are emulsifiers in bile; cortisol, which is a hormone that regulates our physiological response to stress; and testosterone and estrogen, which are hormones necessary for reproduction.

> **cholesterol** A sterol, produced by the liver and consumed in the diet, which is needed to build cell membranes and make hormones and other essential molecules.

In the diet, cholesterol is found only in foods from animal sources. Plant foods do not contain cholesterol unless it has been added in the course of cooking or processing. Plants do contain other sterols, however, and these **plant sterols** have a role similar to that of cholesterol in animals: They help form plant cell membranes. Plant sterols are found in small quantities in most plant foods; when consumed in the diet, they can help reduce cholesterol levels in the body.

CONCEPT CHECK **STOP**

1. **How** are triglycerides and fatty acids related?
2. **What** is the structural difference between saturated and unsaturated fatty acids?
3. **Why** are phospholipids good emulsifiers?
4. **Which** types of food contain the most saturated fat and cholesterol?

5.3 Absorbing and Transporting Lipids

LEARNING OBJECTIVES

1. **Discuss** the steps involved in the digestion and absorption of lipids.
2. **Describe** how lipids are transported in the blood and delivered to cells.
3. **Compare** the functions of LDLs and HDLs.

The fact that oil and water do not mix poses a problem for the digestion and absorption of lipids in the watery environment of the small intestine and their transport in the blood, which is mostly water. Therefore, the body has special mechanisms that allow it to digest, absorb, and transport lipids.

Digestion and Absorption of Lipids

In healthy adults, most fat digestion and absorption occurs in the small intestine (**Figure 5.9**). Here, the bile acids in bile act as emulsifiers, breaking down large lipid droplets into small globules. The triglycerides in the globules can then be digested by enzymes from the pancreas.

Lipid digestion and absorption • Figure 5.9

THE PLANNER

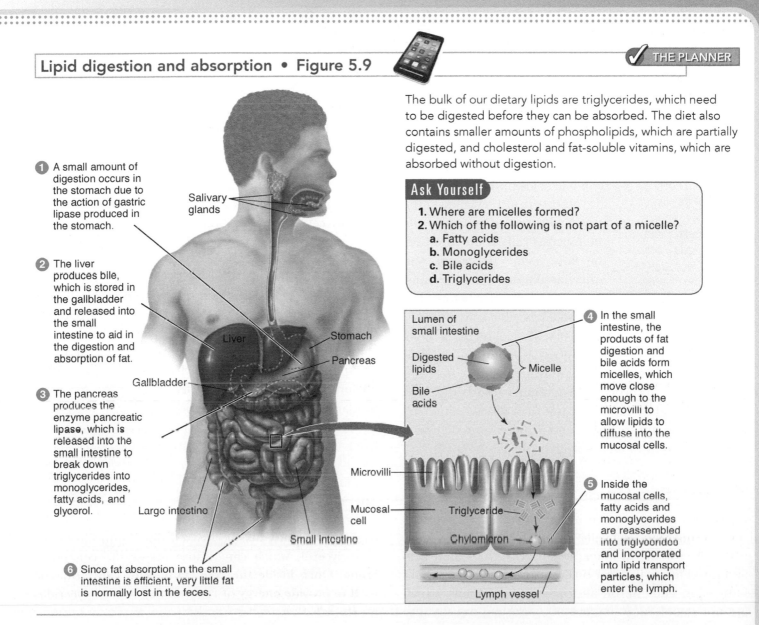

The bulk of our dietary lipids are triglycerides, which need to be digested before they can be absorbed. The diet also contains smaller amounts of phospholipids, which are partially digested, and cholesterol and fat-soluble vitamins, which are absorbed without digestion.

Ask Yourself

1. Where are micelles formed?
2. Which of the following is not part of a micelle?
   a. Fatty acids
   b. Monoglycerides
   c. Bile acids
   d. Triglycerides

1 A small amount of digestion occurs in the stomach due to the action of gastric lipase produced in the stomach.

2 The liver produces bile, which is stored in the gallbladder and released into the small intestine to aid in the digestion and absorption of fat.

3 The pancreas produces the enzyme pancreatic lipase, which is released into the small intestine to break down triglycerides into monoglycerides, fatty acids, and glycerol.

6 Since fat absorption in the small intestine is efficient, very little fat is normally lost in the feces.

Salivary glands

Liver

Gallbladder

Large intestine

Small Intestine

Stomach

Pancreas

4 In the small intestine, the products of fat digestion and bile acids form micelles, which move close enough to the microvilli to allow lipids to diffuse into the mucosal cells.

5 Inside the mucosal cells, fatty acids and monoglycerides are reassembled into triglycerides and incorporated into lipid transport particles, which enter the lymph.

Lumen of small intestine

Digested lipids

Bile acids

Micelle

Microvilli

Mucosal cell

Triglyceride

Chylomicron

Lymph vessel

Lipoprotein structure • Figure 5.10

A lipoprotein consists of a core of triglycerides and cholesterol surrounded by a shell of protein, phospholipids, and cholesterol. Phospholipids orient with their fat-soluble "tails" toward the interior and their water-soluble "heads" toward the outside. This allows the fat-soluble substances in the interior to travel through the aqueous blood.

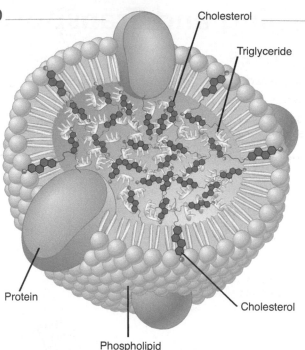

Cholesterol

Triglyceride

Protein

Cholesterol

Phospholipid

---

monoglyceride A glycerol molecule with one fatty acid attached.

micelle A particle that is formed in the small intestine when the products of fat digestion are surrounded by bile acids. It facilitates the absorption of lipids.

The resulting mixture of fatty acids, **monoglycerides**, cholesterol, and bile acids forms smaller droplets called **micelles**, which facilitate absorption (see Figure 5.9). The bile acids in the micelles are also absorbed and returned to the liver to be reused. Once inside the mucosal cells of the intestine, the fatty acids, cholesterol, and other fat-soluble substances must be processed further before they can be transported in the blood.

The fat-soluble vitamins (A, D, E, and K) are absorbed through the same process as other lipids. These vitamins are not digested but must be incorporated into micelles to be absorbed. The amounts absorbed can be reduced if dietary fat is very low or if disease, other dietary components, or medications such as the diet drug Alli®, interfere with fat absorption (see Figure 9.19).

Transporting Lipids in the Blood

Lipids that are consumed in the diet are absorbed into the intestinal mucosal cells. From here, small fatty acids, which are soluble in water, are absorbed into the blood and travel to the liver for further processing. Long-chain fatty acids, cholesterol, and fat-soluble vitamins, which are not soluble in water, are not absorbed directly into the blood and must be packaged for transport. They are covered with a water-soluble envelope of protein, phospholipids, and cholesterol to form particles called **lipoproteins** (**Figure 5.10**). Different types of lipoproteins transport dietary lipids from the small intestine to body cells, from the liver to body cells, and from body cells back to the liver for disposal.

lipoprotein A particle that transports lipids in the blood.

Transport from the small intestine After long-chain fatty acids (from the digestion of triglycerides) have been absorbed into the mucosal cells, they are reassembled into triglycerides. These triglycerides, along with cholesterol and fat-soluble vitamins, are packaged with phospholipids, and protein to form lipoproteins called **chylomicrons**. Chylomicrons are too large to enter the capillaries in the small intestine, so they pass from the intestinal mucosa into the lymph, which then delivers them to the blood (**Figure 5.11**). They circulate in the blood, delivering triglycerides to body cells. To enter the cells, the triglycerides must first be broken down into fatty acids and glycerol, which can diffuse across the cell membrane. Once inside the cells, fatty acids can either be used to provide energy or reassembled into triglycerides for storage.

chylomicron A lipoprotein that transports lipids from the mucosal cells of the small intestine and delivers triglycerides to other body cells.

Lipid transport and delivery • Figure 5.11

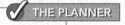

Chylomicrons and very-low-density lipoproteins (VLDLs) transport triglycerides and deliver them to body cells. Low-density lipoproteins (LDLs) transport and deliver cholesterol, and high-density lipoproteins (HDLs) help return cholesterol to the liver for reuse or elimination.

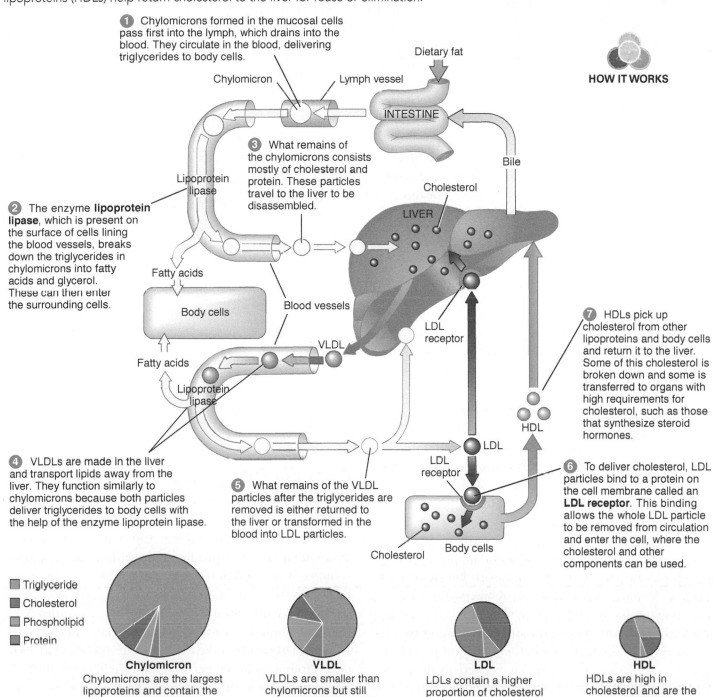

1 Chylomicrons formed in the mucosal cells pass first into the lymph, which drains into the blood. They circulate in the blood, delivering triglycerides to body cells.

2 The enzyme **lipoprotein lipase**, which is present on the surface of cells lining the blood vessels, breaks down the triglycerides in chylomicrons into fatty acids and glycerol. These can then enter the surrounding cells.

3 What remains of the chylomicrons consists mostly of cholesterol and protein. These particles travel to the liver to be disassembled.

4 VLDLs are made in the liver and transport lipids away from the liver. They function similarly to chylomicrons because both particles deliver triglycerides to body cells with the help of the enzyme lipoprotein lipase.

5 What remains of the VLDL particles after the triglycerides are removed is either returned to the liver or transformed in the blood into LDL particles.

6 To deliver cholesterol, LDL particles bind to a protein on the cell membrane called an **LDL receptor**. This binding allows the whole LDL particle to be removed from circulation and enter the cell, where the cholesterol and other components can be used.

7 HDLs pick up cholesterol from other lipoproteins and body cells and return it to the liver. Some of this cholesterol is broken down and some is transferred to organs with high requirements for cholesterol, such as those that synthesize steroid hormones.

HOW IT WORKS

Legend:
- ▢ Triglyceride
- ▢ Cholesterol
- ▢ Phospholipid
- ▢ Protein

Chylomicron
Chylomicrons are the largest lipoproteins and contain the greatest proportion of triglycerides.

VLDL
VLDLs are smaller than chylomicrons but still contain a high proportion of triglycerides.

LDL
LDLs contain a higher proportion of cholesterol than do other lipoproteins.

HDL
HDLs are high in cholesterol and are the densest lipoproteins due to their high protein content.

Ask Yourself

1. Which lipoprotein contains the highest proportion of cholesterol?

2. Which lipoprotein has the highest proportion of triglyceride?

Transport from the liver The liver can synthesize lipids. Lipids are transported from the liver in **very-low-density lipoproteins (VLDLs)**. Like chylomicrons, VLDLs are lipoproteins that circulate in the blood, delivering triglycerides to body cells (see Figure 5.11). When the triglycerides have been removed from the VLDLs, a denser, smaller particle remains. About two-thirds of these particles are returned to the liver, and the rest are transformed in the blood into **low-density lipoproteins (LDLs)**.

low-density lipoprotein(LDL)
A lipoprotein that transports cholesterol to cells.

LDLs are the primary cholesterol delivery system for cells. They contain a higher proportion of cholesterol than do chylomicrons or VLDLs (see Figure 5.11). High levels of LDLs in the blood have been associated with an increased risk for heart disease. For this reason, they are sometimes referred to as "bad cholesterol."

Eliminating cholesterol Because most body cells have no system for breaking down cholesterol, cholesterol must be returned to the liver to be eliminated from the body. This reverse cholesterol transport is accomplished by **high-density lipoproteins (HDLs)** (see Figure 5.11). HDL cholesterol is often called "good cholesterol" because high levels of HDL in the blood are associated with a reduction in the risk of heart disease.

high-density lipoprotein (HDL)
A lipoprotein that picks up cholesterol from cells and transports it to the liver so that it can be eliminated from the body.

CONCEPT CHECK STOP

1. **How** does bile help in the digestion and absorption of lipids?
2. **Why** are lipoproteins needed to transport lipids?
3. **What** is the primary function of LDLs?

5.4 Lipid Functions

LEARNING OBJECTIVES

1. **List** the functions of lipids in the body.
2. **Explain** why we need the right balance of omega-3 and omega-6 fatty acids.
3. **Summarize** how fatty acids are used to provide energy.
4. **Describe** how fat is stored and how it is retrieved from storage.

L ipids are necessary to maintain health. In our diet, fat is needed to absorb fat-soluble vitamins and is a source of essential fatty acids and energy. In our bodies, lipids form structural and regulatory molecules and are broken down to provide ATP. As discussed earlier, cholesterol plays both regulatory and structural roles: It is used to make steroid hormones, and it is an important component of cell membranes and the myelin coating that is necessary for brain and nerve function.

Most lipids in the body are triglycerides stored in **adipose tissue**, which is body fat that lies under the skin and around internal organs (**Figure 5.12**). The triglycerides in our adipose tissue provide a lightweight energy storage molecule, help cushion our internal organs, and insulate us from changes in temperature. Triglycerides are also found in oils that lubricate body surfaces, keeping the skin soft and supple.

Essential Fatty Acids

Humans are not able to synthesize fatty acids that have double bonds in the omega-6 and omega-3 positions (see Figure 5.4b). Therefore, the fatty acids **linoleic acid** (omega-6) and **alpha-linolenic acid (α-linolenic acid)** (omega-3) are considered essential fatty acids. They must be consumed in the diet because they cannot be made in the body. As illustrated in the top portion of **Figure 5.13** they can be used to synthesize longer-chain omega-6 and omega-3 fatty acids. If the diet is low in linoleic acid and/ or α-linolenic acid, longer-chain fatty acids that the body would normally synthesize from them become dietary essentials as well.

Omega-6 and omega-3 fatty acids are important for health. They are needed for the formation of the phospholipids that give cell membranes their structure and functional properties. Therefore, they are essential for growth, development, and fertility, as well as for

Adipose tissue • Figure 5.12

The cells that make up our adipose tissue enlarge when we gain weight (store more triglyceride) and shrink when the amount of stored triglyceride decreases.

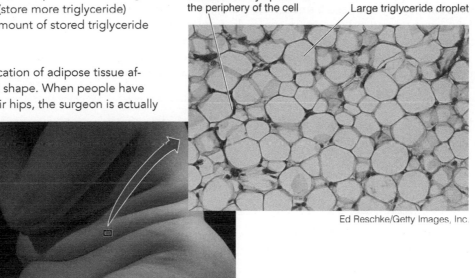

Nucleus and cytoplasm at the periphery of the cell

Large triglyceride droplet

a. The amount and location of adipose tissue affect our body size and shape. When people have liposuction to slim their hips, the surgeon is actually vacuuming out fat cells from the adipose tissue in the region.

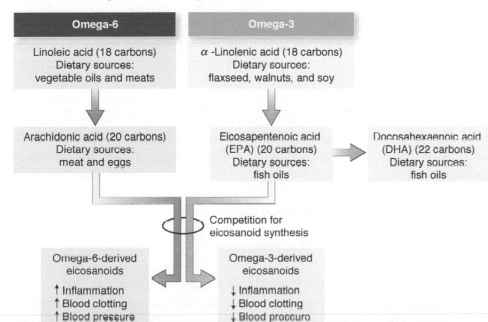

Karen Kasmauski/NG ImageCollection

b. Adipose tissue cells contain large droplets of triglyceride that push the other cell components to the perimeter of the cell. As weight is gained, the triglyceride droplets enlarge.

Ed Reschke/Getty Images, Inc.

maintaining the structure of red blood cells and cells in the skin and nervous system. The omega-3 fatty acid DHA is particularly important in the retina of the eye. Both DHA and the omega-6 fatty acid arachidonic acid are needed to synthesize cell membranes in the central nervous system and are therefore important for normal brain development in infants and young children.

essential fatty acid deficiency A condition characterized by dry, scaly skin and poor growth that results when the diet does not supply sufficient amounts of linoleic acid and α-linolenic acid.

If adequate amounts of linoleic and α-linolenic acid are not consumed, an **essential fatty acid deficiency** will result. Symptoms include scaly, dry skin, liver abnormalities, poor wound healing, impaired vision and hearing, and growth failure in infants. Because the requirement for essential fatty acids is well below the typical intake in the United States, essential fatty acid deficiencies are rare in this country.

Essential fatty acids • Figure 5.13

Omega-6	Omega-3	
Linoleic acid (18 carbons) Dietary sources: vegetable oils and meats	α-Linolenic acid (18 carbons) Dietary sources: flaxseed, walnuts, and soy	
Arachidonic acid (20 carbons) Dietary sources: meat and eggs	Eicosapentenoic acid (EPA) (20 carbons) Dietary sources: fish oils	Docosahexaenoic acid (DHA) (22 carbons) Dietary sources: fish oils

Competition for eicosanoid synthesis

Omega-6-derived eicosanoids

↑ Inflammation
↑ Blood clotting
↑ Blood pressure

Omega-3-derived eicosanoids

↓ Inflammation
↓ Blood clotting
↓ Blood pressure

The omega-6 fatty acid linoleic acid can be used to synthesize **arachidonic acid.** The omega-3 fatty acid α-linolenic acid can be used to synthesize **eicosapentaenoic acid (EPA)** and **docosahexaenoic acid (DHA).** Arachidonic acid and EPA compete for the enzymes that synthesize eicosinoids (see next page). More omega-3-derived eicosinoids, and the functions they provide, will result when more EPA is consumed or synthesized.

Metabolism of fat • Figure 5.14

Triglycerides are broken down to fatty acids and a small amount of glycerol. The fatty acids provide most of the energy stored in a triglyceride molecule. Fatty acids are transported into the mitochondria, where, in the presence of oxygen, they are broken down to form acetyl-CoA, which can be further metabolized to generate ATP. The glycerol molecules, which contain three carbon atoms, can also be used to generate ATP or small amounts of glucose.

HOW IT WORKS

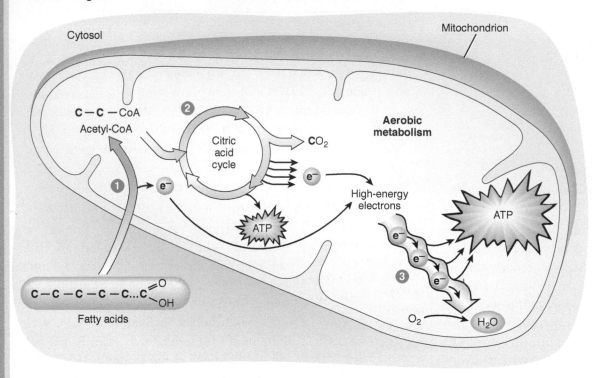

1 Beta-oxidation splits fatty acids into two-carbon units that form acetyl-CoA and releases high-energy electrons (purple balls).

2 If oxygen and enough carbohydrate are available, acetyl-CoA enters the citric acid cycle releasing two molecules of carbon dioxide (CO_2) and more high-energy electrons.

3 In the final step of aerobic metabolism, the high-energy electrons released in β-oxidation and the citric acid cycle combine with oxygen and hydrogen to form water, and their energy is used to generate ATP.

However, deficiencies have occurred in infants and young children consuming low-fat diets and in individuals unable to absorb lipids.

Getting enough essential fatty acids in your diet will prevent deficiency, and the ratio of dietary omega-6 to omega-3 fatty acids also affects your health. This is because the omega-6 and omega-3 polyunsaturated fatty acids made from them are used to make hormone-like molecules called **eicosanoids**. Eicosanoids help regulate blood clotting, blood pressure, immune function, and other body processes. The effect of eicosanoids on these functions depends on the fatty acid from which they are made. For example, when the omega-6 fatty acid arachidonic acid is the starting material, the eicosanoid synthesized increases blood clotting; when the omega-3 fatty acid EPA is the starting material, the eicosanoid made decreases blood clotting. The

eicosanoids
Regulatory molecules that can be synthesized from omega-3 and omega-6 fatty acids.

ratio of dietary omega-6 to omega-3 fatty acids affects the balance of the omega-6 and omega-3 fatty acids in the body and, therefore, the balance of the omega-6- and omega-3-derived eicosanoids produced (see Figure 5.13).

The U.S. diet contains a higher ratio of omega-6 to omega-3 fatty acids than is optimal for health. Increasing consumption of foods that are rich in omega-3 fatty acids increases the proportion of omega-3 eicosanoids. This reduces the risk of heart disease by decreasing inflammation, lowering blood pressure, and reducing blood clotting (see Figure 5.13).[9] The American Heart Association recommends eating two or more servings per week of fish, which is a good source of EPA and DHA, along with plant sources of omega-3 fatty acids, such as walnuts, canola oil, and flaxseed.[10]

Fat as a Source of Energy

Fat is an important source of energy in the body (**Figure 5.14**). Triglycerides that are consumed in the diet can be

Feasting and fasting • Figure 5.15

Feasting: When excess energy is consumed, it is stored as triglycerides in **adipose** tissue.

Chylomicron

VLDL

Fatty acids

Triglycerides — **Adipose tissue**

Fasting: When no food has been eaten for a while, triglycerides from adipose tissue are broken down, releasing fatty acids as an energy source.

C—C—C—C—C...C $\begin{array}{c}=O\\OH\end{array}$

Fatty acids

Used for energy → ATP

When we eat more than we need, excess energy is stored as triglycerides. When we don't eat enough, triglycerides in adipose tissue are broken down, releasing fatty acids, which can be used to provide energy.

Ask Yourself

It is 1 PM, and you have not eaten since 7:30 AM. Where is your body getting energy?

---

either used immediately to fuel the body or stored in adipose tissue. Depositing fat in adipose tissue is an efficient way to store energy because each gram of fat provides 9 Calories, compared with only 4 Calories per gram from carbohydrate or protein. This allows a large amount of energy to be stored in the body without a great increase in body size or weight. For example, even a lean man stores over 50,000 Calories in his adipose tissue.

Throughout the day, as we eat and then go for hours without eating, triglycerides are stored and then retrieved from storage, depending on the body's immediate energy needs. For example, after we have feasted on a meal, some triglycerides will be stored; then, in the small fasts between meals, some of the stored triglycerides will be broken down to provide energy. When the energy consumed in the diet equals the body's energy requirements, the net amount of body fat does not change.

Feasting When we consume more calories than we need, the excess is stored primarily as fat. Excess fat from our diet is packaged in chylomicrons and transported directly from the intestines to the adipose tissue. Because the fatty acids in our body fat come from the fatty acids we eat, what we eat affects the fatty acid composition of our adipose tissue; therefore, if you eat more saturated fat, there will be more saturated fat in your adipose tissue. Excess calories that are consumed as carbohydrate or protein can also be stored as fat, but less efficiently because the absorbed glucose and amino acids must first

go to the liver, where they can be used to synthesize fatty acids, which are then assembled into triglycerides, packaged in VLDLs, and transported in the blood to adipose tissue (**Figure 5.15**).

The ability of the body to store excess triglycerides is theoretically limitless. Cells in your adipose tissue can increase in weight by about 50 times, and new fat cells can be made when existing cells reach their maximum size.

Fasting When you eat fewer calories than you need, your body takes energy from its fat stores. In this situation, an enzyme inside the fat cells receives a signal to break down stored triglycerides. The fatty acids and glycerol that result are released directly into the blood and circulate throughout the body. They are taken up by cells and used to produce ATP (see Figures 5.14 and 5.15).

To be used for energy, fatty acids are broken into two-carbon units that form acetyl-CoA. When oxygen and carbohydrate are available, acetyl-CoA can be used to generate ATP (see Figure 5.14). If there is not enough carbohydrate available in cells to allow the acetyl-CoA to enter the citric acid cycle, it will be used to make *ketones* (see Chapter 4). Many tissues in the body can use ketones as an energy source. During prolonged fasting, even the brain can adapt itself to use ketones to meet about half of its energy needs. For the other half, the brain continues to require glucose. Fatty acids cannot be used to make glucose, and only a small amount of glucose can be made from the glycerol released from triglyceride breakdown.

CONCEPT CHECK STOP

1. **Why** does a deficiency of essential fatty acids cause health problems?

2. **How** does eating fish regularly affect the types of eicosanoids produced in the body?

3. **How** are fatty acids used to produce ATP?

4. **What** happens to excess dietary fat after it has been absorbed?

What affects the risk of heart disease? Table 5.1

Risk factor	How it affects risk
Obesity	Obesity increases blood pressure, blood cholesterol levels, and the risk of developing diabetes. It also increases the amount of work the heart must do to pump blood throughout the body.
Diabetes	High blood glucose damages blood vessel walls, initiating atherosclerosis.
High blood pressure	High blood pressure can damage blood vessel walls, initiating atherosclerosis. It forces the heart to work harder, causing it to enlarge and weaken over time.
Gender	Men and women are both at risk for heart disease, but men are generally affected a decade earlier than are women. This difference is due in part to the protective effect of the hormone estrogen in women. As women age, the effects of menopause—including a decline in estrogen level and a gain in weight—increase heart disease risk.
Age	The risk of heart disease is increased in men age 45 and older and in women age 55 and older.

Nutrition InSight Nutrients, foods, and dietary patterns affect heart disease risk • Figure 5.17

The overall pattern of food intake, often referred to as the total diet, has a greater impact on the risk of heart disease than the individual nutrients we consume.

Individual nutrients and food components

Factors That Increase Risk	Factors That Reduce Risk
Cholesterol	Polyunsaturated fat
Saturated fat	Monosaturated fat
Trans fat	Fiber
Sodium	B vitamins
Excess sugar	Antioxidants
Excess energy	Moderate alcohol

Nutrients are found in foods.

Whole foods

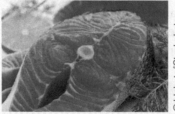
© hlphoto/iStockphoto

Fish is high in omega-3 fatty acids, which reduce the risk of heart disease. In addition to lowering LDL cholesterol and triglyceride levels, omega-3 fatty acids protect against heart disease by decreasing blood clotting, lowering blood pressure, improving the function of the cells lining blood vessels, reducing inflammation, and modulating heartbeats.[16]

Whole foods

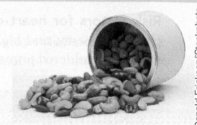
© Donald Erickson/iStockphoto

Nuts are a good source of monounsaturated fat, which lowers LDL cholesterol and makes it less susceptible to oxidation. Nuts are also high in omega-3 fatty acids, fiber, vegetable protein, antioxidants, and plant sterols. Diets containing nuts may improve blood lipids and the functioning of cells lining the artery wall.[17]

Whole foods

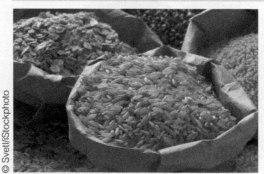
© Svetl/iStockphoto

Oatmeal and brown rice are good sources of soluble fiber, which has been shown to reduce blood cholesterol levels. Whole grains also provide omega-3 fatty acids, B vitamins, and antioxidants, as well as other phytochemicals that may protect against heart disease.[18]

Whole foods

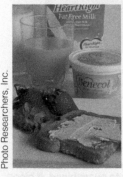
Photo Researchers, Inc.

Plant sterols resemble cholesterol chemically, making it difficult for the digestive tract to distinguish them from cholesterol. Consuming plant sterols reduces cholesterol absorption, lowering total and LDL cholesterol levels.[19] Plant sterols are found in vegetable oils, nuts, seeds, cereals, legumes, and many fruits and vegetables and are added to special margarines, salad dressings, and orange juice.

Whole foods

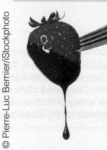
© Pierre-Luc Bernier/iStockphoto

Modest consumption of dark chocolate is associated with reduced risk of heart disease. This is attributed to the phytochemicals in dark chocolate.[20] In addition, most of the fat in chocolate is from stearic acid, a saturated fatty that does not cause an increase in blood levels of LDL cholesterol.

Family history	Individuals with a male family member who exhibited heart disease before age 55 or a female family member who exhibited heart disease before age 65 are considered to be at increased risk. African Americans have a higher risk of heart disease than the general population, in part due to the high incidence of high blood pressure among African Americans.[22]
Smoking	Smoking increases risk. If smoking is stopped, about a third of the excess risk is eliminated within 2 years and risk returns to the level of a nonsmoker within 10 to 14 years following cessation.[23]
Activity	Regular exercise decreases risk by reducing blood pressure, lowering LDL cholesterol, increasing healthy HDL cholesterol levels, reducing the risk of diabetes, and promoting a healthy weight. Adults are advised to engage in 40 minutes of moderate to vigorous-intensity aerobic physical activity 3 to 4 times per week.[15]
Diet	Diet, including the types of lipids, the amounts of fiber and other dietary components, as well as overall dietary pattern can affect the risk of heart disease.
Blood lipid level	High blood levels of LDL cholesterol and triglycerides, and low levels of HDL cholesterol increase risk (see online Appendix F). An individual's specific goal for LDL cholesterol depends on his or her other risk factors for heart disease. Cholesterol-lowering medications, called statins, are recommended for individuals with a high overall risk.[24]

Whole foods

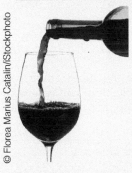

© Florea Marius Catalin/iStockphoto

Moderate alcohol consumption—that is, one drink a day for women and two a day for men (one drink is equivalent to 5 ounces wine, 12 ounces beer, or 1.5 ounces distilled spirits)—reduces blood clotting and increases HDL cholesterol but also raises blood triglyceride levels. Higher alcohol intake increases the risk of heart disease and causes other health and societal problems.

Whole foods

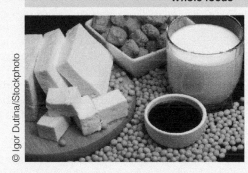

© Igor Dutina/iStockphoto

Soy can lower the risk of heart disease. It has a small LDL cholesterol-lowering effect and is high in healthy polyunsaturated fat, fiber, vitamins, and minerals and low in unhealthy saturated fat.[21]

Foods make up dietary patterns

Dietary patterns

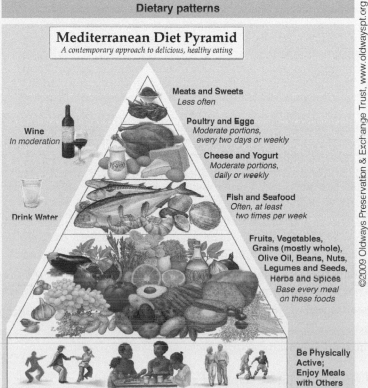

Mediterranean Diet Pyramid
A contemporary approach to delicious, healthy eating

©2009 Oldways Preservation & Exchange Trust, www.oldwayspt.org

Meats and Sweets
Less often

Poultry and Eggs
Moderate portions, every two days or weekly

Wine
In moderation

Cheese and Yogurt
Moderate portions, daily or weekly

Fish and Seafood
Often, at least two times per week

Drink Water

Fruits, Vegetables, Grains (mostly whole), Olive Oil, Beans, Nuts, Legumes and Seeds, Herbs and Spices
Base every meal on these foods

Be Physically Active; Enjoy Meals with Others

Illustration by George Middleton © 2009 Oldways Preservation and Exchange Trust www.oldwayspt.org

In the Mediterranean region, the main source of dietary fat is olive oil, and the typical diet is high in nuts, vegetables, and fruits. Fish is consumed routinely and red meat rarely. Despite a fat intake that is similar to that of the U.S. diet, the incidence of heart disease is much lower. This diet pyramid is based on the dietary patterns of Crete, Greece, and southern Italy around 1960, when the rates of chronic disease in this region were among the lowest in the world. This is one of the dietary patterns recommended in the 2010 Dietary Guidelines.

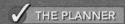
The Issue: Does eating eggs increase your risk of cardiovascular disease?

Dietary recommendations in the United States have been telling us to limit egg consumption since the 1960s. What could be bad about this high-protein, easy-to-prepare food? The problem is that one egg has over 200 mg of cholesterol. An ounce of lean meat has only about 30 mg. The Dietary Guidelines and the American Heart Association recommend limiting dietary cholesterol to less than 300 mg per day. So, is it okay to eat eggs for breakfast?

The cholesterol in our bodies comes from what we eat as well as cholesterol synthesized by our livers. Even if you don't eat any cholesterol, your liver will make all you need. For many people, when they eat cholesterol, their liver production slows, so blood levels don't rise; others are missing this regulation. For them, an increase in dietary cholesterol results in an increase in blood cholesterol. However, the increase is typically due to increases in "good" HDL cholesterol as well as "bad" LDL cholesterol, so the risk of atherosclerosis does not change.[27] Furthermore, the LDL particles that form when dietary cholesterol increases are large. These larger LDL particles are thought to be less of a cardiovascular risk than smaller ones.[27] This suggests that the cholesterol in eggs is not a problem. However, the lipoproteins in these studies were measured in people who were fasting, which may not give the best measure of the effect of dietary cholesterol. Some researchers believe that the harm caused by dietary cholesterol occurs just after a meal when it may affect blood lipid levels, increase the susceptibility of LDL cholesterol to oxidation, and potentiate the adverse effects of dietary saturated fat.[28]

Currently, the vast majority of epidemiological studies do not find a relationship between dietary cholesterol or egg consumption and cardiovascular disease.[27,29] For example, an evaluation of more than 20,000 male physicians participating in the Physicians' Health Study found that eating up to six eggs per week did not affect the risk or incidence of cardiovascular disease.[30] However, eating seven or more eggs per week caused an increased risk of death from cardiovascular disease, and eating any eggs was found to increase the risk of cardiovascular disease in people with type 2 diabetes.[29,30]

Nutrition professionals recognize that it is the overall dietary pattern, not the avoidance of particular foods, that is most important for health and wellness. Eggs are part of the Mediterranean dietary pattern, and this pattern is associated with good cardiovascular health. One large egg contains 6 g of high-quality protein, and unlike many other sources of cholesterol, eggs are low in cholesterol-raising saturated fat (see the accompanying table). Eggs are also a good source of zinc, B vitamins, vitamin A, and iron. The yolk is rich in lutein and zeaxanthin, two phytochemicals that help protect against age-related eye disorders. Eggs may also help you maintain your weight. A recent study found that people who eat an egg-based breakfast eat fewer overall calories during the day than people who have a bagel-based breakfast.[31]

The 2010 Dietary Guidelines has concluded that eating one egg per day is not harmful and does not result in increased risk of cardiovascular disease in healthy individuals. Despite this conclusion, the guidelines continue to recommend limiting dietary cholesterol to less than 300 mg per day, with further reductions to less than 200 mg per day for persons with, or at high risk for, cardiovascular disease.[2] If you eat an egg every day, is your diet likely to exceed 300 mg of cholesterol per day?

Think Critically: What food or foods in this table other than eggs contain more than 50 mg of cholesterol but less than 4 g of saturated fat? How might they impact the risk of cardiovascular disease?

Cholesterol and saturated fat content of foods		
Food	Cholesterol (mg)	Saturated fat (g)
Egg, one	212	1.6
Shrimp, 3 oz, raw	129	0.3
Salmon, 3 oz, cooked	57	0.6
Hamburger patty, 3 oz, broiled	71	7.5
Bacon, 3 oz, pan fried	94	11.7
Pork sausage, 3 oz, cooked	71	7.8
Butter, 2 Tbsp	61	14.6
Milk, whole, 8 fluid oz	24	4.6
Cheese, cheddar, 1 oz	30	6.0
Ice cream, vanilla, ½ cup	32	4.9

reduce risk by lowering blood cholesterol. Replacing foods that are high in cholesterol-raising fats with foods that provide omega-3 fatty acids, monounsaturated fat, soluble fiber, and plant sterols, which have been shown to lower total and LDL cholesterol, can reduce the risk of heart disease (see *Debate: Good Egg, Bad Egg?*).[14]

Nutrients and other dietary components can also affect heart disease risk through mechanisms unrelated to blood cholesterol level. For example, adequate intakes of vitamin B_6, vitamin B_{12}, and folate help protect against heart disease because they help maintain low blood levels of the amino acid homocysteine (discussed further in

Chapter 7). Elevated homocysteine levels are associated with a higher incidence of heart disease.[25] Much of the heart-protective effect of omega-3 fatty acids, such as those found in fish, is due to the eicosanoids made from omega-3 fatty acids; these eicosanoids prevent the growth of atherosclerotic plaque, reduce blood clotting and blood pressure, and decrease inflammation.[16] Plant foods add soluble fiber to the diet, which can reduce blood cholesterol, but in addition they provide vitamins, minerals, and phytochemicals, some of which protect against heart disease because they perform antioxidant functions. **Antioxidants** decrease the oxidation of LDL cholesterol and, therefore, may prevent the development of plaque in artery walls (see Figure 5.16).[26]

antioxidant A substance that decreases the adverse effects of reactive molecules.

Diet and Cancer

Cancer is the second-leading cause of death in the United States. As with heart disease, there is evidence that the risk of cancer can be reduced with changes in diet and activity patterns.[32] Populations consuming diets that are high in fruits and vegetables tend to have a lower risk of cancer than populations with lower intakes. These foods are rich in antioxidants such as vitamin C, vitamin E, and β-carotene. In contrast, in populations that consume diets that are high in fat, particularly animal fats, the incidence of cancer is higher.[33]

The good news is that the same dietary pattern that protects you from cardiovascular disease may also reduce the risk of certain forms of cancer. For example, the Mediterranean diet, which is high in monounsaturated fat from olive oil and omega-3 fatty acids from fish, is associated with a low risk of cancers of the breast, ovary, colon, and

upper digestive and respiratory tracts.[34–36] *Trans* fatty acids, on the other hand, not only raise LDL cholesterol levels but are also believed to increase the risk of breast cancer.[37]

Dietary Fat and Obesity

Excess dietary fat consumption contributes to weight gain and obesity. One reason is that fat contains 9 Calories/gram, more than twice the calorie content of carbohydrate or protein. Therefore, a high-fat meal contains more calories in the same volume than does a lower-fat meal. Because people have a tendency to eat a certain weight or volume of food, consuming meals that are high in fat leads to more calories being consumed.[38,39] Dietary fat may also contribute to weight gain because it is stored very efficiently as body fat.

Despite the fact that fat is fattening, the fat content of the U.S. diet is unlikely to be the sole reason for the high rate of obesity in the United States.[40] Weight gain occurs when energy intake exceeds energy expenditure, regardless of whether the extra energy comes from fat, carbohydrate, or protein. The increasing prevalence of overweight and obesity in the United States and worldwide is likely due to a general increase in calorie intake combined with a decrease in energy expenditure.[2]

CONCEPT CHECK 🛑 STOP

1. **How** does atherosclerotic plaque lead to a heart attack?
2. **What** are three dietary factors that increase the risk of heart disease?
3. **Why** might eating a high-fat diet increase the number of calories you consume?

5.6 Meeting Lipid Needs

LEARNING OBJECTIVES

1. **Discuss** the recommendations for fat and cholesterol intake.
2. **Choose** heart-healthy foods from each section of MyPlate.
3. **Use** food labels to choose foods containing healthy fats.

T he amount of fat the body requires from the diet is small, but a diet that provides only the minimum amount would be very high in carbohydrate, would not be very palatable, and would not necessarily be any healthier than diets with more fat. Therefore, the recommendations for fat intake focus on meeting essential fatty acid needs and

A Case Study on Improving Heart Health

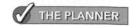
THE PLANNER

Rafael is a financial advisor who spends much of his day sitting at his computer. When he is home with his family, he enjoys watching his children play soccer and basketball but rarely finds time to exercise himself. Based on a cardiovascular disease risk assessment, Rafael's doctor suggests he make some changes. His potential risk factors are given in the table:

Sex	Male
Age	40
Family history	Mother had heart attack at age 60
Height/weight	68 in/160 lb (within healthy range)
Blood pressure	145/90 (elevated)
LDL cholesterol	195 mg/100 mL (elevated)
HDL cholesterol	30 mg/100 mL (low)
Smoker	Yes
Activity level	Sedentary

 1 Which factors in addition to his elevated LDL cholesterol increase Rafael's risk of developing heart disease?

Your answer:

Based on his overall risk analysis, Rafael's doctor tells him he would benefit from a statin, but improving his diet and getting more exercise will further lower his risk. Rafael meets with a dietitian. A diet recall reveals that his breakfast typically consists of bacon and eggs; his lunch is a fast food hamburger, fries, and a soda; and his dinner consists of beef or chicken, a green or orange vegetable, and rice or potatoes.

An analysis of Raphael's diet indicates that his total fat intake is within the recommended range of 20 to 35% of calories, but he consumes more saturated fat than is recommended. He does not consume enough fruits, vegetables, or whole grains. The dietitian suggests that he modify his eating pattern.

 2 Suggest a breakfast and a fast-food lunch that would reduce Rafael's intake of saturated fat and increase his intake of fruits, vegetables, and whole grains.

Your answer:

Based on the dietitian's suggestions, Rafael switches to canola oil and olive oil for cooking at home to increase his monounsaturated fat intake and eats fish or shellfish twice a week to increase his omega-3 intake. Because his new diet has fewer calories and Rafael does not need to lose weight, he starts bringing snacks to work.

3 Which snack is a better choice for Rafael? Why?

Your answer:

© Juanmonino/iStockphoto

© HHLtDave5/iStockphoto

Granola Bar

Nutrition Facts
Serving Size 1 bar (35g)
Servings Per Container 6

Amount Per Serving	
Calories	140
Calories from Fat	30

	% Daily Value*
Total Fat 3.5g	6%
Saturated Fat 2g	10%
Trans Fat 0g	
Cholesterol 0mg	0%
Sodium 130mg	5%
Total Carbohydrate 26g	9%
Dietary Fiber 1g	5%
Sugars 13g	
Protein 2g	

Apple and Peanut Butter

Nutrition Facts
Serving Size 1 medium apple and 1 Tbsp peanut butter

Calories	195

Total Fat	8 g
Saturated Fat	1.3 g
Trans Fat	0 g
Cholesterol	0 mg
Sodium	54 mg
Total Carbohydrate	28 g
Dietary Fiber	5 g
Sugars	19 g
Protein	4 g

(Check your answers in online Appendix L.)

---

choosing the amounts and types of fat that will promote health and prevent disease.

Fat and Cholesterol Recommendations

The DRIs recommend a total fat intake of 20 to 35% of calories for adults. Of this, a small proportion needs to come from the essential fatty acids. The AI for linoleic acid is 12 g/day for women and 17 g/day for men. You can meet your requirement by consuming a half-cup of almonds or 2 tablespoons of corn oil. For α-linolenic acid, the AI is 1.1 g/day for women and 1.6 g/day for men. Your requirement can be met by eating a quarter-cup of

walnuts or 1 tablespoon of ground flaxseed. Consuming these amounts provides the recommended ratio of linoleic to α-linolenic acid of between 5:1 and 10:1.[41]

To reduce the risk of heart disease, the 2010 Dietary Guidelines recommend limiting saturated fat intake to less than 10% of total calories by replacing foods high in saturated fat with sources of mono or polyunsaturated fat (see *Thinking It Through*). Adults with elevated cholesterol would benefit from eating a dietary pattern with only 5 to 7% of calories from saturated fat and keeping *trans* fat intake as low as possible.[2,15] The guidelines recommend limiting cholesterol to less than 300 mg per day for the general

WHAT A SCIENTIST SEES
Looking for Lean Meat

Most fresh meats (whole cuts and ground and chopped products) are required to have a Nutrition Facts label on the package or have the equivalent nutrition information displayed nearby, but the information related to fat content can still be misleading.[42] The terms *lean* and *extra lean* are used to describe the fat content of fresh meats, such as pork chops, poultry, and steaks as well as packaged meats, such as hot dogs and lunch meat. "Lean" means that the meat contains less than 10% fat by weight, and "extra lean" means that it contains less than 5% fat by weight (see online Appendix I). So a package of ground beef like this one that is 85% lean looks like a good choice.

What a scientist sees is that "lean" and "percent lean" are not the same thing. "Percent lean" refers to the weight of the meat that is lean, not the percentage of calories provided by lean meat. So when the label says it is 85% lean, it means that 15% of the weight of the meat is fat, or that there are 15 g of fat in

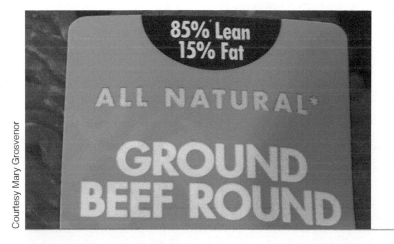

Courtesy Mary Grosvenor

| Fat | Protein | Water |

Percentage by weight   Percentage by calories

The chart on the left shows what percentage of the weight of the ground beef consists of fat, protein, and water. The chart on the right shows the percentage of calories contributed by fat and protein.

100 g (3.5 oz) of raw meat. The % fat must also be listed on the label, but because fat contains 9 Calories/gram, a relatively small percentage of fat by weight can make a large calorie contribution. For example, the 15% fat by weight in the ground beef shown here contributes 63% of the calories in the meat (see chart).

Should you pass on the ground beef and select ground turkey instead? Check the label. If the package is labeled "ground turkey," it may contain skin and leg meat and actually have more fat than the ground beef. Only poultry labeled "ground turkey (or chicken) breast" is made with just the lean breast meat.

Think Critically If you want to purchase ground beef that fits the definition of a "lean" meat, what "percent lean" should you look for on the label?

---

population and suggest that those at high risk for heart disease reduce their cholesterol intake to less than 200 mg/day. Limiting sources of solid fats in the diet will help to reduce intake of saturated fat, *trans* fat, and cholesterol.[2]

Children need more fat than adults to allow for growth and development, so their acceptable ranges of fat intake are higher: 30 to 40% of calories for ages 1 to 3 and 25 to 35% of calories for ages 3 to 18, compared to 20 to 35% for adults. Like adults, adolescents and children over age 2 should consume a diet that is low in saturated fat, cholesterol, and *trans* fat.[2]

Choosing Fats Wisely

The typical U.S. diet falls within the recommended 20 to 35% of calories from fat. However, our intake of cholesterol and saturated fat often exceeds recommendations, and

most people don't get enough omega-3 polyunsaturated fatty acids.[2,4] Our *trans* fat intake is declining because food manufacturers have been replacing partially hydrogenated oils with fats that do not contain synthetic *trans* fat. If the FDA's recent determination that partially hydrogenated oils are not generally recognized as safe is finalized, partially hydrogenated vegetable oils will become food additives and with few exceptions will be banned from the food supply, effectively eliminating synthetic *trans* fat from the diet.[8]

Shifting the sources of dietary fat can improve the proportion of healthy fats in your diet. Limiting fatty cuts of meat, full-fat dairy products, and high-fat processed meats; and trimming the fat from meat, and removing the skin from poultry will reduce your intake of saturated fat and cholesterol (see *What a Scientist Sees*). Avoiding foods such as hard margarines and baked goods that contain hydrogenated fats will limit your intake of *trans* fat. Eating more nuts and avocados and cooking with canola and olive oils will boost your intake of monounsaturated fat, and eating more fish, nuts, and flaxseed will boost your omega-3 intake.

Making wise MyPlate choices Your choices from each food group can have a significant impact on the amounts and types of fats in your diet (**Figure 5.18**). Generally, grains, fruits, and vegetables are low in total fat and saturated fat, and they contain no cholesterol. However, choices from these groups need to be made with care to avoid fats that are added in processing or preparation. Smart choices from the protein group and the dairy group can reduce your intake of unhealthy fats. Oils, butter, margarine, fatty sauces, and salad dressings used in cooking or added at the table are the most concentrated sources

of fat in the diet. Solid fats such as butter, beef fat, and lard are higher in saturated and lower in healthy unsaturated fats than liquid oils. Because solid fats are abundant in the diets of Americans, they contribute significantly to excess calorie intake, so MyPlate considers them to be empty calories. Limiting excess solid fats in the diet will reduce the intake of saturated fatty acids, *trans* fatty acids, and calories. Consuming too many empty calories makes it difficult to meet your nutrient needs without gaining weight. If you consume a 2000-Calorie diet, you can include only about 260 empty Calories. Spreading 1 tablespoon of butter on your morning bagel uses up 100 Calories, over one-third of your empty calorie allowance.

Looking at food labels Food labels are an accessible source of information about the fat content of packaged foods (**Figure 5.19**). The Nutrition Facts panel shows

Healthy MyPlate choices • Figure 5.18

MyPlate recommends limiting intake of solid fats, which includes fats that are high in saturated or *trans* fat, and choosing liquid oils, which are high in mono- and polyunsaturated fats.

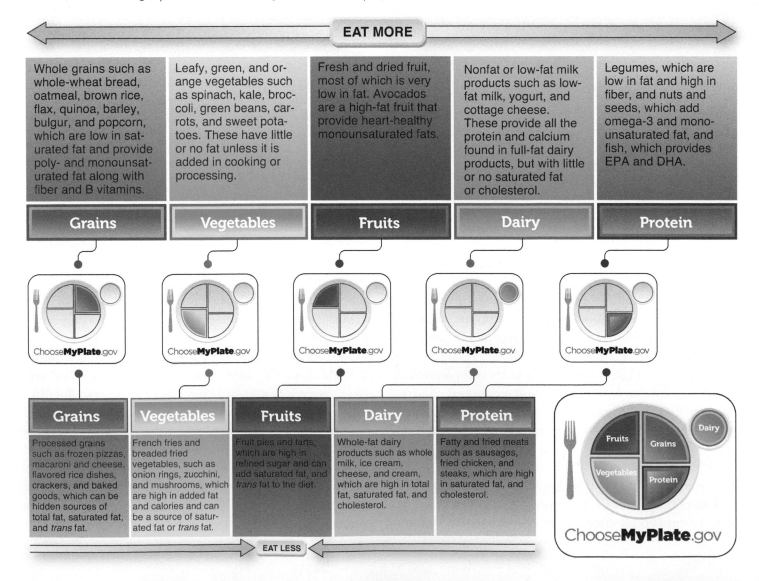

EAT MORE

Grains	Vegetables	Fruits	Dairy	Protein
Whole grains such as whole-wheat bread, oatmeal, brown rice, flax, quinoa, barley, bulgur, and popcorn, which are low in saturated fat and provide poly- and monounsaturated fat along with fiber and B vitamins.	Leafy, green, and orange vegetables such as spinach, kale, broccoli, green beans, carrots, and sweet potatoes. These have little or no fat unless it is added in cooking or processing.	Fresh and dried fruit, most of which is very low in fat. Avocados are a high-fat fruit that provide heart-healthy monounsaturated fats.	Nonfat or low-fat milk products such as low-fat milk, yogurt, and cottage cheese. These provide all the protein and calcium found in full-fat dairy products, but with little or no saturated fat or cholesterol.	Legumes, which are low in fat and high in fiber, and nuts and seeds, which add omega-3 and mono-unsaturated fat, and fish, which provides EPA and DHA.

ChooseMyPlate.gov

Grains	Vegetables	Fruits	Dairy	Protein
Processed grains such as frozen pizzas, macaroni and cheese, flavored rice dishes, crackers, and baked goods, which can be hidden sources of total fat, saturated fat, and *trans* fat.	French fries and breaded fried vegetables, such as onion rings, zucchini, and mushrooms, which are high in added fat and calories and can be a source of saturated fat or *trans* fat.	Fruit pies and tarts, which are high in refined sugar and can add saturated fat, and *trans* fat to the diet.	Whole-fat dairy products such as whole milk, ice cream, cheese, and cream, which are high in total fat, saturated fat, and cholesterol.	Fatty and fried meats such as sausages, fried chicken, and steaks, which are high in saturated fat, and cholesterol.

ChooseMyPlate.gov

EAT LESS

Lipids on food labels • Figure 5.19

a. The Nutrition Facts and ingredient list help identify the types and sources of lipids in packaged foods. By noting the grams of fat and the total number of calories, you can determine the percentage of calories from fat in a product as follows:

1. Multiply the grams of fat by 9 Calories/gram. For example, this product provides 8 g of fat:

    8 g × 9 Calories/gram = 72 Calories from fat

2. Divide Calories from fat by total Calories and multiply by 100 to obtain the percentage. For example, this food contains 160 Calories/serving and 72 Calories from fat:

    72 Calories ÷ 160 Calories × 100 = 45% of Calories from fat

The Nutrition Facts panel lists Calories from fat; grams of total fat, saturated fat, and *trans* fat; and milligrams of cholesterol in a serving. The amount of monounsaturated and polyunsaturated fat is voluntarily included on the labels of some products.

Understanding how to use food labels can help you make more informed choices about the lipids in the foods you eat.

Chocolate Chip Cookies

Nutrition Facts
Serving Size 3 Cookies (33g)
Servings Per Container About 13

Amount Per Serving	
Calories 160	Calories from Fat 70

	% Daily Value*
Total Fat 8g	12%
Saturated Fat 3g	15%
Trans Fat 0g	
Polyunsat Fat 2.5g	
Monounsat Fat 2g	
Cholesterol 0mg	0%
Sodium 110mg	5%
Potassium 45mg	1%
Total Carbohydrate 22g	7%
Dietary Fiber Less than 1gram	3%
Sugars 11g	
Protein 2g	

Vitamin A 0%	•	Vitamin C 0%
Calcium 0%	•	Iron 4%

*Percent Daily Values are based on a 2,000 calorie diet. Your daily values may be higher or lower depending on your calorie needs:

	Calories:	2,000	2,500
Total Fat	Less than	65g	80g
Sat Fat	Less than	20g	25g
Cholesterol	Less than	300mg	300mg
Sodium	Less than	2,400mg	2,400mg
Potassium	Less than	3,500mg	3,500mg
Total Carbohydrate		300g	375g
Dietary Fiber		25g	30g

INGREDIENTS: ENRICHED FLOUR (WHEAT FLOUR, NIACIN, REDUCED IRON, THIAMINE MONONITRATE (VITAMIN B1), FOLIC ACID, SEMISWEET CHOCOLATE CHIPS (SUGAR, CHOCOLATE, COCOA BUTTER, DEXTROSE, SOY LECITHIN AN EMULSIFIER), SUGAR, SOY BEAN OIL AND/OR PARTIALLY HYDROGENATED COTTONSEED OIL, HIGH FRUCTOSE CORN SYRUP, LEAVENING (BAKING SODA AND/OR AMMONIUM PHOSPHATE), SALT, WHEY (FROM MILK), NATURAL AND ARTIFICIAL FLAVOR, CARAMEL COLOR.
CONTAINS: WHEAT, SOY, MILK

Changes proposed to the Nutrition Facts panel would eliminate *Calories from Fat*.

A % Daily Value is listed for total fat, saturated fat, and cholesterol. This allows consumers to tell how a food fits the recommendations. Generally, ≤ 5% of the Daily Value is low, and ≥ 20% is high. There are no Daily Values for *trans*, polyunsaturated, and monounsaturated fats.

If the product has less than 0.5 g of *trans* fat per serving, the Nutrition Facts panel will list the amount of *trans* fat as 0, even if partially hydrogenated oil is an ingredient.

Ask Yourself

If you eat two servings of these cookies, what percentage of your recommended saturated fat intake will it provide? (Assume that you eat 2000 Calories per day.)

a. 12%
b. 13%
c. 24%
d. 30%

The Daily Values recommend consuming less than 30% of calories as fat, no more than 300 mg of cholesterol per day, and no more than 10% of calories as saturated fat. It is recommended that *trans* fat intake be limited to the amounts present naturally in meats and dairy products (≤ 0.5% of calories).

The sources of fat in a product are listed in the ingredient list with the other ingredients, in order of prominence by weight.

Fat free: Contains < 0.5 g fat per serving

Reduced fat: Contains at least 25% less fat per serving than the regular or reference product

Low fat: Contains ≤ 3 g fat per serving

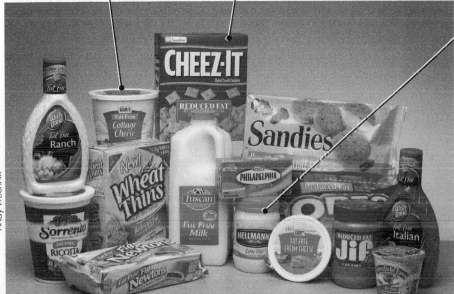

b. Food labeling regulations have developed standard definitions for descriptors such as "low fat" and "low cholesterol," and such terms can be used only in ways that will not confuse the consumer. For example, because saturated fat in the diet raises blood cholesterol, to be labeled "low cholesterol," a food must contain ≤ 20 mg cholesterol per serving and ≤ 2 g saturated fat per serving. No descriptors have been defined for *trans* fat.

149

the amounts of total fat, saturated fat, cholesterol, and *trans* fat, and the ingredient list indicates the source of the fat—for example, whether a food contains corn oil, soybean oil, coconut oil, or partially hydrogenated vegetable oil. Nutrient content claims such as "low fat," "fat free," and "low cholesterol" on food labels can also be used to identify foods that help you meet the recommendations for fat intake. Health claims can help you choose foods that will meet your nutritional goals. For example, foods that are low in saturated fat and cholesterol may state that they help reduce the risk of heart disease (online Appendix I).

The Role of Fat Replacers

People often choose low-fat and reduced-fat products in order to reduce the total amount of fat in their diets. Some of these foods, such as low-fat and nonfat milk and yogurt, are made by simply removing the fat, but in other products, the fat is replaced with ingredients that mimic the taste and texture of the fat. Some reduced-fat foods contain added sugars to improve the taste and texture. Some contain soluble fiber or modified proteins that simulate fat, and others contain fats that have been altered to reduce or prevent absorption (**Figure 5.20**).[43]A problem with nonabsorbable fats is that they

Fat replacers • Figure 5.20

Carbohydrates and proteins added to replace fat add calories to foods. In some cases, so much is added that the low-fat food is not much lower in calories than the original product. Some fat replacers are made from fats that have been modified to reduce how well they can be digested and absorbed. The calories they provide depend on how much is absorbed.

The artificial fat Olestra (sucrose polyester) is made from sucrose with fatty acids attached. Olestra cannot be digested by either human enzymes or bacterial enzymes in the gastrointestinal tract. Therefore, it is excreted in the feces without being absorbed.

Soluble fibers such as pectins and gums are often used in baked goods, as well as salad dressings, sauces, and ice cream, to mimic the texture that fat provides. They reduce the amount of fat in a product and at the same time add soluble fiber.

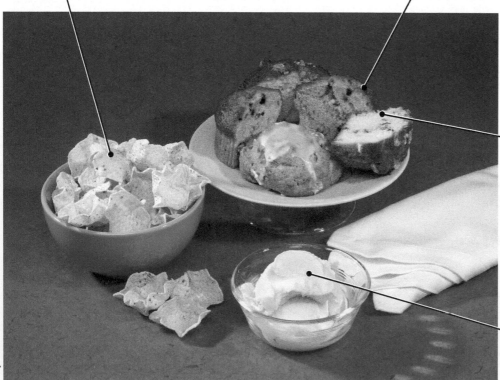

The sugar sucrose is usually added to low-fat and nonfat baked goods to improve flavor and add volume. Sucrose adds 4 Calories per gram.

Protein-based fat replacers are made from milk and egg proteins processed to form millions of microscopic balls that slide over each other, mimicking the creamy texture of fat.[43] They are used in frozen desserts, cheese foods, and other products but cannot be used for frying because they break down at high temperatures.

Andy Washnik

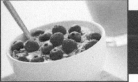
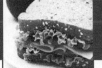
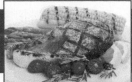

© Sara Winter/iStockphoto   © Jill Chen/iStockphoto   © Steve Mcsweeny/iStockphoto

WHAT SHOULD I EAT?

Fats and Cholesterol

Limit your intake of cholesterol, *trans* fat, and saturated fat
- Choose low-fat milk and yogurt.
- Trim the fat from your meat and serve chicken and fish but don't eat the skin.
- Cut in half your usual amount of butter and use soft rather than stick margarine.
- Watch your fast-food choices—choose grilled chicken over burgers and skip the special sauce.

Increase your proportion of polyunsaturated and monounsaturated fats
- Snack on nuts and seeds.
- Add olives and avocados to your salads.
- Use olive, peanut, or canola oil for cooking and salad dressing.
- Use corn, sunflower, or safflower oil for baking.

Up your omega-3 intake
- Sprinkle ground flaxseeds on your cereal or yogurt.
- Have a serving of mackerel, lake trout, sardines, tuna, or salmon.
- Pick a leafy green vegetable with dinner.
- Add walnuts to your salad or cereal.

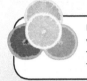

Use iProfile to find the varieties of nuts and fish that are highest in omega-3 fatty acids.

---

reduce the absorption of the fat-soluble substances in the diet, including the fat-soluble vitamins, A, D, E, and K. To avoid depleting these vitamins, products made with the nonabsorbable fat substitute Olestra have been fortified with them. However, these products are not fortified with β-carotene and other fat-soluble substances that may be important for health. Another potential problem with Olestra is that it can cause abdominal cramping and loose stools in some individuals because it passes into the colon without being digested.

Will using low-fat and reduced-fat products improve your diet? Some low-fat foods make an important contribution to a healthy diet. Low-fat dairy products are recommended because they provide all the essential nutrients contained in the full-fat versions but have fewer calories and less saturated fat and cholesterol. Using these products increases the nutrient density of the diet as a whole. However, not all reduced-fat foods are nutrient dense. Low-fat baked goods often have more sugar than the full-fat versions because extra sugar is needed to add volume and make up for the flavor that is lost when the fat is removed. Some are just lower-fat versions of nutrient-poor choices, such as cookies and chips. If these reduced-fat desserts and snack foods replace whole grains, fruits, and vegetables, the resulting diet could be low in fat but also

low in fiber, vitamins, minerals, and phytochemicals (see *What Should I Eat?*).

Using low-fat foods does not necessarily transform a poor diet into a healthy one or improve overall diet quality, but if used appropriately, fat-modified foods can be part of a healthy diet.[43] For example, if a low-fat salad dressing replaces a full-fat version, it allows you to enhance the appeal of a nutrient-rich salad without as much added fat and calories from the dressing. Low-fat products can also be used in conjunction with weight-loss diets because they are often lower in calories. But check the label. Although most are lower in calories, they are by no means calorie free and cannot be consumed liberally without adding calories to the diet and possibly contributing to weight gain.

CONCEPT CHECK   STOP

1. **How** much fat is recommended in a healthy diet?

2. **Which** food groups contribute the most foods that are high in saturated fat and cholesterol?

3. **How** can labels help you identify foods that are low in saturated and *trans* fat?

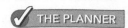

Summary

1 Fats in Our Food 126

- Fat adds calories, texture, and flavor to foods. Some of the fats we eat are visible, but others are hidden.

- Over the past 40 years, Americans have changed the sources of fat in their diets, but the number of grams of fat consumed daily has changed little, as seen in this graph, and the incidence of obesity and other chronic diseases has continued to rise.

U.S. food intake in the 1970s and today • Figure 5.2c

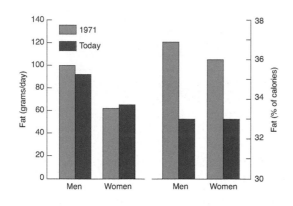

- The structure of fatty acids affects their chemical properties and functions in the body. Each carbon atom in the carbon chain of a **saturated fatty acid** is attached to as many hydrogen atoms as possible, so no carbon–carbon double bonds form. Saturated fatty acids are found primarily in animal products. Exceptions include saturated plant oils often called **tropical oils**. A **monounsaturated fatty acid** contains one carbon–carbon double bond. A **polyunsaturated fatty acid** contains more than one carbon–carbon double bond. The location of the first double bond determines whether it is an **omega-3** or **omega-6 fatty acid**. The orientation of hydrogen atoms around a carbon–carbon double bond distinguishes *cis* fatty acids from ***trans* fatty acids. Hydrogenation** transforms some carbon–carbon double bonds to the *trans* configuration.

- A **phospholipid** contains a **phosphate group** and two fatty acids attached to a backbone of glycerol. One end of the molecule is water soluble, and one end is fat soluble. Phospholipids therefore make good **emulsifiers**. In the human body, they are an important structural component of cell membranes and **lipoproteins**.

- **Sterols,** of which **cholesterol** is the best known, are made up of multiple chemical rings. Cholesterol is made by the body and consumed in animal foods in the diet. In the body, it is a component of cell membranes and is used to synthesize vitamin D, bile acids, and some hormones.

2 Types of Lipids 127

- **Lipids** are a diverse group of organic compounds, most of which do not dissolve in water. **Triglycerides**, commonly referred to as fat, are the type of lipid that is most abundant in our food and in our **adipose tissue**. As shown here, a triglyceride contains three **fatty acids** attached to a molecule of glycerol.

Triglycerides • Figure 5.3

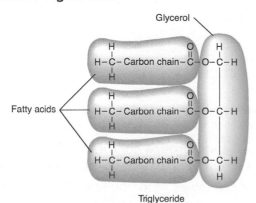

3 Absorbing and Transporting Lipids 133

- In the small intestine, muscular churning mixes chyme with bile from the gallbladder to break fat into small globules. This allows pancreatic lipase to access triglycerides for digestion. The products of triglyceride digestion, cholesterol, phospholipids, and other fat-soluble substances combine with bile to form **micelles**, as depicted depicted at the top of the next page, which facilitate the absorption of these materials.

- Lipids absorbed from the intestine are packaged with protein to form **chylomicrons.** The triglycerides in chylomicrons are broken down by **lipoprotein lipase** on the surface of cells lining the blood vessels. The fatty acids released are taken up by surrounding cells, and what remains is taken up by the liver.

- **Very-low-density lipoproteins (VLDLs)** are synthesized by the liver. With the help of lipoprotein lipase, they deliver triglycerides to body cells. **Low-density lipoproteins (LDLs)** deliver cholesterol to tissues by binding to **LDL receptors** on the cell surface. **High-density lipoproteins (HDLs)** help remove cholesterol from cells and transport it to the liver for disposal.

Lipid digestion and absorption • Figure 5.9

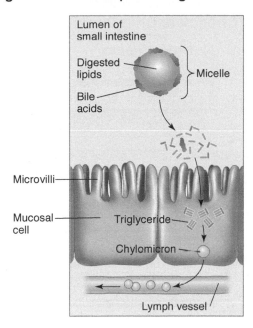

Feasting and fasting • Figure 5.15

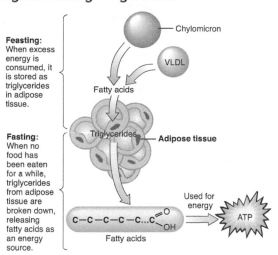

5 Lipids in Health and Disease 140

- **Atherosclerosis** is a disease characterized by the formation of **atherosclerotic plaque** in the artery wall. It starts with an injury to the artery wall that triggers **inflammation**, leading to plaque formation. A key event in the process is the oxidation of LDL cholesterol in the artery wall. **Oxidized LDL cholesterol** promotes inflammation and is taken up by macrophages, as depicted here, forming **foam cells** that deposit in the artery wall. High blood levels of LDL cholesterol are a risk factor for heart disease and high blood HDL cholesterol levels protect against heart disease. The risk of atherosclerosis is also increased by diabetes, high blood pressure, and obesity.

Development of atherosclerosis • Figure 5.16

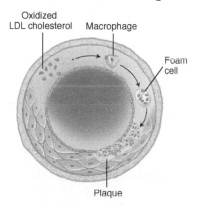

4 Lipid Functions 136

- Dietary fat is needed for the absorption of fat-soluble vitamins and to provide essential fatty acids. In the body, triglycerides in adipose tissue provide a concentrated source of energy and insulate the body against shock and temperature changes. **Essential fatty acids** are needed for normal structure and function of cell membranes, particularly those in the retina and central nervous system. Omega-6 and omega-3 polyunsaturated fatty acids are used to synthesize **eicosanoids**, which help regulate blood clotting, blood pressure, immune function, and other body processes. The ratio of dietary omega-6 to omega-3 fatty acids affects the balance of omega-6 and omega-3 eicosanoids made and hence their overall physiological effects.

- Throughout the day triglycerides are continuously stored in adipose tissue and then broken down to release fatty acids, as shown in the illustration, depending on the immediate energy needs of the body. To generate ATP from fatty acids, the carbon chain is broken into two carbon units that form acetyl-CoA, which can then be metabolized in the presence of oxygen.

- Diets high in saturated fat, *trans* fat, and cholesterol increase the risk of heart disease. Diets high in omega-6 and omega-3 polyunsaturated fatty acids, monounsaturated fatty acids, certain B vitamins, and plant foods containing fiber, antioxidants, and phytochemicals reduce the risk of heart disease. The total dietary and lifestyle pattern is more important than any individual dietary factor in reducing heart disease risk.

- Diets high in fat correlate with an increased incidence of certain types of cancer. In general, the same types of lipids and other dietary components that protect you from heart disease will also protect you from certain forms of cancer.
- Fat contains 9 Calories per gram. A high-fat diet may therefore increase energy intake and promote weight gain, but it is not the primary cause of obesity. Consuming more energy than expended leads to weight gain, regardless of whether the energy is from fat, carbohydrate, or protein.

6 Meeting Lipid Needs 145

- The DRIs recommend that adults consume a diet that provides 20 to 35% of energy from fat and is low in cholesterol, saturated fat, and *trans* fat. The Dietary Guidelines recommend limiting saturated fatty acid intake to less than 10% of total calories, limiting cholesterol to 300 mg per day, and avoiding *trans* fat. It is recommended that individuals with heart disease or a high risk of heart disease limit their intake even further.
- The U.S. diet is not too high in fat, but it often does not contain the healthiest types of fats. To reduce saturated fat and cholesterol intake, limit solid fats and choose liquid oils, fish, and nuts and seeds often. Use food labels like the one shown here to avoid processed foods that are high in saturated and *trans* fat. A diet based on whole grains, fruits, vegetables, and lean meats and low-fat dairy products will meet the recommendations for fat intake.

Lipids on food labels • Figure 5.19a

Chocolate Chip Cookies

Nutrition Facts
Serving Size 3 Cookies (33g)
Servings Per Container About 13

Amount Per Serving	
Calories 160	*Calories from Fat* 70
	% Daily Value*
Total Fat 8g	**12%**
Saturated Fat 3g	**15%**
Trans Fat 0g	
Polyunsat Fat 2.5g	
Monounsat Fat 2g	
Cholesterol 0mg	**0%**
Sodium 110mg	**5%**
Potassium 45mg	**1%**
Total Carbohydrate 22g	**7%**
Dietary Fiber Less than 1gram	**3%**
Sugars 11g	
Protein 2g	

- Fat replacers are used to create reduced-fat products with taste and texture similar to the original. Some low-fat products are made by using mixtures of carbohydrates or proteins to simulate the properties of fat, and some use lipids that are modified to reduce their digestion and absorption. Products containing fat replacers can help reduce fat and energy intake when used in moderation as part of a balanced diet.

Key Terms

- adipose tissue 136
- alpha-linolenic acid (α-linolenic acid) 136
- antioxidant 145
- arachidonic acid 137
- atherosclerosis 140
- atherosclerotic plaque 141
- cardiovascular disease 140
- cholesterol 132
- chylomicron 134
- docosahexaenoic acid (DHA) 137
- eicosanoids 138
- eicosapentaenoic acid (EPA) 137
- emulsifier 131
- essential fatty acid 130
- essential fatty acid deficiency 137
- fasting 139
- fat 124
- fatty acid 127
- feasting 139
- foam cell 140
- high-density lipoprotein (HDL) 136
- hydrogenation 130
- inflammation 140
- LDL receptor 135
- lecithin 131
- linoleic acid 136
- lipid bilayer 131
- lipids 127
- lipoprotein 134
- lipoprotein lipase 135
- low-density lipoprotein (LDL) 136
- macrophage 140
- micelle 134
- monoglyceride 134
- monounsaturated fatty acid 128
- omega-3 fatty acid 129
- omega-6 fatty acid 129
- oxidized LDL cholesterol 140
- partially hydrogenated oils 130
- phosphate group 131
- phospholipid 128
- plant sterol 132
- polyunsaturated fatty acid 129
- saturated fat 127
- saturated fatty acid 129
- sterol 128
- *trans* fat 127
- *trans* fatty acid 129
- triglyceride 127
- tropical oil 130
- unsaturated fat 127
- unsaturated fatty acid 129
- very-low-density lipoprotein (VLDL) 136

What is happening in this picture?

This hand belongs to an individual with familial hypercholesterolemia, a rare genetic disease in which the LDL receptors on cells do not function properly. It causes cholesterol levels so high that the cholesterol deposits in body tissues, seen here as raised lumps.

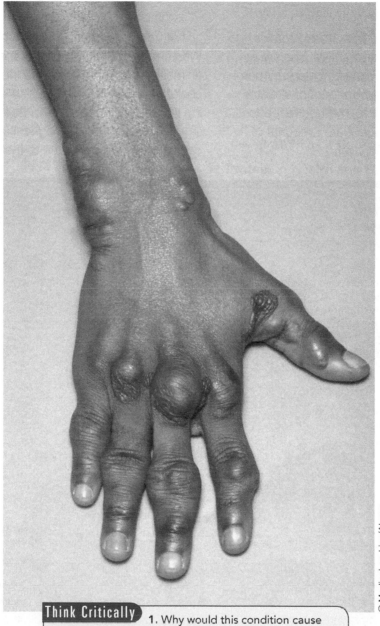

© Medical-on-Line/Alamy

Think Critically
1. Why would this condition cause elevated blood cholesterol?
2. How would this condition affect the risk of developing heart disease?

THE PLANNER ✓

Review your Chapter Planner on the chapter opener and check off your completed work.

6.1 Proteins in Our Food

LEARNING OBJECTIVES

1. **Describe** the types of foods that provide the most concentrated sources of protein.

2. **Compare** the nutrients in plant sources of protein with those in animal sources of protein.

When we think of protein, we usually think of a steak, a plate of scrambled eggs, or a glass of milk. These animal foods provide the most concentrated sources of protein in our diet, but plant foods such as grains, nuts, and **legumes** are also important sources of dietary protein. The proteins found in plants are made up of different combinations of **amino acids** than proteins found in animals. Because of this difference, most plant proteins are not used as efficiently as animal proteins to build proteins in the human body. Nevertheless, a diet that includes a variety of plant proteins can easily meet most people's protein needs.

The sources of protein in your diet have an impact not only on the amount of protein and variety of amino acids available to your body but also on what other nutrients you are consuming (**Figure 6.1**). Animal products provide B vitamins and readily absorbable sources of minerals, such as iron, zinc, and calcium. They are low in fiber, however, and are often high in saturated fat and cholesterol—a nutrient mix that increases the risk of heart disease.

Plant sources of protein provide B vitamins except vitamin B_{12} and supply iron, zinc, and calcium, but often these minerals are less absorbable than they are from animal products. Plant foods are generally excellent sources of fiber, phytochemicals, and unsaturated fats—dietary substances that promote health. Recommendations for a healthy diet, including the Dietary Guidelines and MyPlate, suggest that our diets be based on whole grains, vegetables, and fruits and include smaller amounts of meats and dairy products. Following these guidelines will provide plenty of protein from a mixture of plant and animal sources.

> **legume** The starchy seed of a plant that produces bean pods; includes peas, peanuts, beans, soybeans, and lentils.

> **amino acids** The building blocks of proteins. Each amino acid contains an amino group, an acid group, and a unique side chain.

CONCEPT CHECK STOP

1. **Which** is higher in protein: an egg or a cup of rice?

2. **How** do the nutrients provided by meat and milk differ from those in grains and legumes?

Animal versus plant proteins • Figure 6.1

Animal sources of protein, such as those on the left, add saturated fat and cholesterol to the diet. Plant sources of protein, such as those on the right, are rich in fiber, phytochemicals, and monounsaturated and polyunsaturated fats.

© ACE STOCK LIMITED/Alamy

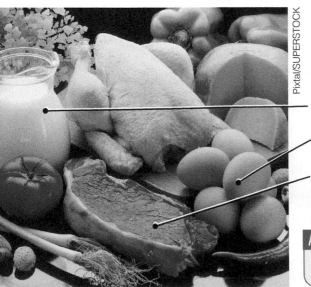

Pixtal/SUPERSTOCK

1 cup milk: 8 grams protein

One egg: 7 grams protein

3 ounces meat: over 20 grams protein

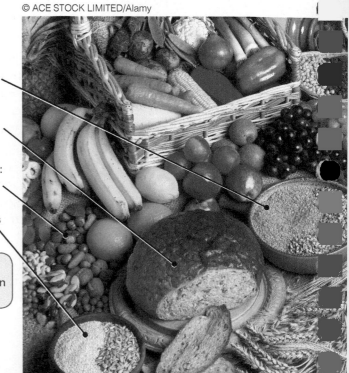

½ cup legumes: 6–10 grams protein

1 slice bread: about 2 grams protein

¼ cup nuts or seeds: 5–10 grams protein

½ cup rice, pasta, or cereal: 2–3 grams protein

Ask Yourself

Why might a diet high in animal protein increase the risk of heart disease?

The Structure of Amino Acids and Proteins

LEARNING OBJECTIVES

1. **Describe** the general structure of an amino acid and of a protein.
2. **Distinguish** between essential and nonessential amino acids.
3. **Discuss** how the order of amino acids in a polypeptide chain affects protein structure.
4. **Explain** how a protein's structure is related to its function.

What do the proteins in a lamb chop, a kidney bean, and your thigh muscle have in common? They are all constructed of amino acids linked together to form one or more folded, chainlike strands. Twenty amino acids are commonly found in proteins. Each kind of protein contains a different number, combination, and sequence of amino acids. These differences give proteins their specific functions in living organisms and their unique characteristics in foods.

Amino Acid Structure

Each amino acid consists of a central carbon atom that is bound to a hydrogen atom; an amino group, which contains nitrogen; an acid group; and a side chain (**Figure 6.2a**). The nitrogen in amino acids distinguishes protein from carbohydrate and fat; all three contain carbon, hydrogen, and oxygen, but only protein contains nitrogen. The side chains of amino acids vary in size and structure; they give different amino acids their unique properties.

> **essential amino acid (or indispensable) amino acid** An amino acid that cannot be synthesized by the body in sufficient amounts to meet its needs and therefore must be included in the diet.

Nine of the amino acids needed by the adult human body must be consumed in the diet because they cannot be made in the body (see Figure 6.2a). If the diet is deficient in one or more of these **essential amino acids** (also called **indispensable amino acids**), the body cannot make new proteins without breaking down existing proteins to provide the needed amino acids. The other 11 amino acids that are commonly found in protein are **nonessential**, or **dispensable**, **amino acids** because they can be made in the body.

Under certain conditions, some of the nonessential amino acids cannot be synthesized in sufficient amounts to meet the body's needs. These are therefore referred to as **conditionally essential amino acids**. For example, the amino acid tyrosine can be made in the body from the essential amino acid phenylalanine. In individuals who have the inherited disease **phenylketonuria (PKU)**, phenylalanine cannot be converted into tyrosine, so tyrosine is an essential amino acid for these individuals (see *What a Scientist Sees* on page 161).

> **phenylketonuria (PKU)** A genetic disease in which the amino acid phenylalanine cannot be metabolized normally, causing it to build up in the blood. If untreated, the condition results in brain damage.

Protein Structure

To form proteins, amino acids are linked together by **peptide bonds**, which join the acid group of one amino acid to the amino group of another amino acid (**Figure 6.2b**). Many amino acids bonded together constitute a **polypeptide**. A protein is made up of one or more polypeptide chains that are folded into three-dimensional shapes.

> **polypeptide** A chain of amino acids linked by peptide bonds that is part of the structure of a protein.

The order and chemical properties of the amino acids in a polypeptide determine its final shape because the folding of the chain occurs in response to forces that attract or repel amino acids from one another or from water. The folded polypeptide chain may constitute the final protein, or it may join with several other folded polypeptide chains to form the final structure of the protein (see Figure 6.2b).

The shape of a protein is essential to its function. For example, the elongated shape of the protein collagen, found in connective tissue, helps it give strength to tendons and ligaments. The spherical shape of the protein hemoglobin contributes to the proper functioning of red blood cells, and the linear shape of muscle proteins allows them to overlap and shorten muscles during contraction.

Amino acids all have the same basic structure. How they are linked together in the polypeptide chain determines the three-dimensional shape and function of the protein.

Amino acid

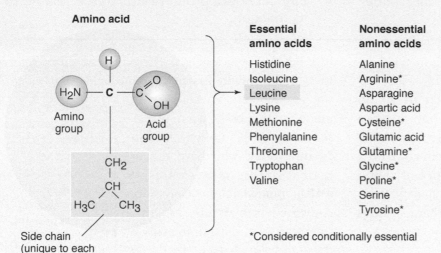

Amino group

Acid group

Side chain (unique to each amino acid)

Essential amino acids	Nonessential amino acids
Histidine	Alanine
Isoleucine	Arginine*
Leucine	Asparagine
Lysine	Aspartic acid
Methionine	Cysteine*
Phenylalanine	Glutamic acid
Threonine	Glutamine*
Tryptophan	Glycine*
Valine	Proline*
	Serine
	Tyrosine*

*Considered conditionally essential

a. All "amino" "acids" have a similar structure that includes an amino group and an acid group, giving them their name, but each has a different side chain. Of the 20 amino acids in proteins 9 are considered dietary essentials because they cannot be made in the body.

b. Amino acids linked by peptide bonds are called **peptides**. When two amino acids are linked, they form a **dipeptide**; three form a **tripeptide**. Many amino acids bonded together constitute a polypeptide. Polypeptide chains may contain hundreds of amino acids. The final structure of a protein molecule consists of one or more folded polypeptide chains.

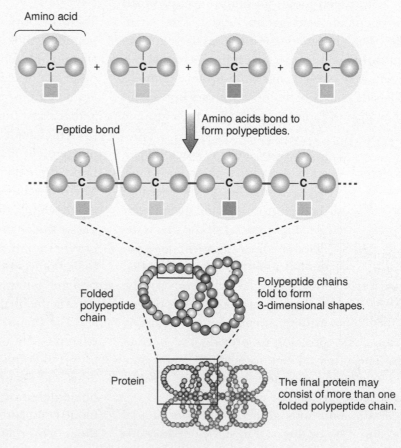

Amino acid

Peptide bond

Amino acids bond to form polypeptides.

Folded polypeptide chain

Polypeptide chains fold to form 3-dimensional shapes.

Protein

The final protein may consist of more than one folded polypeptide chain.

WHAT A SCIENTIST SEES
Phenylketonuria

The warning on this can of diet soda probably doesn't mean much unless you have the genetic disease phenylketonuria (PKU). Individuals with PKU must limit their intake of the amino acid phenylalanine. Usually this means limiting their consumption of high-protein foods. When a scientist looks at this label, she recognizes that the artificial sweetener aspartame in this soda is the source of the phenylalanine. The breakdown of aspartame in the digestive tract releases phenylalanine, which cannot be properly metabolized by individuals with PKU. If they consume large amounts of this amino acid, compounds called phenylketones build up in their blood. In infants and young children, phenylketones interfere with brain development, and in pregnant women they cause birth defects in the baby. To prevent these effects, individuals with PKU must consume a diet that provides just enough phenylalanine to meet the body's needs but not so much that phenylketones build up in their blood.

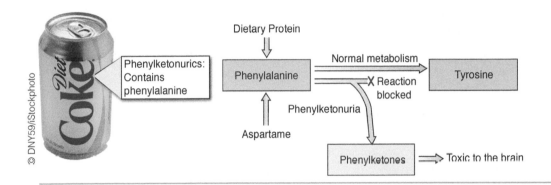

Think Critically Why do you think this warning appears on diet soda labels but not on labels for high-protein foods such as meat and milk?

Protein denaturation • Figure 6.3

When an egg is cooked, the heat denatures the protein, causing the polypeptide chains to unfold. The protein in a raw egg white forms a clear, viscous liquid, but when heat denatures it, the cooked egg white becomes white and firm and cannot be restored to its original form. The denaturation of proteins in our food also creates other characteristics we desire. For example, whipped cream is made when mechanical agitation denatures the protein in cream.

When the shape of a protein is altered, the protein no longer functions normally. For example, when the enzyme salivary amylase, which is a protein, enters the stomach, the acid causes the structure of the protein to change, and it no longer functions in the digestion of starch. This change in structure is called **denaturation**, referring to a change from the natural. Proteins in food are often denatured during processing and cooking (**Figure 6.3**).

> **denaturation**
> Alteration of a protein's three-dimensional structure.

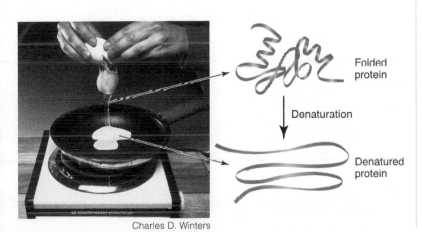

Folded protein

Denaturation

Denatured protein

Charles D. Winters

CONCEPT CHECK   STOP

1. **Which** chemical elements are found in all amino acids?

2. **What** determines whether an amino acid is essential in the diet?

3. **What** determines the shape of a protein?

4. **How** does denaturation affect the function of proteins?

Protein digestion and absorption • Figure 6.4

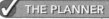

Protein must be broken down into small peptides and amino acids to be absorbed into the mucosal cells.

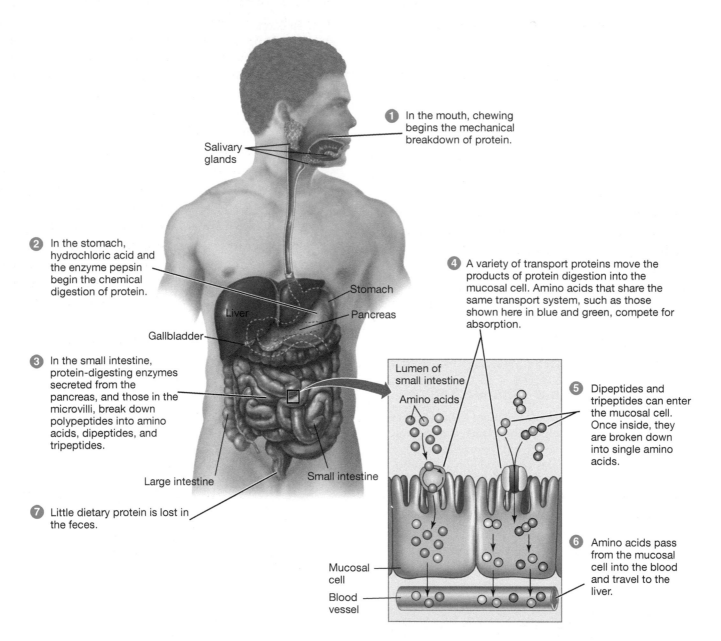

1 In the mouth, chewing begins the mechanical breakdown of protein.

Salivary glands

2 In the stomach, hydrochloric acid and the enzyme pepsin begin the chemical digestion of protein.

4 A variety of transport proteins move the products of protein digestion into the mucosal cell. Amino acids that share the same transport system, such as those shown here in blue and green, compete for absorption.

Stomach

Liver

Pancreas

Gallbladder

3 In the small intestine, protein-digesting enzymes secreted from the pancreas, and those in the microvilli, break down polypeptides into amino acids, dipeptides, and tripeptides.

Lumen of small intestine

Amino acids

5 Dipeptides and tripeptides can enter the mucosal cell. Once inside, they are broken down into single amino acids.

Large intestine

Small intestine

7 Little dietary protein is lost in the feces.

Mucosal cell

Blood vessel

6 Amino acids pass from the mucosal cell into the blood and travel to the liver.

Think Critically

When you eat a burger, do the muscle protein molecules from the cow end up in your muscles? Why or why not?

6.3 Protein Digestion and Absorption

LEARNING OBJECTIVES

1. **Describe** the process of protein digestion.
2. **Discuss** how amino acids are absorbed.

Proteins must be digested before their amino acids can be absorbed into the body (**Figure 6.4**). The chemical digestion of protein begins in the acid environment of the stomach. Here, hydrochloric acid denatures proteins, opening up their folded structure to make the polypeptide chains more accessible for breakdown by enzymes. Stomach acid also activates the protein-digesting enzyme *pepsin*, which breaks some of the peptide bonds in the polypeptide chains, leaving shorter polypeptides. Most protein digestion occurs in the small intestine, where polypeptides are broken into even smaller peptides and amino acids by protein-digesting enzymes produced in the pancreas and small intestine. Single amino acids, dipeptides, and tripeptides are absorbed into the mucosal cells of the small intestine.

Because protein must be broken down in order to be absorbed, proteins consumed in the diet enter the body as a collection of individual amino acids, not as functioning proteins. Supplements of specific proteins therefore do not retain their function in the body. For example, an enzyme supplement advertised to destroy free radicals, eliminate toxins, or enhance muscle growth will not provide these functions in the body because the amino acids that make up the enzyme, not the enzyme itself, are what enters the body. Supplements of enzymes that function in the GI tract, such as lactase, taken to prevent the symptoms of lactose intolerance, retain enzyme activity long enough to break down the lactose in the intestine but are also eventually digested to amino acids, which are then absorbed.

Amino acids from protein digestion enter your body by crossing from the lumen of the small intestine into the mucosal cells and then into the blood. This process involves one of several energy-requiring amino acid transport systems. Amino acids with similar structures use the same transport system (see Figure 6.4). As a result, amino acids may compete with one another for absorption. If there is an excess of any one of the amino acids sharing a transport system, more of it will be absorbed, slowing the absorption of competing amino acids. This competition for absorption is usually not a problem because foods contain a variety of amino acids, none of which are present in excessive amounts. However, when people consume amino acid supplements, the supplemented amino acid may overwhelm the transport system, reducing the absorption of other amino acids that share the same transport system. For example, weight lifters often take supplements of the amino acid arginine. Because arginine shares a transport system with lysine, large doses of arginine can inhibit the absorption of lysine, upsetting the balance of amino acids in the body.

CONCEPT CHECK STOP

1. **Where** does the chemical digestion of protein begin?
2. **Why** might supplementing one amino acid reduce the absorption of other amino acids?

6.4 Protein Synthesis and Functions

LEARNING OBJECTIVES

1. **Discuss** the steps involved in synthesizing proteins.
2. **Explain** what is meant by the term *limiting amino acid*.
3. **Name** four general functions provided by body proteins.
4. **Describe** the conditions under which the body uses protein to provide energy.

As discussed earlier, proteins are made from amino acids. Amino acids are also used to make other nitrogen-containing molecules, including neurotransmitters; the units that make up DNA and RNA; the skin pigment melanin; the vitamin niacin; creatine phosphate, which is used to fuel muscle contraction; and histamine, which causes blood vessels to dilate. In some situations, amino acids from proteins are also used to provide energy or synthesize glucose or fatty acids.

The amino acids available for these functions come from the proteins consumed in the diet and from the breakdown of body proteins. These amino acids are referred to collectively as the **amino acid pool** (**Figure 6.5**). There is not actually a "pool" in the body

amino acid pool
All the amino acids in body tissues and fluids that are available for use by the body.

containing a collection of amino acids, but these molecules are available in body fluids and cells to provide the raw materials needed to synthesize proteins and other molecules.

Synthesizing Proteins

The instructions for making proteins are contained in the nucleus of the cell in stretches of DNA called

gene A length of DNA that contains the information needed to synthesize a polypeptide chain.

genes. When a protein is needed, the process of protein synthesis begins, and the information contained in the gene is used to make the necessary protein (**Figure 6.6**).

Regulating protein synthesis Both the types of proteins made and when they are made are carefully regulated by increasing or decreasing **gene expression**. When a gene is expressed, the protein it codes for is made. Not all genes are expressed in all cells or at all times; only the proteins that are needed are made at any given time. Which genes are expressed is also affected by genetic background and by the nutrients and other food

components we consume (see *Debate: Is Personalized Nutrition the Best Approach to Reducing Chronic Disease?* on page 166).

The regulation of gene expression allows the body to save energy and resources. For example, when your diet is high in iron, expression of the gene that codes for the protein ferritin, which stores iron, izs increased. This causes more ferritin to be synthesized and allows the body to store extra iron in this protein. When the diet is low in iron, the production of ferritin is suppressed so that the body doesn't waste amino acids and energy making large amounts of a protein that it doesn't need.

Limiting amino acids During the synthesis of a protein, a shortage of one amino acid can stop the process. This is similar to an assembly line, where if one part is missing, the line stops; a different part cannot be substituted. If the missing amino acid is a nonessential amino acid, it can be made in the body, and protein

synthesis can continue. Most non-essential amino acids are made through a process called **transamination**, which involves transferring the amino group from one amino acid to a carbon-containing molecule to form the needed amino acid (**Figure 6.6a**). If the

transamination
The process by which an amino group from one amino acid is transferred to a carbon compound to form a new amino acid.

missing amino acid is an essential amino acid, the body cannot make the amino acid, but it can break down its own protein to obtain it, allowing protein synthesis to proceed (**Figure 6.6b**). If an amino acid cannot be supplied, protein synthesis will stop.

Amino acid pool • Figure 6.5

Amino acids enter the available pool from the diet and from the breakdown of body proteins. Of the approximately 300 g of protein synthesized by the body each day, only about 100 g are made from amino acids consumed in the diet. The other 200 g are produced using amino acids recycled from protein broken down in the body. Amino acids in the pool can be used to synthesize body proteins and other nitrogen-containing molecules, to provide energy, or to synthesize glucose or fatty acids.

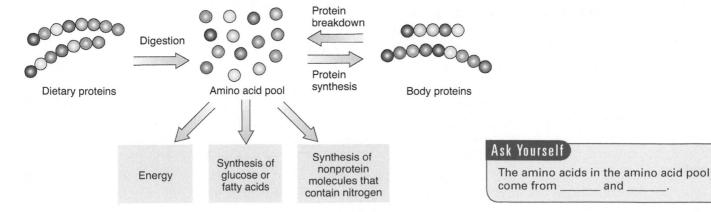

Dietary proteins → Digestion → Amino acid pool → Protein synthesis → Body proteins ; Protein breakdown

Energy ; Synthesis of glucose or fatty acids ; Synthesis of nonprotein molecules that contain nitrogen

Ask Yourself
The amino acids in the amino acid pool come from _____ and _____.

Protein is synthesized from amino acids. All of the amino acids in the protein must be available for protein synthesis to proceed.

a. Amino acids come from protein in the diet and from the breakdown of body proteins. Some can be made in the body by transamination.

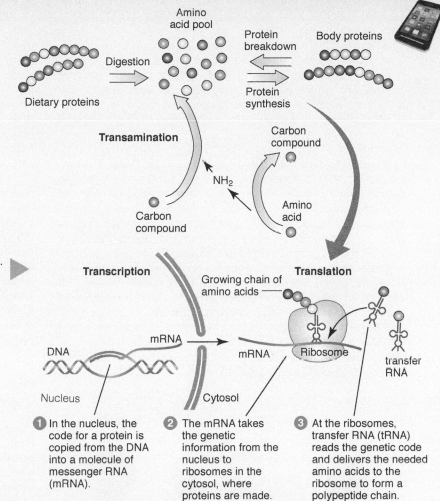

b. The instructions for protein synthesis come from genes. The process of protein synthesis involves **transcription** and **translation**.

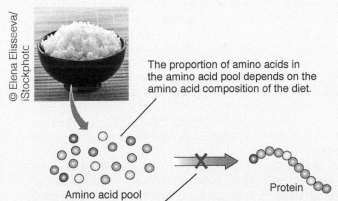

The proportion of amino acids in the amino acid pool depends on the amino acid composition of the diet.

Amino acid pool

A shortage of the amino acid represented by the orange spheres limits the ability to synthesize a protein that is high in this amino acid.

Protein

① In the nucleus, the code for a protein is copied from the DNA into a molecule of messenger RNA (mRNA).

② The mRNA takes the genetic information from the nucleus to ribosomes in the cytosol, where proteins are made.

③ At the ribosomes, transfer RNA (tRNA) reads the genetic code and delivers the needed amino acids to the ribosome to form a polypeptide chain.

c. Amino acids needed for protein synthesis come from the amino acid pool. If the protein to be made requires more of a particular amino acid than is available, that amino acid limits protein synthesis and is referred to as the *limiting amino acid*.

© Elena Elisseeva/iStockphoto

The essential amino acid that is present in shortest supply relative to the body's need for it is called the **limiting amino acid** because lack of this amino acid limits the ability to synthesize protein (**Figure 6.6c**). Different food sources of protein provide different combinations of amino acids. The limiting amino acid in a food is the one supplied in the lowest amount relative to the body's need. For example, lysine is the limiting amino acid in wheat, whereas methionine is the limiting amino acid in beans. When the diet provides adequate amounts of all the essential amino acids needed to synthesize a specific protein, synthesis of

> **limiting amino acid** The essential amino acid that is available in the lowest concentration relative to the body's need.

the polypeptide chains that make up the protein can be completed (see Figure 6.6b).

Proteins Provide Structure and Regulation

When you think of the protein in your body, you probably think of muscle, but muscle contains only a few of the many types of proteins found in your body. There are more than 500,000 proteins in the human body, each with a specific function. Some perform important structural roles, and others help regulate specific body processes.

Structural proteins are found in skin, hair, ligaments, and tendons (**Figure 6.7a** on page 167). Proteins also provide structure to individual cells, where they are an

Is Personalized Nutrition the Best Approach to Reducing Chronic Disease?

✓ THE PLANNER

The Issue: The concept of personalized nutrition suggests that you could be prescribed a diet based on your genetic makeup that could prevent, moderate, or cure the chronic diseases for which you are at risk. But genetics are not the only factor in determining your disease risk. So is an individualized diet prescription a better path to health than choosing an overall healthy diet?

Our health is determined by many factors, including environment, lifestyle, and genetics. We have control over lifestyle factors that affect our disease risk, such as what we eat and how much we exercise. We don't have control over our genetic background. Nutrigenomics suggests that we can reduce our risk of disease by tailoring our diets to our individual genetic makeup (see figure and Chapter 1)[1] This new science predicts that someday we may to go to the doctor's office, have our genes analyzed, and then have specific foods and dietary supplements prescribed to optimize our health and prevent diseases to which we are susceptible.

Current nutrition guidelines are designed to improve and maintain the health of almost all healthy people in the population. Yet, we know that different people respond differently to the same diet, so dietary advice that is good for the majority of people may not be optimum for everyone. Modern medicine is already practicing nutrigenomics at a very basic level; dietitians design special diets based on patients' existing medical conditions. People with elevated blood lipids are instructed to reduce their intake of saturated fat and increase their fiber intake, those with high blood pressure are shown how to reduce their salt intake, and people with diabetes are taught how to manage blood sugar levels by modifying their carbohydrate intake.

Proponents of nutrigenomics suggest that reviewing an individual's genetic analysis will permit the development of more personalized dietary recommendations and these will prevent or improve outcomes for a variety of chronic diseases.[2] These diets could be customized to take into consideration not only individual genetic variation, but also life stage, dietary preferences, and other aspects of health status.[3] Some propose that if followed, these personalized dietary recommendations may supplement and even replace prescription drugs.

Would the benefit of these individualized diet plans justify the expense of the genetic analyses? Some argue that this approach is unlikely to improve individual or public health.[4] Many people fail to follow current population-wide guidelines for a healthy diet, not because they lack the knowledge, money, or motivation to do so, but simply because they choose not to. Therefore, it is unlikely that individuals will follow personalized guidelines any better or that genetic test results will motivate them to eat a healthier diet.[5,6] The priority for public health dollars should not be to fine-tune diet prescriptions, but to find out what will make people change their diets and live healthier lives.

Other concerns with nutrigenomics are the ethics of widespread genetic testing and the possibility that commercial interests will drive nutrigenomics rather than any benefits to public health.[6] People who strictly adhere to their diet prescriptions will certainly benefit, but the big beneficiaries of personalized diet prescriptions could be biotech companies, which would profit from genetic testing needed to establish disease profiles, and the food industry, which would benefit from the creation and sale of functional foods to prevent disease.[4] There is also concern that personalized nutrition will be very costly; perhaps reserved for those with money and education.[3]

In the future, will we select breakfast cereals and dietary supplements based on our genes? Will these choices, which target the prevention of some potential chronic diseases, increase the risk of others? Will following personalized dietary prescriptions make us healthier than just choosing an overall healthy diet? In choosing foods based on nutrigenomics will we lose track of the pleasure we get from food and the cultural and social roles that food plays in our lives?

Zoe's genetic background

Nathan's genetic background

Zoe's individualized diet

Nathan's individualized diet

Optimal health

Think Critically: If genetic testing determines that you are at low risk of type 2 diabetes, does this mean that you can eat as much refined sugar as you want? Why or why not?

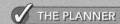

The proteins that are part of the human body perform a myriad of structural and regulatory roles.

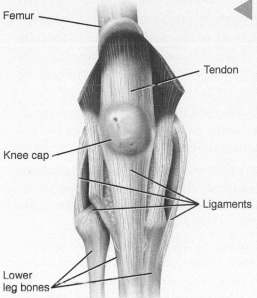

Femur — Tendon — Knee cap — Ligaments — Lower leg bones

a. Collagen is the most abundant protein in the body. It is the major protein in ligaments, which hold our bones together, and in tendons, which attach muscles to bones, and it forms the protein framework of bones and teeth.

b. Enzymes, such as this one, are protein molecules. Almost all the chemical reactions occurring within the body require the help of enzymes. Each enzyme has a structure or shape that allows it to interact with the specific molecules in the reaction it accelerates. Without enzymes, metabolic reactions would occur too slowly to support life.

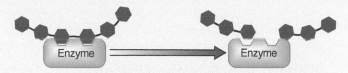

Enzyme → Enzyme

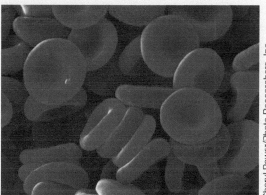

Cheryl Power/Photo Researchers, Inc.

c. Proteins help transport materials throughout the body and into and out of cells. The protein hemoglobin, which gives these red blood cells their color, shuttles oxygen to body cells and carries away carbon dioxide.

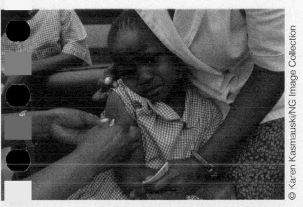

© Karen Kasmauski/NG Image Collection

e. Proteins help us move. The proteins actin and myosin in the arm and leg muscles of this rock climber are able to slide past each other to contract the muscles. A similar process causes contraction in the heart muscle and in the muscles of the digestive tract, blood vessels, and body glands.

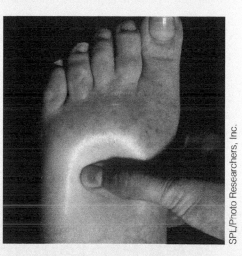

SPL/Photo Researchers, Inc.

d. Proteins help protect us from disease. This child is being immunized against measles. The vaccine contains a small amount of dead or inactivated measles virus. It does not make the child sick, but it does stimulate her immune system to make proteins called *antibodies*, which help destroy the measles virus and prevent the child from contracting the disease.

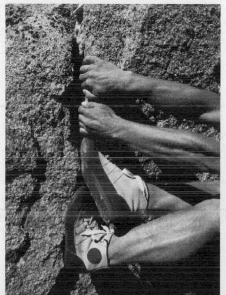

Gordon Wiltsie/NG Image Collection

f. Proteins help regulate fluid balance through their effect on *osmosis*. Blood proteins help hold fluid in the blood because they contribute to the number of dissolved particles in the blood. If protein levels in the blood fall too low, water leaks out of the blood vessels and accumulates in the tissues, causing swelling known as **edema**, shown here. Proteins also regulate fluid balance because some are membrane transporters, which pump dissolved substances from one side of a membrane to the other.

integral part of the cell membrane, cytosol, and organelles. Proteins such as enzymes, which speed up biochemical reactions (**Figure 6.7b**), and transport proteins that travel in the blood or help materials cross membranes, regulate processes throughout the body (**Figure 6.7c**).

Proteins are an important part of the body's defense mechanisms. Skin, which is made up primarily of protein, is the first barrier against infection and injury. Foreign particles such as dirt or bacteria that are on the skin cannot enter the body and can be washed away. If the skin is broken and blood vessels are injured, blood-clotting proteins help prevent too much blood from being lost. If a foreign material does get into the body, *antibodies*, which are immune system proteins, help destroy it (**Figure 6.7d**).

Some proteins have contractile properties, which allow muscles to move various parts of the body (**Figure 6.7e**). Others are hormones, which regulate biological processes. The hormones insulin, growth hormone, and glucagon are made from amino acids. These protein hormones act rapidly because they affect the activity of proteins that are already present in the cell.

Proteins also help regulate fluid balance (**Figure 6.7f**) and prevent the level of acidity in body fluids from deviating from the normal range. The chemical reactions of metabolism require a specific level of acidity, or pH, to function properly. Inside the body, pH must be maintained at a relatively neutral level in order to allow metabolic reactions to proceed normally. If the pH changes, these reactions slow or stop. Proteins both within cells and in the blood help prevent large changes in pH.

Protein as a Source of Energy

In addition to all the essential functions performed by body proteins, under some circumstances, proteins can be broken down and their amino acids used to provide energy or synthesize glucose or fatty acids (**Figure 6.8**). When the diet does not provide enough energy to meet the body's needs, such as during starvation or when consuming a low-calorie weight-loss diet, body protein is used to provide energy. Because our bodies do not store protein, functional body proteins, such as enzymes and muscle proteins, must be broken down to yield amino acids, which can then be used as fuel or to make glucose. This ensures that cells have a constant energy supply but also robs the body of the functions performed by these proteins.

Amino acids are also used for energy when the amount of protein consumed in the diet is greater than that needed to make body proteins and other molecules. This occurs in most Americans every day because our typical diet contains more protein than we need. The body first uses amino acids from the diet to make body proteins and other nitrogen-containing molecules. Then, because extra amino acids can't be stored, they are metabolized to provide energy. When your diet includes more energy and protein than you need, amino acids can be converted into fatty acids, which are stored as triglycerides, thus contributing to weight gain.

CONCEPT CHECK 🛑 STOP

1. **How** does the body know in what order to assemble the amino acids when making a protein?

2. **Why** does protein synthesis stop when the supply of an amino acid is limited?

3. **What** type of protein speeds up chemical reactions?

4. **When** is protein used as an energy source?

6.5 Protein in Health and Disease

LEARNING OBJECTIVES

1. **Distinguish** kwashiorkor from marasmus.

2. **Explain** why protein-energy malnutrition is more common in children than in adults.

3. **Discuss** the potential risks associated with high-protein diets.

4. **Explain** how a dietary protein can trigger a food allergy.

W e need to eat protein to stay healthy. If we don't eat enough of it, less-essential body proteins are broken down, and their amino acids are used to synthesize proteins that are critical for survival. For example, when the diet is deficient in protein, muscle protein is broken down to provide amino acids to make hormones and enzymes for which there is an immediate need. If protein deficiency

Producing ATP from amino acids • Figure 6.8

Amino acids from dietary or body protein can be used to produce ATP. First, the amino group (NH_2) must be removed through a process called **deamination**. The remaining compound, composed of carbon, hydrogen, and oxygen, can then be broken down to produce ATP or used to make glucose or fatty acids.

1 The amino group is removed by deamination and converted into the waste product **urea**. Urea is removed from the blood by the kidneys and excreted in the urine.

2 Deamination of some amino acids results in three-carbon molecules that can be used to synthesize glucose.

3 Deamination of some amino acids results in acetyl-CoA that enters the citric acid cycle.

4 Deamination of some amino acids forms molecules that enter the citric acid cycle directly.

5 The acetyl-CoA derived from the breakdown of amino acids can be used to synthesize fatty acids. This occurs when calories and protein are consumed in excess of needs.

6 In the final step of aerobic metabolism, the energy released from the amino acid molecules is transferred to ATP.

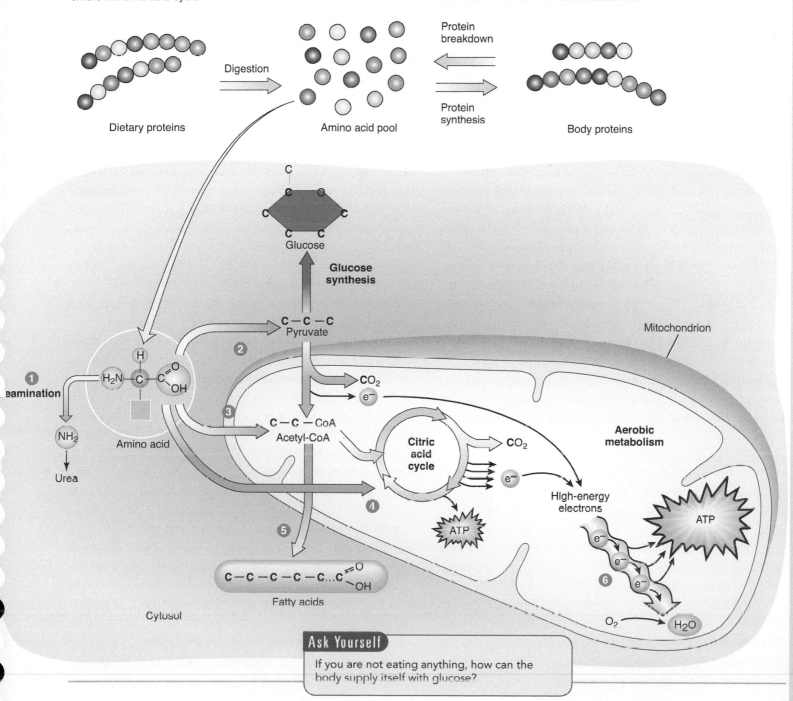

Dietary proteins

Digestion

Amino acid pool

Protein breakdown

Protein synthesis

Body proteins

Glucose

Glucose synthesis

C — C — C
Pyruvate

Mitochondrion

CO_2

e^-

C — C — CoA
Acetyl-CoA

1 eamination

H

H_2N — C — C⚬O
                    OH

Amino acid

NH_2

Urea

Citric acid cycle

CO_2

Aerobic metabolism

e^-

High-energy electrons

ATP

e^-

e^-

ATP

e^-

C — C — C — C — C...C⚬O
                         OH

Fatty acids

Cytosol

O_2

H_2O

Ask Yourself

If you are not eating anything, how can the body supply itself with glucose?

continues, eventually so much body protein is lost that all life-sustaining functions cannot be supported. In some cases, too much protein or the wrong proteins can also contribute to health problems.

Protein Deficiency

Protein deficiency is a great concern in the developing world but generally not a problem in economically developed societies, where plant and animal sources of protein are abundant (**Figure 6.9a**). Usually, protein deficiency occurs along with a general lack of food and other nutrients. The term **protein-energy malnutrition (PEM)** is used to refer to a continuum of conditions ranging from pure protein deficiency, called **kwashiorkor**, to an overall energy deficiency, called **marasmus**.

Protein deficiency occurs when the diet is very low in protein or when protein needs are high, as they are in young children. Hence, kwashiorkor is typically a disease found in children (**Figure 6.9b**). The word *kwashiorkor* comes from the Ga language of coastal Ghana. It means "the disease that the first child gets when a second child is born."[7] When the new baby is born, the older child is no longer breast-fed. Rather than receiving protein-rich breast milk, the young child is fed a watered-down version of the diet eaten by the rest of the family. This diet is low in protein and often high in fiber and difficult to digest. The child, even if he or she is able to obtain adequate calories from the diet, may not be able to eat a large enough quantity to get adequate protein. Because children are growing, their protein needs per unit of body weight are higher than those of adults, and a deficiency occurs more quickly. Although kwashiorkor only occurs in those whose diet is deficient in protein, it is associated with, or even triggered by, infectious diseases.

At the other end of the continuum of protein-energy malnutrition is marasmus, meaning "to waste away" (**Figure 6.9c**). Marasmus is caused by starvation; the diet doesn't supply enough calories or nutrients to meet the body's needs. Marasmus may have some of the same symptoms as kwashiorkor, but there are differences. In kwashiorkor, some fat stores are retained because energy intake is adequate. In marasmus, individuals appear emaciated because their stores of body fat have been depleted to provide energy. Although they are most common in children, both marasmus and kwashiorkor can occur in individuals of all ages.

High-Protein Diets and Health

The recent popularity of high-protein, low-carbohydrate diets for weight loss (see Chapters 4 and 9) has raised questions about whether consuming too much protein can be harmful. As protein intake increases, so does the production of protein-breakdown products, such as urea (see Figure 6.8), which must be eliminated from the body by the kidneys. This increases the workload of the kidneys, which may speed the progression of renal failure in people with kidney disease.[8] It is not clear whether a high-protein diet increases the likelihood of developing kidney disease in those with normal kidney function.[9] Because high-protein diets increase the amount of wastes that must be excreted in urine, they also increase water loss. Although not a concern for most people, this can be a problem if the kidneys are not able to concentrate urine, as is the case for infants. Feeding a newborn an infant formula that is too high in protein increases the amount of water lost in the urine and can lead to dehydration.

It has also been suggested that the amount and source of protein in the diet affect calcium status and bone health.[10] Adequate protein is essential for healthy bones, but too much protein has been shown to increase the amount of calcium lost in the urine. Some studies suggest that the amount of calcium lost in the urine is greater when protein comes from animal rather than vegetable sources.[10] These findings have contributed to a widely held belief that high-protein diets (especially diets that are high in animal protein) result in bone loss. However, clinical studies do not support the idea that animal protein has a detrimental effect on bone health or that bone is lost to provide the extra calcium lost in the urine.[11,12] In fact, when calcium intake is adequate, high-protein diets are associated with greater bone mass and fewer fractures.[11]

The increase in urinary calcium excretion associated with high-protein diets has led to speculation that a high-protein intake may increase the risk of kidney stones. Kidney stones are deposits of calcium and other substances in the kidneys and urinary tract. Higher concentrations of calcium and acid in the urine increase the likelihood

protein-energy malnutrition (PEM) A condition characterized by loss of muscle and fat mass and an increased susceptibility to infection that results from the long-term consumption of insufficient amounts of energy and/or protein to meet the body's needs.

kwashiorkor A form of protein-energy malnutrition in which only protein is deficient.

marasmus A form of protein-energy malnutrition in which a deficiency of energy in the diet causes severe body wasting.

Protein-energy malnutrition • Figure 6.9

Protein-energy malnutrition affects the health of children in many parts of the world.

a. Protein-energy malnutrition is uncommon in the United States and other developed nations, but in developing countries, it is a serious public health problem that results in high infant and child mortality. The highest prevalence is in sub-Saharan Africa and south Asia.

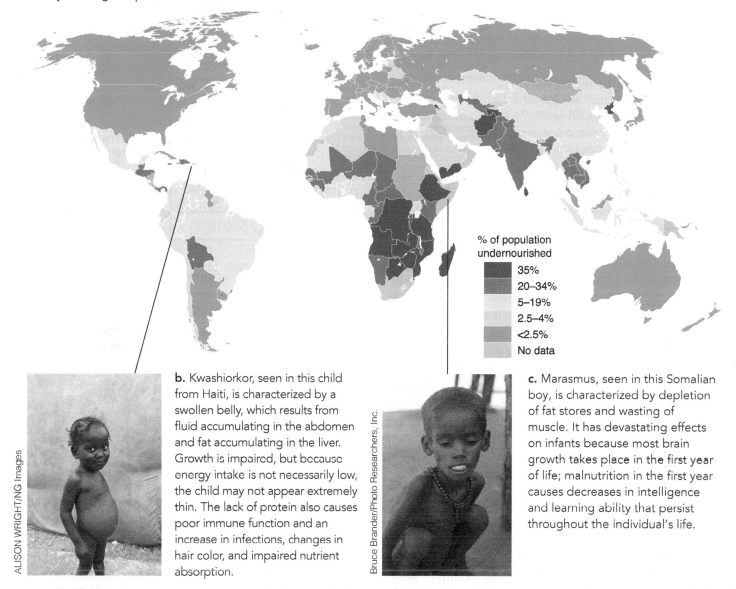

% of population undernourished
- 35%
- 20–34%
- 5–19%
- 2.5–4%
- <2.5%
- No data

ALISON WRIGHT/NG Images

Bruce Brander/Photo Researchers, Inc.

b. Kwashiorkor, seen in this child from Haiti, is characterized by a swollen belly, which results from fluid accumulating in the abdomen and fat accumulating in the liver. Growth is impaired, but because energy intake is not necessarily low, the child may not appear extremely thin. The lack of protein also causes poor immune function and an increase in infections, changes in hair color, and impaired nutrient absorption.

c. Marasmus, seen in this Somalian boy, is characterized by depletion of fat stores and wasting of muscle. It has devastating effects on infants because most brain growth takes place in the first year of life; malnutrition in the first year causes decreases in intelligence and learning ability that persist throughout the individual's life.

that the calcium will be deposited, forming these stones. Epidemiological studies suggest that diets that are rich in animal protein and low in fluid contribute to the formation of kidney stones.[13]

The best-documented concern with high-protein diets is related more to the rest of the diet than to the amount of protein consumed. Typically, high-protein diets are also high in animal products; this dietary pattern is high in saturated fat and cholesterol and low in fiber, and it therefore increases the risk of heart disease. These diets are also typically low in grains, vegetables, and fruits, a pattern associated with an increased risk of certain types of cancer.[14]

Proteins and Food Allergies and Intolerances

When a protein from the diet is absorbed without being completely digested, it can trigger a **food allergy**. The first time the protein

> **food allergy** An adverse immune response to a specific food protein.

Protein needs per unit of body weight decrease as growth slows. During the first year of life, growth is rapid, so a large amount of protein is required per unit of body weight. As growth rate slows during childhood and adolescence, requirements per unit of body weight decrease, but continue to be greater than adult requirements, until age 19.

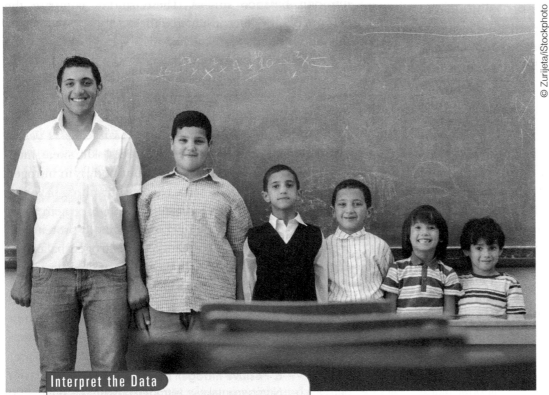

© Zurijeta/iStockphoto

Interpret the Data

What is the RDA for a 2-year-old child who weighs 14 kg?

a. 14 g/day   b. 15.4 g/day
c. 11.2 g/day   d. 21 g/day

Recommended Protein Intake

Most of us eat more protein than we need: Adult males in the United States consume almost 100 g of protein/day and adult females about 68 grams.[17] The RDA for protein for adults is 0.8 g/kg of body weight. For a person weighing 70 kg (154 lb), the RDA is 56 g of protein/day. RDAs have also been developed for each of the essential amino acids;[18] these are not a concern in typical diet planning but this information is important for the development of solutions for intravenous feeding.

Protein recommendations are expressed per unit of body weight because protein is needed to maintain and repair the body. The more a person weighs, the more protein he or she needs for those purposes. Because children are small, they need less total protein than adults do,

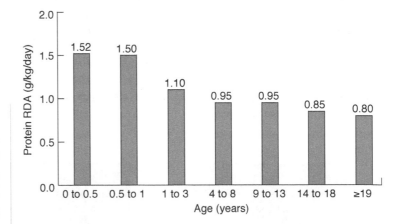

but because new protein must be synthesized for growth to occur, protein requirements per unit of body weight are much greater for infants and children than for adults (**Figure 6.12**). To calculate protein needs per day, multiply weight in kilograms (which equals weight in pounds multiplied by 0.45) by the recommended amount for the individual's age.

Protein needs are increased during pregnancy and lactation. Additional protein is needed during pregnancy to support the expansion of maternal blood volume, the growth of the uterus and breasts, the formation of the placenta, and the growth and development of the fetus. The RDA for pregnant women is 25 g of protein/day higher than the recommendation for nonpregnant women. An extra 25 g/day is also needed during lactation to provide protein for the production of breast milk.

The RDA for protein is not different for older adults, but because there is a decrease in energy needs with aging, the diet must be higher in protein relative to calories than in younger adults. There is also increasing evidence that older adults may benefit from a diet with more protein.[19] Declining muscle mass is a problem that affects health and the ability to maintain independence in the elderly. Protein intake that meets or, many believe, exceeds the current RDA, along with strength-training exercise, may delay loss of muscle mass and help maintain physical function and optimal health.[19]

Extreme stresses on the body, such as infections, fevers, burns, or surgery, increase the amount of protein that is broken down. For the body to heal and rebuild, the amount of protein lost must be replaced. The extra amount needed for healing depends on the injury. A severe infection may increase the body's protein needs by about 30%; a serious burn can increase protein requirements by 200 to 400%.

Although most athletes can meet their protein needs by consuming the RDA of 0.8 g/kg of body weight, endurance athletes and strength athletes benefit from higher protein intakes (**Figure 6.13**).[20] Athletes often think

Protein needs of athletes • Figure 6.13

Athletes who participate in endurance events and those engaged in muscle building need extra protein.

a. Endurance athletes need extra protein because some protein is used for energy and to maintain blood glucose during endurance events, such as triathlons and long-distance cross country skiing. Endurance athletes may benefit from the daily consumption of 1.2 to 1.4 g/kg of body weight.[20]

b. Strength athletes, such as weight lifters and body builders, need extra protein because it provides the raw materials needed for muscle growth; 1.2 to 1.7 g/kg/day is recommended.[20]

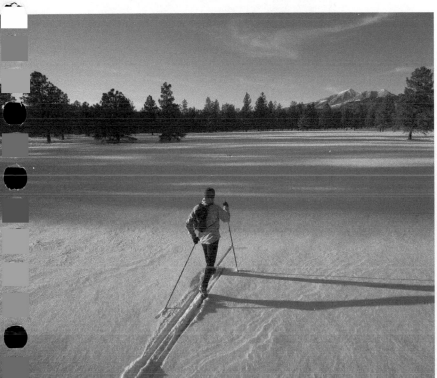

JOHN BURCHAM/NG Images

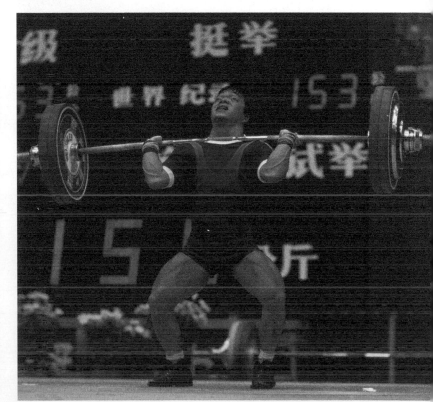

Michael Nichols/NG Image Collection

they need supplements to meet their higher protein needs (**Figure 6.14**). However, supplements tend to be an expensive way to increase protein intake. Because athletes typically need to consume more calories than nonathletes to meet their energy needs, they also consume more dietary protein and can easily meet their protein needs through diet alone.

In addition to the RDA, the DRIs include a recommendation for protein intake as a percentage of calories: The Acceptable Macronutrient Distribution Range for protein is 10 to 35% of calories.[18] This range allows for different food preferences and eating patterns. A protein intake in this range will meet protein needs and allow sufficient intakes of other nutrients to promote health. A diet that provides 10% of calories from protein will meet the RDA but is a relatively low-protein diet compared with typical eating patterns in the United States. The upper end of this healthy range—35% of calories—is a relatively high-protein diet, about twice as much protein as the average American eats. This amount of protein is not harmful, but if the diet is this high in protein, it is probably high in animal products, which tend to be high in saturated fat and cholesterol. Therefore, unless protein sources are chosen carefully, a diet that contains 35% protein would tend to include more saturated fat and cholesterol than would a diet with the same number of calories that contains only 10% protein. For example, a 2500-Calorie diet that provides 35% of calories from protein would include the animal protein equivalent of a 16-oz steak and 2 quarts of milk daily.

Protein and amino acid supplements • Figure 6.14

Protein and amino acid supplements are rarely needed to meet protein needs. Nonetheless, supplements are marketed to boost total protein intake and to add individual amino acids.

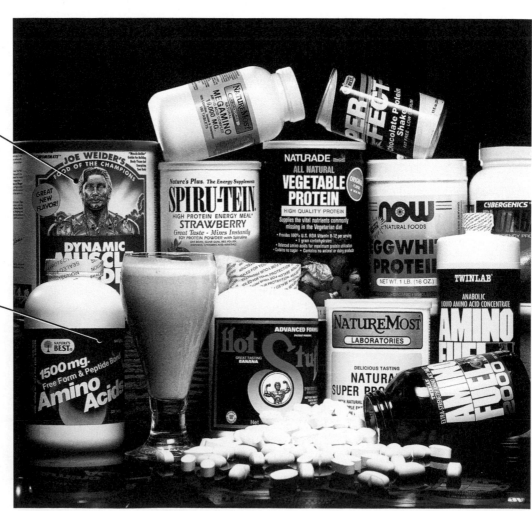

Protein supplements are marketed to promote proper immune function, make hair healthy, and stimulate muscle growth, but increasing protein intake above the level required for good health does not protect you from disease, make your hair shine, or give you larger biceps.

Many promises are made about amino acid supplements, from aiding sleep to enhancing athletic performance. There is weak evidence to support some of these claims, but consuming large amounts of one amino acid may interfere with the absorption of others. Due to insufficient research, no ULs have been set for amino acids.

Choosing Protein Wisely

To evaluate protein intake, it is important to consider both the amount and the quality of protein in the diet. **Protein quality** is a measure of how good the protein in a food is at providing the essential amino acids the body

Protein complementation • Figure 6.15

The amino acids in grains, nuts, or seeds complement the amino acids in legumes to provide complete proteins.

a. As a general rule, legumes are deficient in methionine and cysteine but high in lysine. Grains, nuts, and seeds are deficient in lysine but high in methionine and cysteine. So, when rice is eaten with beans, the meal provides enough of all the amino acids needed by the body.

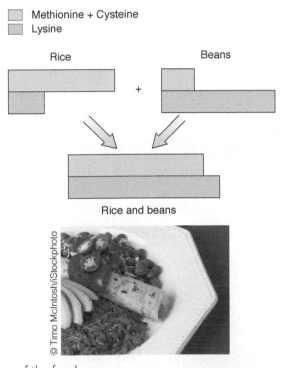

Methionine + Cysteine
Lysine

Rice   +   Beans

Rice and beans

© Timo McIntosh/iStockphoto

b. Many of the food combinations consumed in traditional diets take advantage of complementary plant proteins, such as lentils and rice or chickpeas and rice in India, rice and beans in Mexico and South America, hummus (chickpeas and sesame seeds) in the Middle East, and bread and peanut butter (peanuts are a legume) in the United States.

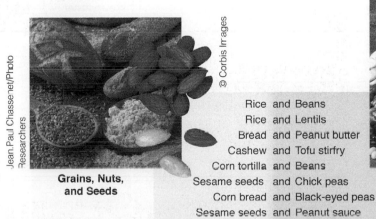

Jean.Paul Chassenet/Photo Researchers

Grains, Nuts, and Seeds

© Corbis Images

Rice and Beans
Rice and Lentils
Bread and Peanut butter
Cashew and Tofu stirfry
Corn tortilla and Beans
Sesame seeds and Chick peas
Corn bread and Black-eyed peas
Sesame seeds and Peanut sauce
Nuts and Soy beans
Rice and Tofu

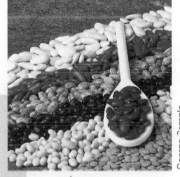

Legumes

George Semple

needs to synthesize proteins (see online Appendix K for methods used to measure protein quality). Because animal amino acid patterns are similar to those of humans, the animal proteins in our diet generally provide a mixture of amino acids that better matches our needs than the amino acid mixtures provided by plant proteins. Animal proteins also tend to be digested more easily than plant proteins; only protein that is digested can contribute amino acids to meet the body's requirements.[21] Because they are easily digested and supply essential amino acids in the proper proportions for human use, foods of animal origin are generally sources of **high-quality protein**, or **complete dietary protein**. When your diet contains high-quality protein, you don't have to eat as much total protein to meet your needs.

Compared to animal proteins, plant proteins are usually more difficult to digest and are lower in one or more of the essential amino acids. They are therefore generally referred to as **incomplete dietary protein**. Exceptions include quinoa and soy protein, which are both high-quality plant proteins.

Complementary proteins If you get your protein from a single source and that source is an incomplete protein, it will be difficult to meet your body's protein needs. However, combining proteins that are limited in different amino acids can supply a complete mixture of essential amino acids. For example, legumes are limited in methionine but high in lysine. When legumes are consumed with grains, which are high in methionine and low in lysine, the combination provides all the needed amino acids (**Figure 6.15a**). Vegetarian diets rely on this technique, called **protein complementation**, to meet protein needs. By eating plant proteins that have complementary amino acid patterns, a person can meet his or her essential amino acid requirements without consuming any animal proteins. Many vegetarian meals include complementary proteins (**Figure 6.15b**). However, complementary proteins do not have to be consumed in the same meal; eating an assortment of plant foods throughout the day can provide enough of all the essential amino acids.[22]

protein complementation The process of combining proteins from different sources so that they collectively provide the proportions of amino acids required to meet the body's needs.

MyPlate and Dietary Guidelines recommendations MyPlate and the Dietary Guidelines include recommendations regarding both animal and plant sources of protein to meet your need for protein and essential amino acids (**Figure 6.16**). The MyPlate food groups that provide the most protein per serving are the dairy and protein groups; 1 cup of milk provides about 8 g of protein, 1 ounce of meat or fish about 7 g, ½ cup of beans or ¼ cup of nuts, or seeds provides 6 to 10 g. Each serving from the

Choosing healthy protein sources • Figure 6.16

The protein group and the dairy group of MyPlate provide the most concentrated sources of protein. Nuts, dry beans, and peas are the most concentrated sources of plant protein. When you eat dry beans or peas, you can count them in either the vegetables group or the protein group. There is very little protein in fruits.

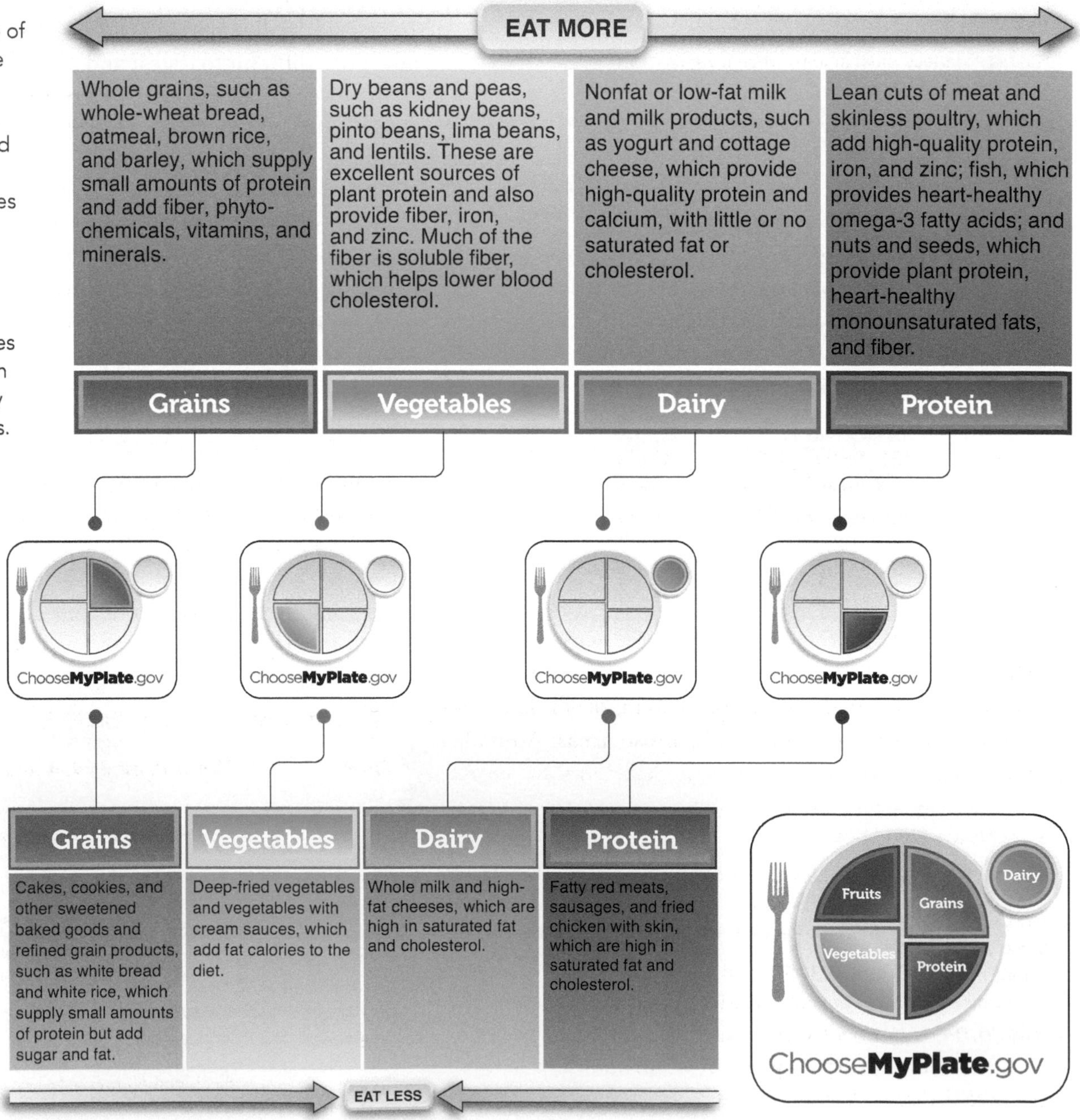

EAT MORE

Grains	Vegetables	Dairy	Protein
Whole grains, such as whole-wheat bread, oatmeal, brown rice, and barley, which supply small amounts of protein and add fiber, phytochemicals, vitamins, and minerals.	Dry beans and peas, such as kidney beans, pinto beans, lima beans, and lentils. These are excellent sources of plant protein and also provide fiber, iron, and zinc. Much of the fiber is soluble fiber, which helps lower blood cholesterol.	Nonfat or low-fat milk and milk products, such as yogurt and cottage cheese, which provide high-quality protein and calcium, with little or no saturated fat or cholesterol.	Lean cuts of meat and skinless poultry, which add high-quality protein, iron, and zinc; fish, which provides heart-healthy omega-3 fatty acids; and nuts and seeds, which provide plant protein, heart-healthy monounsaturated fats, and fiber.

ChooseMyPlate.gov

Grains	Vegetables	Dairy	Protein
Cakes, cookies, and other sweetened baked goods and refined grain products, such as white bread and white rice, which supply small amounts of protein but add sugar and fat.	Deep-fried vegetables and vegetables with cream sauces, which add fat calories to the diet.	Whole milk and high-fat cheeses, which are high in saturated fat and cholesterol.	Fatty red meats, sausages, and fried chicken with skin, which are high in saturated fat and cholesterol.

ChooseMyPlate.gov

EAT LESS

WHAT SHOULD I EAT?

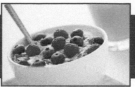 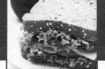 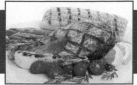

Protein Sources

Get protein without too much saturated fat
- Eat more fish.
- Have a grilled chicken sandwich rather than a burger.
- Choose lean cuts of red meat, such as round steaks and loin chops.
- Grill, roast, or broil so the fat will end up in the pan or the fire.
- Choose low-fat milk, yogurt, and cheese.

Eat both animal and plant proteins
- Have your beef or chicken in a stir-fry with lots of vegetables.
- Serve a small portion of meat over noodles.
- Add nuts and seeds to snacks and salads.
- Have a meatless meal at least once a week.
- Try a veggie burger.

Go with beans
- Have some hummus.
- Order beans in your burrito.
- Snack on edamame or roasted soybeans.
- Choose baked beans rather than potatoes.

Use iProfile to look up the protein content of your favorite vegetarian entree.

---

grains group and the vegetables group provides 2 to 4 g, so choosing the recommended number of servings from these groups will provide a significant proportion of your protein needs. To assure an overall healthy diet, the 2010 Dietary Guidelines recommend that we choose a variety of protein foods, including seafood, lean meat and poultry, eggs, beans, soy products, and unsalted nuts and seeds. They recommend increasing consumption of seafood and low-fat or fat-free dairy products and replacing protein foods that are high in solid fats with those that are lower in solid fats and calories (see *What Should I Eat?*).

Vegetarian Diets

In many parts of the world, diets based on plant proteins, called **vegetarian diets**, have evolved mostly out of necessity because animal sources of protein are limited, either physically or economically, in those areas. Animals require more land and resources to raise and are more expensive to purchase than are plants. The developing world relies primarily on plant foods to meet protein needs. For example, in rural Mexico, most of the protein in the diet comes from beans, rice, and tortillas (corn), and in India, protein comes from lentils and rice. As a population's economic prosperity rises, the proportion of animal foods in its diet typically increases, but in developed countries, people eat vegetarian diets for a variety of reasons other than economics, such as health, religion, personal ethics, or environmental awareness. **Vegan diets** eliminate all animal products, but there are other types of vegetarian diets that are less restrictive (**Table 6.1**).

> **vegetarian diet** A diet that includes plant-based foods and eliminates some or all foods of animal origin.

> **vegan diet** A plant-based diet that eliminates all animal products.

Benefits of vegetarian diets A vegetarian diet can be a healthy, low-cost alternative to the traditional American meat-and-potatoes diet. Vegetarians have been shown to have lower body weight relative to height and a reduced incidence of obesity and of other chronic diseases, such as diabetes, cardiovascular disease, high blood pressure, and some types of cancer.[22] The lower body weight of

Types of vegetarian diets   Table 6.1

Diet	What it excludes and includes
Semivegetarian	Excludes red meat but may include fish and poultry, as well as dairy products and eggs.
Pescetarian	Excludes all animal flesh except fish.
Lacto-ovo vegetarian	Excludes all animal flesh but does include eggs and dairy products such as milk and cheese.
Lacto vegetarian	Excludes animal flesh and eggs but does include dairy products.
Vegan	Excludes all food of animal origin.

vegetarians is a result of lower energy intake, primarily due to higher intake of fiber, which makes the diet more filling. The reductions in the risk of other chronic diseases may be due to lower body weight and to the fact that these diets are lower in saturated fat and cholesterol, which increase disease risk. Or it could be that vegetarian diets are higher in whole grains, legumes, nuts, vegetables, and fruits, which add fiber, vitamins, minerals, antioxidants, and phytochemicals—substances that have been shown to lower disease risk. It is likely that the total dietary pattern, rather than a single factor, is responsible for the health-promoting effects of vegetarian diets (see *Thinking It Through*).

In addition to reducing disease risks, diets that rely more heavily on plant protein than on animal protein are more economical. For example, a vegetarian stir-fry over rice costs about half as much as a meal of steak and potatoes. Yet both meals provide a significant portion of the day's protein requirement. A small steak, a baked potato with sour cream, and a tossed salad provides about 50 g of protein, whereas a dish of rice with tofu and vegetables provides about 30 g.

Risks of vegetarian diets Despite the health and economic benefits of vegetarian diets, a poorly planned vegetarian diet can cause nutrient deficiencies. Protein deficiency is a risk when vegan diets that contain little high-quality protein are consumed by small children or by adults with increased protein needs, such as pregnant women and those recovering from illness or injury. Most people can easily meet their protein needs with lacto and lacto-ovo vegetarian diets. These diets contain high-quality animal proteins from eggs or milk, which complement the limiting amino acids in the plant proteins.

Vitamin and mineral deficiencies are a greater concern for vegetarians than is protein deficiency.[22] Of primary concern to vegans is vitamin B_{12}. Because this B vitamin is found almost exclusively in animal products, vegans must take vitamin B_{12} supplements or consume foods fortified with vitamin B_{12} to meet their needs for this nutrient. Another nutrient of concern is calcium. Dairy products are the major source of calcium in the North American diet, so diets that eliminate these foods must include plant sources of calcium such as greens and tofu. Likewise, because much of the dietary vitamin D comes from fortified milk, this vitamin must be made in the body from exposure to sunlight or consumed in other sources. Iron and zinc may be deficient in vegetarian diets because they exclude red meat, which is an excellent source of these minerals, and iron and zinc are poorly absorbed from plant sources. Because dairy products are low in iron and zinc, lacto-ovo and lacto vegetarians as well as vegans are at risk for deficiencies of these minerals. Vegan diets may also be low in iodine and the omega-3 fatty acids EPA and DHA (see Chapter 5).[22] **Table 6.2** provides suggestions for how vegans can meet the need for the nutrients just discussed.

Meeting nutrient needs with a vegan diet[22]   Table 6.2

Nutrient at risk	Sources in vegan diets
Protein	Soy-based products, legumes, seeds, nuts, grains, and vegetables.
Vitamin B_{12}	Products fortified with vitamin B_{12}, such as soy beverages, rice milk*, almond milk*, and breakfast cereals; fortified nutritional yeast; dietary supplements.
Calcium	Tofu processed with calcium; broccoli, kale, collard and mustard greens, bok choy, and legumes; products fortified with calcium, such as soy beverages, rice milk*, almond milk*, grain products, and orange juice.
Vitamin D	Sunshine; products fortified with vitamin D, such as soy beverages, rice milk*, almond milk*, breakfast cereals, and margarine.
Iron	Legumes, tofu, dark-green leafy vegetables, dried fruit, whole grains, iron-fortified grain products (absorption is improved when iron-containing foods are consumed with vitamin C found in citrus fruit, tomatoes, strawberries, and dark-green vegetables).
Zinc	Whole grains, wheat germ, legumes, nuts, tofu, and fortified breakfast cereals.
Iodine	Iodized salt, sea vegetables (seaweed), and foods grown near the sea.
Omega-3 fatty acids	Canola oil, flaxseed and flaxseed oil, soybean oil, walnuts, and sea vegetables (seaweed), which provide fatty acids that can be used to synthesize EPA and DHA; DHA-rich microalgae.

*Most rice milk and almond milk products are low in protein (about 1 g per serving) but fortified with vitamin B_{12}, calcium, and vitamin D.

A Case Study on Choosing a Healthy Vegetarian Diet

Simon is 26 years old and weighs 154 pounds. A year ago, he decided to stop eating meat because he thought it would make his diet healthier. Now that he is studying nutrition, he has become concerned that his vegetarian diet may not be as healthy as he thought. Simon records his food intake for one day and then uses iProfile to assess his nutrient intake. His analysis reveals that his diet provides 2900 Calories, 78 g of protein, and 43 g of saturated fat.

 1 Does Simon's diet provide enough protein to meet his RDA of 0.8 g of protein per kilogram of body?

Your answer:

 2 How does the percentage of calories from saturated fat in Simon's diet compare with recommendations?

Your answer:

3 This is a photo of Simon's typical lunch. Why is it high in saturated fat?

Your answer:

 4 Vegetarian diets are often deficient in calcium, vitamin D, zinc, and iron. Assuming Simon eats plenty of dairy products and enriched grains, is his diet likely to be low in any of these?

Your answer:

 5 Suggest a dinner meal for Simon that would be low in saturated fat and provide the nutrients that may be lacking in his diet.

Your answer:

 6 To reduce his saturated fat intake, Simon wants to try a vegan lunch. Suggest a vegan sandwich Simon could have that makes use of complementary plant proteins.

Your answer:

(Check your answers in online Appendix L)

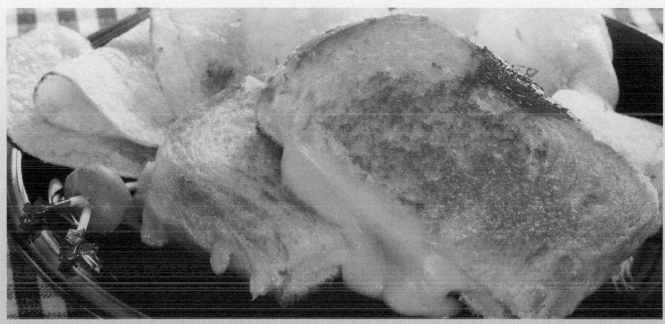

Rosemary Buffoni/iStockphoto

Planning vegetarian diets Well-planned vegetarian diets, including vegan diets, can meet nutrient needs at all stages of the life cycle, from infancy, childhood, and adolescence to early, middle, and late adulthood, and during pregnancy and lactation.[22] One way to plan a healthy vegetarian diet is to modify the selections from MyPlate. The food choices and recommended amounts from the grains, vegetables, and fruits groups should stay the same for vegetarians. Including 1 cup of dark-green and colorful vegetables daily will help meet iron and calcium needs. The dairy group and the protein group include foods of animal origin. Vegetarians who consume eggs and milk can still choose these foods. Those who avoid all animal foods can choose dry beans, nuts and seeds, and soy products from the protein group. Fortified soymilk and protein-enriched rice milk can be substituted for dairy foods. To obtain adequate vitamin B_{12}, vegans must take supplements or use products fortified with vitamin B_{12}. Obtaining plenty of omega-3 fatty acids from foods such as canola oil, nuts, and flaxseed ensures adequate synthesis of the long-chain omega-3 fatty acids DHA and EPA.

CONCEPT CHECK

1. **What** circumstances result in a positive nitrogen balance?

2. **Why** is the quality of animal protein generally considered to be higher than that of plant protein?

3. **What** could you serve with rice to increase the overall protein quality of the meal?

4. **Why** are vegans at risk for vitamin B_{12} deficiency?

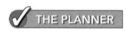

Summary

1 Proteins in Our Food 158

- Dietary protein comes from both animal and plant sources. Animal sources of protein are generally good sources of iron, zinc, and calcium but are high in saturated fat and cholesterol. Plant sources of protein, such as the grains, nuts, and legumes shown in the photo, are higher in unsaturated fat, fiber, and phytochemicals.

Animal vs. plant proteins • Figure 6.1b

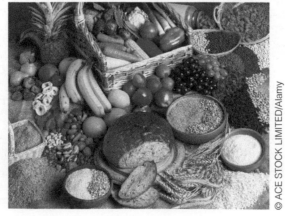

© ACE STOCK LIMITED/Alamy

2 The Structure of Amino Acids and Proteins 159

- **Amino acids** are the building blocks from which proteins are made. Each amino acid contains an amino group, an acid group, and a unique side chain. The amino acids that the body is unable to make in sufficient amounts are called **essential amino acids** and must be consumed in the diet.

- Proteins are made by linking amino acids by **peptide bonds**, as shown here, to form **polypeptides**. Polypeptide chains fold to create unique three-dimensional protein structures. The shape of a protein determines its function.

Amino acid and protein structure • Figure 6.2b

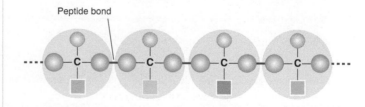

Peptide bond

3 Protein Digestion and Absorption 163

• Digestion breaks dietary protein into small **peptides** and amino acids that can be absorbed. Because amino acids that share the same transport system, such as those pictured here in green and blue, compete for absorption, an excess of one can inhibit the absorption of another.

Protein digestion and absorption • Figure 6.4

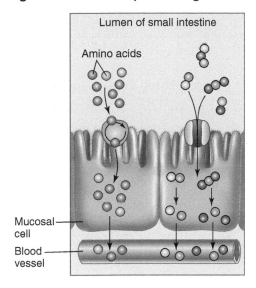

4 Protein Synthesis and Functions 163

• Amino acids are used to synthesize proteins and other nitrogen-containing molecules. **Genes** located in the nucleus of the cell code for the order of amino acids in the **polypeptide** chains that make up proteins. Regulatory mechanisms ensure that proteins are made only when they are needed. For a protein to be synthesized, all the amino acids it contains must be available. The essential amino acid present in shortest supply relative to need, depicted here as the orange balls, is called the **limiting amino acid**.

Protein synthesis • Figure 6.6c

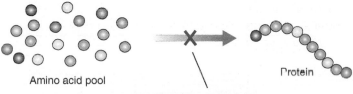

Amino acid pool

A shortage of the amino acid represented by the orange spheres limits the ability to synthesize a protein that is high in this amino acid.

Protein

• In the body, protein molecules form structures, regulate body functions, transport molecules through the blood and in and out of cells, function in the immune system, and aid in muscle contraction, fluid balance, and acid balance.

• When the diet is deficient in energy or when the diet contains more protein than needed, amino acids are used as an energy source and to synthesize glucose or fatty acids. Before amino acids can be used for these purposes, the amino group must be removed via **deamination**.

5 Protein in Health and Disease 168

• **Protein-energy malnutrition (PEM)** is a health concern primarily in developing countries. **Kwashiorkor**, shown here, occurs when the protein content of the diet is deficient but energy is adequate. It is most common in children. **Marasmus** occurs when total energy intake is deficient.

Protein-energy malnutrition • Figure 6.9a

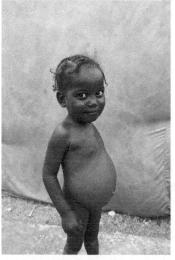

ALISON WRIGHT/NG Images

• High-protein diets increase the production of urea and other waste products that must be excreted in the urine and therefore can increase water losses. High protein intakes increase urinary calcium losses, but when calcium intake is adequate, high-protein diets are associated with greater bone mass and fewer fractures. Diets high in animal proteins and low in fluid are associated with an increased risk of kidney stones. High-protein diets can be high in saturated fat and cholesterol.

• If proteins are absorbed without being completely digested, they can trigger an immune system reaction, resulting in a **food allergy**. Some amino acids and proteins can also cause **food intolerances**.

6 Meeting Protein Needs 173

- Protein requirements are determined by looking at **nitrogen balance**, the amount of nitrogen consumed as dietary protein compared with the amount excreted as protein waste products.

- For healthy adults, the RDA for protein is 0.8 g/kg of body weight. Growth, pregnancy, lactation, illness, injury, and certain types of physical exercise increase requirements. Recommendations for a healthy diet are to ingest 10 to 35% of calories from protein.

- Animal proteins are considered **high-quality proteins** because their amino acid composition matches that needed to synthesize body proteins. Most plant proteins are limited in one or more of the essential amino acids needed to make body protein; therefore, they are considered **incomplete proteins**. The **protein quality** of plant sources can be increased through **protein complementation**. As illustrated here, it combines proteins with different limiting amino acids to supply enough of all the essential amino acids.

Protein complementation • Figure 6.15b

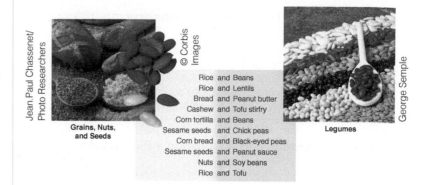

Grains, Nuts, and Seeds

Rice	and	Beans
Rice	and	Lentils
Bread	and	Peanut butter
Cashew	and	Tofu stirfry
Corn tortilla	and	Beans
Sesame seeds	and	Chick peas
Corn bread	and	Black-eyed peas
Sesame seeds	and	Peanut sauce
Nuts	and	Soy beans
Rice	and	Tofu

Legumes

- Compared with meat-based diets, **vegetarian diets** are lower in saturated fat and cholesterol and higher in fiber, certain vitamins and minerals, antioxidants, and phytochemicals. People consuming **vegan diets** must plan their diets carefully to meet their needs for vitamin B_{12}, calcium, vitamin D, iron, zinc, iodine, and omega-3 fatty acids.

Key Terms

- amino acid 158
- amino acid pool 164
- celiac disease 172
- conditionally essential amino acid 159
- deamination 169
- denaturation 161
- dipeptide 160
- edema 167
- essential, or indispensable, amino acid 159
- food allergy 171
- food intolerance or food sensitivity 172

- gene 164
- gene expression 164
- high-quality protein or complete dietary protein 177
- hydrolyzed protein or protein hydrolysate 172
- incomplete dietary protein 177
- kwashiorkor 170
- legume 158
- limiting amino acid 165
- marasmus 170

- monosodium glutamate (MSG) 172
- MSG symptom complex or Chinese restaurant syndrome 172
- nitrogen balance 173
- nonessential, or dispensable, amino acid 159
- peptide bond 159
- peptide 160
- phenylketonuria (PKU) 159
- polypeptide 159
- protein complementation 178

- protein-energy malnutrition (PEM) 170
- protein quality 177
- transamination 164
- transcription 165
- translation 165
- tripeptide 160
- urea 169
- vegan diet 179
- vegetarian diet 179

What is happening in this picture?

Sickle cell anemia is an inherited disease caused by an abnormality in the gene for the protein hemoglobin. It causes red blood cells to take on a sickle shape.

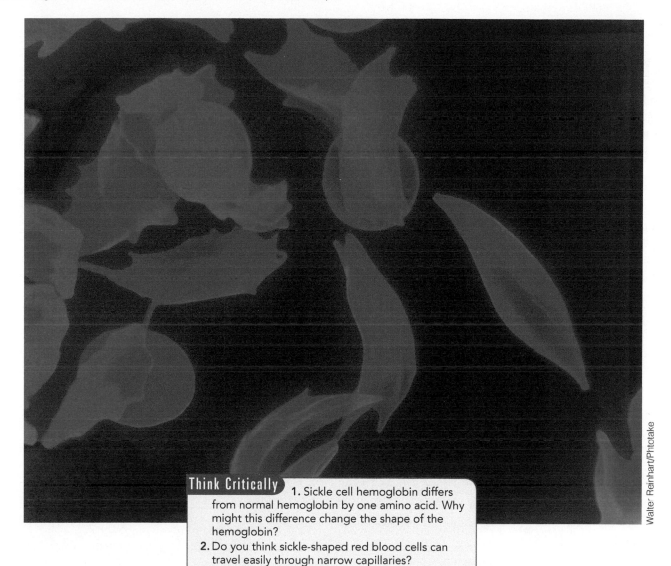

Walter Reinhart/Phtotake

Think Critically

1. Sickle cell hemoglobin differs from normal hemoglobin by one amino acid. Why might this difference change the shape of the hemoglobin?

2. Do you think sickle-shaped red blood cells can travel easily through narrow capillaries?

3. How might this disorder affect the ability to get oxygen to the body's cells?

THE PLANNER ✓

Review your Chapter Planner on the chapter opener and check off your completed work.

7 Vitamins

Multiple sclerosis (MS) is a degenerative neurological disease in which the protective layer around nerves (the myelin sheath) becomes damaged. Although this disease occurs around the world, more cases are reported in northern and southern latitudes than near the equator, prompting investigators to wonder what factors might contribute to such a distribution.

At the extreme northern edge of the Scottish mainland lies an archipelago called the Orkney Islands. These islands have the largest concentration of MS in the world. One in every 170 women suffers from the condition. The reasons proposed for this remarkable number of cases range from a genetic trait inherited from Norse settlers to a deficiency of vitamin D. This vitamin can be made in the body when exposure to sunlight is plentiful, but in northern Scotland sunlight is limited by short winter days and frequent cloud cover. Interestingly enough, rickets, also caused by a lack of vitamin D, is making a comeback in northern parts of Scotland and England.

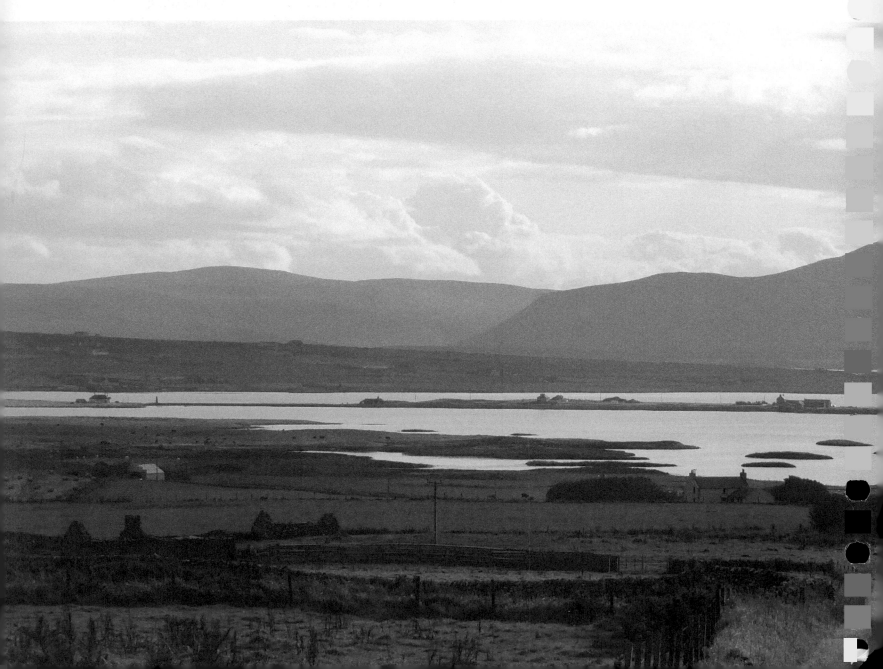

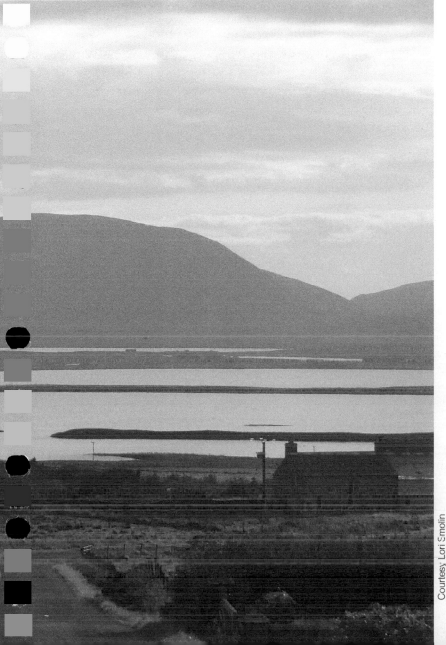

Populations enduring sun-starved northern winters have traditionally acquired vitamin D from a diet rich in fish and eggs. But as consumption of these foods has declined in favor of a more modern diet high in processed foods, vitamin D deficiency has increased. Health authorities in the United Kingdom are proposing fortifying milk with vitamin D, a common practice in the United States, to ensure consumers are getting enough to promote better health and perhaps prevent disease.

Courtesy Lori Smolin

CHAPTER OUTLINE

CHAPTER PLANNER ✔

❑ Stimulate your interest by reading the opening story and looking at the visual.
❑ Scan the Learning Objectives in each section:
   p. 188 ❑   p. 196 ❑   p. 214 ❑   p. 230 ❑
❑ Read the text and study all figures and visuals. Answer any questions.

Analyze key features

❑ What a Scientist Sees, p. 190 ❑   p. 227 ❑
❑ Process Diagram, p. 191 ❑   p. 193 ❑   p. 208 ❑
   p. 216 ❑   p. 220 ❑
❑ Debate, p. 233 ❑
❑ Nutrition InSight, p. 192 ❑   p. 202 ❑   p. 218 ❑   p. 222 ❑
❑ Thinking It Through, p. 217 ❑
❑ Stop: Answer the Concept Checks before you go on:
   p. 195 ❑   p. 214 ❑   p. 229 ❑   p. 235 ❑

End of chapter and online review:

❑ Review the Summary, Key Terms, and online links to Additional Resources.
❑ Answer the online Critical and Creative Thinking Questions.
❑ Answer What is happening in this picture?
❑ Complete the Self-Test and check your answers.

7.1 A Vitamin Primer

LEARNING OBJECTIVES

1. **Discuss** the dietary sources of vitamins.
2. **Describe** how bioavailability affects vitamin requirements.
3. **Explain** the function of coenzymes.
4. **Describe** the vitamin information provided on food labels.

Vitamins are organic compounds that are essential in the diet in small amounts to promote and regulate body processes necessary for growth, reproduction, and the maintenance of health. When a vitamin is lacking in the diet, deficiency symptoms occur. When the vitamin is restored to the diet, the symptoms resolve.

Vitamins have traditionally been assigned to two groups, based on their solubility in water or fat. This chemical characteristic allows generalizations to be made about how the vitamins are absorbed, transported, excreted, and stored in the body. The **water-soluble vitamins** include the B vitamins and vitamin C. The **fat-soluble vitamins** include vitamins A, D, E, and K (**Figure 7.1**).

Vitamins in Our Food

Almost all foods contain some vitamins, and all the food groups contain foods that are good sources of a variety of vitamins (**Figure 7.2**). The amount of a vitamin in a food depends on the amount that is naturally present in the food, what is added to it, and how the food is processed, prepared, and stored.

Fortification adds nutrients to foods. Sometimes nutrients are added to foods to comply with government fortification programs that mandate such additions in order to prevent vitamin or mineral deficiencies and promote health in the population (see *What a Scientist Sees*, page 200). For example, grains are enriched with B vitamins and iron to prevent deficiencies, and milk is fortified with vitamin D to promote bone health. In other cases, manufacturers add nutrients with the goal of increasing product sales.

The vitamins in foods can be damaged by exposure to light or oxygen, washed away during preparation, or destroyed by cooking. Thus, processing steps used by food producers can cause nutrient losses, as can cooking and storage methods used at home (**Figure 7.3**).

The vitamins • Figure 7.1

The vitamins were initially named alphabetically, in approximately the order in which they were identified. The B vitamins were first thought to be a single chemical substance but were later found to be many different vitamins and for this reason they were distinguished by numbers. Vitamins B_6 and B_{12} are the only ones that are still routinely referred to by their numbers.

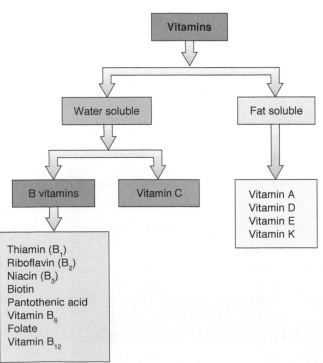

Vitamins

Water soluble — Fat soluble

Water soluble → B vitamins, Vitamin C

Fat soluble → Vitamin A, Vitamin D, Vitamin E, Vitamin K

B vitamins:
Thiamin (B_1)
Riboflavin (B_2)
Niacin (B_3)
Biotin
Pantothenic acid
Vitamin B_6
Folate
Vitamin B_{12}

Vitamins on MyPlate • Figure 7.2

Vitamins are found in foods from all the food groups, as well as in oils, but some groups are low or lacking in specific vitamins. For example, grains, fruits, and vegetables lack vitamin B_{12}, and grains, dairy, and protein foods are low in vitamin C.

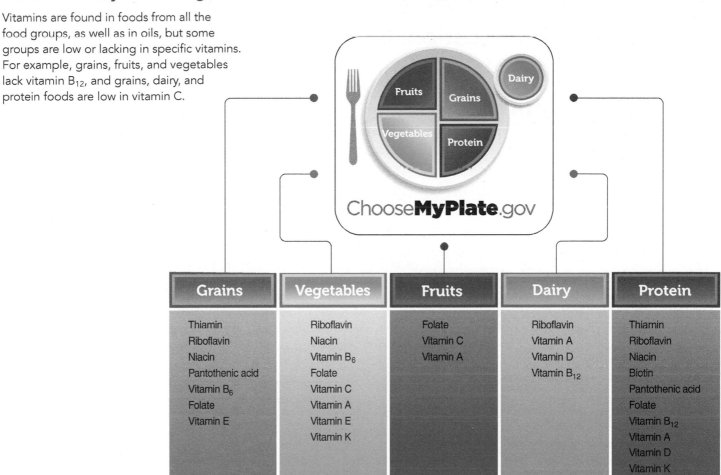

ChooseMyPlate.gov

Grains	Vegetables	Fruits	Dairy	Protein
Thiamin	Riboflavin	Folate	Riboflavin	Thiamin
Riboflavin	Niacin	Vitamin C	Vitamin A	Riboflavin
Niacin	Vitamin B_6	Vitamin A	Vitamin D	Niacin
Pantothenic acid	Folate		Vitamin B_{12}	Biotin
Vitamin B_6	Vitamin C			Pantothenic acid
Folate	Vitamin A			Folate
Vitamin E	Vitamin E			Vitamin B_{12}
	Vitamin K			Vitamin A
				Vitamin D
				Vitamin K

Which choice is highest in vitamins? • Figure 7.3

Because heat, light, air, and the passage of time all cause foods to lose nutrients, most of us try to purchase fresh produce, but is fresh always best?

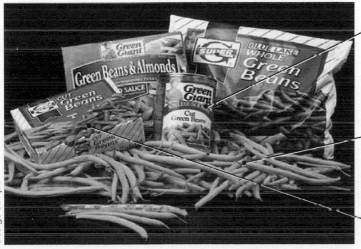

George Semple

The high temperatures used in canning reduce nutrient content. However, because canned foods keep for a long time, do not require refrigeration, and are often less expensive than fresh or frozen foods, they provide an available, affordable source of nutrients that may be the best choice in some situations.

Sometimes "fresh" produce is lower in nutrients than you would expect because it has spent a week in a truck, traveling to your store, several days on a shelf, and maybe another week in your refrigerator.

Frozen foods are often frozen in the field in order to minimize nutrient losses. Thus, frozen fruits and vegetables may supply more vitamins than "fresh" ones.

A Vitamin Primer **189**

WHAT A SCIENTIST SEES
Fortification: Benefits and Risks

Fortified Breakfast Cereal

Nutrition Facts

Serving Size   1 Cup (50g/1.8 oz.)
Servings Per Container   About 10

Amount Per Serving	Cereal	Cereal with 1/2 Cup Vitamins A&D Fat-Free Milk
Calories	180	220
Calories from Fat	5	5

		% Daily Value**
Total Fat 0.5g*	1%	1%
Saturated Fat 0g	0%	0%
Trans Fat 0g		
Cholesterol 0mg	0%	0%
Sodium 280mg	12%	14%
Potassium 100mg	3%	9%
Total Carbohydrate 35g	12%	14%
Dietary Fiber 2g	9%	9%
Sugars 7g		
Other Carbohydrate 26g		
Protein 3g		

Vitamin A	15%	20%
Vitamin C	25%	25%
Calcium	0%	15%
Iron	100%	100%
Vitamin D	10%	25%
Vitamin E	100%	100%
Thiamin	100%	100%
Riboflavin	100%	110%
Niacin	100%	100%
Vitamin B$_6$	100%	100%
Folic Acid	100%	100%
Vitamin B$_{12}$	100%	110%
Pantothenate	100%	100%
Phosphorus	10%	20%
Magnesium	8%	10%
Zinc	100%	100%
Copper	4%	6%

The Nutrition Facts panel on a box of breakfast cereal shows an abundance of vitamins and minerals, many of which have been added through fortification. A consumer sees an easy way to meet nutrient needs. A scientist sees both the health benefits and the risks of fortification.

Fortification began as a way to address nutrient deficiencies. In the early 1900s, the niacin deficiency disease *pellagra* caused more than 3000 deaths annually in the southern United States. In 1938, bakers voluntarily began enriching flour with B vitamins, a move that led to a decline in mortality from pellagra (see graph).[1] By 1943, enrichment of flour was becoming mandatory. Other government-supported fortification programs in the United States have helped to prevent vitamin A and D deficiencies.

Not all fortification is mandated by the government. Scientists recognize that indiscriminate fortification of foods, such as snack bars, beverages, and breakfast cereals, can increase the risk of nutrient toxicities. A recent analysis of nutrient intakes in toddlers and preschoolers showed that a significant percentage had intakes of preformed vitamin A, folate, and zinc that exceeded the ULs. Much of the excess zinc is likely to be from fortified breakfast cereals.[2]

Think Critically Should the government regulate all fortification of food?

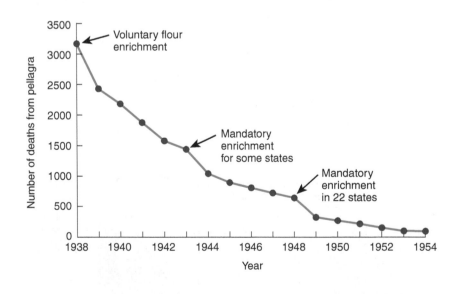

Vitamin losses can be minimized through food preparation methods that reduce exposure to heat and light, which destroy some vitamins, and to water, which washes away water-soluble vitamins (**Table 7.1**).

Vitamin Bioavailability

About 40 to 90% of the vitamins in food are absorbed, primarily from the small intestine (**Figure 7.4**). The composition of the diet and conditions in the digestive

Tips for preserving the vitamins in your food	Table 7.1

- Store food away from heat and light and eat it soon after purchasing it.
- Cut fruits and vegetables as close as possible to the time when they will be cooked or served.
- Don't soak vegetables.
- Cook vegetables with as little water as possible by microwaving, pressure-cooking, roasting, grilling, stir-frying, or baking rather than boiling them.
- If foods are cooked in water, use the cooking water to make soups and sauces so that you can retrieve some of the nutrients.
- Don't rinse rice before cooking, in order to avoid washing away water-soluble vitamins.

tract and the rest of the body influence vitamin **bioavailability**. For example, fat-soluble vitamins are absorbed along with dietary fat. If the diet is very low in fat, absorption of these vitamins is impaired.

bioavailability The extent to which the body can absorb and use a nutrient.

Once they have been absorbed into the blood, vitamins must be transported to the cells. Most of the water-soluble vitamins are bound to blood proteins for transport. Fat-soluble vitamins are incorporated into chylomicrons for transport from the small intestine. The bioavailability of a vitamin depends on the availability of these transport systems.

Vitamin absorption • Figure 7.4

THE PLANNER

Most vitamin absorption takes place in the small intestine. The mechanism by which a vitamin is absorbed and transported affects its bioavailability.

HOW IT WORKS

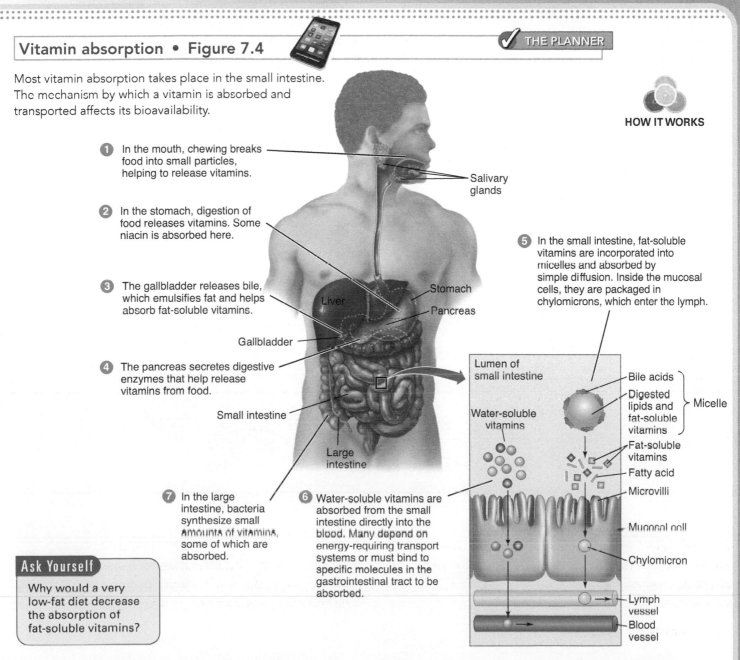

1 In the mouth, chewing breaks food into small particles, helping to release vitamins.

2 In the stomach, digestion of food releases vitamins. Some niacin is absorbed here.

3 The gallbladder releases bile, which emulsifies fat and helps absorb fat-soluble vitamins.

4 The pancreas secretes digestive enzymes that help release vitamins from food.

5 In the small intestine, fat-soluble vitamins are incorporated into micelles and absorbed by simple diffusion. Inside the mucosal cells, they are packaged in chylomicrons, which enter the lymph.

6 Water-soluble vitamins are absorbed from the small intestine directly into the blood. Many depend on energy-requiring transport systems or must bind to specific molecules in the gastrointestinal tract to be absorbed.

7 In the large intestine, bacteria synthesize small amounts of vitamins, some of which are absorbed.

Salivary glands
Stomach
Liver
Pancreas
Gallbladder
Small intestine
Large intestine

Lumen of small intestine
Water-soluble vitamins
Bile acids
Digested lipids and fat-soluble vitamins } Micelle
Fat-soluble vitamins
Fatty acid
Microvilli
Mucosal cell
Chylomicron
Lymph vessel
Blood vessel

Ask Yourself

Why would a very low-fat diet decrease the absorption of fat-soluble vitamins?

PROCESS DIAGRAM

While each vitamin has unique functions, many have complementary roles in supporting health.

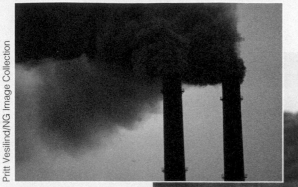

Pritt Vesilind/NG Image Collection

Vitamin C, vitamin E, and provitamin A are antioxidants that can help protect us from molecules that cause oxidative damage.

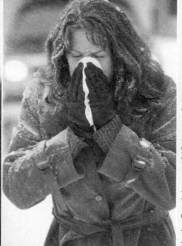

Alaska Stock Images/NG Image Collection

Vitamin A and vitamin D are needed for normal growth and development.

The B vitamins thiamin, riboflavin, niacin, biotin, pantothenic acid, and vitamin B_6 are needed to produce ATP from carbohydrate, fat, and protein.

Courtesy Lori Smolin

Vitamins A, B_6, C, and D, as well as folate, are needed for healthy immune function, and thus help protect us from infection.

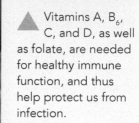

Folate, vitamin B_6, and vitamin B_{12} are important for protein and amino acid metabolism.

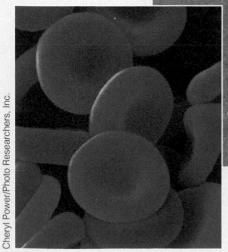

Cheryl Power/Photo Researchers, Inc.

Folate, vitamin B_6, vitamin B_{12}, and vitamin K are needed to keep blood healthy.

Vitamins A, D, K, and C are needed for bone health.

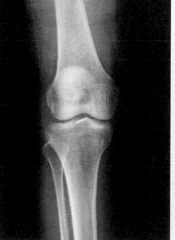

© stockdevil /iStockphoto

provitamin or **vitamin precursor** A compound that can be converted into the active form of a vitamin in the body.

Some vitamins are absorbed in an inactive form called either a **provitamin** or a **vitamin precursor**. To perform vitamin functions, provitamins must be converted into active vitamin forms once they are inside the body. How much of each provitamin can be converted into the active vitamin and the rate at which this process occurs affect the amount of a vitamin available to function inside the body.

Vitamin Functions

Vitamins promote and regulate the body's activities. Each vitamin has one or more important functions (Figure 7.5). For example, vitamin A is needed for vision as well as normal growth and development. Vitamin K is needed for blood clotting and bone health. Often more than one vitamin is needed to ensure the health of a particular organ or system. Some vitamins act in a similar manner to do their jobs. For example, all the B vitamins act as **coenzymes** (Figure 7.6).

A few vitamins function as **antioxidants**, substances that protect against **oxidative damage**. Oxidative damage is caused when reactive oxygen molecules

coenzyme An organic nonprotein substance that binds to an enzyme to promote its activity.

antioxidant A substance that decreases the adverse effects of reactive molecules on normal physiological function.

Coenzymes • Figure 7.6

Coenzymes are needed for enzyme activity. They act as carriers of electrons, atoms, or chemical groups that participate in the reaction. All the B vitamins are coenzymes, but there are also coenzymes that are not dietary essentials and therefore are not vitamins.

HOW IT WORKS

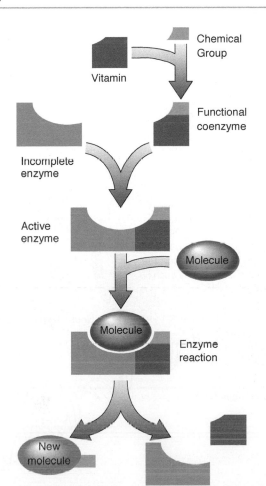

❶ The vitamin combines with a chemical group to form the functional coenzyme (active vitamin).

❷ The functional coenzyme combines with the incomplete enzyme to form the active enzyme.

❸ The active enzyme binds to one or more molecules and accelerates the chemical reaction to form one or more new molecules.

❹ The new molecules are released, and the enzyme and coenzyme (vitamin) can be reused or separated.

PROCESS DIAGRAM

A Vitamin Primer 193

steal electrons from other compounds, causing changes in their structure and function. Reactive oxygen molecules such as **free radicals** can be generated by normal oxygen-requiring reactions inside the body, such as cellular respiration, or can come from environmental sources such as air pollution or cigarette smoke. Free radicals cause damage by snatching electrons from DNA, proteins, carbohydrates, or unsaturated fatty acids. This loss of electrons results in changes in the structure and function of these molecules. Antioxidants act by reducing the formation of or destroying free radicals and other reactive oxygen molecules before they can do damage (**Figure 7.7**).

Some antioxidants are produced in the body; others, such as vitamin C, vitamin E, and the mineral selenium, are consumed in the diet.[3]

Meeting Vitamin Needs

The right amounts and combinations of vitamins and other nutrients are essential to health. Despite our knowledge of what vitamins do and how much of each we need, not everyone consumes the right amounts. In developing countries, vitamin deficiencies remain a major public health problem. In industrialized countries, thanks to the more varied food supply, along with fortification, vitamin-deficiency diseases have been almost eliminated. In these countries, concern now focuses on

How antioxidants work • Figure 7.7

Many antioxidants, including vitamin C, function by donating electrons to free radicals. A donated electron stabilizes the free radical so that it is no longer reactive and cannot steal electrons from important molecules in and around cells.

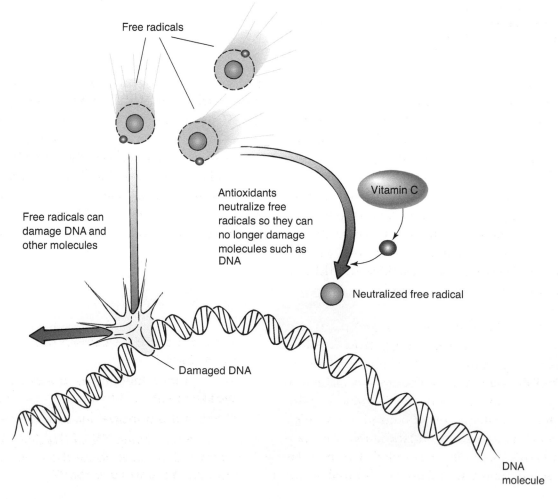

Free radicals

Antioxidants neutralize free radicals so they can no longer damage molecules such as DNA

Vitamin C

Free radicals can damage DNA and other molecules

Neutralized free radical

Damaged DNA

DNA molecule

As a general guideline, if the % Daily Value is 20% or more, the food is an excellent source of that nutrient; if it is 10 to 19%, the food is a good source; and if it is 5% or less, the food is a poor source of that nutrient.

Orange Juice

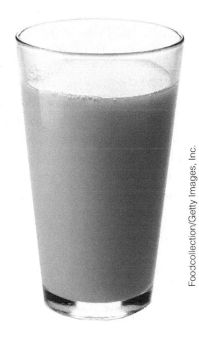

Foodcollection/Getty Images, Inc.

Nutrition Facts

Serving Size 8 fl oz (250 mL)
Servings Per Container 8

Amount Per Serving

Calories 110	Calories from Fat 0

	%Daily V alue**
Total Fat 0g	**2%**
Sodium 0mg	**0%**
Potassium 450mg	**13%**
Total Carbohydrate 26g	**9%**
Sugars 7g	
Protein 2g	

Vitamin C 120%	•	Calcium	2%
Thiamin	10%	• Riboflavin	4%
Niacin	4%	• Vitamin B$_6$	6%
Folate	15%	• Magnesium	6%

Not a significant source of saturated fat, cholesterol, dietary fiber, vitamin A and iron.

*Percent Daily Values are based on a 2,000 calorie diet.

To determine the exact amount of a vitamin in a food, look up the Daily Value (see Appendix I) and multiply it by the % Daily Value on the label.

Interpret the Data

The Daily Value for vitamin C is 60 mg. Based on the information on this label, how many milligrams of vitamin C are in 4 fluid ounces of orange juice?
a. 36   **b.** 60   **c.** 72   **d.** 120

meeting the needs of high-risk groups, such as children and pregnant women; determining the consequences of marginal deficiencies, such as the effect of low vitamin D on the risk of multiple sclerosis; and evaluating the risks of consuming large amounts of certain vitamins.

The RDAs and AIs of the DRIs recommend amounts that provide enough of each of the vitamins to prevent deficiency and promote health (see Chapter 2). Because more is not always better when it comes to nutrient intake, the DRIs have also established ULs as a guide to amounts that avoid the risk of toxicity (see Appendix A).

Food labels can help identify packaged foods that are good sources of vitamins. Current labels are required to list the amounts of vitamin A and vitamin C in foods as a percentage of the Daily Values (**Figure 7.8**). The proposed changes to food labels will require that they list, vitamin D, which is a vitamin of concern in today's diet. Both the amount in micrograms and the amount as a percentage of the Daily Value will be included. The amounts of vitamin A and vitamin C would not be required on the

proposed food label because they are no longer considered nutrients at risk in the American diet, but amounts and Daily Values for these and other vitamins could be provided voluntarily. Fresh fruits, vegetables, and fish, which are excellent sources of many vitamins, do not carry food labels. The FDA has therefore asked that grocery stores voluntarily provide nutrition information for the raw fruits, vegetables, and fish that are most frequently purchased, and about 75% of stores comply.[4]

CONCEPT CHECK   STOP

1. **What** food groups contain the greatest variety of vitamins?

2. **Why** might a low-fat diet affect the bioavailability of fat-soluble vitamins?

3. **What** is the principal function of coenzymes?

4. **What** does having 5% of the Daily Value for vitamin C indicate about the amount of that vitamin in a particular food?

7.2 The Water-Soluble Vitamins

LEARNING OBJECTIVES

1. **Discuss** the role of thiamin, riboflavin, and niacin in producing ATP.
2. **Explain** why vitamin B_6 is important for amino acid metabolism.
3. **Compare** the functions of folate and vitamin B_{12}.
4. **Relate** the role of vitamin C in the body to the symptoms of scurvy

The water-soluble vitamins include the B vitamins and vitamin C. The B vitamins are directly involved in transferring the energy in carbohydrate, fat, and protein to ATP, the high-energy molecule that is used to fuel the body. Vitamin C is needed to synthesize connective tissue and to protect us from damage by oxidation.

Because water-soluble vitamins are not stored to any great extent, supplies of most of these vitamins are rapidly depleted. For this reason, water-soluble vitamins must be consumed regularly. Nevertheless, it takes more than a few days to develop deficiency symptoms, even when one of these vitamins is completely eliminated from the diet. For years, we thought that because most water-soluble vitamins are not stored in the body and are excreted in the urine, high doses were not harmful. However, we now recognize that high doses of some of these vitamins are toxic.

Thiamin

Thiamin, the first of the B vitamins to be discovered, is sometimes called vitamin B_1. **Beriberi**, the disease that results from a deficiency of this vitamin, flourished in East Asian countries for over 1000 years. It came to the attention of Western medicine in colonial Asia in the 19th century. The disease became such a problem that the Dutch East India Company sent a team of scientists to determine its cause. A young physician named Christian Eijkman worked on this problem for over 10 years. His success came as a result of a twist of fate. He ran out of food for his experimental chickens and, instead of the usual brown rice, fed them

> **beriberi** A thiamin deficiency disease that may manifest in one of two forms: dry beriberi, which causes weakness and nerve degeneration, or wet beriberi, which causes heart changes.

How thiamin functions • Figure 7.9

The role of thiamin in producing ATP from glucose and synthesizing neurotransmitters has been linked to the neurological symptoms of the thiamin deficiency disease, beriberi.

a. Thiamin is needed to convert pyruvate into acetyl-CoA. Acetyl-CoA can continue through cellular respiration to produce ATP. Acetyl-CoA is also needed to synthesize the neurotransmitter acetylcholine.

b. In Sri Lanka, the word *beriberi* means "I cannot," referring to the extreme weakness and depression that are the earliest symptoms of the disease. These symptoms may result from the inability of nerve cells to produce ATP from glucose. Other neurological symptoms, such as poor coordination, tingling sensations, and paralysis, may be related to the body's inability to synthesize certain neurotransmitters when thiamin is deficient.

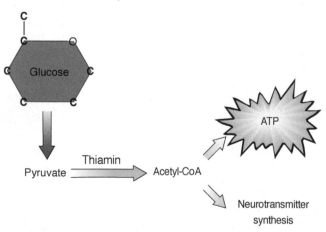

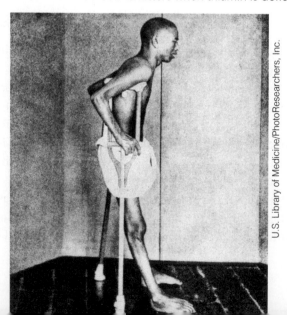

U.S. Library of Medicine/PhotoResearchers, Inc.

Ask Yourself

How would a deficiency of thiamin affect the amounts of ATP and neurotransmitters available?

white rice. Shortly thereafter, the chickens displayed beri-beri-like symptoms. When he fed them brown rice again, their health was restored. These events provided evidence that beriberi was not caused by a poison or a microorganism, as had previously been thought, but rather by something that was missing from the diet.

Knowledge gained from Eijkman's studies made it possible to prevent and cure beriberi by feeding people a diet adequate in thiamin; however, the vitamin itself was not isolated until 1926. We now know that polishing the bran layer off rice kernels to make white rice removes the thiamin-rich portion of the grain. Therefore, in populations where white rice was the staple of the diet, beriberi became a common health problem. The incidence of beriberi in eastern Asia increased dramatically in the late 1800s due to the rising popularity of polished rice.

Thiamin is a coenzyme that is needed for the breakdown of glucose to provide energy. It is particularly important for nerve function because glucose is the energy source for nerve cells. In addition to its role in energy metabolism, thiamin is needed for the synthesis of **neurotransmitters**, the metabolism of other sugars and certain amino acids, and the synthesis of ribose and deoxyribose, sugars that are part of the structure of RNA (ribonucleic acid) and DNA, respectively.

When thiamin intake is deficient, neurological symptoms such as impaired motor and sensory reflexes (dry beriberi), or cardiovascular systems such as a rapid heart rate, enlargement of the heart, and accumulation of fluid in the tissues (wet beriberi) occur. The neurological symptoms of dry beriberi can be related to the functions of thiamin (**Figure 7.9**), but it is not clear why thiamin deficiency causes the cardiovascular symptoms seen with wet beriberi.[5]

Thiamin deficiency can also result in **Wernicke–Korsakoff syndrome**, which causes confusion, loss of coordination, vision changes, and hallucinations and can progress to coma and death. It occurs most often in alcoholics because alcohol decreases thiamin absorption and diets high in alcohol are typically low in micronutrients. It has also been identified in those with eating disorders, in those on long-term intravenous nutrition, and in individuals who have undergone gastric bypass surgery.[6]

Thiamin is abundant in pork, legumes, and seeds. In addition to being found in the bran layer of brown rice and other whole grains, thiamin is added to enriched grains (**Figure 7.10**).

> **neurotransmitter**
> A chemical substance produced by a nerve cell that can stimulate or inhibit another cell.

Meeting thiamin needs • Figure 7.10

A large proportion of the thiamin consumed in the United States comes from enriched grain products that we consume in abundance, such as pasta, rice dishes, baked goods, and breakfast cereals. The dashed lines indicate the RDAs for adult men and women, which are 1.2 mg/day and 1.1 mg/day, respectively.

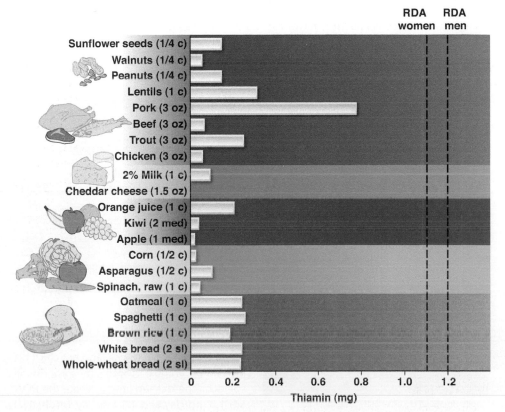

Although thiamin is needed to provide energy, unless the diet is deficient in thiamin, increasing thiamin intake does not increase the ability to produce ATP. There is no UL for thiamin because no toxicity has been reported when an excess of this vitamin is consumed from either food or supplements.[5]

Riboflavin

Riboflavin is a B vitamin that provides a visible indicator of excessive consumption; the excess is excreted in the urine, turning it a bright fluorescent yellow. The color may surprise you, but it is harmless. No adverse effects of high doses of riboflavin from either foods or supplements have been reported.

Riboflavin forms two active coenzymes that serve as electron carriers. They function in the reactions needed to produce ATP from carbohydrate, fat, and protein. Riboflavin is also involved directly or indirectly in converting a number of other vitamins, including folate, niacin, vitamin B_6, and vitamin K, into their active forms.

One of the best sources of riboflavin in the diet is milk (**Figure 7.11**). When riboflavin is deficient, injuries heal poorly because new cells cannot grow to replace the damaged ones. The tissues that grow most rapidly, such as the skin and the linings of the eyes, mouth, and tongue, are the first to be affected. Deficiency causes symptoms such as cracking of the lips and at the corners of the mouth; increased sensitivity to light; burning, tearing, and itching

Meeting riboflavin needs • Figure 7.11

Riboflavin is found in a variety of foods but can be destroyed by exposure to light.

a. Ever wonder why milk doesn't come in glass bottles anymore? The reason is that riboflavin is destroyed by light. Cloudy plastic containers block some of the light, but opaque ones, such as cardboard containers, are the most effective. Exposure to light can also cause an "off" flavor and losses of vitamins A and D.[7]

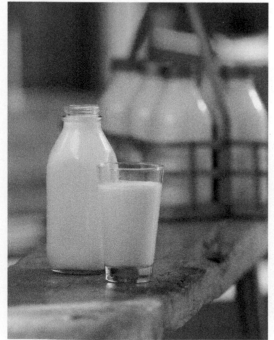

Jupiter Images/FoodPix /Getty Images, Inc.

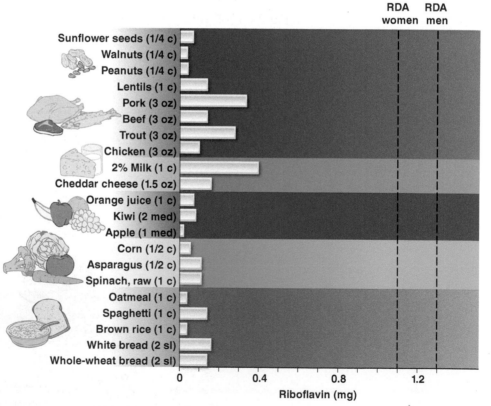

b. Major dietary sources of riboflavin include dairy products, red meat, poultry, fish, whole grains, and enriched breads and cereals. Vegetable sources include asparagus, broccoli, mushrooms, and leafy green vegetables such as spinach. The dashed lines indicate the RDAs for adult men and women, which are 1.3 mg/day and 1.1 mg/day, respectively.[5]

of the eyes; and flaking of the skin around the nose, eyebrows, and earlobes.

A deficiency of riboflavin usually occurs in conjunction with deficiencies of other B vitamins because the same foods are also sources of those vitamins and because riboflavin is needed to convert other vitamins into their active forms. Some of the symptoms seen in cases of riboflavin deficiency therefore reflect deficiencies of these other nutrients as well.

Niacin

In the early 1900s, psychiatric hospitals in the southeastern United States were filled with patients with the niacin-deficiency disease **pellagra** (**Figure 7.12**). **Niacin** is a B vitamin that forms coenzymes essential for glucose metabolism

pellagra A disease resulting from niacin deficiency, which causes dermatitis, diarrhea, dementia, and, if not treated, death.

Tracking down the cause of pellagra • Figure 7.12

In 1914, Dr. Joseph Goldberger was appointed by the U.S. Public Health Service to investigate the pellagra epidemic in the South. He unraveled the mystery of its cause by using the scientific method.

Observation
Goldberger observed that individuals in institutions such as hospitals, orphanages, and prisons suffered from pellagra, but the staff did not. If pellagra were an infectious disease, both populations would be equally affected.

Hypothesis
Goldberger hypothesized that pellagra was due to a deficiency in the diet.

Experiments
Experimental design: Goldberger and coworkers added nutritious foods, including meat, milk, and vegetables, to the diets of children in two orphanages.

Results: Those consuming the healthier diets recovered from pellagra. Those without the disease who ate the new diet did not contract pellagra, supporting the hypothesis that it was caused by a dietary deficiency.

Experimental design: Goldberger and colleagues fed 11 volunteers a diet believed to be lacking in the dietary substance that prevents pellagra.

Results: Six of the eleven developed symptoms of pellagra after 5 months of consuming the experimental diet, supporting the hypothesis that it was caused by a dietary deficiency.

Continued experiments: Human and animal studies by a number of scientists lead to the identification of nicotinic acid, better known as the water-soluable B vitamin niacin, in 1937, as the dietary component that cures and prevents pellagra.

Theory
Pellagra is caused by a deficiency of the B vitamin niacin.

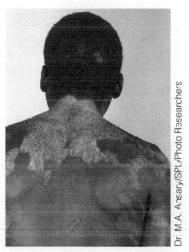

This photograph illustrates the cracked, inflamed skin that is characteristic of pellagra. The rash most commonly appears on areas of the skin that are exposed to sunlight or other stresses.

Dr. M.A. Ansary/SPL/Photo Researchers

Sources of niacin • Figure 7.13

Niacin needs can be met by consuming foods that are sources of niacin and foods that contain tryptophan, which can be converted to niacin.

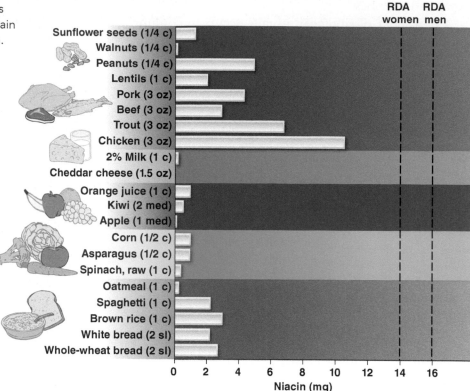

a. Meat, fish, peanuts, and whole and enriched grains are the best sources of niacin. Other sources include legumes and wheat bran. The dashed lines indicate the RDAs for adult men and women, which are 16 mg NE/day and 14 mg NE/day, respectively.

Think Critically Using the values in this graph, plan a dinner that provides 100% of the RDA of niacin for women.

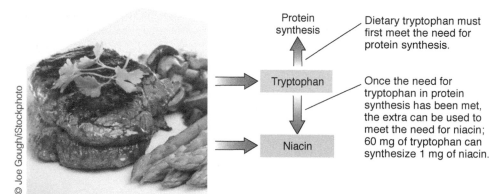

The diet provides food sources of both niacin and tryptophan.

Protein synthesis

Dietary tryptophan must first meet the need for protein synthesis.

Tryptophan

Once the need for tryptophan in protein synthesis has been met, the extra can be used to meet the need for niacin; 60 mg of tryptophan can synthesize 1 mg of niacin.

Niacin

b. The essential amino acid tryptophan, found in dietary protein, can be used to synthesize niacin but only after the body's need for tryptophan in protein synthesis has been met. Values given in food composition tables and databases do not include the amount of niacin that could be made from the tryptophan in a food.

and the synthesis of fatty acids and cholesterol. The need for niacin is so widespread in metabolism that a deficiency causes major changes throughout the body. The early symptoms of pellagra include fatigue, decreased appetite, and indigestion. These are followed by symptoms that can be remembered as the three Ds: dermatitis, diarrhea, and dementia. If left untreated, niacin deficiency results in a fourth D—death.

Meats and grains are good sources of niacin. Niacin can also be synthesized in the body from the essential amino acid tryptophan (**Figure 7.13**). Tryptophan, however, is used to make niacin only if enough of it is available

to first meet the needs of protein synthesis. When the diet is low in tryptophan, it is not used to synthesize niacin. Because some of the requirement for niacin can be met through the synthesis of niacin from tryptophan, the RDA is expressed as **niacin equivalents (NEs)**. One NE is equal to 1 mg of niacin or 60 mg of tryptophan, the amount needed to make 1 mg of niacin.[5]

Niacin deficiency was rampant in the South in the early 1900s because the local diet among the poor was based on corn. Corn is low in tryptophan, and the niacin found naturally in corn is bound to other molecules and therefore is not well absorbed. Today, as a result of the enrichment of grains with an available form of niacin, pellagra is rare in the United States, but it remains a problem in areas of Africa where the diet is based on corn.[8] Despite the corn-based diet in Mexico and Central American countries, pellagra is uncommon in those countries, in part because the treatment of corn with limewater, as is done during the making of tortillas, enhances the bioavailability of niacin. The diet in these regions also includes legumes, which provide both niacin and a source of tryptophan for the synthesis of niacin.

There is no evidence of any adverse effects from consuming the niacin that occurs naturally in foods, but niacin supplements can be toxic. Excess niacin supplementation can cause flushing of the skin, a tingling sensation in the hands and feet, a red skin rash, nausea, vomiting, diarrhea, high blood sugar levels, abnormalities in liver function, and blurred vision. The UL for adults is 35 mg/day. Doses of 50 mg/day or greater of one form of niacin are used as a drug to treat elevated blood cholesterol; this amount should be consumed only when prescribed by a physician.

Biotin

The B vitamin **biotin** is a coenzyme that functions in energy metabolism and glucose synthesis. It is also important in the metabolism of fatty acids and amino acids. Good sources of biotin in the diet include cooked eggs,

Raw eggs and biotin bioavailability • Figure 7.14

Raw egg whites contain a protein called avidin that tightly binds biotin and prevents its absorption. Even if you were not concerned with biotin deficiency, raw eggs should never be eaten because they can contain harmful bacteria. Thoroughly cooking eggs kills bacteria and denatures avidin so that it cannot bind biotin.

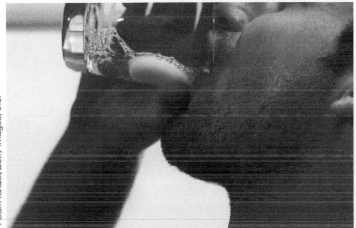

A Carmichael/Getty Images, Inc.

liver, yogurt, and nuts. Fruit and meat are poor sources. Bacteria in the gastrointestinal tract synthesize biotin, and some of this is absorbed into the body and helps meet our biotin needs. An AI of 30 μg/day has been established for adults.[5]

Although biotin deficiency is uncommon, it has been observed in people with malabsorption and those taking certain medications for long periods.[5] Eating raw eggs can also cause biotin deficiency (**Figure 7.14**). Biotin deficiency in humans causes nausea, thinning hair, loss of hair color, a red skin rash, depression, lethargy, hallucinations, and tingling of the extremities. High doses of biotin have not resulted in toxicity symptoms; there is no UL for biotin.

Pantothenic Acid

Pantothenic acid, which gets its name from the Greek word *pantothen* (meaning "from everywhere"), is a B vitamin that is widely distributed in foods. It is particularly abundant in meat, eggs, whole grains, and legumes, and it is found in lesser amounts in milk, vegetables, and fruits.

In addition to being "from everywhere" in the diet, pantothenic acid seems to be needed everywhere in the body. It is part of coenzyme A (CoA), which is needed for the breakdown of carbohydrates, fatty acids, and amino acids, as well as for the modification of proteins and the synthesis of neurotransmitters, steroid hormones, and hemoglobin. Pantothenic acid is also needed to form a molecule that is essential for the synthesis of cholesterol and fatty acids.

The wide distribution of pantothenic acid in foods makes deficiency rare in humans. The AI is 5 mg/day for adults. Pantothenic acid is relatively nontoxic, and there are insufficient data to establish a UL.[5]

Vitamin B$_6$

Vitamin B$_6$ is a B vitamin that is particularly important for amino acid and protein metabolism. It is needed to synthesize nonessential amino acids, make neurotransmitters, synthesize hemoglobin, convert tryptophan into niacin, and break down glycogen to release glucose into the blood. There are three forms of vitamin B$_6$: pyridoxal, pyridoxine, and pyridoxamine. These can be converted into the active coenzyme **pyridoxal phosphate**, which is needed for the activity of more than 100 enzymes involved in the metabolism of protein, carbohydrate, and fat.

Vitamin B$_6$ deficiency leads to poor growth, skin lesions, decreased immune function, anemia, and neurological symptoms. Because vitamin B$_6$ is needed for amino acid metabolism, the onset of a deficiency can be hastened by a diet that is low in vitamin B_6 but high in protein. Many of the symptoms can be linked to the biochemical reactions that depend on this vitamin coenzyme (**Figure 7.15**). For example, poor growth, skin lesions, and decreased antibody formation may occur with a diet that is low in vitamin B_6 because of the central role of vitamin B_6 in protein and energy metabolism. Anemia and neurological symptoms can be linked to the role of vitamin B_6 in hemoglobin synthesis and myelin formation, respectively.

Meat and fish are excellent animal sources of vitamin B_6, and whole grains and legumes are good plant sources. Refined grain products such as white rice and white

Nutrition InSight | Vitamin B_6 functions and deficiency symptoms • Figure 7.15

The functions of vitamin B_6 in amino acid metabolism, myelin formation, and red and white blood cell synthesis help explain the symptoms that occur when this vitamin is deficient.

a. The coenzyme form of vitamin B_6 (pyridoxal phosphate) is needed for a number of reactions that are essential to amino acid synthesis, the breakdown of amino acids for energy, and the use of amino acids for the synthesis of glucose and neurotransmitters.

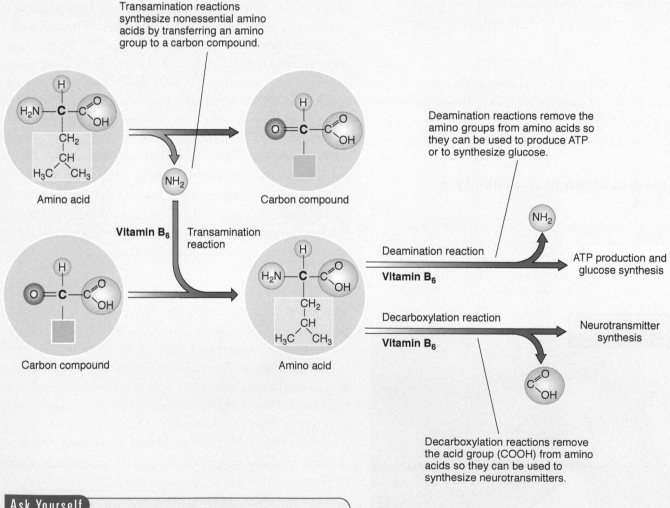

Transamination reactions synthesize nonessential amino acids by transferring an amino group to a carbon compound.

Deamination reactions remove the amino groups from amino acids so they can be used to produce ATP or to synthesize glucose.

Decarboxylation reactions remove the acid group (COOH) from amino acids so they can be used to synthesize neurotransmitters.

Ask Yourself

What functions of vitamin B_6 might explain why a deficiency of this vitamin interferes with nerve function?

bread are not good sources of vitamin B_6 because the vitamin is lost during refining but is not added back through enrichment (**Figure 7.16**). It is, however, added to many fortified breakfast cereals, making these good sources of the vitamin. Vitamin B_6 is destroyed by heat and light, so it can easily be lost during processing.

No adverse effects have been associated with high intake of vitamin B_6 from foods, but large doses found in supplements can cause severe nerve impairment. To prevent nerve damage, the UL for adults is set at 100 mg/day from food and supplements.[5] Despite the potential for toxicity, high-dose supplements of vitamin B_6 containing 100 mg/dose

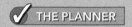

b. Vitamin B_6 is needed for the synthesis of lipids that are part of the **myelin** coating on nerves. Myelin is essential for nerve transmission. The role of vitamin B_6 in myelin formation and neurotransmitter synthesis may explain the neurological symptoms that occur with deficiency, such as numbness and tingling in the hands and feet, depression, headaches, confusion, and seizures.

c. Vitamin B_6 is needed to synthesize hemoglobin, the oxygen-carrying protein in red blood cells. When vitamin B_6 is deficient, hemoglobin cannot be made; the result is a type of anemia characterized by small, pale red blood cells. Vitamin B_6 is also needed to form white blood cells, which are part of the immune system, so deficiency reduces immune function.

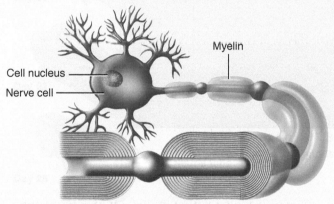

Myelin

Cell nucleus

Nerve cell

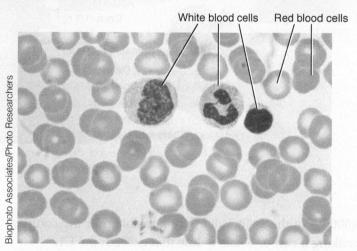

White blood cells   Red blood cells

Biophoto Associates/Photo Researchers

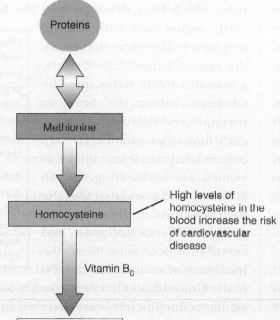

Proteins

Methionine

Homocysteine

High levels of homocysteine in the blood increase the risk of cardiovascular disease

Vitamin B_6

Cysteine

d. If vitamin B_6 status is low, homocysteine, which is formed from the amino acid methionine, cannot be converted to the amino acid cysteine, so levels rise. Even a mild elevation in blood homocysteine levels has been shown to increase the risk of cardiovascular disease.[9]

The Water-Soluble Vitamins 203

Folate deficiency and macrocytic anemia • Figure 7.18

Folate is needed for DNA replication. Without folate, developing red blood cells cannot divide. Instead, they just grow bigger. The abnormally large immature red blood cells, called megaloblasts, then mature into abnormally large red blood cells called macrocytes. Fewer red blood cells are produced, and they often contain less hemoglobin, resulting in what is called macrocytic anemia.

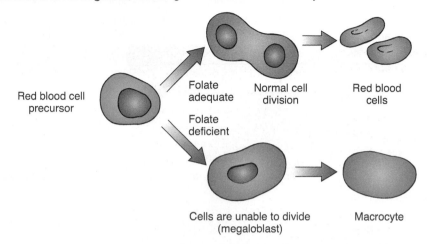

Red blood cell precursor

Folate adequate

Normal cell division

Red blood cells

Folate deficient

Cells are unable to divide (megaloblast)

Macrocyte

(**Figure 7.18**). Other symptoms of folate deficiency include poor growth, problems with nerve development and function, diarrhea, and inflammation of the tongue.

Low folate status may also increase the risk of developing heart disease. Folate's connection with heart disease has to do with the metabolism of homocysteine. Elevated levels of homocysteine have been associated with increased risk of heart disease. Folate and vitamins B_{12} and B_6 are all needed to prevent homocysteine levels from rising (**Figure 7.19**). Despite this, supplementation with these vitamins has failed to exert significant effects on cardiovascular risk.[9]

Population groups most at risk of folate deficiency include pregnant women and premature infants (because of their rapid rates of cell division and growth), the elderly (because of their limited intake of foods high in folate), alcoholics (because alcohol inhibits the absorption of folate), and tobacco smokers (because smoke inactivates folate in the cells lining the lungs).[5]

Asparagus, oranges, legumes, liver, and yeast are excellent food sources of folate (**Figure 7.20**). Whole grains are a fair source, and, as discussed earlier, folic acid is added to enriched grain products, including enriched breads, flours, corn meal, pasta, grits, and rice.

B vitamins and homocysteine metabolism • Figure 7.19

Folate and vitamin B_{12} are both needed to convert homocysteine to methionine. When either folate, vitamin B_{12}, or, as discussed earlier, vitamin B_6 are deficient, homocysteine levels rise, increasing the risk of developing cardiovascular disease.

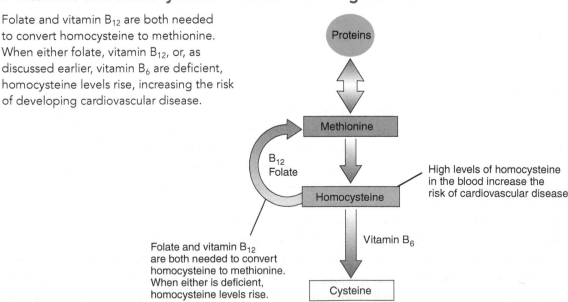

Proteins

Methionine

B_{12}
Folate

Homocysteine

High levels of homocysteine in the blood increase the risk of cardiovascular disease

Folate and vitamin B_{12} are both needed to convert homocysteine to methionine. When either is deficient, homocysteine levels rise.

Vitamin B_6

Cysteine

Meeting folate needs • Figure 7.20

The word folate comes from the Latin for *foliage*, because leafy greens, such as spinach, are good sources of this vitamin. Legumes, nuts, enriched grains, and orange juice are also good sources. Whole grains and many vegetables are fair sources. Only small amounts of folate are found in meats, cheese, milk, and most fruits. The dashed line indicates the RDA for adult men and women, which is 400 µg/day.

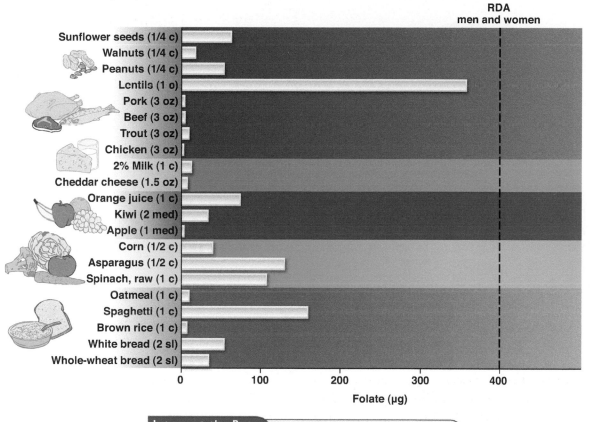

Interpret the Data

Which three of the foods shown here provide the most folate? Are any of these foods fortified?

Because supplementing folic acid early in pregnancy has been shown to reduce neural tube defects in the fetus, it is recommended that women who are capable of becoming pregnant consume 400 µg of synthetic folic acid from fortified foods and/or supplements in addition to the food folate consumed in a varied diet.[5] To get 400 µg of folic acid, women of childbearing age would need to eat four to six servings of fortified grain products each day or take a supplement containing folic acid.

Although there is no known folate toxicity, a high intake from fortified foods or supplements could potentially mask the early symptoms of vitamin B_{12} deficiency, allowing it to go untreated. Based on this concern, a UL for adults has been set at 1000 µg/day of folic acid from supplements and/or fortified foods.

Vitamin B_{12}

In the early 1900s, **pernicious anemia** amounted to a death sentence. There was no cure. In the 1920s, researchers George Minot and William Murphy pursued their belief that pernicious anemia could be cured by something in the diet. They discovered that they could restore patients' health by feeding them about 4 to 8 ounces of slightly cooked liver at every meal. Today we know that eating liver cured pernicious anemia because liver is a concentrated source of **vitamin B_{12}**. Individuals with pernicious anemia lack a protein produced in the

> **pernicious anemia** A macrocytic anemia resulting from vitamin B_{12} deficiency that occurs when dietary vitamin B_{12} cannot be absorbed due to a lack of intrinsic factor.

Vitamin B₁₂ absorption • Figure 7.21

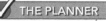

The body stores and reuses vitamin B₁₂ more efficiently than it does most other water-soluble vitamins, so deficiency is typically caused by poor absorption rather than by low intake alone. Absorption of adequate amounts of vitamin B₁₂ from food depends on the presence of stomach acid, protein-digesting enzymes, and intrinsic factor.

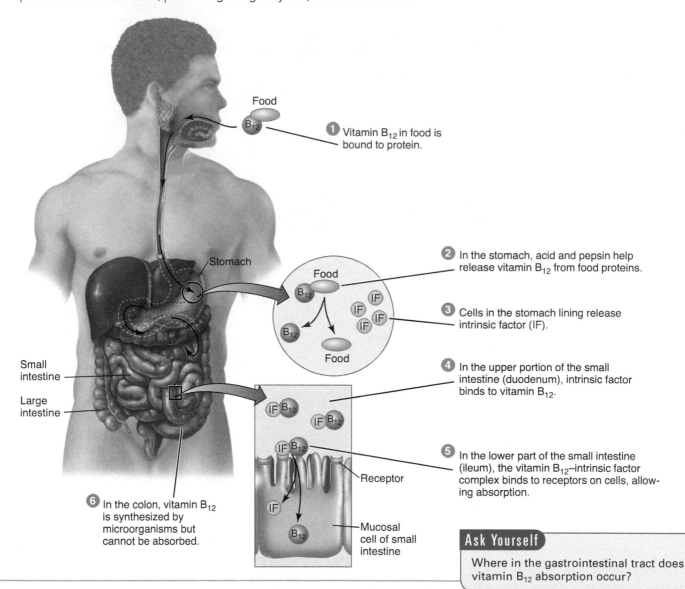

Food

① Vitamin B₁₂ in food is bound to protein.

Stomach

Food

② In the stomach, acid and pepsin help release vitamin B₁₂ from food proteins.

③ Cells in the stomach lining release intrinsic factor (IF).

Food

Small intestine

Large intestine

④ In the upper portion of the small intestine (duodenum), intrinsic factor binds to vitamin B₁₂.

⑤ In the lower part of the small intestine (ileum), the vitamin B₁₂–intrinsic factor complex binds to receptors on cells, allowing absorption.

Receptor

⑥ In the colon, vitamin B₁₂ is synthesized by microorganisms but cannot be absorbed.

Mucosal cell of small intestine

Ask Yourself

Where in the gastrointestinal tract does vitamin B₁₂ absorption occur?

---

stomach, called **intrinsic factor**, that enhances vitamin B₁₂ absorption (**Figure 7.21**). Eating large amounts of liver was an effective treatment because a small proportion of dietary B₁₂ can be absorbed by passive diffusion even when intrinsic factor is absent. Today, pernicious anemia is treated with injections or mega-doses of vitamin B₁₂ rather than with plates full of liver.

> **intrinsic factor** A protein produced in the stomach that aids in the absorption of vitamin B₁₂.

Vitamin B₁₂, also known as **cobalamin**, is necessary for the production of ATP from certain fatty acids, to maintain the myelin coating on nerves (see Figure 7.15b), and for a reaction that converts homocysteine to methionine and converts folate to the form that is active for DNA synthesis (**Figure 7.22**). When vitamin B₁₂ is deficient, homocysteine levels rise, and folate is trapped in an inactive form. Without adequate active folate, DNA synthesis slows, red blood cells do not divide normally, and macrocytic anemia develops. Lack of vitamin B₁₂ also leads to

The relationship between folate and vitamin B₁₂ • Figure 7.22

When vitamin B₁₂ is deficient it causes what is called a secondary folate deficiency; folate is available, but the B₁₂ deficiency prevents it from being activated. The folic acid provided by supplements and fortified foods does not need to be activated. This has raised concerns that our folic acid-fortified food supply will prevent folate-deficiency symptoms, such as macrocytic anemia, from occurring when B₁₂ is deficient and allow the B₁₂ deficiency to go unnoticed.

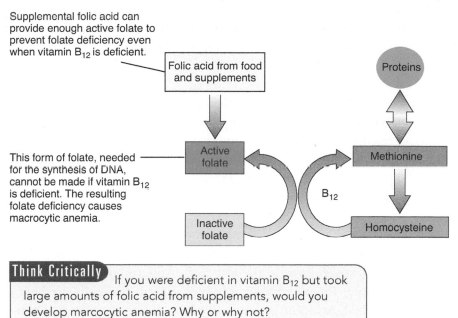

Supplemental folic acid can provide enough active folate to prevent folate deficiency even when vitamin B₁₂ is deficient.

Folic acid from food and supplements

This form of folate, needed for the synthesis of DNA, cannot be made if vitamin B₁₂ is deficient. The resulting folate deficiency causes macrocytic anemia.

Active folate

Inactive folate

Proteins

Methionine

B₁₂

Homocysteine

Think Critically If you were deficient in vitamin B₁₂ but took large amounts of folic acid from supplements, would you develop marcocytic anemia? Why or why not?

degeneration of the myelin that coats nerves including those in the spinal cord and brain, resulting in symptoms such as numbness and tingling, abnormalities in gait, memory loss, and disorientation. If not treated, vitamin B₁₂ deficiency can cause irreversible nerve damage and eventually death.

Vitamin B₁₂ is found naturally only in animal products (**Figure 7.23**). Therefore, meeting vitamin B₁₂

Meeting vitamin B₁₂ needs • Figure 7.23

Animal foods provide vitamin B₁₂, but plant foods do not unless they have been fortified with it or contaminated by bacteria, soil, insects, or other sources of B₁₂. The dashed line indicates the RDA for adult men and women of all ages, which is 2.4 µg/day. No toxic effects have been reported for vitamin B₁₂ intakes of up to 100 µg/day from food or supplements. Insufficient data are available to establish a UL for vitamin B₁₂.[5]

Interpret the Data

What food groups provide vitamin B₁₂?

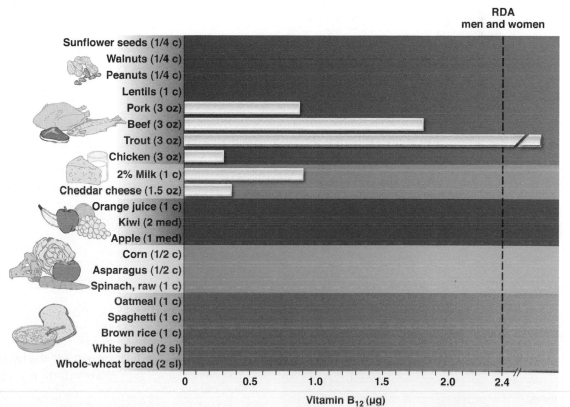

RDA
men and women

Sunflower seeds (1/4 c)
Walnuts (1/4 c)
Peanuts (1/4 c)
Lentils (1 c)
Pork (3 oz)
Beef (3 oz)
Trout (3 oz)
Chicken (3 oz)
2% Milk (1 c)
Cheddar cheese (1.5 oz)
Orange juice (1 c)
Kiwi (2 med)
Apple (1 med)
Corn (1/2 c)
Asparagus (1/2 c)
Spinach, raw (1 c)
Oatmeal (1 c)
Spaghetti (1 c)
Brown rice (1 c)
White bread (2 sl)
Whole-wheat bread (2 sl)

0   0.5   1.0   1.5   2.0   2.4

Vitamin B₁₂ (µg)

needs is a concern among vegans—those who consume no animal products. Vegans must consume supplements or foods fortified with vitamin B_{12} in order to meet their needs for this vitamin.[14] Vitamin B_{12} deficiency is also a concern in older adults because of a condition called **atrophic gastritis**, which reduces the secretion of

> **atrophic gastritis**
> An inflammation of the stomach lining that results in reduced secretion of stomach acid, microbial overgrowth, and, in severe cases, a reduction in the production of intrinsic factor.

stomach acid. Without sufficient stomach acid, the enzymes that release the vitamin B_{12} bound to proteins in food cannot function properly, so vitamin B_{12} remains bound to the food proteins and cannot be absorbed (see Figure 7.21). In addition, lack of stomach acid allows large numbers of microbes to grow in the gut and compete for available vitamin B_{12},

reducing the amount absorbed. Atrophic gastritis affects 10% to 30% of adults over age 50. To ensure adequate

vitamin B_{12} absorption, it is recommended that individuals over age 50 meet their RDA by consuming foods fortified with vitamin B_{12} or taking vitamin B_{12} supplements.[5] The vitamin B_{12} in these products is not bound to proteins, so it is absorbed even when stomach acid levels are low.

Vitamin C

Vitamin C, also called **ascorbic acid**, is best known for its role in the synthesis and maintenance of **collagen** (**Figure 7.24**). Collagen, the most abundant protein in the body, can be thought of as the glue that holds the body together. It forms the base of all connective tissue. It is the framework for bones and teeth; it is the main component of ligaments, tendons, and the scars that bind a wound together; and it gives structure to the walls of blood vessels. When vitamin C is lacking, collagen cannot be formed and maintained, and the symptoms

Vitamin C function and deficiency • Figure 7.24

A deficiency of vitamin C results in the inability to form healthy collagen, which leads to the symptoms of scurvy.

a. A reaction requiring vitamin C is essential for the formation of bonds that hold adjacent collagen strands together and give the protein strength. Like all other body proteins, collagen is continuously being broken down and reformed. Without vitamin C, the bonds cross-linking adjacent collagen molecules cannot be formed, so the collagen that is broken down is replaced with abnormal collagen.

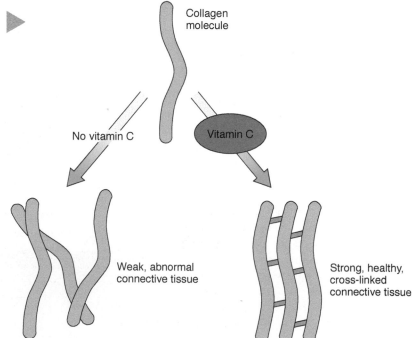

Collagen molecule

No vitamin C

Vitamin C

Weak, abnormal connective tissue

Strong, healthy, cross-linked connective tissue

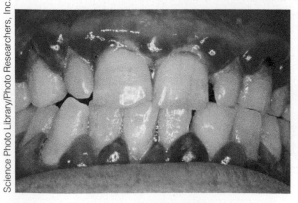

Science Photo Library/Photo Researchers, Inc.

b. When vitamin C intake is below 10 mg/day, the symptoms of scurvy begin to appear. The gums become inflamed, swell, and bleed. The teeth loosen and eventually fall out. The capillary walls weaken and rupture, causing bleeding under the skin and into the joints. This causes raised red spots on the skin, joint pain and weakness, and easy bruising. Wounds do not heal, old wounds may reopen, and bones fracture. People with scurvy become tired and depressed, and they suffer from hysteria.

of **scurvy** appear. In the 17th and 18th centuries, sailors were far more likely to die of scurvy than to be killed in shipwrecks or battles.

In addition to its role in the synthesis and maintenance of collagen, vitamin C functions in reactions that synthesize neurotransmitters, hormones, bile acids, and carnitine, which is needed for the breakdown of fatty acids. It is also an antioxidant that acts in the blood and other body fluids. Because its antioxidant properties help maintain the immune system, the ability to fight infection is decreased when this vitamin is deficient. Vitamin C's antioxidant action also regenerates the active antioxidant form of vitamin E and enhances iron absorption in the small intestine by keeping iron in its more readily absorbed form.

Citrus fruits are an excellent source of vitamin C. A large orange contains enough vitamin C to meet the RDA of 90 mg/day for men and 75 mg/day for women.[3] Other fruits and vegetables are also good sources of this vitamin (**Figure 7.25**).

Vitamin C is destroyed by oxygen, light, and heat, so it is readily lost in cooking. This loss is accelerated in low-acid foods and by the use of copper or iron cooking utensils. Although most Americans consume enough vitamin C to prevent severe deficiency, marginal vitamin C deficiency is a concern for individuals who consume few fruits and vegetables. Cigarette smoking increases the requirement for vitamin C because the vitamin is used to break down compounds in cigarette smoke. It is recommended that cigarette smokers consume an extra 35 mg of vitamin C daily—an amount that can easily be supplied by a half-cup of broccoli.[3]

One-third of the population of the United States takes vitamin C supplements—usually in the hope that they will prevent the common cold. Although vitamin C does not prevent colds or reduce their severity, regular vitamin C supplementation may help reduce the duration

Meeting vitamin C needs • Figure 7.25

Fruits that are high in vitamin C include citrus fruits, strawberries, kiwis, and cantaloupe. Vegetables in the cabbage family, such as broccoli, cauliflower, bok choy, and Brussels sprouts, as well as dark-green vegetables, green and red peppers, okra, tomatoes, and potatoes, are also good sources of vitamin C. Meat, fish, poultry, eggs, dairy products, and grains are poor sources.

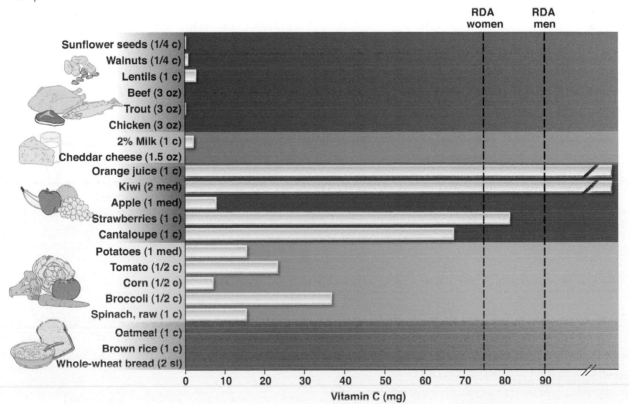

of cold symptoms.[15] It has also been suggested that vitamin C supplements reduce the risk of cardiovascular disease and cancer, but there is insufficient evidence to support this claim.[3]

Taking high doses of supplemental vitamin C can cause diarrhea, nausea, and abdominal cramps. In susceptible individuals, high-dose supplements may increase the risk of kidney stone formation because vitamin C can be metabolized to a compound found in some types of kidney stones.[16] In individuals who are unable to regulate iron absorption, taking vitamin C supplements, which increase iron absorption, increases the risk that toxic amounts of iron will accumulate in the body. For those with sickle cell anemia, excess vitamin C can worsen symptoms. In those taking medication to reduce blood clotting, taking more than 3000 mg/day of vitamin C can interfere with the effectiveness of the medication. In large doses, chewable vitamin C supplements can dissolve tooth enamel. The UL for vitamin C has been set at 2000 mg/day from food and supplements.[3]

Choline and Other Vitamin-Like Compounds

There are a number of substances that perform vitamin-like functions in the body, but are not classified as vitamins because adequate amounts can be synthesized in the body so that they are not required in the diet. For example, carnitine is needed to transport fatty acids into the mitochondria where they are broken down to produce ATP. Lipoic acid functions as a coenzyme, and inositol is important for membrane function. Choline is discussed below because a dietary recommendation has been established.

Choline is a water-soluble substance that you may see included in supplements called "vitamin B complex." It is needed for the synthesis of the neurotransmitter acetylcholine, the structure and function of cell membranes, lipid transport, and homocysteine metabolism. It can be synthesized to a limited extent by humans. Although it is not currently classified as a vitamin, it is recognized as an essential nutrient. Deficiency during pregnancy can interfere with brain development in the fetus, and deficiency in adults causes fatty liver and muscle damage.[17] The DRIs have set AIs for this compound: 550 mg/day for men and 425 mg/day for women.[5]

Choline is found in many foods, with large amounts in egg yolks, liver, meat and fish, wheat germ, and nuts.[18] Because the average daily choline intake in the United States exceeds the recommended intake, a deficiency is unlikely in healthy humans in this country.

Excess choline intake can cause a fishy body odor, sweating, reduced growth rate, low blood pressure, and liver damage. The amounts needed to cause these symptoms are much higher than can be obtained from foods. The UL for choline for adults is 3.5 g/day.[5]

A summary of the water-soluble vitamins and choline is provided in **Table 7.2**.

A summary of the water-soluble vitamins and choline		Table 7.2					
Vitamin	**Sources**	**Recommended intake for adults**	**Major functions**	**Deficiency diseases and symptoms**	**Groups at risk of deficiency**	**Toxicity**	**UL**
Thiamin (vitamin B₁, thiamin mononitrate)	Pork, whole and enriched grains, seeds, nuts, legumes	1.1–1.2 mg/day	Coenzyme in glucose and energy metabolism; needed for neurotransmitter synthesis and normal nerve function	Beriberi: weakness, apathy, irritability, nerve tingling, poor coordination, paralysis, heart changes	Alcoholics, those living in poverty	None reported	ND
Riboflavin (vitamin B₂)	Dairy products, whole and enriched grains, dark-green vegetables, meats	1.1–1.3 mg/day	Coenzyme in energy and lipid metabolism	Inflammation of the mouth and tongue, cracks at corners of the mouth	None	None reported	ND

Vitamin	Sources	Recommended intake for adults	Major functions	Deficiency diseases and symptoms	Groups at risk of deficiency	Toxicity	UL
Niacin (nicotinamide, nicotinic acid, vitamin B$_3$)	Beef, chicken, fish, peanuts, legumes, whole and enriched grains; can be made from tryptophan	14–16 mg NE/day	Coenzyme in energy metabolism and lipid synthesis and breakdown	Pellagra: diarrhea, dermatitis on areas exposed to sun, dementia	Those consuming a limited diet based on corn; alcoholics	Flushing nausea, rash, tingling extremities	35 mg/day from fortified foods and supplements
Biotin	Liver, egg yolks; synthesized in the gut	30 μg/day	Coenzyme in glucose synthesis and energy and fatty acid metabolism	Dermatitis, nausea, depression, hallucinations	Those consuming large amounts of raw egg whites; alcoholics	None reported	ND
Pantothenic acid (calcium pantothenate)	Meat, legumes, whole grains; widespread in foods	5 mg/day	Coenzyme in energy metabolism and lipid synthesis and breakdown	Fatigue, rash	Alcoholics	None reported	ND
Vitamin B$_6$ (pyridoxine, pyridoxal phosphate, pyridoxamine)	Meat, fish, poultry, legumes, whole grains, nuts and seeds	1.3–1.7 mg/day	Coenzyme in protein and amino acid metabolism, neurotransmitter and hemoglobin synthesis, many other reactions	Headache, convulsions, other neurological symptoms, nausea, poor growth, anemia	Alcoholics	Numbness, nerve damage	100 mg/day
Folate (folic acid, folacin, pteroyglutamic acid)	Leafy green vegetables, legumes, seeds, enriched grains, orange juice	400 μg DFE/day	Coenzyme in DNA synthesis and amino acid metabolism	Macrocytic anemia, inflammation of tongue, diarrhea, poor growth, neural tube defects	Pregnant women, alcoholics	Masks B$_{12}$ deficiency	1000 μg/day from fortified food and supplements
Vitamin B$_{12}$ (cobalamin, cyano-cobala-min)	Animal products	2.4 μg/day	Coenzyme in folate and homocysteine metabolism; myelin maintenance and nerve function	Pernicious anemia, macrocytic anemia, nerve damage	Vegans, elderly, people with stomach or intestinal disease	None reported	ND
Vitamin C (ascorbic acid, ascorbate)	Citrus fruit, broccoli, strawberries, greens, peppers	75–90 mg/day	Coenzyme in collagen (connective tissue) synthesis; hormone and neurotransmitter synthesis; antioxidant	Scurvy: poor wound healing, bleeding gums, loose teeth, bone fragility, joint pain, pinpoint hemorrhages	Alcoholics, elderly people	GI distress, diarrhea	2000 mg/day
Choline*	Egg yolks, organ meats, wheat germ, meat, fish, nuts, synthesis in the body	425–550 mg/day	Synthesis of cell membranes and neurotransmitters	Fatty liver, muscle damage, abnormal prenatal development	None	Sweating, low blood pressure, liver damage	3500 mg/day

*Choline is technically not a vitamin, but recommendations have been made for its intake.
Note: UL, Tolerable Upper Intake Level; NE, niacin equivalent; DFE, dietary folate equivalent; ND, not determined due to insufficient data.

1. **Why** do people think B vitamin supplements give them energy?
2. **What** is the role of vitamin B$_6$ in amino acid metabolism?
3. **How** can folate and vitamin B$_{12}$ deficiency both cause macrocytic anemia?
4. **What** is the role of vitamin C in collagen formation?

7.3 The Fat-Soluble Vitamins

LEARNING OBJECTIVES

1. **Explain** the roles of vitamin A in keeping eyes healthy.
2. **Relate** the functions of vitamin D to the symptoms that occur when it is deficient in the body.
3. **Describe** the function of vitamin E.
4. **Discuss** how vitamin K is involved in blood clotting.

The fat-soluble vitamins—A, D, E, and K—are found along with fats in foods. They require special handling for absorption into and transport through the body. Because excesses of these vitamins can be stored in the liver and fatty tissues, intakes can vary without a risk of deficiency as long as average intake over a period of weeks or months meets the body's needs. Their solubility in fat, however, limits their routes of excretion and therefore increases the risk of toxicity.

Vitamin A

Did you ever hear that eating carrots would help you see in the dark? It turns out to be true. Carrots are a good source of **beta-carotene** (β-carotene), a provitamin that can be converted into vitamin A in your body. **Vitamin A** is needed for vision and healthy eyes.

Vitamin A in the diet Vitamin A is found both preformed and in provitamin form in our diet. Preformed

> **retinoids** Chemical forms of preformed vitamin A. includes retinol, retinal, and retinoic acid.

vitamin A compounds are known as **retinoids**. Three retinoids are active in the body: retinal, retinol, and retinoic acid. Retinal and retinoic acid are formed in the body from retinol consumed in the diet. **Carotenoids** are yellow-orange pigments found in plants, some of which are vitamin A precursors; once inside the body, they can be converted into retinoids (**Figure 7.26a**). Beta-carotene is the most potent vitamin A precursor. **Alpha-carotene** (α-**carotene**), found in dark-green vegetables, carrots, and squash, and **beta-cryptoxanthin** (β-**cryptoxanthin**), found in papaya, sweet red peppers, and winter squash, are also provitamin A carotenoids, but they are not converted into retinoids as efficiently as β-carotene. Carotenoids that are not converted into retinoids may function as antioxidants and thus may play a role in protecting against cancer and heart disease.

> **carotenoids** Yellow, orange, and red pigments synthesized by plants and many microorganisms. Some can be converted to vitamin A.

You can meet your needs for vitamin A by eating animal products, such as eggs and dairy products, that are sources of retinol, and by eating fruits and vegetables that are sources of provitamin A carotenoids (**Figure 7.26b**). Because carotenoids are not absorbed as well as retinol and are not completely converted into vitamin A in the body, you get less functional vitamin A from this form. To account for this difference, **retinol activity equivalents (RAEs)** are used to express the amount of usable vitamin A in foods; 1 RAE is the amount of retinol, β-carotene, α-carotene, or β-cryptoxanthin that provides vitamin A activity equal to 1 μg of retinol (see online Appendix K).[19]

Both carotenoids and retinol are bound to proteins in food. To be absorbed, they must be released from protein by pepsin and other protein-digesting enzymes. In the small intestine, they combine with bile acids and other dietary fats in order to be absorbed. The fat content of the diet can affect the amount of vitamin A absorbed. When dietary fat intake is very low (less than 10 g/day),

Meeting vitamin A needs • Figure 7.26

Vitamin A needs can be met by consuming plant sources of provitamin A carotenoids as well as animal sources of the preformed vitamin.

a. Carrots and broccoli are plentiful in β-carotene. Most orange and yellow vegetables and fruits such as squash and apricots, are also good sources, as are other dark-green vegetables, in which the yellow–orange pigment is masked by green chlorophyll. ▶

b. Eating ½ cup of cooked carrots can provide enough vitamin A for the entire day. The dashed lines indicate the RDA for adult men and women, which are 900 µg/day and 700 µg/day, respectively. No specific recommendations have been made for intakes of carotenoids; their intake is considered only with regard to the amount of retinol they provide. ▼

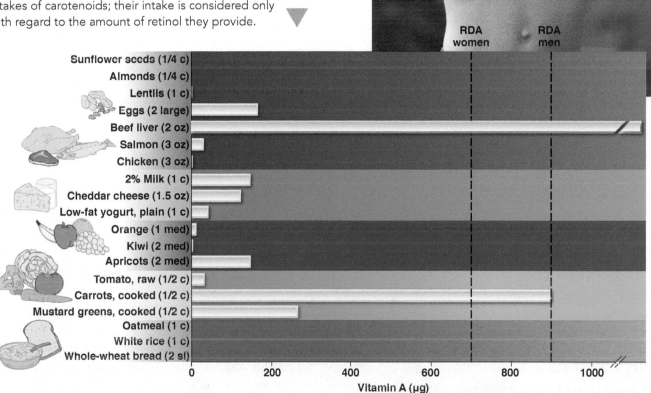

Skip Brown/NG Image Collection

vitamin A absorption is impaired. This is rarely a problem in the United States and other industrialized countries, where typical fat intake is greater than 50 g/day. However, in developing countries, vitamin A deficiency may occur not only because the diet is low in vitamin A but also because the diet is too low in fat for the vitamin to be absorbed efficiently. Diseases that cause fat malabsorption can also interfere with vitamin A absorption and cause deficiency.

Protein and zinc status are also important for healthy vitamin A status. To move from liver stores to other body tissues, vitamin A must be bound to a protein called **retinol-binding protein**. When protein is deficient, the amount of retinol-binding protein made is inadequate, so vitamin A cannot be transported to the tissues where it is needed. Likewise, when zinc is deficient, a vitamin A deficiency may occur because zinc is needed to make proteins involved in vitamin A transport and metabolism.

Vitamin A functions and deficiency Vitamin A is needed for vision and eye health because it is involved in the perception of light and because it is needed for normal **cell differentiation**, the process whereby immature cells change in structure and function to become specialized.

Vitamin A helps us see light because retinal is part of **rhodopsin**, a visual pigment in the eye. When light strikes rhodopsin, it initiates a series of events that break apart rhodopsin and cause a nerve signal to be sent to the brain, which allows us to perceive the light (**Figure 7.27**). After the light stimulus has passed, rhodopsin is re-formed. Because some retinal is lost in these reactions, it must be replaced by vitamin A from the blood. If blood levels of vitamin A are low, as they are in someone who is vitamin A deficient, there is a

The visual cycle • Figure 7.27

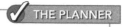 THE PLANNER

Looking into the bright headlights of an approaching car at night is temporarily blinding for all of us, but for someone with vitamin A deficiency, the blindness lasts a lot longer. This occurs because of the role of vitamin A in the visual cycle.

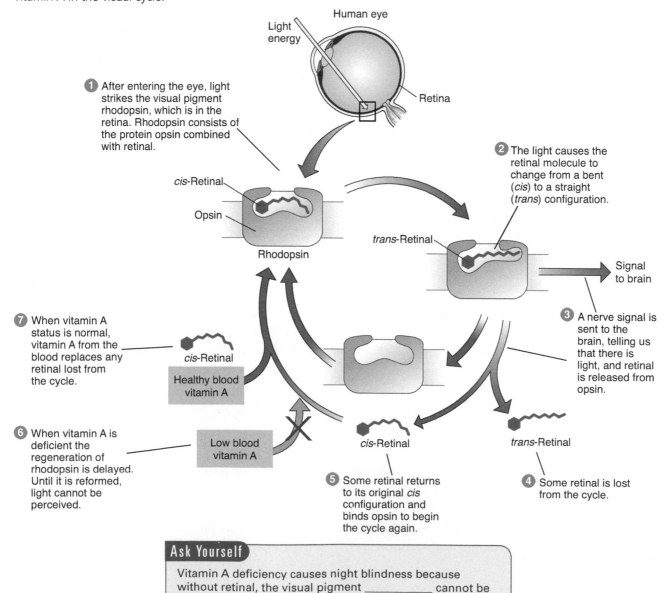

Human eye

Light energy

Retina

1 After entering the eye, light strikes the visual pigment rhodopsin, which is in the retina. Rhodopsin consists of the protein opsin combined with retinal.

2 The light causes the retinal molecule to change from a bent (*cis*) to a straight (*trans*) configuration.

cis-Retinal

Opsin

Rhodopsin

trans-Retinal

Signal to brain

3 A nerve signal is sent to the brain, telling us that there is light, and retinal is released from opsin.

7 When vitamin A status is normal, vitamin A from the blood replaces any retinal lost from the cycle.

cis-Retinal

Healthy blood vitamin A

6 When vitamin A is deficient the regeneration of rhodopsin is delayed. Until it is reformed, light cannot be perceived.

Low blood vitamin A

cis-Retinal

trans-Retinal

5 Some retinal returns to its original *cis* configuration and binds opsin to begin the cycle again.

4 Some retinal is lost from the cycle.

Ask Yourself

Vitamin A deficiency causes night blindness because without retinal, the visual pigment _____ cannot be formed.

A Case Study on Vitamins and Fast Food

John lives on his own, goes to school, and works part time. He eats breakfast at home and usually takes a sandwich for lunch; dinner is always fast food. He recently heard that fast food is low in some vitamins, particularly vitamin A. To check on his vitamin A intake, John uses iProfile to look up the nutrient content of his favorite fast-food meals.

1 Which of the meals shown here is higher in vitamin A? Which ingredients are sources of the vitamin?

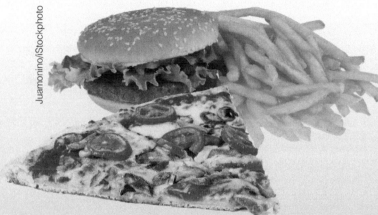

Juamonino/iStockphoto

Konstantin Papadakis/iStockphoto

Your answer:

John doesn't want to give up his fast food, so he looks at his other meals to make sure they provide enough vitamin A. For breakfast, he has Cheerios with milk, toast with jelly, and coffee, and for lunch, he packs a ham and cheese sandwich on whole-wheat bread, potato chips, an apple, and a soda.

2 Which foods in John's breakfast and lunch are good sources of vitamin A?

Answer: The cereal is fortified with vitamin A, and the milk and cheese also contain vitamin A. The bread, meat, chips and soda contain little or none. Together, these foods provide only about 400 μg of vitamin A.

3 Suggest foods that John could add to his lunch that would allow him to meet the RDA for a 20-year-old male.

Your answer:

4 John also discovers that his diet is low in vitamin C. Suggest one fruit and one vegetable that he could add to his breakfast and/or lunch that would provide half of his vitamin C needs.

Your answer:

(Check your answers in online Appendix L.)

---

delay in the regeneration of rhodopsin. This delay causes difficulty seeing in dim light, a condition called **night blindness**. Night blindness is one of the first and most easily reversible symptoms of vitamin A deficiency. If the deficiency progresses, more serious and less reversible symptoms can occur.

Vitamin A deficiency is uncommon in developed countries, but many Americans may have marginal deficiencies.[19] Intakes below the RDA can be caused by poor food choices even when the food supply is plentiful. In the United States, intake of fruits and vegetables, many of which are excellent sources of provitamin A, does not meet recommendations. A typical fast-food meal of a hamburger and French fries provides almost no vitamin A (see *Thinking It Through*).

gene expression
The events of protein synthesis in which the information coded in a gene is used to synthesize a protein or a molecule of RNA.

Vitamin A affects cell differentiation through its role in **gene expression**: It can increase or decrease the expression of certain genes. When a specific gene is expressed, it instructs the cell to make a particular protein. Proteins have structural and regulatory functions within cells and throughout the body. Altering the expression of specific genes increases (or decreases) the production of certain proteins and thereby affects various cellular and body functions. By affecting gene expression, vitamin A can determine what type of cell an immature cell will become.

Vitamin A is necessary for the maintenance of epithelial tissue, which covers internal and external body surfaces. The skin and the linings of the eyes, intestines,

Vitamin A deficiency causes blindness by interfering with the maintenance of epithelial tissue. This deficiency is a threat to the sight, health, and lives of millions of children in the developing world.

The lining of the eye normally contains cells that secrete mucus, which lubricates the eye. When these cells die, immature cells differentiate to become new mucus-secreting cells that replace the dead ones. Without vitamin A, the immature cells can't differentiate normally, and instead of mucus-secreting cells, they become cells that produce a hard protein called keratin.

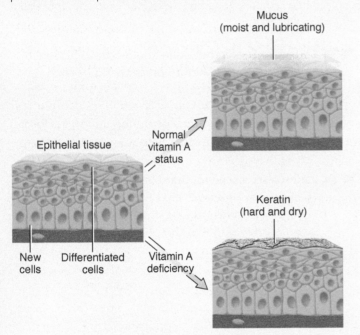

Mucus
(moist and lubricating)

Epithelial tissue

Normal
vitamin A
status

New cells

Differentiated cells

Vitamin A
deficiency

Keratin
(hard and dry)

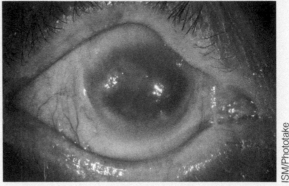

ISM/Phototake

▲ When mucus-secreting cells are replaced by keratin-producing cells, the surface of the eye becomes dry and cloudy. As xerophthalmia progresses, the drying of the cornea results in ulceration and infection. If left untreated, the damage is irreversible and causes permanent blindness.

Interpret the Data

On which continents is clinical vitamin A deficiency most prevalent?

It is estimated that more than 250 million preschool children worldwide are vitamin A deficient and that 250,000 to 500,000 children go blind annually due to vitamin A deficiency. Children with clinical vitamin A deficiency have poor appetites, are anemic, are more susceptible to infections, and are more likely to die in childhood.[20]

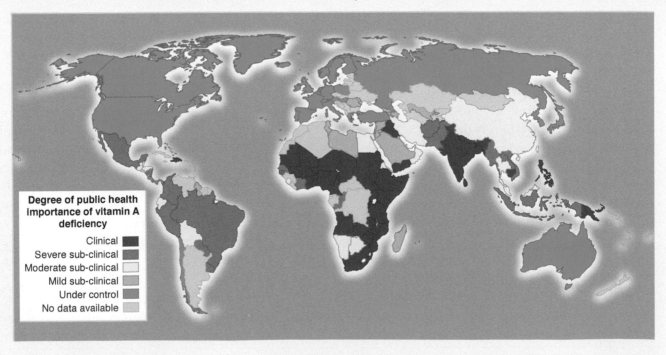

Degree of public health importance of vitamin A deficiency

- Clinical
- Severe sub-clinical
- Moderate sub-clinical
- Mild sub-clinical
- Under control
- No data available

lungs, vagina, and bladder are all epithelial tissue. When vitamin A is deficient, epithelial cells do not differentiate normally because vitamin A is not there to regulate the production of particular proteins. All epithelial tissue is affected by vitamin A deficiency, but that in the eye is particularly susceptible (**Figure 7.28**). The eye disorders associated with vitamin A deficiency are collectively known as **xerophthalmia**. Night blindness is an early stage of xeropthalmia and can be treated by increasing vitamin A intake. If left untreated, xerophthalmia affects the epithelial lining of the eye and can result in permanent blindness.

> **xerophthalmia** A spectrum of eye conditions resulting from vitamin A deficiency that may lead to blindness.

The ability of vitamin A to regulate the growth and differentiation of cells makes it essential throughout life for normal reproduction, growth, and immune function. In the developing embryo, vitamin A is needed to direct cells to differentiate and to form the shapes and patterns needed for the development of a complete organism. In growing children, vitamin A affects the activity of cells that form and break down bone; a deficiency early in life can cause abnormal jawbone growth, resulting in crooked teeth and poor dental health. In the immune system, vitamin A is needed for the differentiation that produces the different types of immune cells. When vitamin A is deficient, the activity of specific immune cells cannot be stimulated; the result is increased susceptibility to infections.

Vitamin A toxicity Preformed vitamin A is toxic in large doses, causing symptoms such as nausea, vomiting, headache, dizziness, blurred vision, and lack of muscle coordination (**Figure 7.29a**). Excess vitamin A is a particular concern for pregnant women because it may contribute to birth defects. Derivatives of vitamin A that are used to treat acne (Retin-A and Accutane) should never be used by pregnant women because they cause birth defects. High intakes of vitamin A have also been found to cause liver damage and increase the incidence of bone fractures.[21,22] The UL is set at 2800 µg/day of preformed vitamin A for 14- to 18-year-olds and 3000 µg/day for adults.[19]

Because preformed vitamin A can be toxic, dietary supplements typically contain β-carotene. Carotenoids are not toxic because when consumed in high doses, their absorption from the diet decreases, and their conversion to active vitamin A is limited. However, large daily intakes of carotenoids from supplements or the diet can lead to a harmless condition known as **hypercarotenemia** (**Figure 7.29b**). β-carotene supplements have also been associated with an increase in lung cancer in

> **hypercarotenemia** A condition caused by the accumulation of carotenoids in the adipose tissue, causing the skin to appear yellow-orange.

Vitamin A toxicity • Figure 7.29

Only preformed vitamin A is toxic.

a. Although foods generally do not naturally contain large enough amounts of nutrients to be toxic, polar bear liver contains about 100,000 µg of vitamin A in just 1 ounce— enough to have caused vitamin A toxicity in Arctic explorers. Polar bear liver is not a common dish at most dinner tables, but supplements of preformed vitamin A also have the potential to deliver a toxic dose.

b. β-carotene supplements or regular consumption of large amounts of carrot juice can cause hypercarotenemia. The hand on the right illustrates this harmless buildup of carotenoids in the adipose tissue, which makes the skin look yellow-orange, particularly on the palms of the hands and the soles of the feet.

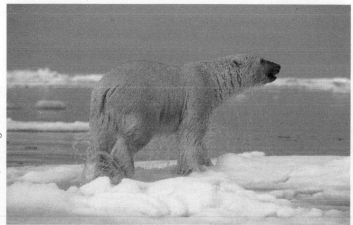

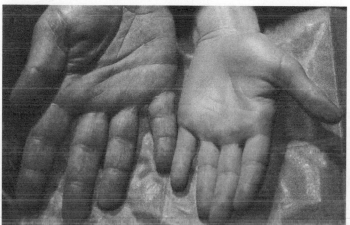

From A. Mazzone and A. Dal Canton, The New England Journal of Medicine, 2002; 347-222-223

Vitamin D activation and function • Figure 7.30

In order to function, vitamin D from food and from synthesis in the skin must be activated.

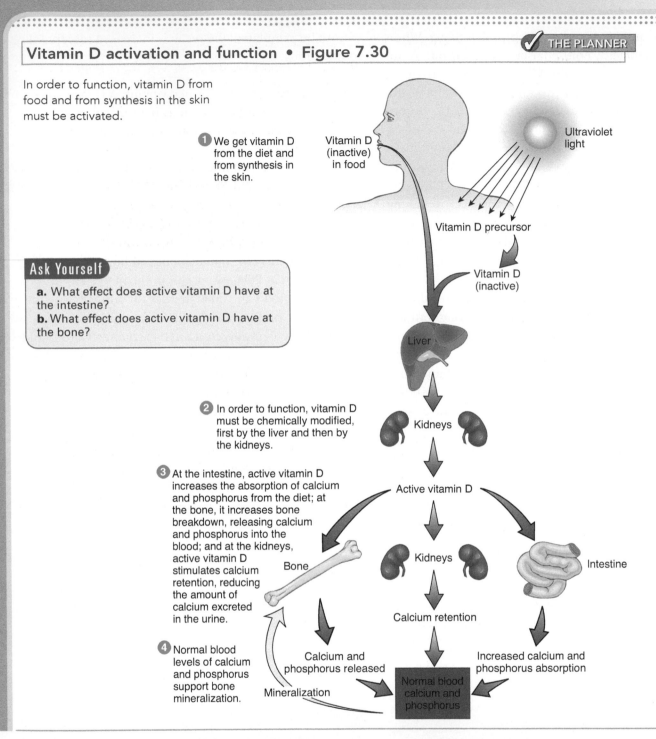

1 We get vitamin D from the diet and from synthesis in the skin.

Vitamin D (inactive) in food

Ultraviolet light

Vitamin D precursor

Vitamin D (inactive)

Ask Yourself

a. What effect does active vitamin D have at the intestine?
b. What effect does active vitamin D have at the bone?

Liver

2 In order to function, vitamin D must be chemically modified, first by the liver and then by the kidneys.

Kidneys

3 At the intestine, active vitamin D increases the absorption of calcium and phosphorus from the diet; at the bone, it increases bone breakdown, releasing calcium and phosphorus into the blood; and at the kidneys, active vitamin D stimulates calcium retention, reducing the amount of calcium excreted in the urine.

Active vitamin D

Bone

Kidneys

Intestine

Calcium retention

4 Normal blood levels of calcium and phosphorus support bone mineralization.

Calcium and phosphorus released

Mineralization

Normal blood calcium and phosphorus

Increased calcium and phosphorus absorption

cigarette smokers.[23] Therefore, smokers are advised to avoid β-carotene supplements. There is no UL for carotenoids, and the small amounts found in standard-strength multivitamin supplements are not likely to be harmful for any group.

Vitamin D

Vitamin D is known as the sunshine vitamin because it can be made in the skin with exposure to ultraviolet (UV) light. Because vitamin D can be made in the body, it is essential in the diet only when exposure to sunlight is limited or the body's ability to synthesize it is reduced.

Vitamin D, whether from the diet or from synthesis in the skin, is inactive until it is modified by biochemical reactions in both the liver and the kidney (**Figure 7.30**). Active vitamin D is needed to maintain normal levels of the minerals calcium and phosphorus in the blood. Calcium is important for bone health, but it is also needed for proper functioning of nerves, muscles, glands, and other tissues. Blood levels of calcium are regulated so that a steady supply of the mineral is available when and where it is needed.

When calcium levels in the blood drop too low, the body responds immediately to correct the problem. The

> **parathyroid hormone (PTH)** A hormone released by the parathyroid gland that acts to increase blood calcium levels.

response starts with the release of **parathyroid hormone (PTH)**, which stimulates the activation of vitamin D by the kidneys. Active vitamin D enters the blood and travels to its major target tissues—intestine, bone, and kidneys—where it acts to increase calcium and phosphorus levels in the blood (see Figure 7.29). The functions of vitamin D, like vitamin A, are due to its role in gene expression. In the intestine, it increases the production of proteins needed for the absorption of calcium. In the bone, it increases the production of proteins that are needed for the differentiation of cells that break down bone.

Vitamin D deficiency When vitamin D is deficient, only about 10 to 15% of the calcium in the diet can be absorbed. Without adequate calcium, bone structure be-

> **rickets** A vitamin D deficiency disease in children, characterized by poor bone development due to inadequate calcium absorption.
>
> **osteomalacia** A vitamin D deficiency disease in adults, characterized by loss of minerals from bone, bone pain, muscle aches, and an increase in bone fractures.

comes abnormal. In children, vitamin D deficiency causes **rickets**; it is characterized by narrow rib cages known as pigeon breasts and by bowed legs (**Figure 7.31**). In adults, vitamin D deficiency causes a condition called **osteomalacia**. Bone deformities do not occur with osteomalacia because adults are no longer growing, but the bones are weakened because not enough calcium is available to form the mineral deposits needed to maintain healthy bone. Insufficient bone mineralization leads to fractures of the weight-bearing

bones, such as those in the hips and spine. This lack of calcium in bones can precipitate or exacerbate **osteoporosis**, which is a loss of total bone mass, not just minerals (discussed further in Chapter 8). Osteomalacia is common in adults with kidney failure because the conversion of vitamin D to the active form is reduced in these patients.

Over the past decade, it has been recognized that vitamin D may have functions that affect tissues other than bone. Vitamin D deficiency has been suggested to

Rickets • Figure 7.31

The vitamin D deficiency disease rickets causes short stature and bone deformities. The characteristic bowed legs occur because the bones are too weak to support the body. It is most common in children with poor diets and little exposure to sunlight, in those with disorders that affect fat absorption, and in vegan children who do not receive adequate exposure to sunlight.

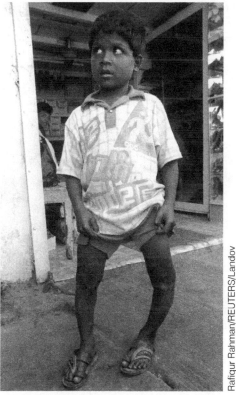

Rafiqur Rahman/REUTERS/Landov

contribute to the development of cancer, cardiovascular disease, type 2 diabetes, and autoimmune disorders.[24] However, the current evidence that vitamin D provides health benefits beyond bone health is mixed and inconclusive.[25, 26]

Meeting vitamin D needs Vitamin D is not very widespread in the diet. It is found naturally in liver, egg yolks, and oily fish such as salmon (**Figure 7.32a**). Foods fortified with vitamin D include milk, milk substitutes, margarine, and some yogurts, cheeses, and breakfast cereals. National surveys indicate that average vitamin D intake is below recommendations, but average blood levels of vitamin D are above the level needed for good bone health. This dichotomy suggests that vitamin D synthesis from sun exposure contributes enough vitamin D to allow the majority of the population to meet vitamin D needs even when intake is below recommendations.[25] Anything that interferes with the transmission of UV radiation to Earth's surface or its penetration into the skin will affect

Limited food sources as well as factors that reduce the amount of sunlight that reaches the skin make it difficult for many people to meet their vitamin D needs.

a. Only a few foods are natural sources of vitamin D. Without adequate sun exposure, supplements, or fortified foods, it is difficult to meet the body's needs for this vitamin, particularly for vegans. The dashed line indicates the RDA for ages 1 to 70, which is 600 IU (15 µg)/day. It would take about 5 cups of vitamin D–fortified milk to provide this much vitamin D.

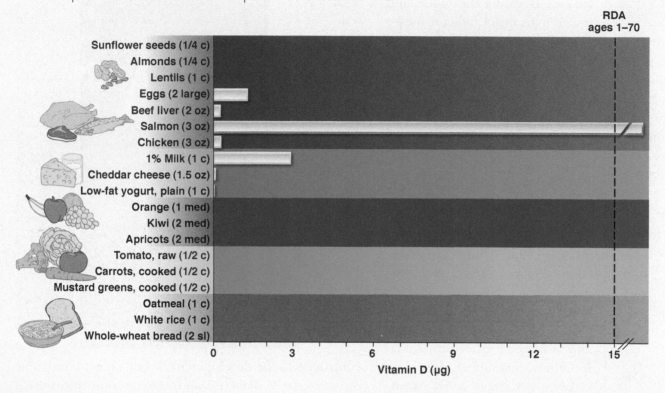

b. The angle at which the sun strikes the Earth affects the body's ability to synthesize vitamin D in the skin. During the winter at latitudes greater than about 40 degrees north or south, there is not enough UV radiation to synthesize adequate amounts. However, during the spring, summer, and fall at 42 degrees latitude, as little as 5 to 10 minutes of midday sun exposure three times weekly can provide a light-skinned individual with adequate vitamin D.[27]

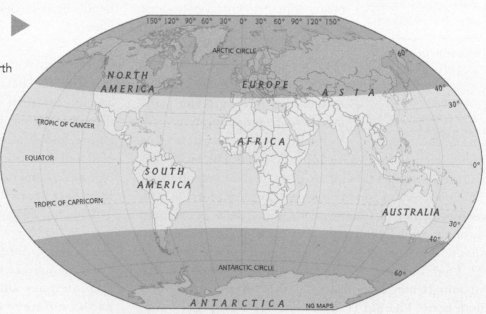

c. Sunscreen with an SPF of 15 decreases vitamin D synthesis by 99%.[28] Sunscreen is important for reducing the risk of skin cancer, but some time in the sun without sunscreen may be needed to meet vitamin D needs. In the summer, children and active adults usually spend enough time outdoors without sunscreen to meet their vitamin D requirements. ▼

d. Dark skin pigmentation prevents UV light rays from penetrating into the layers of the skin where vitamin D is formed and reduces the body's ability to make vitamin D in the skin by as much as 99%. Dark-skinned individuals living in temperate climates have a higher rate of vitamin D deficiency than do those living near the equator. ▼

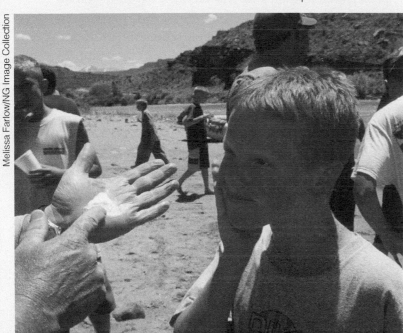

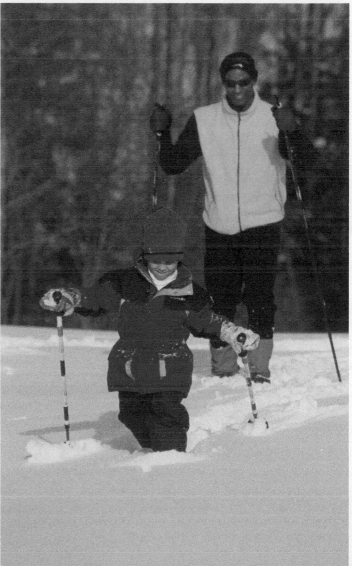

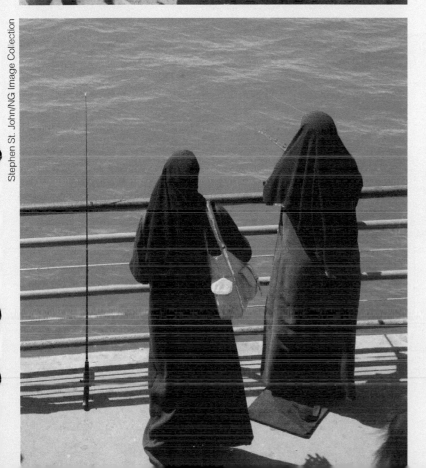

◄ **e.** Concealing clothing worn by certain cultural and religious groups prevents sunlight from striking the skin. This explains why vitamin D deficiency occurs in women and children in some of the sunniest regions of the world. The elderly also typically cover their skin with clothing when they are outdoors. Risk of vitamin D deficiency in elderly people is further compounded because they consume a diet that is low in vitamin D, and the ability to synthesize vitamin D in the skin declines with age.

The Fat-Soluble Vitamins **223**

the synthesis of vitamin D. Therefore, living at higher latitudes, staying indoors, and keeping the skin covered when outdoors increase the risk of vitamin D deficiency (**Figure 7.32b–d**).

The RDA for vitamin D is expressed both in International Units (IUs) and in µg. The amount of vitamin D listed on dietary supplement labels is given in IUs. One IU is equal to 0.025 µg of vitamin D (40 IU = 1 µg of vitamin D; see online Appendix K). The RDA for vitamin D for children and adults 70 and under is set at 600 IU (15 µg)/day—an amount that ensures that vitamin D levels in the blood are high enough to support bone health even when sun exposure is minimal.[25] Due to physiological changes that occur with aging, such as less efficient vitamin D synthesis in the skin, the amount of vitamin D needed to reduce the risk of fractures is higher in older adults. The RDA for adults older than 70 is 800 IU (20 µg)/day.

Too much vitamin D in the body can cause high calcium concentrations in the blood and urine, deposition of calcium in soft tissues such as the blood vessels and kidneys, and cardiovascular damage. Synthesis of vitamin D from exposure to sunlight does not produce toxic amounts because the body regulates vitamin D

formation. The UL for ages 9 and older for vitamin D is 4000 IU (100 µg)/day.[25]

Vitamin E

Vitamin E is an antioxidant that protects lipids throughout the body by neutralizing reactive oxygen compounds before they can cause damage (**Figure 7.33**). Vitamin E protects membranes in red blood cells, white blood cells, nerve cells, and lung cells, where it is particularly important because oxygen concentrations in the lungs are high.[29] Vitamin E can also defend cells against damage caused by heavy metals, such as lead and mercury, and toxins, such as carbon tetrachloride, benzene, and a variety of drugs.

Vitamin E deficiency Because vitamin E is needed to protect cell membranes, a deficiency causes those membranes to break down. Red blood cells and nerve tissue are particularly susceptible. With a vitamin E deficiency, red blood cell membranes may rupture, causing a type of anemia called **hemolytic anemia**. This is most common in premature infants. All newborn infants have low blood vitamin E levels because there is little transfer of

The antioxidant role of vitamin E • Figure 7.33

By neutralizing free radicals, vitamin E guards not only cell membranes, as shown here, but also body proteins, DNA, and cholesterol.

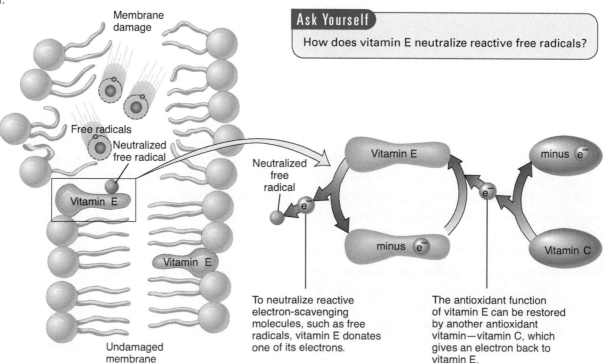

Ask Yourself

How does vitamin E neutralize reactive free radicals?

Membrane damage

Free radicals

Neutralized free radical

Vitamin E

Undamaged membrane

Neutralized free radical

Vitamin E

minus e⁻

minus e⁻

Vitamin C

To neutralize reactive electron-scavenging molecules, such as free radicals, vitamin E donates one of its electrons.

The antioxidant function of vitamin E can be restored by another antioxidant vitamin—vitamin C, which gives an electron back to vitamin E.

WHAT SHOULD I EAT?

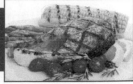
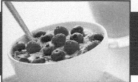

© Sara Winter/iStockphoto   © Jill Chen/iStockphoto   © Steve Mcsweeny/iStockphoto

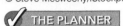

Vitamins

THE PLANNER

Focus on foliage for folate, vitamin A, and vitamin K

- Snack on an orange—you'll get your folate as well as vitamin C.
- Add beans—such as lentils and kidneys—to soups and tacos.
- Munch on a hidden source of β-carotene by eating something dark green.
- Have a salad with a heaping helping of leafy greens to add folate, vitamin K, and β-carotene.

B (vitamin) sure

- Don't forget the whole grains—you'll get vitamin B_6 as well as fiber.
- Enrich your diet with some enriched grains.
- Have a bowl of fortified breakfast cereal for B_{12} insurance.
- Enjoy lean meats, poultry, and fish to get a B_6 and B_{12} boost.

Get your antioxidants

- Snack on nuts and seeds and cook with canola oil to increase your vitamin E intake.
- Try for five different colors of fruits and veggies each day.
- Add carrot sticks to your lunch or snack to increase your vitamin A intake.
- Savor some strawberries and kiwis for dessert—they are loaded with vitamin C.

Soak up some D

- Exercise outside to stay fit and make some vitamin D.
- Have three servings of fortified dairy per day to boost your intake of vitamin D.

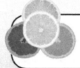

Use iProfile to calculate your vitamin C intake for a day.

---

this vitamin from mother to fetus until the last weeks of pregnancy. The levels are lower in premature infants because they are born before much vitamin E has been transferred from the mother. To prevent vitamin E deficiency in premature infants, special formulas for these infants contain higher amounts of vitamin E.

Vitamin E deficiency is rare in adults, occurring only when other health problems interfere with fat absorption, which reduces vitamin E absorption. In such cases, the vitamin E deficiency is usually characterized by symptoms associated with nerve degeneration, such as poor muscle coordination, weakness, and impaired vision.

The antioxidant role of vitamin E suggests that it may help reduce the risk of heart disease, cancer, Alzheimer's disease, macular degeneration, and a variety of other chronic diseases associated with oxidative damage. Particular attention has been paid to its possible benefits in guarding against heart disease. In addition to the potential for vitamin E to protect against cardiovascular disease through its antioxidant function, there is evidence that it may also have anti-inflammatory functions and be involved in modulating the immune response, regulating genes that affect cell growth and cell death, and detoxifying harmful substances.[90] Studies examining the

relationship between blood levels of vitamin E or vitamin E intake and the incidence of cardiovascular disease have been mixed, and studies investigating the effect of vitamin E supplements on the incidence of cardiovascular disease and other chronic diseases in humans have failed to provide evidence of any benefits.[31, 32] The best approach is to get plenty of dietary vitamin E; however, most Americans do not consume enough vitamin E to meet the RDA (see *What Should I Eat?*).[33]

Meeting vitamin E needs Nuts, seeds, and plant oils are the best sources of vitamin E; fortified products such as breakfast cereals also make a significant contribution to our vitamin E intake (**Figure 7.34**). The need for vitamin E increases as polyunsaturated fat intake increases because polyunsaturated fats are particularly susceptible to oxidative damage; fortunately, polyunsaturated oils are one of the best sources of dietary vitamin E. However, because vitamin E is sensitive to destruction by oxygen, metals, light, and heat, when vegetable oils are repeatedly used for deep-fat frying, most of the vitamin E in them is destroyed.

The chemical name for vitamin E is **tocopherol**. Several forms of vitamin E occur naturally in food, but the body

Meeting vitamin E needs • Figure 7.34

Dietary sources of vitamin E include sunflower seeds, nuts, peanuts, and refined plant oils such as canola, safflower, and sunflower oils. Vitamin E is also found in leafy green vegetables, such as spinach and mustard greens, and in wheat germ and fortified breakfast cereals. The dashed line represents the RDA for adults of 15 mg α-tocopherol/day.

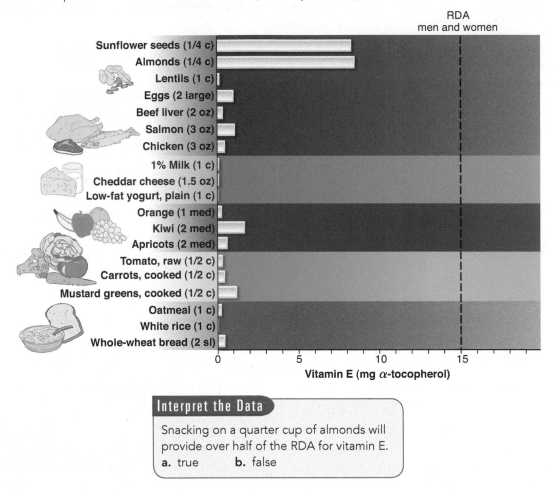

Interpret the Data

Snacking on a quarter cup of almonds will provide over half of the RDA for vitamin E.

a. true   **b.** false

can use only the **alpha-tocopherol (α-tocopherol)** form to meet vitamin E requirements. Therefore, the RDA is expressed as mg α-tocopherol. Synthetic α-tocopherol used in supplements and fortified foods provides only half as much vitamin E activity as the natural form. Supplement labels often express vitamin E content in IUs. Appendix K (online) contains information for converting IUs into mg α-tocopherol.

There is no evidence of adverse effects from consuming large amounts of vitamin E naturally present in foods. The amounts typically contained in supplements are also safe for most people; however, large doses can interfere with blood clotting, so individuals taking blood-thinning medications should not take vitamin E supplements. The UL is 1000 mg/day from supplemental sources.[3]

Vitamin K

Blood is a fluid that flows easily through your blood vessels, but when you cut yourself, blood must solidify or clot to stop your bleeding. **Vitamin K** is needed in the production of several blood proteins, called clotting factors, that cause blood to clot (**Figure 7.35**). The *K* in vitamin K comes from the Danish word for coagulation, *koagulation*, which means "blood clotting." Abnormal blood coagulation is the major symptom of vitamin K deficiency. Without vitamin K, even a bruise or small scratch could cause you to bleed to death (see *What a Scientist Sees*).

Vitamin K is also needed for the synthesis of several proteins involved in bone formation and breakdown, inhibition of blood vessel calcification, and regulation cell growth.[34] Because of the roles of these vitamin

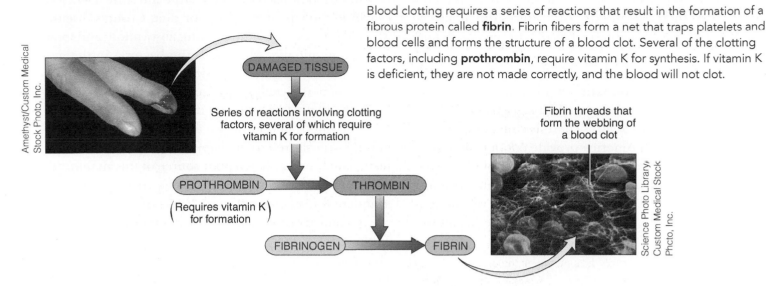

Blood clotting requires a series of reactions that result in the formation of a fibrous protein called **fibrin**. Fibrin fibers form a net that traps platelets and blood cells and forms the structure of a blood clot. Several of the clotting factors, including **prothrombin**, require vitamin K for synthesis. If vitamin K is deficient, they are not made correctly, and the blood will not clot.

DAMAGED TISSUE

Series of reactions involving clotting factors, several of which require vitamin K for formation

PROTHROMBIN → THROMBIN
(Requires vitamin K for formation)

FIBRINOGEN → FIBRIN

Fibrin threads that form the webbing of a blood clot

WHAT A SCIENTIST SEES
Anticoagulants Take Lives and Save Them

Consumers see warfarin as a way to eliminate some unwanted houseguests. A scientist sees that this rat poison can also be used to save lives. Warfarin is an anticoagulant, which means it prevents blood from clotting. It acts by blocking the activation of vitamin K. When rats eat warfarin, minor bumps and scrapes cause them to bleed to death. Dicoumarol, a derivative of warfarin, was first isolated from moldy clover hay in 1940. At that time, cows across the Midwest were bleeding to death because they were being fed this moldy hay during the winter months.

Blood clot formation is essential to survival, but blood clots in the arteries cause heart attacks and strokes and are responsible for killing about half a million Americans annually. Scientists have taken advantage of what they learned about dicoumarol and vitamin K and used it to save human lives. Dicoumarol was the first anticoagulant used to treat humans that could be taken orally rather than by injection. In the 1950s, the more potent anticoagulant warfarin, also known by the brand name Coumadin, was developed. It was used to treat President Eisenhower when he had a heart attack in 1955, and this "rat poison" is still used to prevent blood clots and treat heart attack patients today.

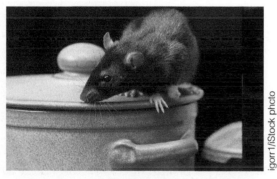

Inactive vitamin K

Warfarin

Warfarin inhibits the formation of active vitamin K so blood does not clot.

Active vitamin K

Synthesis of blood-clotting proteins

Normal blood clotting

Think Critically Why might patients taking warfarin need to avoid vitamin K supplements?

The drug warfarin blocks the activation of vitamin K. Without vitamin K, several blood-clotting factors cannot be produced.

K-dependent proteins, mild vitamin K deficiency is believed to be responsible for a reduction in bone mineral density that increases the risk of fractures due to osteoporosis as well as an increased risk of atherosclerosis and cancer.[34]

Vitamin K is used more rapidly than other fat-soluble vitamins, so a constant supply is necessary. Only a small number of foods provide a significant amount of vitamin K (**Figure 7.36**). There is concern that typical intakes in North America provide enough vitamin K for normal blood coagulation, but not enough for adequate synthesis of other vitamin K-dependent proteins. Evidence is accumulating that the current recommendations may not be high enough to provide for all the functions of vitamin K.[34, 35]

A frank deficiency is rare in adults because vitamin K is synthesized by bacteria in the large intestine. Deficiency can be precipitated by a poor diet; Crohn's disease, which damages the colon, limiting absorption; and long-term antibiotic use, which kills the bacteria in the gastrointestinal tract that synthesize the vitamin. Newborns are at risk of deficiency because when a baby is born, no bacteria are present in the GI tract to synthesize vitamin K. In addition, newborns are at risk because little vitamin K is transferred to the baby from the mother before birth, and breast milk is a poor source of this vitamin. To ensure normal blood clotting, infants are typically given a vitamin K injection within six hours of birth.

A summary of the fat-soluble vitamins is provided in **Table 7.3**.

Meeting vitamin K needs • Figure 7.36

Leafy green vegetables, such as spinach, broccoli, brussels sprouts, kale, and turnip greens, and some vegetable oils are good sources of vitamin K. The dashed lines indicate the AIs for adult men and women, which are 120 μg/day and 90 μg/day, respectively.

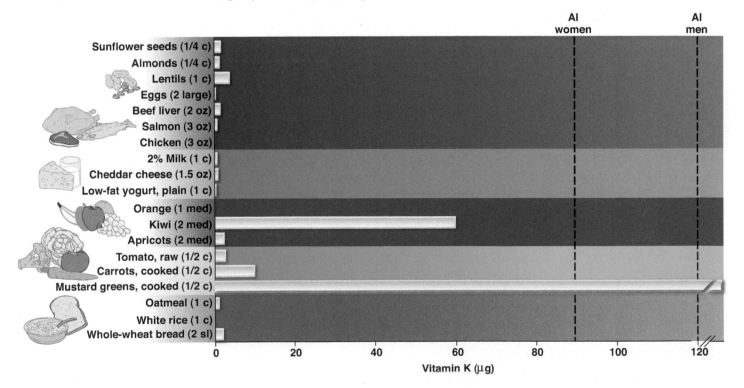

A summary of the fat-soluble vitamins   Table 7.3

Vitamin	Sources	Recommended intake for adults	Major functions	Deficiency diseases and symptoms	Groups at risk of deficiency	Toxicity	UL
Vitamin A (retinol, retinal, retinoic acid, vitamin A acetate, vitamin A palmitate, retinyl palmitate, provitamin A, carotene, β-carotene, carotenoids)	Retinol: liver, fish, fortified milk and margarine, butter, eggs; carotenoids: carrots, leafy greens, sweet potatoes, broccoli, apricots, cantaloupe	700–900 μg/day	Vision, health of cornea and other epithelial tissue, cell differentiation, reproduction, immune function	Xerophthalmia: night blindness, dry cornea, eye infections; poor growth, dry skin, impaired immune function	People living in poverty (particularly children and pregnant women), people who consume very low-fat or low-protein diets	Headache, vomiting, hair loss, liver damage, skin changes, bone pain, fractures, birth defects	3000 μg/day of preformed vitamin A
Vitamin D (calciferol, cholecalciferol, calcitriol, ergocalciferol, dihydroxy vitamin D)	Egg yolk, liver, fish oils, tuna, salmon, fortified milk, synthesis from sunlight	600–800 IU/day (15–20 μg/day)	Absorption of calcium and phosphorus, maintenance of bone	Rickets in children: abnormal growth, misshapen bones, bowed legs, soft bones; osteomalacia in adults: weak bones and bone and muscle pain	Some breast-fed infants; children and elderly people (especially those with dark skin and little exposure to sunlight); people with kidney disease	Calcium deposits in soft tissues, growth retardation, kidney damage	4000 IU/day (100 μg/day)
Vitamin E (tocopherol, alpha-tocopherol)	Vegetable oils, leafy greens, seeds, nuts, peanuts	15 mg/day	Antioxidant, protects cell membranes	Broken red blood cells, nerve damage	People with poor fat absorption, premature infants	Inhibition of vitamin K activity	1000 mg/day from supplemental sources
Vitamin K (phylloquinones, menaquinone)	Vegetable oils, leafy greens, synthesis by intestinal bacteria	90–120 μg/day	Synthesis of blood-clotting proteins and proteins needed for bone health and cell growth	Hemorrhage	Newborns (especially premature), people on long-term antibiotics	Anemia, brain damage	ND

Note: UL, Tolerable Upper Intake Level; ND, not determined due to insufficient evidence.

CONCEPT CHECK

1. How does vitamin A help us see in the dark?
2. Why do the leg bones bow when children are vitamin D deficient?

3. How does vitamin E protect membranes?
4. What is the role of vitamin K in blood clotting?

Meeting Needs with Dietary Supplements

LEARNING OBJECTIVES

1. **List** some population groups that may benefit from taking vitamin and/or mineral supplements.
2. **Explain** how the safety of dietary supplements is monitored.
3. **Evaluate** the safety of a dietary supplement using a Supplement Facts panel.

Currently, 66% of all adult Americans consider themselves supplement users.[36] We take supplements for a variety of reasons—to energize ourselves, to protect ourselves from disease, to cure illnesses, to lose weight, to enhance what we obtain from the foods we eat, and simply to ensure against deficiencies. These products may be beneficial and even necessary under some circumstances for some people, but they also have the potential to cause harm.

Some dietary supplements contain vitamins and minerals, some contain herbs and other plant-derived substances, and some contain compounds that are found in the body but are not essential in the diet. While supplements can help us obtain adequate amounts of specific nutrients, they do not provide all the benefits of foods. A pill that meets a person's vitamin needs does not provide the energy, protein, minerals, fiber, or phytochemicals supplied by food sources of these vitamins.

Who Needs Vitamin/Mineral Supplements?

Eating a variety of foods is the best way to meet nutrient needs, and most healthy adults who consume a reasonably good diet do not need supplements.[37] In fact, an argument against the use of supplements is that supplement use gives people a false sense of security, causing them to pay less attention to the nutrient content of the foods they choose. For some people, however, taking supplements may be the only way to meet certain nutrient needs because of low intakes, increased needs, or excess losses (**Table 7.4**).

Herbal Supplements

Technically, an herb is a nonwoody, seed-producing plant that dies at the end of the growing season. However, the term *herb* is generally used to refer to any botanical or plant-derived substance. Throughout history, folk medicine has used herbs to prevent and treat disease. Today, herbs and herbal supplements are still popular (**Figure 7.37**).

Groups for whom dietary supplements are recommended[38] **Table 7.4**	
Group	**Recommendation**
Dieters	People who consume fewer than 1200 Calories/day should take a multivitamin/multimineral supplement.
Vegans and those who eliminate all dairy foods	To obtain adequate vitamin B_{12}, people who do not eat animal products need to take supplements or consume vitamin B_{12}–fortified foods. Because dairy products are an important source of calcium and vitamin D, those who do not consume dairy products may benefit from taking supplements that provide calcium and vitamin D.
Infants and children	Supplemental fluoride, vitamin D, and iron are recommended under certain circumstances.
Young women and pregnant women	Women of childbearing age should consume 400 μg of folic acid daily from either fortified foods or supplements. Supplements of iron and folic acid are recommended for pregnant women, and multivitamin/multimineral supplements are usually prescribed during pregnancy.
Older adults	Because of the high incidence of atrophic gastritis in adults over age 50, vitamin B_{12} supplements or fortified foods are recommended. It may also be difficult for older adults to meet the RDAs for vitamin D and calcium, so supplements of these nutrients are often recommended.
Individuals with dark skin pigmentation	People with dark skin may be unable to synthesize enough vitamin D to meet their needs for this vitamin and may therefore require supplements.
Individuals with restricted diets	Individuals with health conditions that affect what foods they eat or how nutrients are used may require vitamin and mineral supplements.
People taking medications	Medications may interfere with the body's use of certain nutrients.
Cigarette smokers and alcohol users	People who smoke heavily require more vitamin C and possibly vitamin E than do nonsmokers.[3,39] Alcohol consumption inhibits the absorption of B vitamins and may interfere with B vitamin metabolism.

Popular herbal supplements • Figure 7.37

Ginkgo biloba, St. John's wort, ginseng, garlic, and Echinacea are among the best-selling herbal supplements in the United States today.

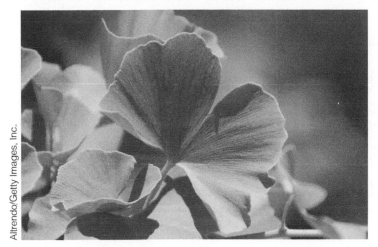

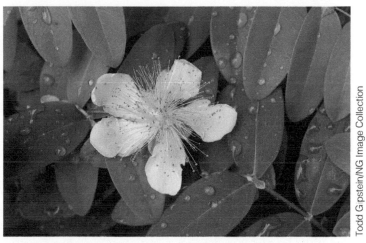

Ginkgo biloba, also called "maidenhair," is marketed to enhance memory and to treat a variety of circulatory ailments. *Ginkgo biloba* extract does not appear to enhance cognitive function in healthy adults, and evidence that it can reduce the incidence of dementia or protect against cognitive decline in the elderly is inconsistent.[41–43] Side effects include headaches and gastrointestinal symptoms.[44] *Ginkgo biloba* also interacts with a number of medications. It can cause bleeding when combined with warfarin or aspirin, elevated blood pressure when combined with a thiazide diuretic, and coma when combined with the antidepressant trazodone.[45]

St. John's wort, taken to promote mental well-being, contains low doses of the chemical found in the antidepressant drug fluoxetine (Prozac). The results of clinical trials suggest that it may be beneficial for the treatment of depression.[46] Side effects include nausea and sensitivity to sunlight. St John's wort should not be used in conjunction with prescription antidepressant drugs, and it has been found to interact with many different medications, including anticoagulants, heart medications, birth control pills, immunosuppressants, antibiotics, and medications used to treat HIV infection.[47]

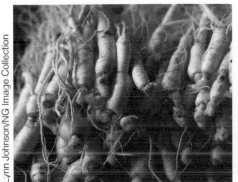

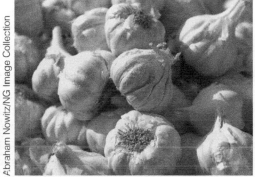

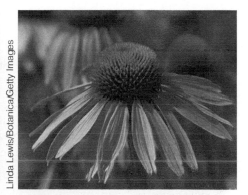

Ginseng has been used in Asia for centuries for its energizing, stress-reducing, and aphrodisiac properties. Today it is popular because it is suggested to improve mental and physical performance, augment immune function, and enhance sexual function. Although ginseng contains substances that have antioxidant, anti-inflammatory, and immunostimulating effects, there is little evidence that it has any health benefits.[48] Adverse effects include diarrhea, headache, and insomnia.

Hippocrates recommended garlic for treating pneumonia and other infections, as well as cancer and digestive disorders. Although it is no longer recommended for those purposes, recent research has shown that garlic may cause a modest reduction in blood cholesterol and triglyceride levels.[49] Even though we often spice our food with garlic, garlic supplements are not safe for everyone. They interfere with drugs used to treat HIV infection and can increase the risk of bleeding, so they should be used with caution before having surgery or dental work.[50]

Native Americans used petals of the Echinacea plant as a treatment for colds, flu, and infections. Today, the plant's root is typically used, and it is a popular herbal cold remedy. Echinacea is believed to act as an immune system stimulant; studies are mixed as to whether it is beneficial in either preventing or treating the common cold.[51] Although side effects have not been reported, allergies are possible.

Potential benefits and side effects of common herbal ingredients **Table 7.5**

Product	Suggested benefit and uses	Side effects
Astragalus (bei qi, huang qi, ogi, hwang ki, milk vetch)	May enhance immune function	Can interact with drugs that suppress the immune system and affect blood sugar levels and blood pressure
Bitter orange (Seville orange, sour orange, Zhi shi)	May relieve heartburn and nasal congestion, stimulate appetite, and promote weight loss	Increased heart rate and blood pressure, fainting, heart attack, stroke
Cat's Claw (uña de gato)	Suggested for relief of arthritis and stimulation of the immune system	Headache, dizziness, vomiting; Should not be taken by individuals who are pregnant
Chamomile	May relieve gastrointestinal upset and promote relaxation and sleep	Allergic reactions
Dandelion (lion's tooth, blowball)	May relieve minor digestive problems, increase urine production, and support liver and kidney health	Upset stomach and diarrhea, allergic reactions
Echinacea (purple coneflower, coneflower)	Proposed to enhance immune system and prevent or treat colds and other upper respiratory infections.	Allergic reactions
Ephedra (Ma Huang, Chinese ephedra)	May relieve colds and nasal congestion, aid in weight loss, increase energy, and enhance athletic performance	High blood pressure, irregular heartbeat, heart attack, stroke, death; banned by the FDA, but the ban does not apply to traditional Chinese herbal remedies or to products like herbal teas regulated as conventional foods
Ginger	Suggested for relief of motion sickness and nausea	Gas, bloating, heartburn, nausea
Ginkgo (*Ginkgo biloba*, maidenhair tree, fossil tree)	May improve memory and mental function, improve circulation	Gastrointestinal distress, headache, dizziness, allergic skin reactions
Ginseng (Asian ginseng, Chinese ginseng)	Suggested to increase sense of well-being and stamina, improve mental and physical performance, enhance immune function, improve sexual function, and lower blood glucose and blood pressure	Headache, insomnia, gastrointestinal upset with prolonged use
Hawthorn	Hypothesized to strengthen heart muscle	Possible drug interactions
Hoodia (Kalahari cactus, Xhoba)	May suppress appetite	Safety unknown; potential risks, side effects, and interactions with medicines and other supplements have not been studied
Kava (kava kava, awa, kava pepper)	Suggested for relief of anxiety, stress, insomnia, and menopausal symptoms	Liver damage, including hepatitis and liver failure (which can cause death); FDA has issued a warning that using kava supplements has been linked to a risk of severe liver damage
Milk thistle (Mary thistle, holy thistle)	May protect against liver disease, improve liver function	Gastrointestinal upset, allergic reactions, low blood sugar
Red clover (cow clover, meadow clover, wild clover)	May relieve menopausal symptoms, breast pain associated with menstrual cycles, and symptoms of prostate enlargement; lower blood cholesterol	Headache, nausea, rash
Saw palmetto (American dwarf palm tree, cabbage palm)	May improve urinary flow with enlarged prostate	Mild stomach discomfort
St. John's wort (hypericum, Klamath weed, goatweed)	Suggested to improve mental well-being; relieve depression, anxiety, and/or sleep disorders	Increased sensitivity to sunlight, anxiety, dry mouth, dizziness, gastrointestinal symptoms, fatigue, headache, sexual dysfunction; interactions with many medications, including antidepressants, birth control pills, digoxin, warfarin, and seizure-control drugs
Valerian (all-heal, garden heliotrope)	Mild sedative, relief of sleep disorders and anxiety	Gastrointestinal upset, headache, and tiredness possible with prolonged use
Yohimbe (yohimbe bark)	Suggested aphrodisiac; may reduce sexual dysfunction, including erectile dysfunction in men	High blood pressure, increased heart rate, headache, anxiety, dizziness, nausea, vomiting, tremors, and sleeplessness

Sources: National Center for Complementary and Alternative Medicine, *Herbs at a Glance*, http://nccam.nih.gov/health/herbsataglance.htm; Office of Dietary Supplements, *Dietary Supplement Fact Sheets*, http://ods.od.nih.gov/factsheets/list-all; and Office of Dietary Supplements, *Botanical Supplement Fact Sheets*, http://ods.od.nih.gov/factsheets/list-Botanicals/.

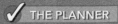
The Issue: Herbal supplements are popular as "natural" remedies. Are these products a helpful addition to traditional health care, or are they a health risk?

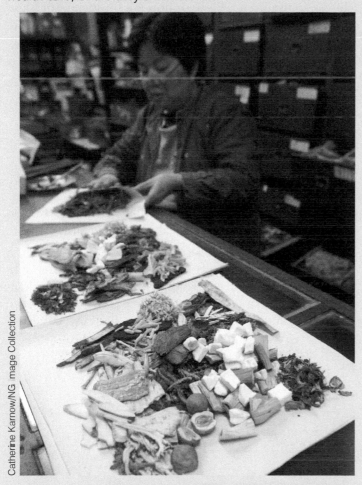

Catherine Karnow/NG image Collection

Many cultures, including the ancient Greeks and Native Americans, have used herbal products to treat everything from coughs, constipation, and poison ivy to arthritis and heart ailments. Today, about one in six Americans uses herbs to treat maladies or boost health.[52] These products are affordable and widely available, and they do not require prescriptions. Advocates of herbal supplements feel that this availability allows people more control of their own health care. Opponents fear that self-dosing with herbs may lead to toxic reactions and prevent people from seeking traditional medical care and proven treatments. How effective and safe are herbal supplements?

Herbs have demonstrated physiological effects. In fact, some of the prescription drugs used today were derived from plants. Aspirin comes from willow bark; digitalis, a drug prescribed for certain heart conditions, comes from foxglove flowers. Herbs are made from all or part of the plant, so the amounts of active ingredients are affected by growing conditions, harvesting, and processing, and they vary with the brand and batch.[53] In contrast, drugs are purified compounds and are tested to ensure consistent amounts in each pill. Advocates believe that having a mixture of compounds is an advantage because some ingredients can enhance the effects of others. Opponents argue that these interactions may be negative, diminishing the effect of one of the active ingredients.

Proponents of herbal supplements argue that most herbal medicines are well tolerated and have fewer unintended consequences than prescription drugs. Prescription drugs are certainly not without side effects, but because of the levels of regulation, we are assured that a prescribed drug is an effective treatment, and any side effects are documented. Herbal products, like other dietary supplements, do not require FDA approval before they are marketed. Opponents believe that this lack of regulation allows adulterated and/or dangerous products to enter the marketplace. A study that tested the quality of herbal supplements found that a third of those tested did not contain the botanical listed on the label and almost 60% were contaminated with substances not included on the label.[54] Some botanical compounds themselves are toxic. The FDA has issued warnings about ingredients such as comfrey, kava, and aristolochic acid; and it took ephedra off the market.[55] Because herbal products are made from unpurified plant material, there is also a risk of contamination with pesticides, microbes, metals, and other toxins.[56]

Another concern when people self-dose with herbs is that the herbs may interact with drugs and cause unwanted side effects.[53] For example, *gingko biloba* and garlic can interfere with blood clotting and so should not be used with blood-thinning medication or before surgery. St. John's wort may interact with anesthetics and antidepressants, and Echinacea can limit the effect of some steroids.[57] Prescription drugs come with instructions and warnings about potential side effects; in addition, a physician or pharmacist considers the other medications and conditions that may alter the safety and effectiveness of the drug, and a prescribing physician monitors patient health. This is not the case with dietary supplements.

Herbs are medicines, and like taking other medications, taking herbs has some advantages and risks. Whether herbal supplements are helpful or harmful depends on the supplement, the dose, and the consumer.

Think Critically: Would you purchase a remedy from the selection of herbs at the shop shown in the photo? Why or why not?

They are readily available and relatively inexpensive, and they can be purchased without a trip to the doctor or a prescription. Although these features are appealing to consumers who want to manage their own health, some herbs may be toxic, either alone or in combination with other herbs and drugs (**Table 7.5**). They should not be taken to replace prescribed medication without the knowledge of your physician (see *Debate: Are Herbal Supplements Helpful or Harmful?*).[40]

Choose Supplements with Care

Using dietary supplements can be part of an effective strategy to promote good health, but supplements are not a substitute for a healthy diet, and they are not without risks. The Dietary Supplement Health and Education Act (DSHEA) of 1994 defined the term *dietary supplement* and created standards for labeling these products (see Chapter 2). However, it left most of the responsibility for manufacturing practices and safety in the hands of manufacturers.

To help ensure that dietary supplements contain the right ingredients and the right amount per dose, the FDA established "current Good Manufacturing Practice" regulations for dietary supplements. These regulations require manufacturers to test their products to ensure identity, purity, strength, and composition.[58]

Supplement manufacturers are responsible for ensuring product safety and efficacy, but these products do not require FDA approval before they are marketed. If a problem arises with a specific product, the FDA must prove that the supplement represents a risk before it can require the manufacturer to remove the supplement from the market. The only dietary supplements that do require pre-market review by the FDA are those containing an ingredient that was not sold in the United States before October 15, 1994. Prior to marketing a supplement containing an ingredient not sold before this date,

the manufacturer must notify the FDA of its intention to market the product and must provide safety data. Ingredients sold prior to this date are presumed to be safe, based on their history of safe use by humans.

Because supplements are not regulated as strictly as drugs, consumers need to use care and caution if they choose to use them. A safe option is a multivitamin/multimineral supplement that does not exceed 100% of the Daily Values. Although there is little evidence that the average person benefits from such a supplement, there is also little evidence of harm. Here are a number of suggestions that will help you when choosing or using dietary supplements:

- **Consider why you want it.** If you are taking it to prevent a deficiency, does it provide the specific nutrients or other substances you need?

- **Compare product costs.** Just as more isn't always better, more expensive is not always better either.

- **Make sure it is safe.** Does the supplement contain a potentially toxic level of any nutrient or other substance? Are you taking the dose recommended on the label? For any nutrients that exceed 100% of the Daily Value, check to see if they exceed the UL. Does it contain any nonvitamin/nonmineral ingredients? If so, have any of them been shown to be toxic to someone like you (**Figure 7.38**)?

Check the Supplement Facts • Figure 7.38

This Supplement Facts panel is from a supplement marketed to reduce appetite and therefore promote weight loss. Would you recommend it? Why or why not?

Supplement Facts

Serving Size: 2 Capsules
Servings Per Container: 60

	Amount Per Serving	DV%
Vitamin C (as ascorbic acid)	60mg	100%
Pantothenic Acid (as calcium, pantothenate)	20mg	200%
Vitamin B-6 (as pyridoxine HCL)	8mg	400%
Niacin	5mg	25%
Folate (as folic acid)	100mcg	25%
Zinc (as zinc gluconate)	5mg	33%
Copper (as copper gluconate)	500mcg	25%
NADH (Nicotinamide Adenine Dinucleotide)	1000mcg	*
Hoodia Gordonii Extract (20:1 Extract- Equal to 2000 mg of whole plant)	100mg	*
5-Hydroxytryptophan (Griffonia Simplicifolia)	25mg	*
N, N Dimethylglycine	50mg	*
Trimethylglycine	75mg	*
L-Phenylalanine	600mg	*
Decaffinated Green Tea Extract (Total Catechins 130mg, Epigaliocatechin Galiate (EGCG) 70mg)	175mg	*
Salvia Scalarea Extract	50mg	*
Choline (as bitartrate)	75mg	*

*Daily Value (DV, not established)

Recommended Use: As a dietary supplement take two capsules before breakfast on a empty stomach (or before exercise) and two capsules at mid-afternoon preferably with 8 oz of water.

This supplement contains more than 100% of the Daily Value for vitamin B_6. Does this amount exceed the UL?

This supplement contains many ingredients that are not vitamins or minerals and therefore have no Daily Value or UL. The ones shown in blue are herbs. Are they safe when taken in these amounts?

- **Check the expiration date.** Some nutrients degrade over time, so expired products will have a lower nutrient content than is shown on the label. This is particularly true if the product has not been stored properly.

- **Consider your medical history.** Do you have a medical condition that recommends against certain nutrients or other ingredients? Are you taking prescription medication that an ingredient in the supplement may interact with? Check with a physician, dietitian, or pharmacist to help identify these interactions.

- **Approach herbal supplements with caution.** If you are pregnant, ill, or taking medications, consult your physician before taking herbs. Do not give them to children. Do not take combinations of herbs. Do not use herbs for long periods. Stop taking any product that causes side effects.

- **Report harmful effects.** If you suffer a harmful effect or an illness that you think is related to the use of a supplement, seek medical attention and go to the FDA Reporting Web site, at www.fda.gov/safety/medwatch/howtoreport/ for information about how to proceed.

CONCEPT CHECK

1. **Why** is it recommended that vegans and older adults take vitamin B$_{12}$ supplements?
2. **Who** regulates the safety of dietary supplements?
3. **How** can the UL be used when evaluating a dietary supplement?

✓ THE PLANNER

Summary

1 A Vitamin Primer 188

- **Vitamins** are essential organic nutrients that do not provide energy and are required in small quantities in the diet to maintain health. Vitamins are classified by their solubility in either water or fat, as illustrated here. Vitamins are present naturally in foods and are also added through fortification and enrichment.

The vitamins • Figure 7.1

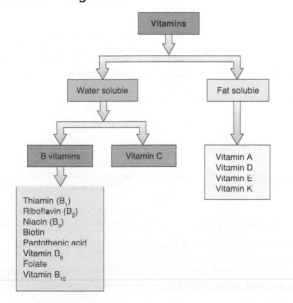

- Vitamin **bioavailability** is affected by the composition of the diet, conditions in the digestive tract, and the ability to transport and activate the vitamin once it has been absorbed.

- Vitamins promote and regulate body activities. The B vitamins act as **coenzymes**. Some vitamins are **antioxidants**, which protect the body from **oxidative damage** by **free radicals**.

- In developing countries, vitamin deficiencies remain a major public health problem. They are less common in industrialized countries due to enrichment, fortification, and a more varied food supply.

2 The Water-Soluble Vitamins 196

- **Thiamin** is a coenzyme that is particularly important for glucose metabolism and **neurotransmitter** synthesis; a deficiency of thiamin, called **beriberi**, causes nervous system abnormalities and cardiovascular changes. Thiamin is found in whole and enriched grains.

- **Riboflavin** coenzymes are needed for ATP production and for the utilization of several other vitamins. Milk is one of the best food sources of riboflavin.

- **Niacin** coenzymes are needed for the breakdown of carbohydrate, fat, and protein and for the synthesis of fatty acids and cholesterol. A deficiency results in **pellagra**, which is characterized by dermatitis, diarrhea, and dementia. The amino acid tryptophan can be converted into niacin. High doses lower blood cholesterol but can cause toxicity symptoms.

- **Biotin** is needed for the synthesis of glucose and for energy, fatty acid, and amino acid metabolism. Some of our biotin need is met by bacterial synthesis in the gastrointestinal tract.

- **Pantothenic acid** is part of coenzyme A. It is required for the production of ATP from carbohydrate, fat, and protein and for the synthesis of cholesterol and fat. It is widespread in the food supply.

- **Vitamin B$_6$** is particularly important for amino acid and protein metabolism. Deficiency causes numbness and tingling, anemia, and may increase the risk of heart disease because it is needed to keep levels of homocysteine low. Food sources include meats and whole grains. Large doses of vitamin B$_6$ can cause nervous system abnormalities.

- **Folate** is necessary for the synthesis of DNA, so it is especially important for rapidly dividing cells. Folate deficiency prevents red blood cell precursor cells from dividing, as shown here, resulting in **macrocytic anemia**. Low levels of folate before and during early pregnancy are associated with an increased incidence of **neural tube defects**. Food sources include liver, legumes, oranges, leafy green vegetables, and fortified grains. A high intake of folate can mask some of the symptoms of vitamin B$_{12}$ deficiency.

Folate deficiency and macrocytic anemia • Figure 7.18

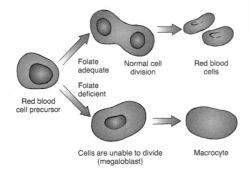

- Absorption of **vitamin** B$_{12}$ requires stomach acid and **intrinsic factor**. Without intrinsic factor, only tiny amounts of vitamin B$_{12}$ are absorbed, and **pernicious anemia** occurs. Vitamin B$_{12}$ is needed for the metabolism of folate and fatty acids and to maintain **myelin**. Deficiency results in macrocytic anemia and nerve damage. Vitamin B$_{12}$ is found almost exclusively in animal products. Deficiency is a concern in vegans and in older individuals with **atrophic gastritis**.

- **Vitamin C** is necessary for the synthesis of **collagen**, hormones, and neurotransmitters. Vitamin C deficiency, called **scurvy**, is characterized by poor wound healing, bleeding, and other symptoms related to the improper formation and maintenance of collagen. Vitamin C is also a water-soluble antioxidant. The best food sources are citrus fruits.

A **retinoids** are found in liver, eggs, fish, and fortified dairy products. High intakes are toxic and have been linked to birth defects and bone loss. Provitamin A **carotenoids**, such as β-**carotene**, are found in yellow-orange fruits and vegetables such as mangoes, carrots, and apricots, as well as leafy greens. Some carotenoids are antioxidants. Carotenoids are not toxic, but a high intake can give the skin a yellow-orange appearance.

- **Vitamin D** can be made in the skin by exposure to sunlight, as depicted here, so dietary needs vary depending on the amount synthesized. Vitamin D is found in fish oils and fortified milk. It is essential for maintaining proper levels of calcium and phosphorus in the body. A deficiency in children results in **rickets**; in adults, vitamin D deficiency causes **osteomalacia**.

- **Vitamin E** functions primarily as a fat-soluble antioxidant. It is necessary for reproduction and protects cell membranes from oxidative damage. It is found in nuts, plant oils, green vegetables, and fortified cereals.

- **Vitamin K** is essential for blood clotting and is important for bone health. Because vitamin K deficiency is a problem in newborns, they are routinely given vitamin K injections at birth. Warfarin, a substance that inhibits vitamin K activity, is used medically as an anticoagulant. Vitamin K is found in plants and is synthesized by bacteria in the gastrointestinal tract.

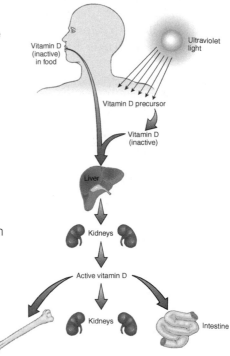

Vitamin D activation and function • Figure 7.30

3 The Fat-Soluble Vitamins 214

- **Vitamin A** is a fat-soluble vitamin needed in the visual cycle and for growth and **cell differentiation**. Its role in **gene expression** makes it essential for maintenance of epithelial tissue, reproduction, and immune function. Vitamin A deficiency causes blindness and death. Preformed vitamin

4 Meeting Needs with Dietary Supplements 230

- About half the adult population in the United States takes some type of dietary supplement. Vitamin and mineral supplements are recommended for dieters, vegetarians, pregnant women and women of childbearing age, older adults, and other nutritionally vulnerable groups.

- Herbal supplements are currently popular. These products, which are made from plants (such as the St. John's wort shown to the right) may have beneficial physiological actions, but their dosage is not regulated, and they can be toxic either on their own or in combination with other herbs or medications or in people with certain medical conditions.

- Manufacturers are responsible for the consistency and safety of supplements before they are marketed. The FDA regulates dietary supplement labeling and can monitor their safety once they are being sold. When choosing a dietary supplement, it is important to carefully consider both the potential risks and benefits of the product.

Popular herbal supplements: St. John's wort • Figure 7.37

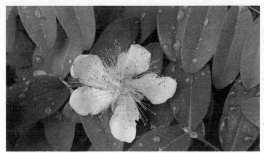

Todd Gipstein/NG Image Collection

Key Terms

- alpha-carotene (α-carotene) 214
- alpha-tocopherol (α-tocopherol) 226
- antioxidant 193
- ascorbic acid 210
- atrophic gastritis 210
- beriberi 196
- beta-carotene (β-carotene) 214
- beta-cryptoxanthin (β-cryptoxanthin) 214
- bioavailability 191
- biotin 201
- carotenoids 214
- cell differentiation 216
- choline 212
- cobalamin 208
- coenzyme 193

- collagen 210
- dietary folate equivalent (DFE) 205
- fat-soluble vitamin 188
- fibrin 227
- folate 204
- folic acid 204
- free radical 194
- gene expression 217
- hemolytic anemia 224
- hypercarotenemia 219
- intrinsic factor 208
- macrocytic anemia 205
- myelin 203
- neural tube defect 204
- neurotransmitter 197
- niacin 199
- niacin equivalent (NE) 200

- night blindness 217
- osteomalacia 221
- osteoporosis 221
- oxidative damage 193
- pantothenic acid 201
- parathyroid hormone (PTH) 221
- pellagra 199
- pernicious anemia 207
- prothrombin 227
- provitamin or vitamin precursor 193
- pyridoxal phosphate 201
- retinoids 214
- retinol activity equivalent (RAE) 214
- retinol-binding protein 215
- rhodopsin 216
- riboflavin 198

- rickets 221
- scurvy 211
- spina bifida 205
- thiamin 196
- tocopherol 225
- vitamin 188
- vitamin A 214
- vitamin B_6 201
- vitamin B_{12} 207
- vitamin C 210
- vitamin D 220
- vitamin E 224
- vitamin K 226
- water-soluble vitamin 188
- Wernicke-Korsakoff syndrome 197
- xerophthalmia 219

What is happening in this picture?

These children, who live in Russia, are being exposed to UV radiation to prevent vitamin D deficiency.

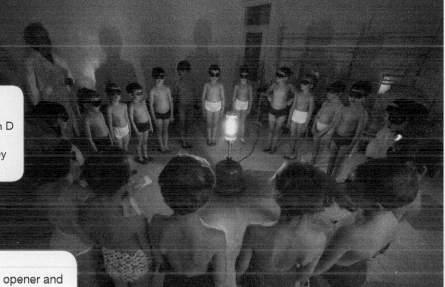

Dean Conger/NG Image Collection

Think Critically
1. Why does this treatment help them meet their need for vitamin D?
2. Why are children in Russia at risk for vitamin D deficiency?
3. What else could be done to ensure that they get adequate amounts of vitamin D?

THE PLANNER ✓

Review your Chapter Planner on the chapter opener and check off your completed work.

Water and Minerals

It is in the water of Earth's first seas that scientists propose life itself originally appeared. These primitive seas were not plain water but rather a complex mixture of minerals, organic compounds, and water. Over time, as simple organisms developed greater complexity, many left this mineral-rich external marine environment behind. To survive, they needed to bring with them a similar internal environment. Within our bodies today, minerals and water make up an "internal sea" that allows the chemistry of life to function.

Getting the right amounts of minerals and water remains essential to survival. Inadequate and excessive intakes of certain minerals are world health problems contributing to such conditions as high blood pressure, bone fractures, anemia, and increased risk of infection. Getting enough clean, fresh water may prove to be an

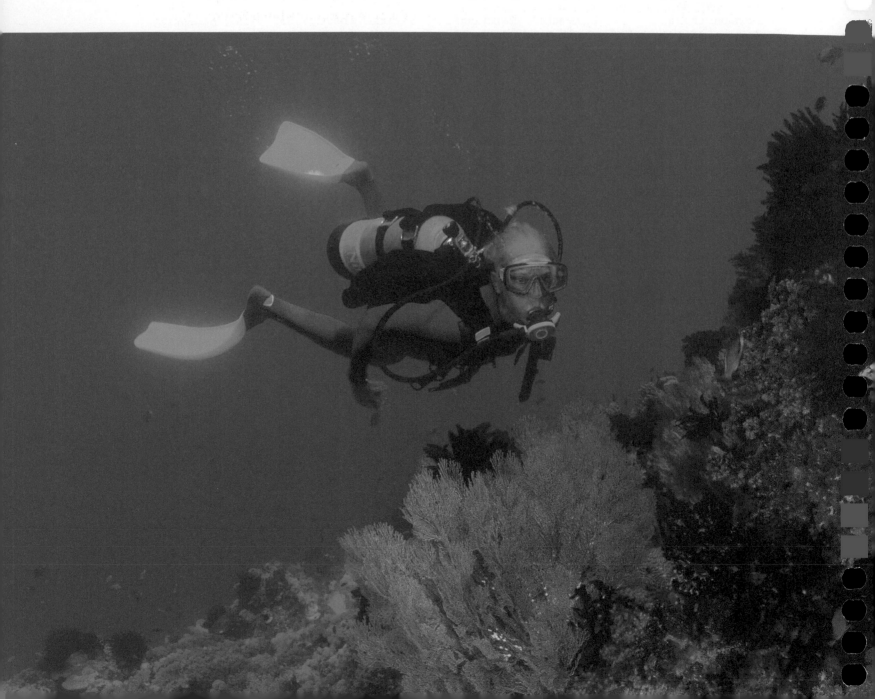

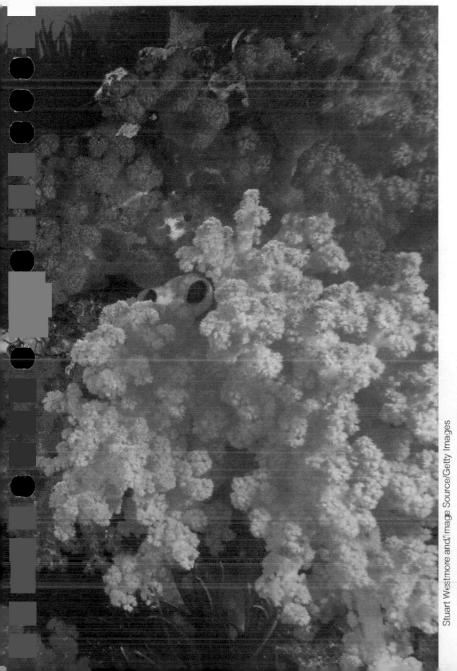

even greater challenge to human survival than meeting mineral needs. Pollution and population growth are making fresh water an increasingly rare commodity: Approximately one in eight people around the world lack access to a safe water supply.[1] In the United States clean water is accessible to most, but the huge aquifers beneath the surface are diminishing. The water crisis may make shrinking oil supplies seem like a minor inconvenience for the simple reason that without water, we die.

Stuart Westmore and Image Source/Getty Images

CHAPTER OUTLINE

CHAPTER PLANNER ✔

- ❏ Stimulate your interest by reading the introduction and looking at the visual.
- ❏ Scan the Learning Objectives in each section:
  p. 240 ❏   p. 247 ❏   p. 251 ❏   p. 259 ❏   p. 269 ❏
- ❏ Read the text and study all figures and visuals. Answer any questions.

Analyze key features:

- ❏ Process Diagram, p. 242 ❏   p. 243 ❏   p. 251 ❏   p. 253 ❏
- ❏ Debate, p. 246 ❏
- ❏ InSight, p. 250 ❏   p. 254 ❏   p. 260 ❏   p. 272 ❏   p. 278 ❏
- ❏ What a Scientist Sees, p. 262 ❏
- ❏ Thinking It Through, p. 273 ❏
- ❏ Stop: Answer the Concept Checks before you go on:
  p. 247 ❏   p. 251 ❏   p. 259 ❏   p. 268 ❏   p. 283 ❏

End of chapter and online review:

- ❏ Review the Summary, Key Terms, and online links to Additional Resources.
- ❏ Answer the online Critical and Creative Thinking Questions.
- ❏ Answer What is happening in this picture?
- ❏ Complete the online Self-Test and check your answers.

8.1 Water

LEARNING OBJECTIVES

1. **Describe** how osmosis affects water distribution.
2. **Explain** the role of the kidneys in regulating the amount of water in the body.
3. **List** five functions of water in the body.
4. **Discuss** factors that increase water needs.

Water is an overlooked but essential nutrient. Lack of sufficient water in the body causes deficiency symptoms more rapidly than does a deficiency of any other nutrient. These symptoms can be alleviated almost as rapidly as they appeared by drinking enough water to restore the body's water balance.

Water in the Body

In adults, water accounts for about 60% of body weight. Water is found in different proportions in different tissues. For example, about 75% of muscle weight is water, whereas only about 25% of the weight of bone is due to water. Water is found both inside cells (intracellular) and outside cells (extracellular) in the blood, the lymph, and the spaces between cells (**Figure 8.1**). The cell membranes that separate the intracellular and extracellular spaces are not watertight; water can pass right through them.

The distribution of water between various intra- and extracellular spaces depends on differences in the concentrations of dissolved substances, or **solutes**, such as

Water distribution • Figure 8.1

About two-thirds of the water in the body is intracellular (located inside the cells). The other one-third is extracellular (located outside the cells). The extracellular portion includes the water in the blood and lymph, the water between cells, and the water in the digestive tract, eyes, joints, and spinal cord. The distribution of water between intracellular and extracellular spaces is affected by blood pressure and the force generated by osmosis.

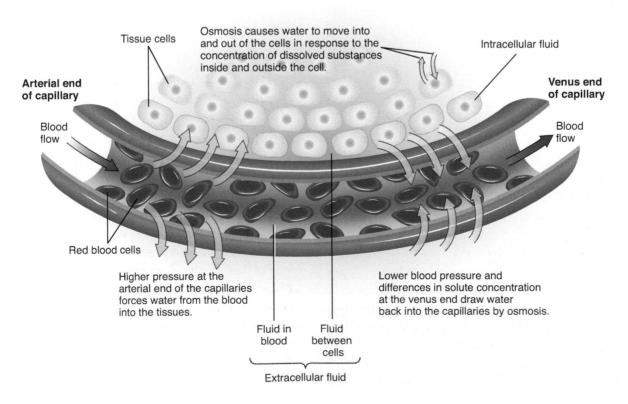

Tissue cells

Osmosis causes water to move into and out of the cells in response to the concentration of dissolved substances inside and outside the cell.

Intracellular fluid

Arterial end of capillary

Venus end of capillary

Blood flow

Blood flow

Red blood cells

Higher pressure at the arterial end of the capillaries forces water from the blood into the tissues.

Lower blood pressure and differences in solute concentration at the venus end draw water back into the capillaries by osmosis.

Fluid in blood

Fluid between cells

Extracellular fluid

Water balance • Figure 8.2

To maintain water balance, intake from food, drink, and water produced by metabolism must equal water output from evaporation, sweat, urine, and feces. This figure illustrates approximate amounts of water that enter and leave the body daily in a typical woman who is in water balance. Increases in temperature or activity increase evaporative losses. If losses from evaporation and sweat remain constant, increasing water consumption proportionately increases urinary excretion.

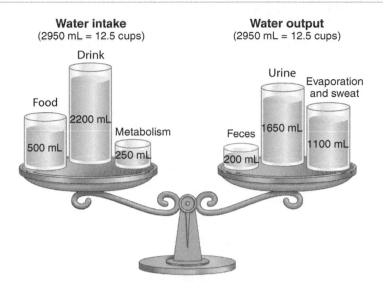

Water intake
(2950 mL = 12.5 cups)

Drink

Food

2200 mL

500 mL

Metabolism

250 mL

Water output
(2950 mL = 12.5 cups)

Urine

Evaporation and sweat

Feces

1650 mL

1100 mL

200 mL

proteins, sodium, potassium, and other small molecules. The concentration differences of these substances drive *osmosis*, the diffusion of water in a direction that equalizes the concentration of dissolved substances on either side of a membrane (see Chapter 3). Water is also moved by

> **blood pressure**
> The amount of force exerted by the blood against the walls of arteries.

blood pressure, which forces water from the capillary blood vessels into the spaces between the cells of the surrounding tissues (see Figure 8.1). The body regulates the amount of water in cells and in different extracellular spaces by adjusting the concentration of dissolved particles and relying on osmosis to move the water.

Water Balance

The amount of water in the body remains relatively constant over time. Because water cannot be stored in the body, water intake and output must be balanced to maintain the right amount. Most of the water we consume comes from water and other liquids that we drink. Solid foods also provide water; most fruits and vegetables are over 80% water, and even roast beef is about 50% water. A small amount of water is also produced in the body as a by-product of metabolic reactions. We lose water from our bodies in urine and feces, through evaporation from the lungs and skin, and in sweat (**Figure 8.2**).

The amount of water lost in the urine varies with water intake and the amount of waste that needs to be

excreted in the urine. In a healthy person, the amount of water lost in the feces is small—usually less than a cup per day. This is remarkable because every day about 9 L (38 cups) of fluid enters the gastrointestinal tract from liquids we consume and from secretions from the cells and organs of the gastrointestinal tract, but more than 95% of this is absorbed before the feces are eliminated. However, in cases of severe diarrhea, large amounts of water can be lost via this route, compromising health.

We are continuously losing water from our skin and respiratory tract due to evaporation. The amount of water lost through evaporation varies greatly, depending on body size, activity level, and environmental temperature and humidity. In a temperate climate, an inactive person loses about 1 liter (L) (4 cups) per day; the amount increases with increases in activity, environmental temperature, and body size, as well as when humidity is low.

In addition to being lost through evaporation, water is lost through sweat when we exercise or when the environment is hot. More sweat is produced as exercise intensity increases and as the environment becomes hotter and more humid. An individual doing light work at a temperature of 84°F will lose about 2 to 3 L of sweat per day. Strenuous exercise in a hot environment can increase this to 2 to 4 L in an hour.[2] Clothing that permits the evaporation of sweat helps keep the body cool and therefore decreases the amount of sweat produced.

Regulating water intake When water losses increase, intake must increase to keep body water at a healthy

Stimulating water intake • Figure 8.3

The sensation of thirst motivates fluid intake in order to restore water balance.

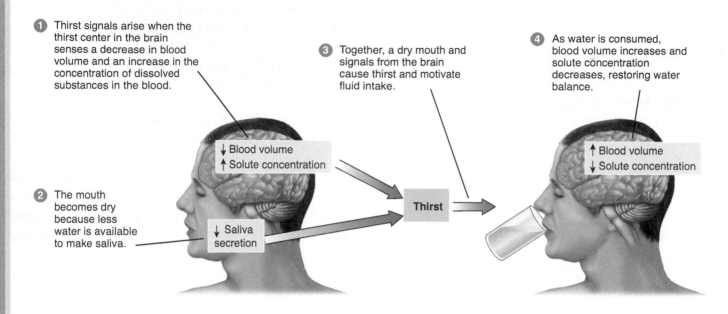

1 Thirst signals arise when the thirst center in the brain senses a decrease in blood volume and an increase in the concentration of dissolved substances in the blood.

2 The mouth becomes dry because less water is available to make saliva.

↓ Blood volume
↑ Solute concentration

↓ Saliva secretion

3 Together, a dry mouth and signals from the brain cause thirst and motivate fluid intake.

Thirst

4 As water is consumed, blood volume increases and solute concentration decreases, restoring water balance.

↑ Blood volume
↓ Solute concentration

level. The need to consume water is signaled by the sensation of **thirst**. Thirst is caused by dryness in the mouth as well as by signals from the brain (**Figure 8.3**). It is a powerful urge but often lags behind the need for water, and we don't or can't always drink when we are thirsty. Therefore, thirst alone cannot be relied on to maintain water balance.

Regulating water loss: The kidneys To maintain water balance, the kidneys regulate water loss in urine. The kidneys typically produce about 1 to 2 L (4 to 8 cups) of urine per day, but urine production varies, depending on the amount of water consumed and the amount of waste that needs to be excreted. Wastes that must be eliminated in the urine include urea and other nitrogen-containing molecules (produced by protein breakdown), ketones (from incomplete fat breakdown), sodium, and other minerals.

The kidneys function like a filter. As blood flows through them, water molecules and other small molecules move through the filter and out of the blood, while blood cells and large molecules are retained in the

blood. Some of the water and other molecules that are filtered out are reabsorbed into the blood, and the rest are excreted in the urine.

The amount of water that is reabsorbed into the blood rather than excreted in the urine depends on conditions in the body. When the solute concentration in the blood is high, as it would be in someone who has exercised strenuously and not consumed enough water, a hormone called **antidiuretic hormone (ADH)** signals the kidneys to reabsorb water, reducing the amount lost in the urine (**Figure 8.4**). This reabsorbed water is returned to the blood, maintaining body water and preventing the concentration of dissolved particles from increasing further. When the solute concentration in the blood is low, as it might be after someone has guzzled several glasses of water, ADH levels decrease. With less ADH, the kidneys reabsorb less water, and more water is excreted in the urine, allowing the solute concentration in the blood to increase to its normal level. The amount of sodium in the blood, blood volume, and blood pressure also play a role in regulating body water (as discussed later in the chapter).

Even though the kidneys work to control how much water is lost, their ability to concentrate urine is limited so there is a minimum amount of water that must be lost to excrete dissolved wastes. If there are a lot of wastes to be excreted, more water must be lost.

The Functions of Water

Water doesn't provide energy, but it is essential to life. Water in the body serves as a medium for and participant in metabolic reactions, helps regulate acid–base balance, transports nutrients and wastes, provides protection, and helps regulate body temperature.

Water in metabolism and transport Water is an excellent **solvent**; glucose, amino acids, minerals, proteins, and many other molecules dissolve in water. The chemical reactions of metabolism that support life take place in water. Water also participates in a number of reactions that join small molecules together or break apart large ones. Some of the reactions in which water participates help maintain the proper level of acidity in the body. Water is the primary constituent of blood, which flows through our bodies, delivering oxygen and nutrients to cells and transporting waste products to the lungs and kidneys for excretion.

Water as protection Water bathes the cells of the body and lubricates and cleanses internal and external body surfaces. Water in tears lubricates the eyes and washes away dirt; water in synovial fluid lubricates the joints; and water in saliva lubricates the mouth, helping us chew and swallow food. Because water resists compression, it cushions the joints and other parts of the body against shock.

Regulating urinary water losses • Figure 8.4

✓ THE PLANNER

The kidneys help regulate water balance by adjusting the amount of water lost in the urine in response to the release of antidiuretic hormone (ADH).

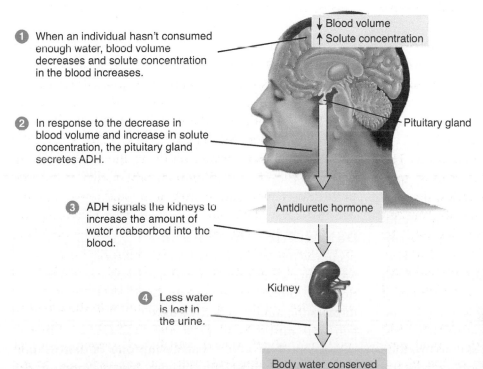

1 When an individual hasn't consumed enough water, blood volume decreases and solute concentration in the blood increases.

2 In response to the decrease in blood volume and increase in solute concentration, the pituitary gland secretes ADH.

3 ADH signals the kidneys to increase the amount of water reabsorbed into the blood.

4 Less water is lost in the urine.

↓ Blood volume
↑ Solute concentration

Pituitary gland

Antidiuretic hormone

Kidney

Body water conserved

Ask Yourself

What would happen to ADH levels and urine volume if someone consumed a lot of extra water?

Water helps cool the body • Figure 8.5

Hot weather and strenuous activity increase blood flow to the surface of the body. Shunting blood to the skin allows heat to be transferred from the blood to the surroundings. Evaporation of sweat cools the skin and the blood near the surface of the skin.

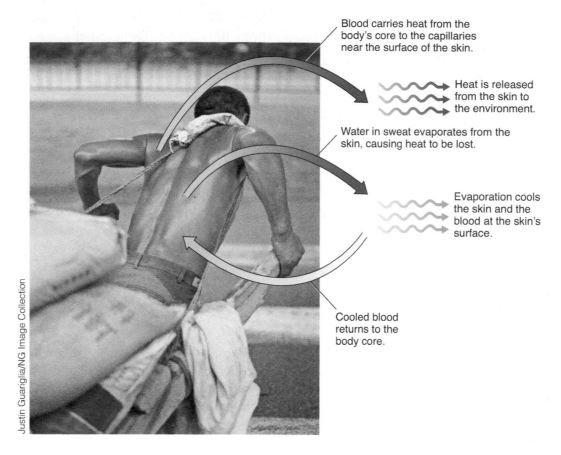

Blood carries heat from the body's core to the capillaries near the surface of the skin.

Heat is released from the skin to the environment.

Water in sweat evaporates from the skin, causing heat to be lost.

Evaporation cools the skin and the blood at the skin's surface.

Cooled blood returns to the body core.

Justin Guariglia/NG Image Collection

The cushioning effect of water in the amniotic sac protects a fetus as it grows inside the uterus.

Water and body temperature The fact that water holds heat and changes temperature slowly helps keep body temperature constant, but water is also actively involved in temperature regulation (**Figure 8.5**). The water in blood helps regulate body temperature by increasing or decreasing the amount of heat lost at the surface of the body. When body temperature starts to rise, the blood vessels in the skin dilate, causing more blood to flow close to the surface, where it can release some of the heat to the surrounding air. Cooling is aided by the production of sweat. When body temperature increases, the brain triggers the sweat glands in the skin to produce sweat, which is mostly water. As sweat evaporates from the skin, additional heat is lost, cooling the body.

Water in Health and Disease

Without food, you could probably survive for about 8 weeks, but without water, you would last only a few days. Too much water can also be a problem if it changes the osmotic balance, disrupting the distribution of water within the body.

Dehydration Dehydration occurs when water loss exceeds water intake. It causes a reduction in blood volume, which impairs the ability to deliver oxygen and nutrients to cells and remove waste products. Early symptoms of dehydration include thirst, headache, fatigue, loss of appetite, dry eyes and mouth, and dark-colored urine (**Figure 8.6**).

> **dehydration** A state that occurs when not enough water is present to meet the body's needs.

Are you at risk for dehydration? • Figure 8.6

Urine color is an indication of whether you are drinking enough. Pale yellow urine indicates you are well hydrated. The darker the urine, the greater the level of dehydration.

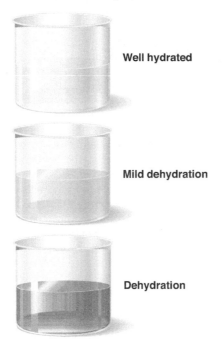

Well hydrated

Mild dehydration

Dehydration

Dehydration affects physical and cognitive performance. As dehydration worsens, it causes nausea, difficulty concentrating, confusion, and disorientation. The milder symptoms of dehydration disappear quickly after water or some other beverage is consumed, but if left untreated, dehydration can become severe enough to require medical attention (**Figure 8.7**). A water loss amounting to about 10 to 20% of body weight can be fatal. Athletes are at risk for dehydration because they may lose large amounts of water in sweat. Older adults are at risk because the thirst mechanism becomes less sensitive with age. Infants are at risk because their body surface area relative to their weight is much greater than that of adults, so they lose proportionately more water through evaporation; also, their kidneys cannot concentrate urine efficiently, so they lose more water in urine. In addition, they cannot tell us they are thirsty.

Water intoxication It is difficult to consume too much water under normal circumstances. However, overhydration, or **water** intoxication, can occur under some conditions (see Chapter 10). When there is too much water relative to the amount of sodium in the body, the concentration of sodium in the blood drops—a condition called **hyponatremia**. When this occurs, water moves

out of the blood vessels and into the tissues by osmosis, causing them to swell. Swelling in the brain can cause disorientation, convulsions, coma, and death. The early symptoms of water intoxication may be similar to those of dehydration: nausea, muscle cramps, disorientation, slurred speech, and confusion. It is important to determine whether the symptoms are due to dehydration or water intoxication because while drinking water will alleviate dehydration, it will worsen the symptoms of water intoxication.

Rehydration saves lives • Figure 8.7

Dehydration due to diarrhea is a major cause of child death in the developing world. Replacing fluids and electrolytes in the right combinations can save lives. In some cases, oral rehydration therapy is sufficient. Drinking mixtures made by simply dissolving a large pinch of salt (1/2 tsp) and a fistful of sugar (2 Tbsp) in 1 L of clean water can restore the body's water balance by promoting the absorption of water and sodium. In severe cases of diarrhea, administration of intravenous fluids, as seen in this hospital in Bangladesh, is needed to restore hydration.

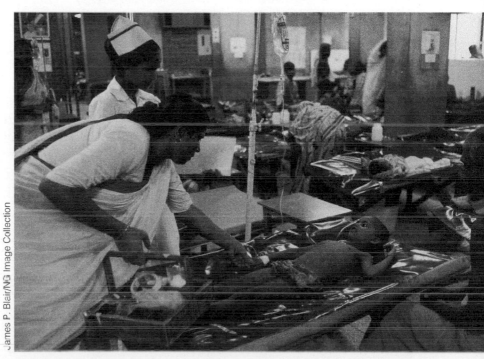

James P. Blair/NG Image Collection

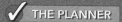
The Issue: Americans consume about 29 gallons of bottled water per person per year.[3] We choose it because it is convenient and because we think it tastes better and is safer than tap water. But the cost to our pocketbooks and our environment is high. Should we be drinking from the tap instead?

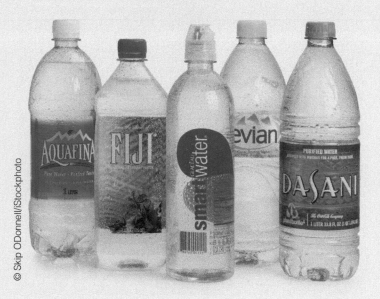

© Skip ODonnell/iStockphoto

It is easy to grab a bottle of water, and most bottled water has no chlorine or other unpleasant aftertaste. Words like *pure, crisp,* and *fresh tasting* on the label lead consumers to buy bottled water because they think it is better than water that comes from the tap. But much of the bottled water sold in the United States is tap water or tap water that has been filtered, disinfected, or otherwise treated. By definition, bottled water can be any water, as long as it has no added ingredients (except antimicrobial agents or fluoride). Labels may help you distinguish: Distilled water and purified water are treated tap water; artesian water, spring water, well water, and mineral water come from underground sources.

Is bottled water safer than tap water? Municipal (tap) water is regulated by the Environmental Protection Agency (EPA), and bottled water sold in interstate commerce is regulated by the Food and Drug Administration (FDA). The FDA uses most of the EPA's tap water standards, so it would make sense that tap water and bottled water would be equally safe. However, tap water advocates argue that tap water may actually be safer. A certified outside laboratory tests municipal water supplies every year, while bottled water companies are permitted to do their own tests for purity.[4] Tap water must also be filtered and disinfected; there are no federal filtration or disinfection requirements for bottled water.

Contamination is a safety concern for both bottled water and tap water. A study of contaminants in bottled water found that 10 popular brands contained a total of 38 chemical pollutants—everything from caffeine and Tylenol to bacteria, radioactive isotopes, and fertilizer residue.[5] Sounds scary, but bottled water advocates argue that public drinking water may also fall short of pollutant standards. Since 2004, testing by water utilities has found over 300 pollutants in tap water. Some of these are substances that are regulated and were found at levels above guidelines, but more than half of the chemicals detected are not subject to health or safety regulations and can legally be present in any amount. [6]

One of the strongest arguments against bottled water is the cost, both to the consumer and the environment. Bottled water typically costs about $3.79 per gallon—1900 times the cost of public tap water. Bottled water drinkers may feel that the added cost is worth it because of the advantages in terms of taste and convenience. Opponents argue that even if you can afford it, the planet can't. Globally, bottled water generates 1.5 million tons of plastic waste per year and consumes oil, which is used to produce the bottles as well as the gasoline and jet fuel needed to transport it.[7] About three-quarters of the water bottles produced in the United States are not recycled.[4] Bottled water proponents argue that despite the large amount of plastic waste, discarded water bottles still represent less than 1% of total municipal waste. And even though bottled water production is more energy-intensive than the production of tap water, it comprises only a small share of total U.S. energy demand.[4]

So which is better? In the United States, bottled water and tap water are both generally safe. If you recycle your bottle, does it matter which you choose?

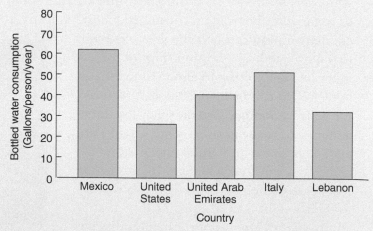

This graph compares the per capita bottled water consumption in the United States and several other countries.

Think Critically: What factors might increase a country's per capita consumption of bottled water?

Meeting Water Needs

The AI for water is 3.7 L/day for men and 2.7 L/day for women. As discussed above, however, the amount of water you need each day varies, depending on your activity level, the environmental temperature, and the humidity. Diet can also affect water needs because more water is lost when more waste must be excreted in the urine. A high-protein diet increases water needs because the urea produced from protein breakdown is excreted in the urine. A low-calorie diet increases water needs because as body fat and protein are broken down to fuel the body, ketones and urea are produced and must be excreted in the urine. A high-salt diet increases water needs because eliminating the excess sodium in the urine increases water losses. A high-fiber diet increases water needs because more water is held in the intestines and is lost in the feces.

In the United States, beverages provide about 80% of the body's requirement for water—about 3 L (13 cups) for men and 2.2 L (9 cups) for women.[8] The rest comes from the water consumed in food. Most beverages, whether water, milk, juice, or soda, help meet the overall need for water (see *Debate: Is Bottled Water Better?*). Beverages containing caffeine, such as coffee, tea, and cola, increase water losses in the short term because caffeine is a **diuretic**.

However, the increase in water loss is small, so the net amount of water that caffeinated beverages add to the body is similar to the amount contributed by noncaffeinated beverages. Alcohol is also a diuretic; the overall effect it has on water balance depends on the relative amounts of water and alcohol in the beverages being consumed.[8] Most adults in the United States consume adequate amounts of water in the their diet, from water and other beverages; however low water intake is a concern for older adults: 83% of men and 95% of women 71 years and older have intakes below the AI.[9]

> **diuretic** A substance that increases the amount of urine passed from the body.

CONCEPT CHECK

1. **How** does osmosis affect the distribution of water in the body?
2. **What** is the role of ADH?
3. **How** does water help cool the body?
4. **Why** do water needs increase when you exercise more?

8.2 An Overview of Minerals

LEARNING OBJECTIVES

1. **Define** minerals in terms of nutrition.
2. **Describe** factors that affect mineral bioavailability.
3. **Discuss** the functions of minerals in the body.

Minerals are found in the ground on which we walk, the jewels we wear on our fingers, and even some of the makeup we wear on our faces. But perhaps the most significant impact of minerals on our lives comes from their importance in our nutritional health. You need to consume more than 20 **minerals** in your food to stay healthy. Some of these make up a significant portion of your body weight; others are found in minute quantities. If more than 100 milligrams of a mineral is required in the diet each day, an amount equivalent in weight to about two drops of water, the mineral is considered a **major mineral**; these include sodium, potassium, chloride, calcium, phosphorus, magnesium, and sulfur. Minerals that are needed in smaller amounts are referred to as **trace minerals**; these include iron, copper, zinc, selenium, iodine, chromium, fluoride, manganese, molybdenum, and others. Just because you need more of the major minerals than of the trace minerals doesn't mean that one group is more important than the other. A deficiency of a trace mineral is just as damaging to your health as a deficiency of a major mineral.

> **mineral** In nutrition, an element needed by the body to maintain structure and regulate chemical reactions and body processes.

> **major mineral** A mineral required in the diet in an amount greater than 100 mg/day or present in the body in an amount greater than 0.01% of body weight.

> **trace mineral** A mineral required in the diet in an amount of 100 mg or less per day or present in the body in an amount of 0.01% of body weight or less.

Minerals on MyPlate • Figure 8.8

Minerals are found in all the MyPlate food groups, but some groups are particularly good sources of specific minerals. Eating a variety of foods, including fresh fruits, vegetables, nuts, legumes, whole grains and cereals, milk, seafood, and lean meats can maximize your diet's mineral content.

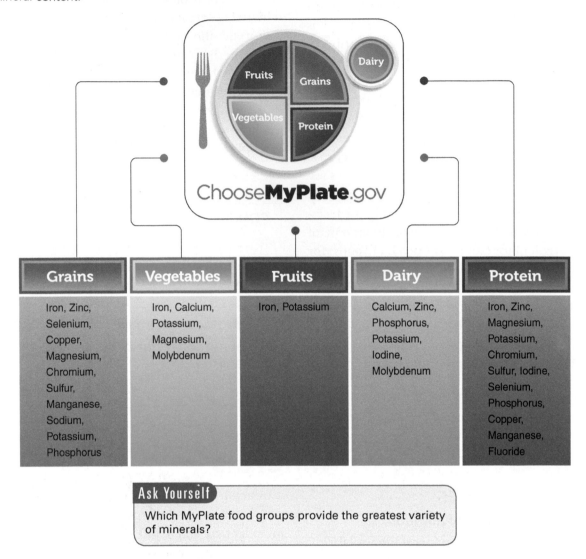

ChooseMyPlate.gov

Grains	Vegetables	Fruits	Dairy	Protein
Iron, Zinc, Selenium, Copper, Magnesium, Chromium, Sulfur, Manganese, Sodium, Potassium, Phosphorus	Iron, Calcium, Potassium, Magnesium, Molybdenum	Iron, Potassium	Calcium, Zinc, Phosphorus, Potassium, Iodine, Molybdenum	Iron, Zinc, Magnesium, Potassium, Chromium, Sulfur, Iodine, Selenium, Phosphorus, Copper, Manganese, Fluoride

Ask Yourself

Which MyPlate food groups provide the greatest variety of minerals?

Minerals in Our Food

Minerals in the diet come from both plant and animal sources (**Figure 8.8**). Some minerals are present as functioning components of the plant or animal and are therefore present in consistent amounts. For instance, the iron content of beef is predictable because iron is part of the muscle protein that gives beef its red color. In other foods, some minerals are present as contaminants from the soil or from processing. For example, plants grown in an area where the soil is high in selenium are higher in selenium than plants grown in other areas, and milk from dairies that

use sterilizing solutions that contain iodine is a source of iodine. Minerals are also added to food intentionally during processing. Sodium is added to soups and crackers as a flavor enhancer; iron is added to refined grain products as part of the enrichment process; and calcium, iron, and other minerals are typically added to fortified breakfast cereals.

Processing can also remove minerals from foods. For example, when vegetables are cooked, the cells are broken down, and potassium is lost in the cooking water. When the skins of fruits and vegetables or the bran and germ of grains are detached, magnesium, iron, selenium, zinc, and copper are lost.

Mineral Bioavailability

The bioavailability of the minerals that we consume in foods varies. For some minerals, such as sodium, we absorb almost all that is present in our food, but for others, we absorb only a small percentage. For instance, we typically absorb only about 25% of the calcium in our diet, and iron absorption may be as low as 5%. How much of a particular mineral is absorbed may vary from food to food, meal to meal, and person to person.

In general, the minerals in animal products are better absorbed than those in plant foods. The difference in absorption is due in part to the fact that plants contain substances such as phytates (also called phytic acid), tannins, oxalates, and fiber that bind minerals in the gastrointestinal tract and can reduce absorption (**Figure 8.9**). The North American diet generally does not contain enough of any of these components to cause a mineral deficiency, but diets in developing countries may. For example, in some populations, the phytate content of the diet is high enough to cause a zinc deficiency.

> **ion** An atom or a group of atoms that carries an electrical charge.

The presence of one mineral can also interfere with the absorption of another. For example, mineral **ions** that carry the same charge compete for absorption in the gastrointestinal tract. Calcium, magnesium, zinc, copper, and iron all carry a 2+ charge, so a high intake of one may reduce the absorption of another. Although this is generally not a problem when whole foods are consumed, a large dose of one mineral from a dietary supplement may interfere with the absorption of other minerals.

The body's need for a mineral may also affect how much of that mineral is absorbed. For instance, if plenty of iron is stored in your body, you will absorb less of the iron you consume. Life stage can also affect absorption; for example, calcium absorption doubles during pregnancy, when the body's needs are high.

Mineral Functions

Minerals contribute to the body's structure and help regulate body processes. Many serve more than one function. For example, we need calcium to keep our bones strong as well as to maintain normal blood pressure, allow muscles to contract, and transmit nerve signals from cell to cell. Some minerals help regulate water balance, others help regulate energy metabolism, and some affect growth and development through their role in

---

Compounds that interfere with mineral absorption • Figure 8.9

Plant foods such as these contain substances that can reduce mineral absorption when consumed in large amounts.

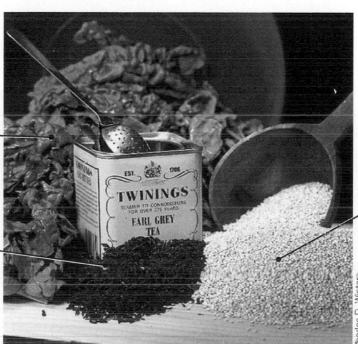

Oxalates, found in spinach, rhubarb, beet greens, and chocolate, have been found to interfere with the absorption of calcium and iron.

Tannins, found in tea and some grains, can interfere with the absorption of iron.

Phytates, found in whole grains, bran, and soy products, bind calcium, zinc, iron, and magnesium, limiting the absorption of these minerals. Phytates can be broken down by yeast, so the bioavailability of minerals is higher in yeast-leavened foods such as breads.

Charles D. Winters

Nutrition InSight | Mineral functions • Figure 8.10 ✓ THE PLANNER

While each mineral has unique functions, many have complimentary roles in supporting health.

Selenium, sulfur, zinc, copper, and manganese are needed for the functioning of antioxidant enzymes and molecules that can defend the body against damaging chemicals.

Sodium, potassium, and chloride help regulate fluid balance.

Zinc, iodine, and calcium are needed for normal growth and development.

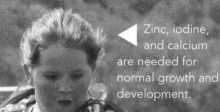

Iron, magnesium, zinc, chromium, selenium, iodine, phosphorus, and calcium are needed to produce ATP to fuel physical activity and to regulate metabolism.

Calcium, sodium, potassium, and chloride are needed for the transmission of nerve impulses and for muscle contraction.

Iron, copper, calcium, zinc, selenium, and magnesium are needed to keep blood healthy and immune function strong.

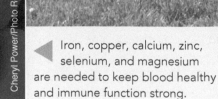

Calcium, phosphorus, magnesium, and fluoride are needed to maintain the health of bones and teeth.

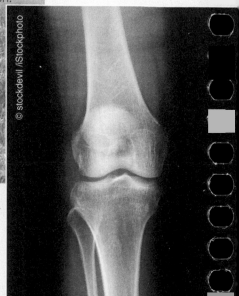

Pritt Vesilind/NG Image Collection

Jason Verschoor/iStockphoto

Amy Myers/iStockphoto

Cheryl Power/Photo Researchers, Inc.

© stockdevil /iStockphoto

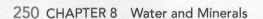

Cofactors • Figure 8.11

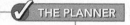

The binding of a cofactor to an enzyme activates the enzyme. For example, zinc is essential for the activity of an enzyme needed for DNA synthesis. Coenzymes, discussed in Chapter 7, are a type of cofactor.

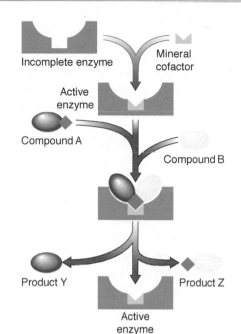

Incomplete enzyme

Mineral cofactor

Active enzyme

Compound A

Compound B

Product Y

Product Z

Active enzyme

HOW IT WORKS

❶ The mineral cofactor combines with the incomplete enzyme to form the active enzyme.

❷ The active enzyme binds to the molecules involved in the chemical reaction (compounds A and B) and accelerates their transformation into the final products (products Y and Z).

❸ The final products are released. The enzyme and cofactor (mineral) can be reused.

---

cofactor An inorganic ion or coenzyme that is required for enzyme activity.

the expression of certain genes (**Figure 8.10**). Many minerals act as **cofactors** needed for enzyme activity (**Figure 8.11**). None of the minerals we require acts in isolation. Instead, they interact with each other as well as with other nutrients and other substances in the body.

CONCEPT CHECK   STOP

1. **How** do minerals differ from vitamins?
2. **How** do phytates, oxalates, and tannins decrease mineral bioavailability?
3. **What** is the function of a cofactor?

8.3 Electrolytes: Sodium, Potassium, and Chloride

LEARNING OBJECTIVES

1. **Explain** how electrolytes function in the body.
2. **Define** hypertension and describe its symptoms and consequences.
3. **Discuss** how diet affects blood pressure.
4. **Contrast** the dietary sources of sodium and potassium.

We think of electrolytes as the things we get by guzzling a sports drink. But what exactly are they, and why do we need them? Electrolytes are ions. Although many substances in the body are electrolytes, in nutrition and in sports drinks,

the term *electrolyte* typically refers to the three principal electrolytes in body fluids: sodium, potassium, and chloride. Sodium and potassium carry a positive charge, and chloride carries a negative charge. In the diet, sodium is most commonly found combined with chloride as **sodium chloride**, what we call either "salt" or "table salt." In our bodies, these electrolytes are important in maintaining fluid balance and allowing nerve impulses to travel throughout our bodies, signaling the activities that are essential for life.

electrolyte A positively or negatively charged ion that conducts an electrical current in solution. Commonly refers to sodium, potassium, and chloride.

Electrolytes in the Body

The concentrations of sodium, potassium, and chloride inside cells differ dramatically from those outside. Potassium is the principal positively charged intracellular ion, sodium is the most abundant positively charged extracellular ion, and chloride is the principal negatively charged extracellular ion.

Functions of electrolytes Electrolytes help regulate fluid balance; the distribution of water throughout the body depends on the concentration of electrolytes and other solutes. Water moves by osmosis in response to differences in solute concentration. So, for example, if the concentration of sodium in the blood increases, water will move into the blood from intracellular and other extracellular spaces to equalize the concentration of sodium and other dissolved substances. A high sodium concentration in the blood also stimulates thirst; water intake helps dilute blood sodium (**Figure 8.12a**).

Sodium, potassium, and chloride are also essential for generating and conducting nerve impulses. Nerve impulses are created by the movement of sodium and potassium ions across the nerve cell membrane. When a nerve cell is at rest, potassium is concentrated inside the nerve cell, and sodium stays outside the cell. Sodium and potassium ions cannot pass freely across the cell membrane. But when a nerve is stimulated, the cell membrane becomes more permeable to sodium, allowing sodium ions to rush into the nerve cell, which initiates a nerve impulse (**Figure 8.12b**).

Regulating electrolyte balance Our bodies are efficient at regulating the concentration of electrolytes, even when dietary intake varies dramatically. Sodium and chloride balance is regulated to some extent by the intake of both salt and water. When sodium chloride intake is high, thirst is stimulated in order to increase water intake. Very low salt intake stimulates a "salt appetite" that causes you to crave salt. The craving that triggers your desire to plunge into a bag of salty chips, however, is not due to this salt appetite. It is a learned preference, not a physiological drive. If you cut back on your salt intake, you will find that your taste buds become more sensitive to the presence of salt, and foods taste saltier.

Electrolyte functions • Figure 8.12

Electrolytes have important roles in fluid balance and nerve conductivity.

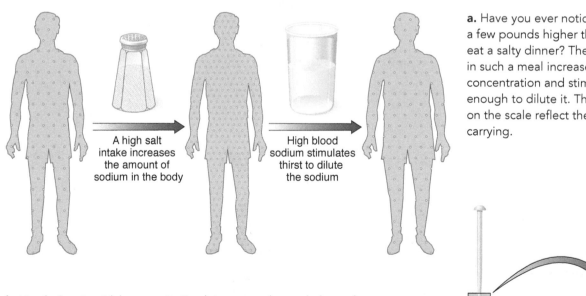

A high salt intake increases the amount of sodium in the body

High blood sodium stimulates thirst to dilute the sodium

a. Have you ever noticed that your weight is a few pounds higher the morning after you eat a salty dinner? The sodium you consume in such a meal increases your blood sodium concentration and stimulates you to drink enough to dilute it. The extra pounds you see on the scale reflect the extra water you are carrying.

b. You feel a pinprick because it stimulates nerves beneath the surface of the skin. This stimulation increases the permeability of the nerve cell membrane to sodium and then to potassium. The sodium rushes in (shown here), initiating a nerve impulse. Potassium then rushes out, restoring the electrical charge across the membrane. The increase in sodium permeability at one spot triggers an increase on the adjacent patch of membrane, spreading the nerve impulse along the nerve to the brain. Once the impulse has passed, the original ion concentrations inside and outside the membrane are restored by a sodium/potassium pump in the membrane so that a new nerve signal can be triggered.

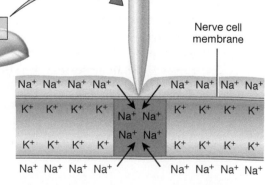

Nerve cell membrane

Regulation of blood pressure • Figure 8.13

When blood pressure decreases, the kidneys help to raise it. As blood pressure increases, these events are inhibited so that blood pressure does not continue to rise.

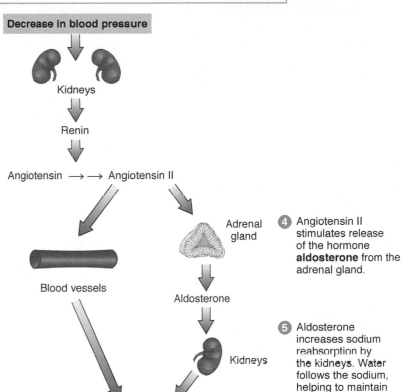

Decrease in blood pressure

1 A decrease in blood pressure triggers the kidneys to release the enzyme renin.

Kidneys

Renin

2 Renin converts angiotensin into angiotensin I, which is activated to angiotensin II.

Angiotensin → → Angiotensin II

3 Angiotensin II increases blood pressure by constricting the walls of blood vessels.

Adrenal gland

4 Angiotensin II stimulates release of the hormone **aldosterone** from the adrenal gland.

Blood vessels

Aldosterone

Kidneys

5 Aldosterone increases sodium reabsorption by the kidneys. Water follows the sodium, helping to maintain blood volume and blood pressure.

Increase in blood pressure

Thirst and salt appetite help ensure that appropriate proportions of sodium chloride and water are taken in, but the kidneys are the primary regulator of sodium, potassium, and chloride concentrations in the body. Excretion of these electrolytes in the urine is decreased when intake is low and increased when intake is high.

Because water follows sodium by osmosis, the ability of the kidneys to conserve sodium provides a mechanism for conserving water in the body. This mechanism also helps regulate blood pressure. When the concentration of sodium in the blood increases, water follows, causing an increase in blood volume. An increase in blood volume can increase blood pressure. When blood pressure decreases, it triggers the production and release of proteins and hormones that stimulate thirst and cause the blood vessels to constrict and the kidneys to retain sodium, and hence water (**Figure 8.13**).

Regulation of blood potassium levels is also important. Even a small increase can be dangerous. If blood potassium levels begin to rise, body cells are stimulated to take up potassium. This short-term regulation prevents the amount of potassium in the extracellular fluid from getting lethally high. Long-term regulation of potassium

balance depends on the release of proteins that cause the kidney to excrete potassium and retain sodium.

Electrolytes in Health and Disease

Electrolyte deficiencies are uncommon in healthy people. Sodium, potassium, and chloride are plentiful in most diets, and the kidneys of healthy individuals are efficient at regulating the amounts of these electrolytes in the body. Acute deficiencies and excesses can occur due to illness or extreme conditions. The health problem most commonly associated with electrolyte imbalance is **hypertension**, or high blood pressure. Hypertension is a serious public health concern in the United States; about one-third of adult Americans ages 20 and older have hypertension. Only about 53% of those with diagnosed hypertension have their blood pressure under control.[10]

> **hypertension** Blood pressure that is consistently elevated to 140/90 millimeters (mm) mercury or greater.

Electrolyte deficiency Deficiencies of any of the electrolytes can lead to electrolyte imbalance, which can cause disturbances in acid–base and fluid balance, poor

Epidemiology and clinical trials have helped identify dietary patterns that are associated with healthy blood pressure.

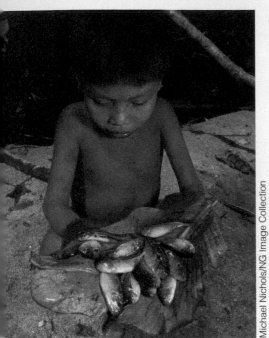

This Yanomami Indian boy lives in the rain forest of Brazil. The Yanomami diet consists of locally grown crops, nuts, insects, fish, and game. It contains less than 1 gram (g) of sodium chloride a day, the lowest salt intake recorded for any population. The Yanomami have very low average blood pressure and no hypertension. Studying the salt intake and blood pressure of the Yanomami and 51 other populations around the world helped to establish a relationship between high salt intake and hypertension.[11]

Michael Nichols/NG Image Collection

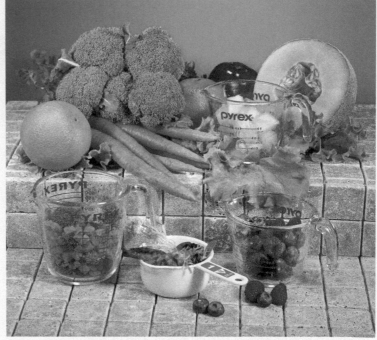

A diet that is high in fruits and vegetables, which are good sources of potassium, magnesium, and fiber, reduces blood pressure compared to a similar diet containing fewer fruits and vegetables.[12] The amounts in the measuring cups shown here, about 2 cups of fruit and 2 1/2 cups of vegetables, represent the amount recommended for a 2000-Calorie diet.

Andy Washnik

appetite, muscle cramps, confusion, apathy, constipation, and, eventually, irregular heartbeat. For example, the sudden death that can occur as a result of fasting, anorexia nervosa, or starvation may be due to irregular heartbeat caused by potassium deficiency. Sodium, chloride, and potassium depletion can occur when losses of these electrolytes are increased by heavy and persistent sweating, chronic diarrhea or vomiting, or kidney disorders that lead to excessive excretion. Medications can also interfere with electrolyte balance. For example, certain diuretic medications that are used to treat high blood pressure cause potassium loss.

Electrolyte toxicity It is not possible for healthy people to consume too much potassium from foods. If, however, supplements are consumed in excess or kidney function is compromised, blood levels of potassium can increase and potentially cause death due to an irregular heartbeat. A high oral dose of potassium generally causes vomiting, but if too much potassium enters the blood, it can cause the heart to stop.

It is difficult to consume more sodium than the body can handle because we usually drink more water when we consume more sodium. Though rare, elevation of blood sodium can result from massive ingestion of salt, such as may occur from drinking seawater or consuming salt tablets. The most common cause of high blood sodium is dehydration, and the symptoms of high blood sodium are similar to those of dehydration.

Hypertension Hypertension, or high blood pressure, has been called "the silent killer" because it has no

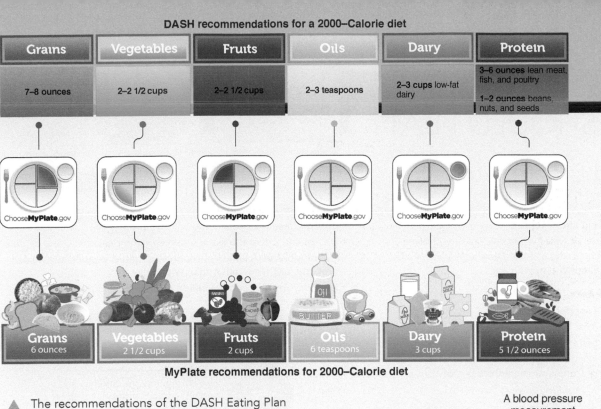

DASH recommendations for a 2000–Calorie diet

Grains	Vegetables	Fruits	Oils	Dairy	Protein
7–8 ounces	2–2 1/2 cups	2–2 1/2 cups	2–3 teaspoons	2–3 cups low-fat dairy	3–6 ounces lean meat, fish, and poultry 1–2 ounces beans, nuts, and seeds

✓ THE PLANNER

Grains 6 ounces	Vegetables 2 1/2 cups	Fruits 2 cups	Oils 6 teaspoons	Dairy 3 cups	Protein 5 1/2 ounces

MyPlate recommendations for 2000–Calorie diet

▲ The recommendations of the DASH Eating Plan (DASH stands for Dietary Approaches to Stop Hypertension) (upper portion of the figure) are similar to those of MyPlate (lower portion). Both recommend eating plenty of fruits and vegetables; choosing whole grains; having beans, nuts, seeds, and fish more often; and choosing lean meats and low-fat dairy products.

Reductions in blood pressure are seen with the DASH diet pattern compared with a typical American eating pattern. Lowering the sodium content of either diet reduces blood pressure.[17] ▶

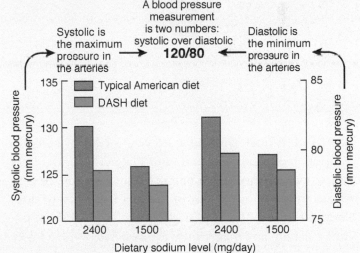

outward symptoms but can lead to atherosclerosis, heart attack, stroke, kidney disease, and early death. It is caused by an increase in blood volume or a narrowing of the blood vessels. Hypertension is a complex disorder resulting from disturbances in one or more of the mechanisms that control body fluid and electrolyte balance.

Elevated blood pressure is treated with diet, exercise, and medication. To allow early treatment and avoid the potentially lethal side effects of elevated blood pressure, people should have their blood pressure monitored regularly. A healthy blood pressure is less than 120/80 mm of mercury. Blood pressure of 120/80 to 139/89 is referred to as **prehypertension**, and blood pressure that is consistently 140/90 mm of mercury or greater indicates hypertension (see online Appendix F).[10]

Some of the risk of developing hypertension is genetic; your risk is increased if you have a family history of the disease. It is more common in African Americans than in Mexican Americans or non-Hispanic whites.[10] Whether you are genetically predisposed to hypertension or not, your risk of developing high blood pressure increases as you grow older and is higher if you are overweight, particularly if the excess fat is in your abdominal region. Lack of physical activity, heavy alcohol consumption, and stress can also increase blood pressure.[13] Regular exercise can prevent or delay the onset of hypertension, and weight loss can help reduce blood pressure in obese individuals. Your risk of developing high blood pressure can also be increased or decreased by your dietary choices **(Figure 8.14)**.

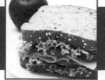
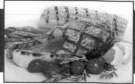

© Sara Winter/iStockphoto   © Jill Chen/iStockphoto   © Steve Mcsweeny/iStockphoto

Water and Electrolytes

✓ THE PLANNER

Stay hydrated
- Drink before, during, and after exercise.
- Guzzle two extra glasses of water when you are outside on a hot day.
- Bring a bottle of water with you in your car.

Boost your potassium intake
- Double your vegetable serving at dinner.
- Take two pieces of fruit for lunch.
- Have orange juice, or better yet, an orange, instead of drinking soda or punch.
- Aim for nine servings of fruits and vegetables per day.

Reduce your sodium intake
- Choose fresh over processed.
- Do not add salt to the water when cooking rice, pasta, and cereals.
- Flavor foods with lemon juice, onions, garlic, pepper, curry, basil, oregano, or thyme rather than with salt.
- Limit salty snacks such as salted potato chips, nuts, popcorn, and crackers.
- Limit condiments such as soy sauce, barbecue sauce, ketchup, and mustard; they are high in sodium.

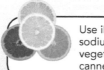

Use iProfile to compare the sodium content of fresh vegetables with that of canned vegetables.

Diet and blood pressure Dietary intake of sodium, chloride, potassium, calcium, and magnesium can affect your blood pressure and your risk of hypertension. In general, as the sodium content of the diet increases, so does blood pressure.[14] In contrast, diets that are high in potassium, calcium, and magnesium are associated with a lower average blood pressure.[15] Other components of the diet, such as the amount of fiber and the type and amount of fat, may also affect your risk of developing hypertension. A dietary pattern, such as the **DASH (Dietary Approaches to Stop Hypertension) Eating Plan**, that incorporates the recommended amounts of each of these can cause a significant reduction in blood pressure and is a dietary pattern recommended by the 2010 Dietary Guidelines. This pattern provides plenty of fiber, potassium, magnesium, and calcium; is low in total fat, saturated fat, and cholesterol; and is lower in sodium than the typical American diet (see online Appendix G). Consuming a diet that follows the DASH pattern lowers blood pressure in individuals with elevated blood pressure even when sodium levels are not severely restricted. Reductions in blood pressure are greater when sodium intake is lower (see Figure 8.14).[16,17]

Meeting Electrolyte Needs

Most people in the United States need to reduce their sodium intake and increase their potassium intake to meet recommendations for a healthy diet (see *What Should I Eat?*). The 2010 Dietary Guidelines recommend a daily sodium intake of less than 2300 mg. This value is the same as the UL for sodium, which is set to avoid the increase in blood pressure seen with higher sodium intakes. For people who are 51 years or older and those of any age who are African American or have hypertension, diabetes, or kidney disease, sodium intake should be reduced to 1500 mg/day. Over 95% of adults in the United States consume more than the UL for sodium; typical sodium intake is about 3400 mg/day.[19] Because salt is 40% sodium and 60% chloride by weight, 3400 mg of sodium represents 8.5 g (8500 mg) of salt per day.

The DRIs recommend a potassium intake of 4700 mg/day; the Daily Value is 3500 mg/day or greater for adults. Usual intake in the United States is about 2600 mg/day; less than 2% of adults meet the DRIs recommended intake of 4700 mg/day.[20] No UL has been set for potassium.

Processing adds sodium • Figure 8.15

Most of the sodium in the American diet comes from processed foods.

a. About 77% of the salt we eat comes from processed foods. Only about 12% comes from salt found naturally in food, while 11% comes from salt added in cooking and at the table. [18]

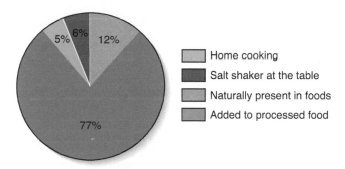

- Home cooking
- Salt shaker at the table
- Naturally present in foods
- Added to processed food

Interpret the Data

According to this pie chart, which of the following will result in the greatest reduction in sodium intake for a typical American?
a. Taking away the salt shaker during meals
b. Reducing the amount of salt added during meal preparation
c. Consuming fewer processed foods

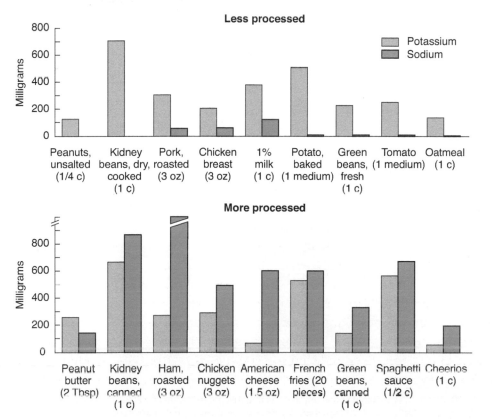

b. Processed foods are generally higher in sodium and may also be lower in potassium than unprocessed foods. Some of the sodium in processed foods comes from salt added for flavoring; some is added as a preservative to inhibit microbial growth. In addition to sodium chloride, sodium bicarbonate, sodium citrate, and sodium glutamate are added to preserve and flavor foods.

One of the reasons our diet is high in salt (sodium chloride) and low in potassium is that we eat a lot of processed foods, which are high in sodium and chloride, and too few fresh unprocessed foods, such as fruits, vegetables, whole grains, and fresh meats, which are high in potassium. Over three-quarters of the salt we eat is from foods that have had salt added during processing and manufacturing (**Figure 8.15**).

You can lower the amount of sodium in your diet by limiting your intake of processed foods and cutting down on the amount of salt added in cooking and at the table. However, even wholesome foods contain a fair amount of sodium; for example a slice of bread contains over 100 mg of sodium. Food labels can help identify low-sodium foods (**Figure 8.16**). Some medications can also contribute a significant amount of sodium. Drug facts labels on over-the-counter medications can help identify those that contain large amounts of sodium. A diet that includes plenty of fruits and vegetables and meets the recommendations of the Dietary Guidelines and MyPlate will easily meet potassium intake recommendations; daily intakes of 8000 to 11,000 mg are not uncommon.[8]

Table 8.1 summarizes information about water, sodium, chloride, and potassium.

Sodium and potassium on food labels • Figure 8.16

The Nutrition Facts panel lists the sodium content of packaged foods in milligrams and as a percentage of the Daily Value. Proposed changes to food labels would include this information for potassium as well. A food that is low in sodium may include on the label the health claim that diets that are low in sodium may reduce the risk of high blood pressure. A food that is low in sodium and a good source of potassium may include the health claim that diets containing foods that are good sources of potassium and low in sodium may reduce the risk of high blood pressure and stroke.

Current food label

The Nutrition Facts section lists the total amount of sodium per serving and the % Daily Value this amount represents.

The Daily Value for sodium for a 2000-Calorie diet is given at the bottom of the label.

Nutrition Facts
Serving Size 1/2 cup (125g)
Servings Per Container about 3½

Amount Per Serving

Calories 50	Calories from Fat 10

	%Daily Value**
Total Fat 1g	**2%**
Saturated Fat 0g	**0%**
Trans Fat 0g	
Cholesterol 0mg	**0%**
Sodium 250mg	**10%**
Potassium 530mg	**15%**
Total Carbohydrate 9g	**3%**
Dietary Fiber 1g	**4%**
Sugars 7g	
Protein 2g	

Vitamin A 10%	•	Vitamin C 25%
Calcium 2%	•	Iron 10%

*Percent Daily Values are based on a 2,000 calorie diet. Your daily values may be higher or lower depending on your calorie needs.

	Calories:	2,000	2,500
Total Fat	Less than	65g	80g
Sat Fat	Less than	20g	25g
Cholesterol	Less than	300mg	300mg
Sodium	Less than	2,400mg	2,400mg
Potassium		3,500mg	3,500mg
Total Carbohydrate		300g	375g
Dietary Fiber		25g	30g

Light Spaghetti Sauce, 250 milligrams (mg) per serving
Regular Spaghetti Sauce, 500 mg per serving

Proposed food label

Potassium information is voluntary on the current label. Proposed changes to food labels would require this information to be included along with the amounts of calcium, iron, and vitamin D.

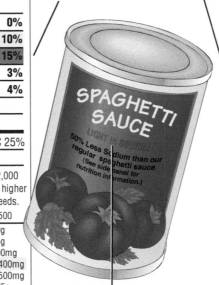

Nutrition Facts
3½ Servings per container

Servings size	1/2 cup (125g)

Amount Per 1/2 cup

Calories	**50**

% DV*	
2%	**Total Fat** 1g
0%	Saturated Fat 0g
	Trans Fat 0g
0%	**Cholesterol** 0mg
10%	**Sodium** 250mg
3%	**Total Carbs** 9g
4%	Dietary Fiber 1g
	Sugars 7g
	Added Sugars 5g
	Protein 2g
0%	Vitamin D 0mcg
2%	Calcium 20mg
10%	Iron 2mg
15%	Potassium 530mg

* Footnote on Daily Values (DV) and calories reference to be inserted here.

"Light in sodium" means that this product contains 50% less sodium than regular spaghetti sauce. Other sodium descriptors seen on food labels include:
Sodium free—a food contains less than 5 mg of sodium per serving
Low sodium—a food contains 140 mg or less of sodium per serving (about 5% of the Daily Value)
Reduced sodium—a food contains at least 25% less sodium than a reference food.

Ask Yourself

If instead of a serving of this spaghetti sauce, which is light in sodium, you ate a serving of regular spaghetti sauce, how much more sodium would you consume?

A summary of water and the electrolytes Table 8.1

Nutrient	Sources	Recommended intake for adults	Major functions	Deficiency diseases and symptoms	Groups at risk of deficiency	Toxicity	UL
Water	Drinking water, other beverages, and food	2.7–3.7 L/day	Solvent, reactant, protector, transporter, regulator of temperature and pH	Thirst, dark-colored urine, weakness, poor endurance, confusion, disorientation	Infants; people with fever, vomiting, or diarrhea; elderly individuals; athletes	Confusion, coma, convulsions	ND
Sodium	Table salt, processed foods	< 2300 mg/day; ideally 1500 mg/day	Major positive extracellular ion, nerve transmission, muscle contraction, fluid balance	Muscle cramps	People consuming too much water compared to sodium, those with vomiting or diarrhea or who sweat excessively	High blood pressure in sensitive people	2300 mg/day
Potassium	Fresh fruits and vegetables, legumes, whole grains, milk, meat	4700 mg/day or more	Major positive intracellular ion, nerve transmission, muscle contraction, fluid balance	Irregular heartbeat, fatigue, muscle cramps	People consuming poor diets high in processed foods, those with vomiting or diarrhea, those taking thiazide diuretics	Abnormal heartbeat	ND
Chloride	Table salt, processed foods	< 3600 mg/day; ideally 2300 mg/day	Major negative extracellular ion, fluid balance	Unlikely	None	None likely	3600 mg/day

Note: UL, Tolerable Upper Intake Level; ND, not determined.

CONCEPT CHECK 🛑 STOP

1. **Why** does eating a salty meal cause your weight to increase temporarily?
2. **Why** is hypertension called "the silent killer"?
3. **What** is the DASH Eating Plan?
4. **Which** types of foods contribute the most sodium to the American diet?

8.4 Major Minerals and Bone Health

LEARNING OBJECTIVES

1. **Describe** factors that affect peak bone mass and the rate of bone loss.
2. **Explain** how blood calcium levels are regulated.
3. **List** foods that are good sources of calcium.
4. **Describe** functions of calcium, phosphorus, and magnesium that are unrelated to their role in bone.

Bones are the hardest, strongest structures in the human body. They support our weight, whether we are stepping off a curb or jumping rope. Age, however, heralds a loss of bone strength. For many people, the loss is so great that the force of stepping off a curb is enough to cause their bones to fracture.

Bone is strong because it is composed of a protein framework, or matrix, that is hardened by deposits of minerals. This matrix consists primarily of the protein

Bone mass and osteoporosis • Figure 8.17

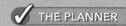
THE PLANNER ✓

Osteoporosis is a major public health problem. In the United States, more than 5 million people over age 50 have osteoporosis, and another 34.5 million are at risk due to low bone mass, called **osteopenia**. [22] Osteoporosis leads to 1.5 million fractures annually, which account for $18 billion per year in direct medical costs. [23]

a. Changes in the balance between bone formation and bone breakdown cause bone mass to increase in children and adolescents and decrease in adults as they grow older. ▼

Both men and women lose bone mass slowly after about age 35.

In growing children, total bone mass increases as the bones grow larger.

Men achieve a higher peak bone mass than do women.

In women, bone loss is accelerated for a span of 5 to 10 years surrounding menopause.

During puberty, bone mass increases rapidly, and sex differences in bone mass appear.

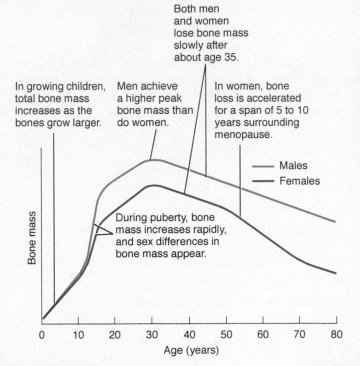

—— Males
—— Females

Bone mass

Age (years)

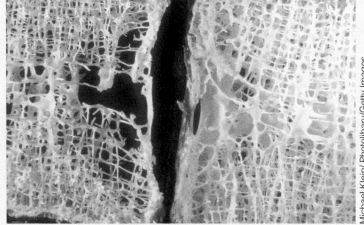

Bone weakened by osteoporosis   Normal bone

Michael Klein/ Photolibary/Getty Images

▲ **b.** The decrease in bone mass and strength that occurs with osteoporosis is illustrated here by comparing osteoporotic bone with normal bone.

Interpret the Data

Based on the information in this graph, why would women over 50 be at greater risk of osteoporosis than men over 50?

Normal spine   Osteoporotic spine

When weakened by osteoporosis, the front edge of the vertebrae collapses more than the back edge, so the spine bends forward.

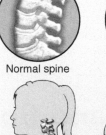
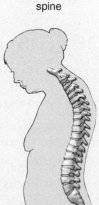
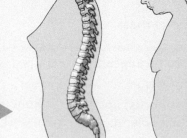
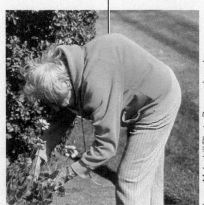

Larry Mulvehill/Photo Researchers, Inc.

c. Spinal compression fractures, shown here, are common and may result in loss of height and a stooped posture (called a "dowager's hump"). ▶

collagen. The mineral portion of bone is composed mainly of calcium associated with phosphorus, but it also contains magnesium, sodium, fluoride, and a number of other minerals. Healthy bone requires adequate dietary protein and vitamin C to maintain the collagen and a sufficient supply of calcium and other minerals to ensure solidity. Adequate vitamin D (discussed in Chapter 7) is needed to maintain appropriate levels of calcium and phosphorus. There is also growing evidence of the importance of vitamin K for bone health.[21]

Bone in Health and Disease

Like other tissues in the body, bone is alive, and it is constantly being broken down and reformed through a process called **bone remodeling**. Most bone is formed early in life. During childhood, bones grow larger; even after growth stops, bone mass continues to increase into young adulthood (**Figure 8.17a**). The maximum amount of bone that you have in your lifetime, called **peak bone mass**, is achieved somewhere between ages 16 and 30. Up to this point, bone formation occurs more rapidly than breakdown, so the total amount of bone increases. After about age 35 to 45, the amount of bone that is broken down begins to exceed the amount that is formed, so total bone mass decreases. Over time, if enough bone is lost, the skeleton is weakened and fractures occur more easily, a condition referred to as **osteoporosis** (**Figure 8.17b** and **c**).

Factors affecting the risk of osteoporosis The risk of developing osteoporosis depends on the level of peak bone mass and the rate at which bone is lost. These variables are affected by genetics, gender, age, hormone levels, and lifestyle factors such as smoking, alcohol consumption, exercise, and diet (**Table 8.2**).

Women have a higher risk of osteoporosis because they have less bone than men and lose it faster as they age. **Age-related bone loss** occurs in both men and women, but women lose additional bone for a period of about 5 to 10 years surrounding **menopause**. This **postmenopausal bone loss** is related to the decline in estrogen level, which increases calcium release from bone and decreases the amount of calcium absorbed in the intestines. A low calcium intake is the most

bone remodeling
The process whereby bone is continuously broken down and reformed to allow for growth and maintenance.

peak bone mass
The maximum bone density attained at any time in life, usually occurring in young adulthood.

osteoporosis
A bone disorder characterized by reduced bone mass, increased bone fragility, and increased risk of fractures.

age-related bone loss Bone loss that occurs in both men and women as they advance in age.

menopause The time in a woman's life when the menstrual cycle ends.

postmenopausal bone loss Accelerated bone loss that occurs in women for about 5 to 10 years surrounding menopause.

Factors affecting the risk of osteoporosis   Table 8.2

Risk factor	How it affects risk
Gender	Fractures due to osteoporosis are about twice as common in women as in men. Men are larger and heavier than women and therefore have a greater peak bone mass. Women lose more bone than men due to postmenopausal bone loss.
Age	Bone loss is a normal part of aging, so the risk of osteoporosis increases with age.
Race	African Americans have denser bones than do Caucasians and Southeast Asians, so their risk of osteoporosis is lower.[22]
Family history	Having a family member with osteoporosis increases risk.
Body size	Individuals who are thin and light have an increased risk because they have a lower peak bone mass.
Smoking	Tobacco use increases risk by reducing bone mass.
Exercise	Weight bearing exercise, such as walking and jogging, throughout life strengthens bone, and increasing weight-bearing exercise at any age can increase your bone density and decrease risk.
Alcohol abuse	Long-term alcohol abuse increases risk by reducing bone formation and interfering with the body's ability to absorb calcium.
Diet	A diet that is lacking in calcium and vitamin D increases the risk of osteoporosis. Low calcium intake during the years of bone formation results in a lower peak bone mass, and low calcium intake in adulthood can accelerate bone loss.

WHAT A SCIENTIST SEES
Soda versus Milk

Carbonated beverages have become a part of U.S. culture. A survey of American adults found that 48% consume soda daily; an average of 2.6 glasses per day.[27] When you grab a can of soda from a vending machine, convenience store, fast-food restaurant, or grocery store, you see a cold, delicious beverage. What a scientist sees is the beverage's nutritional impact. A 12-ounce can of soda contains about 10 teaspoons of sugar and few other nutrients. Replacing a glass of milk with a soda increases the amount of added sugar in the diet by about 40 g and reduces protein, calcium, vitamin A, vitamin D, and riboflavin intake.

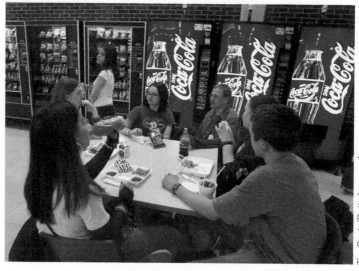

Tim Boyle/Getty Images, Inc.

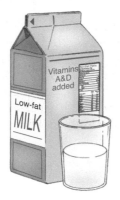
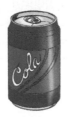

	Low–fat milk	Cola soft drink
Serving size (oz)	12	12
Energy (Cal)	153	150
Protein (g)	12	0
Calcium (mg)	450	0
Phosphorus (mg)	588	45
Riboflavin (mg)	0.6	0
Vitamin A (μg)	216	0
Vitamin D (μg)	3.8	0
Caffeine (mg)	0	40

In recent decades, consumption of sugar-sweetened beverages among children and adolescents has been increasing. Boys aged 12–19 years consume an average of 22 ounces (oz) of sweetened soda per day—more than twice their daily intake of milk (about 10 oz); girls consume an average of about 14 oz of sweetened soda and only about 6 oz of milk per day.[28] Twenty years ago, boys drank more than twice as much milk as soda, and girls drank 50% more milk than soda.[29] Milk is the major source of calcium in the U.S. diet. The reduction in calcium intake that occurs when milk is replaced by soda is of great concern. Teenage girls consume only 60% of the recommended amount of calcium, with soda drinkers consuming almost one-fifth less calcium than those who don't drink soda.[26] Osteoporosis is a major problem among older adults today, and when these adults were children, they drank twice as much milk as kids do today.

Think Critically How do you think the current trend away from milk consumption will affect the incidence of osteoporosis 30 years from now?

significant dietary factor contributing to osteoporosis (see *What a Scientist Sees*).

Some dietary factors can have a negative impact on calcium status and may affect the risk of osteoporosis. High intakes of phytates, oxalates, and tannins can reduce calcium absorption. High intakes of dietary sodium and protein have been found to increase calcium loss in the urine. However, when intakes of calcium and vitamin D are adequate, neither high protein nor high sodium intakes are believed to adversely affect bone health and the risk of osteoporosis. [24-26]

A factor that is associated with a reduced risk of osteoporosis is excess body weight.[30] Having greater body weight, whether that weight is due to an increase in muscle mass or to excess body fat, increases bone mass because it increases the amount of weight the bones must support. In other words, stressing the bones makes them grow stronger. A similar effect is seen in people of all body weights who engage in weight-bearing exercise. In postmenopausal women, excess body fat may also reduce risk because adipose tissue is an important source of estrogen, which helps maintain bone mass and enhances calcium absorption.

Preventing and treating osteoporosis You can't feel your bones weakening, so people with osteoporosis may not know that their bone mass is dangerously low until they are in their 50s or 60s and experience a bone fracture. Once osteoporosis has developed, it is difficult to restore lost bone. Therefore, the best treatment for osteoporosis is to prevent it by achieving a high peak bone mass and slowing the rate of bone loss. During childhood, adolescence, and young adulthood, diet and exercise can help prevent osteoporosis by ensuring maximum peak bone density. A diet that contains adequate amounts of calcium and vitamin D produces greater peak bone mass during the early years and slows bone loss as adults age. Adequate intakes of zinc, magnesium, potassium, fiber, vitamin K, and vitamin C—nutrients that are plentiful in fruits and vegetables—are also important for bone health. Weight-bearing exercise before about age 35 helps to increases peak bone mass, and maintaining an active lifestyle that includes weight-bearing exercise throughout life helps maintain bone density. Limiting smoking and alcohol consumption can also help to increase and maintain bone density.

Osteoporosis is commonly treated with drugs that prevent bone resorption. One class of drugs, called bisphosphonates, inhibits the activity of cells that break down bone. Bisphosphonates have been shown to prevent postmenopausal bone loss, increase bone mineral density, and reduce the risk of fractures.[31] Another class of drugs called selective estrogen receptor modulators (SERMS) provides the benefits of estrogen (reduced bone breakdown and increased calcium absorption), without the negative side effects, such as increasing the risk of heart disease and some types of cancer.

Calcium

In an average person, about 1.5% of body weight is due to calcium, and 99% of this is found in the bones and teeth. The remaining calcium is located in body cells and fluids, where it is needed for release of neurotransmitters, muscle contraction, blood pressure regulation, cell communication, blood clotting, and other essential functions. Neurotransmitter release is critical to nerve function because neurotransmitters relay nerve impulses from one nerve to another and from nerves to other cells. Calcium in muscle cells is essential for muscle contraction because it allows the muscle proteins actin and myosin to interact. Calcium may help regulate blood pressure by controlling the contraction of muscles in the blood vessel walls and signaling the secretion of substances that regulate blood pressure.

Calcium in health and disease The various roles of calcium are so vital to survival that powerful regulatory mechanisms maintain calcium concentrations both inside and outside cells. Slight changes in blood calcium levels trigger the release of hormones that work to keep calcium levels constant. When calcium levels drop, parathyroid hormone (PTH) is released (see Chapter 7). PTH acts in a number of tissues to increase blood calcium levels (**Figure 8.18**). If blood calcium levels become too high, PTH secretion stops, and **calcitonin** is released.

Restoring blood calcium levels • Figure 8.18

Low blood calcium triggers the secretion of PTH from the parathyroid gland. PTH stimulates the release of calcium from bone and causes the kidneys to reduce calcium loss in the urine and to activate vitamin D. Activated vitamin D increases the absorption of calcium from the gastrointestinal tract and acts with PTH to stimulate calcium release from the bone. The overall effect of PTH is to rapidly restore blood calcium levels to normal.

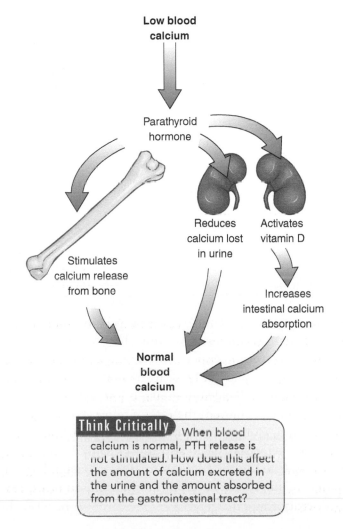

Think Critically When blood calcium is normal, PTH release is not stimulated. How does this affect the amount of calcium excreted in the urine and the amount absorbed from the gastrointestinal tract?

Food sources of calcium • Figure 8.19

Dairy products are an important source of calcium. Fish, such as sardines, that are consumed with the bones are also a good source, as are legumes, almonds, and some dark-green vegetables, such as kale and broccoli. Grains are a moderate source, but because we consume them in large quantities, they make a significant contribution to our calcium intake.

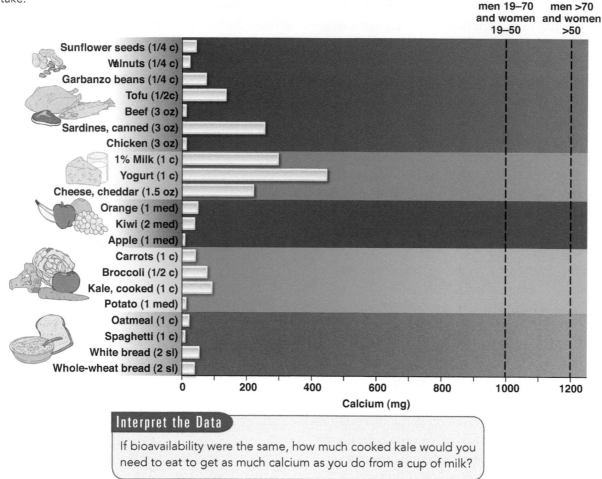

Interpret the Data

If bioavailability were the same, how much cooked kale would you need to eat to get as much calcium as you do from a cup of milk?

Calcitonin is a hormone that acts primarily on bone to inhibit the release of calcium into the blood.

When too little calcium is consumed, the body maintains normal blood levels by breaking down bone to release calcium, a process called **bone resorption**. This process provides a steady supply of calcium and causes no short-term symptoms. Over time, however, inadequate calcium intake can reduce bone mass. Low calcium intake during the years of bone formation results in lower peak bone mass. If calcium intake is low after peak bone mass has been achieved, the rate of bone loss may be increased and, along with it, the risk of osteoporosis.

Too much calcium can also affect health. Because the level of calcium in the blood is finely regulated, elevated blood calcium is rare and is most often caused by cancer and by disorders that increase the secretion of PTH. It can also result from increases in intestinal calcium absorption due to excessive vitamin D intake or high intakes of calcium. Consuming too much calcium from foods is unlikely, but high intakes of calcium from supplements can interfere with the availability of iron, zinc, magnesium, and phosphorus; cause constipation; and contribute to elevated blood and urinary calcium levels. Elevated blood calcium levels can cause symptoms such as loss of appetite, abnormal heartbeat, weight loss, fatigue, frequent urination, and soft tissue calcification. High urinary calcium can damage the kidneys and increase the risk of kidney stones.[32]

The UL for calcium in young adults ages 19 to 50 is 2500 mg/day. In older adults the UL is lower, only 2000 mg/day, based on the occurrence of kidney stones in older age groups.[32] Some postmenopausal women taking supplements may be getting too much calcium and increasing their risk of kidney stones.

Meeting calcium needs For adults ages 19 to 50, 1000 mg/day of calcium is recommended to maintain bone health. Since bone loss is accelerated in women due to menopause, the RDA for women 51 to 70 is set at 1200 mg/day to slow bone loss. For men in this age group it remains at 1000 mg/day. Bone loss and resulting osteoporotic fractures is a concern for both men and women 70 and older, so the RDA for both genders in this age group is 1200 mg/day.[32]

The main source of calcium in the North American diet is dairy products (**Figure 8.19**). Those who do not consume dairy products can meet their calcium needs by consuming dark-green vegetables, fish consumed with bones, foods processed with calcium, and foods fortified with calcium, such as milk substitutes, juices, and breakfast cereals.

In the United States, calcium intake below the RDA is common in women and all adults over 70.[33] Although calcium-rich foods and beverages are the preferred source of calcium, individuals who do not meet their calcium needs through their diet alone can benefit from calcium supplements (**Figure 8.20**). In young individuals,

supplemental calcium can increase peak bone mass. In postmenopausal women, calcium supplements are not effective at increasing bone mass, but in individuals with low dietary calcium intake supplements can help reduce the rate of bone loss. [34]

Whether your calcium comes from foods or from supplements, bioavailability must be considered. Vitamin D is the nutrient that has the most significant impact on calcium absorption. When calcium intake is high, calcium is absorbed by diffusion, but when intake is low to moderate, as it typically is, absorption depends on the active form of vitamin D. When vitamin D is deficient, less than 10% of dietary calcium may be absorbed, compared to the typical 25% when it is present. Other dietary components that affect calcium absorption include acidic foods, lactose, and fat, which increase calcium absorption, and oxalates, phytates, tannins, and fiber, which inhibit calcium absorption. For example, spinach is a high-calcium vegetable, but only about 5% of its calcium is absorbed; the rest is bound by oxalates and excreted in the feces.[35] Vegetables such as broccoli, kale, collard greens, turnip greens, mustard greens, and Chinese cabbage are low in oxalates, so their calcium is more readily absorbed. Chocolate also contains oxalates, but chocolate milk is still a

Calcium supplements • Figure 8.20

If you are not getting enough calcium from foods, a supplement that contains a calcium compound alone or calcium with vitamin D can help you meet your calcium needs. A multivitamin/multimineral supplement will provide only a small amount of the calcium you need. Use the Supplement Facts label to choose an appropriate supplement.

Choose supplements that contain calcium carbonate or calcium citrate. Avoid products that contain aluminum and magnesium. These may actually increase calcium loss.

Choosing a supplement with vitamin D ensures that the vitamin will be available for calcium absorption.

Some antacids are sources of calcium. These are over-the-counter medications, so they carry a Drug Facts panel rather than a Supplement Facts panel.

George Semple

Calcium Is absorbed best when taken in doses of 500 mg or less.

500 mg taken twice a day provides 100% of the RDA for men ages 19 to 70 and women ages 19 to 50.

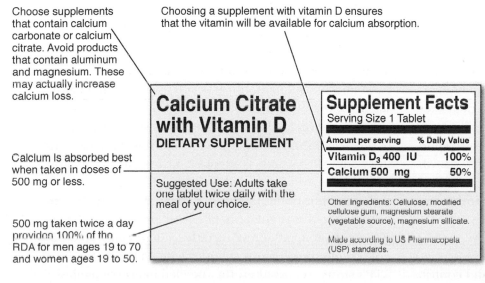

Calcium Citrate with Vitamin D
DIETARY SUPPLEMENT

Suggested Use: Adults take one tablet twice daily with the meal of your choice.

Supplement Facts
Serving Size 1 Tablet

Amount per serving	% Daily Value
Vitamin D₃ 400 IU	100%
Calcium 500 mg	50%

Other Ingredients: Cellulose, modified cellulose gum, magnesium stearate (vegetable source), magnesium sillicate.

Made according to US Pharmacopeia (USP) standards.

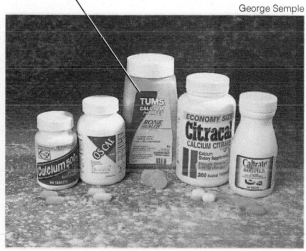

Nonskeletal functions of phosphorus • Figure 8.21

Most of the phosphorus in the body helps form the structure of bones and teeth, but phosphorus also plays an important role in a host of cellular activities.

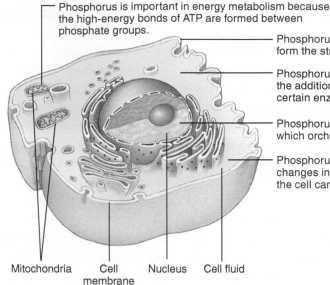

Phosphorus is important in energy metabolism because the high-energy bonds of ATP are formed between phosphate groups.

Phosphorus is a component of phospholipids, which form the structure of cell membranes.

Phosphorus is involved in regulating enzyme activity; the addition of a phosphorus-containing group to certain enzymes can activate or inactivate them.

Phosphorus is a major constituent of DNA and RNA, which orchestrate the synthesis of proteins.

Phosphorus is part of a compound that can prevent changes in acidity so that chemical reactions inside the cell can proceed normally.

Mitochondria   Cell membrane   Nucleus   Cell fluid

good source of calcium because the amount of oxalates from the chocolate added to a glass of milk is small.

Phosphorus

The phosphorus in our bodies is present as part of a chemical group called a phosphate group (see Chapter 5). Most is associated with calcium as part of the hard mineral crystals in bones and teeth. The smaller amount of phosphorus in soft tissues performs an essential role as a structural component of phospholipids, DNA and RNA, and ATP. It is also important in regulating the activity of enzymes and maintaining the proper level of acidity in cells (**Figure 8.21**).

Phosphorus in health and disease Blood levels of phosphorus are not controlled as strictly as calcium levels, but the kidneys help maintain phosphorus levels in a ratio with calcium that allows minerals to be deposited into bone. A deficiency of phosphorus can lead to bone loss, weakness, and loss of appetite. Inadequate phosphorus intake is rare because phosphorus is widely distributed in food. Marginal phosphorus status may be caused by losses due to chronic diarrhea or poor absorption due to overuse of aluminum-containing antacids.

There has been concern that high intake of phosphoric acid (phosphate) used as a flavor enhancer in some soft drinks may interfere with calcium absorption and contribute to bone loss. Cola-type, but not noncola, soft drinks have been associated with lower bone mineral density, but there

is no good evidence that this result is due to phosphate consumption.[36] High dietary phosphorus does not appear to be harmful for healthy adults. The UL for phosphorus is 4000 mg/day for adults, based on an amount associated with the upper limits of normal blood phosphorus levels.[37]

Meeting phosphorus needs The RDA for phosphorus is 700 mg/day for adults; most diets provide this amount.[37] Dairy products such as milk, yogurt, and cheese, as well as meat, cereals, bran, eggs, nuts, and fish, are good sources of phosphorus. Food additives used in baked goods, cheese, processed meats, and soft drinks also provide phosphorus.

Magnesium

Magnesium is far less abundant in the body than are calcium and phosphorus, but it is still essential for healthy bones. About 50 to 60% of the magnesium in the body is in bone, where it helps maintain bone structure. The rest of the magnesium is found in cells and fluids throughout the body. Magnesium is involved in regulating calcium homeostasis and is needed for the action of vitamin D and many hormones, including PTH. Magnesium is important for the regulation of blood pressure and may play a role in maintaining cardiovascular health. In addition, magnesium forms a complex with ATP that stabilizes ATP's structure. It is therefore needed in every metabolic reaction that generates or uses ATP. This includes reactions needed for the release of energy from carbohydrate, fat, and protein; the functioning of the nerves and muscles; and the synthesis of DNA, RNA, and protein, making it particularly important for dividing, growing cells.

Magnesium in health and disease Severe magnesium deficiency can cause nausea, muscle weakness and cramping, irritability, mental derangement, and changes in blood pressure and heartbeat. Although overt magnesium deficiency is rare, the typical intake of magnesium in the United States is below the RDA.[38] Low intakes of magnesium have been associated with a number of chronic diseases, including type 2 diabetes, hypertension, atherosclerosis, and osteoporosis.[38] As discussed earlier, dietary patterns that are high in magnesium are associated with lower blood pressure, and the risk of other types of cardiovascular disease is lower for people with adequate magnesium intake than for those with less magnesium in their diet.[39] Over the last 30 years nutritional messages have focused on increasing calcium intake. This has caused an increase in the ratio of calcium to magnesium in the diet.

There is concern that either our low magnesium intake or the rising ratio of calcium to magnesium may play a role in the development of metabolic syndrome, type 2 diabetes, osteoporosis, and inflammatory disorders.[38]

No toxic effects have been observed from magnesium consumed in foods, but toxicity may occur from drugs containing magnesium, such as milk of magnesia, and supplements that include magnesium. Magnesium toxicity causes nausea, vomiting, low blood pressure, and other cardiovascular changes. The UL for adults and adolescents over age 9 is 350 mg of magnesium from nonfood sources such as supplements and medications.[37]

Meeting magnesium needs Magnesium is found in many foods but in small amounts, so you can't get all you need from a single food (**Figure 8.22**). Enriched grain products are poor sources because magnesium is lost in processing, and it is not added back by enrichment. For example, removing the bran and germ from wheat kernels reduces the magnesium content of 1 cup of white

Sources of magnesium • Figure 8.22

Magnesium is a component of the green pigment chlorophyll, so leafy greens such as spinach and kale are good sources of this mineral. Nuts, seeds, legumes, bananas, and the germ and bran of whole grains are also good sources of magnesium. The dashed lines represent the RDAs of 420 and 320 mg/day for adult men and women over age 30, respectively.[37]

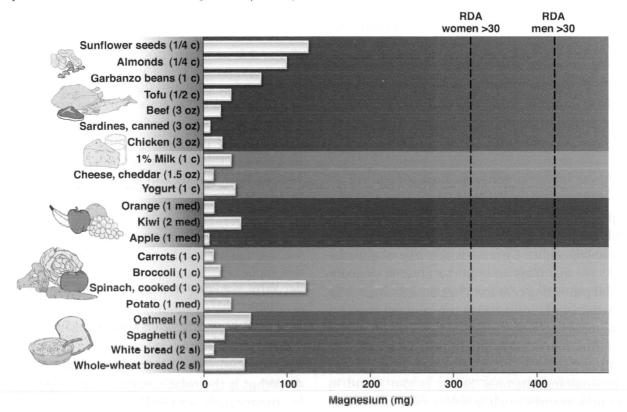

heme iron A readily absorbable form of iron found in meat, fish, and poultry that is chemically associated with certain proteins.

are also involved in drug metabolism and immune function.

Iron absorption and transport The amount of iron absorbed from the intestine depends on the form of the iron and on the dietary components consumed along with it. Much of the iron in meats is heme iron—iron that is part of a chemical complex found in proteins such as hemoglobin and myoglobin. Heme iron is absorbed more than twice as efficiently as the nonheme iron found in plant sources such as leafy green vegetables, legumes, and grains. The amount of nonheme iron absorbed can be enhanced or reduced by the foods and nutrients consumed in the same meal.

Once iron is absorbed, the amount that is delivered to the cells of the body depends to some extent on the body's needs. When the body's iron status is high, less iron is delivered to body cells and more is trapped in the mucosal cells of the small intestine and lost when the cells die and are sloughed into the intestinal lumen. When iron status is low, more iron is transported out of the mucosal cells and delivered to body cells (**Figure 8.23**).[40] This regulation is important because once iron has entered the blood and other tissues, it is not easily eliminated. Even when red blood cells die, the iron in their hemoglobin is not lost from the body; instead, it is recycled and can be incorporated into new red blood cells. Even in healthy individuals, most iron loss occurs through blood loss, including blood lost during menstruation and the small amounts lost from the gastrointestinal tract. Some iron is also lost through the shedding of cells from the intestines, skin, and urinary tract.

Meeting iron needs Iron in the diet comes from both plant and animal sources (**Figure 8.24**). Animal products provide both heme and nonheme iron, but only the less readily absorbed nonheme iron is found in

Iron absorption, uses, and loss • Figure 8.23

The amount of dietary iron that reaches body cells depends on both the amount absorbed into the mucosal cells of the small intestine and the amount transported from the mucosal cells to the rest of the body. The iron that is transported may be used to synthesize iron-containing proteins, such as hemoglobin needed for red blood cell formation, or increase iron stores in the liver or spleen.

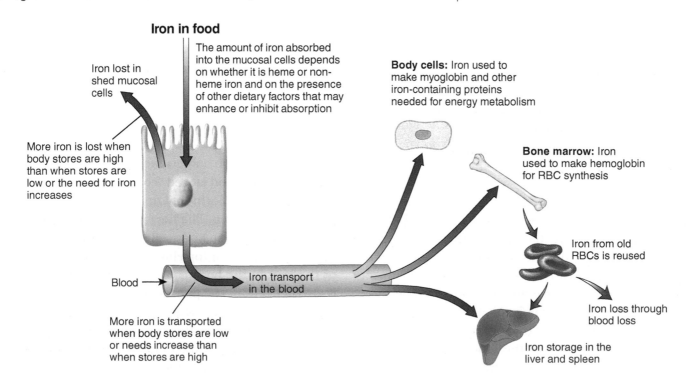

Iron in food

Iron lost in shed mucosal cells

The amount of iron absorbed into the mucosal cells depends on whether it is heme or non-heme iron and on the presence of other dietary factors that may enhance or inhibit absorption

More iron is lost when body stores are high than when stores are low or the need for iron increases

Body cells: Iron used to make myoglobin and other iron-containing proteins needed for energy metabolism

Bone marrow: Iron used to make hemoglobin for RBC synthesis

Iron from old RBCs is reused

Blood

Iron transport in the blood

More iron is transported when body stores are low or needs increase than when stores are high

Iron loss through blood loss

Iron storage in the liver and spleen

Sources of iron • Figure 8.24

The best sources of highly absorbable heme iron are red meats and organ meats such as liver and kidney. Legumes, leafy greens, and whole grains are good sources of nonheme iron; enriched grains are also good sources of nonheme iron because it is added during enrichment. The RDA for adult men and postmenopausal women is 8 mg/day of iron. Due to menstrual losses, the RDA for women of childbearing age is set much higher, 15 mg/day for young women 14 to 18 years and 18 mg/day for women 19 to 50.

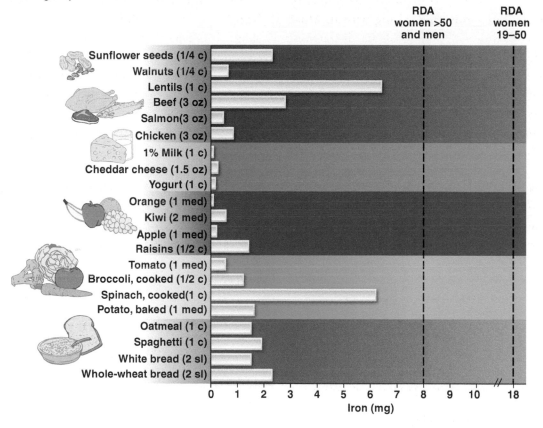

plants. Nonheme iron absorption can be enhanced as much as sixfold if it is consumed along with foods that are rich in vitamin C. Consuming beef, fish, or poultry in the same meal as nonheme iron also increases absorption. For example, a small amount of hamburger in a pot of chili will enhance the body's absorption of iron from the beans. If the pot is made of iron, it increases iron intake because the iron leaches into food. Iron absorption is decreased by fiber, phytates, tannins, and oxalates, which bind iron in the gastrointestinal tract. The presence of other minerals with the same charge, such as calcium, may also decrease iron absorption.

The RDA for iron assumes that the diet contains both plant and animal sources of iron.[41] A separate RDA category has been created for vegetarians. These recommendations are higher, to take into account lower iron

absorption from plant sources. People who have difficulty consuming enough iron can increase their iron intake by choosing foods fortified with iron.

Iron in health and disease When there is too little iron in the body, hemoglobin cannot be produced. When sufficient hemoglobin is not available, the red blood cells that are formed are small and pale, and they are unable to deliver adequate oxygen to the tissues. This condition is known as **iron deficiency anemia**. Symptoms of iron deficiency anemia include fatigue, weakness, headache, decreased work capacity,

> **iron deficiency anemia** An iron deficiency disease that occurs when the oxygen-carrying capacity of the blood is decreased because there is insufficient iron to make hemoglobin.

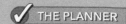

Iron deficiency anemia is the final stage of iron deficiency. It results when there is too little iron to synthesize adequate amounts of hemoglobin. Children and young women are at the greatest risk.

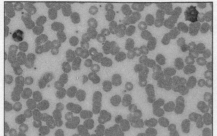

Normal red blood cells

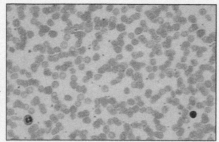

Iron deficiency anemia

B &B Photos/Custom Medical StockPhoto, Inc.

Custom Medical Stock Photo, Inc.

◀ Iron deficiency anemia results in red blood cells that do not contain enough hemoglobin. They are small and pale and unable to transport as much oxygen as red blood cells containing normal amounts of hemoglobin.

Inadequate iron intake first causes a decrease in the amount of stored iron, followed by low iron levels in the blood plasma. It is only after plasma levels drop that there is no longer enough iron to maintain hemoglobin in red blood cells and the symptoms of iron deficiency anemia appear.

▶

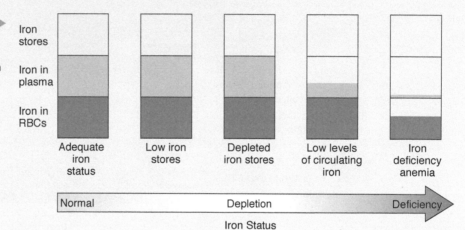

Iron stores

Iron in plasma

Iron in RBCs

Adequate iron status | Low iron stores | Depleted iron stores | Low levels of circulating iron | Iron deficiency anemia

Normal → Depletion → Deficiency

Iron Status

Women of childbearing age lose iron due to menstruation. Pregnant women, infants, children, and teens have increased iron needs due to growth and development.

Demographic

Women of childbearing age, pregnant women, infants, children, adolescents

Dietary

Low total iron, vegetarian diets, dieting

Social/medical

Poverty, intestinal parasites

Diets that are low in meat, which contains the most readily absorbed form of iron (heme iron), and high in phytates and fiber, which reduce iron absorption, increase the risk of deficiency. Low-calorie diets can also reduce iron intake.

Individuals living in poverty are less likely than others to consume adequate iron. Intestinal parasites cause blood loss, which increases iron losses.

◀ The risk of iron deficiency is highest among individuals with greater iron losses, those with greater needs due to growth and development, and those who are unable to obtain adequate dietary iron. In the United States, about 9% of adolescent girls and women of childbearing age and 14% of children between the ages of 1 and 3 years are iron deficient.[42] The incidence is greatest among low-income and minority women and children.

A Case Study on Iron Deficiency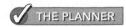

Hanna is a 23-year-old graduate student from South Carolina. She has been working long hours and is always tired. She tries to eat a healthy diet; she has been a lacto-ovo vegetarian for the past six months.

 1 What factors increase Hanna's risk for iron deficiency anemia?

Your answer:

Hanna goes to the health center to see if there is a medical reason for her exhaustion. A nurse draws her blood to check her for anemia. The results of Hanna's blood work are summarized in the figure below.

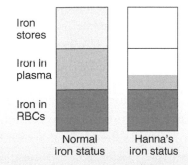

Iron stores
Iron in plasma
Iron in RBCs
Normal iron status
Hanna's iron status

 2 Does Hanna have iron deficiency anemia? Why or why not?

Your answer:

Hanna meets with a dietitian. A diet analysis shows that because she consumes no meat, much of her protein comes from dairy products. She consumes about four servings of dairy, eight servings of whole grains, three fresh fruits, and about a cup of cooked vegetables daily. She drinks four glasses of iced tea daily. Her average iron intake is about 12 mg/day.

 3 Name three dietary factors that put Hanna at risk for iron deficiency.

Your answer:

 4 Suggest two changes Hanna could make to increase her iron intake while sticking with her lacto-ovo vegetarian diet

Your answer:

 5 What could Hanna add to her diet to increase the absorption of the nonheme iron she consumes?

Your answer:

(Check your answers in online Appendix L)

inability to maintain body temperature in a cold environment, changes in behavior, decreased resistance to infection, impaired development in infants, and increased risk of lead poisoning in young children. Anemia is the last stage of iron deficiency (**Figure 8.25**). Earlier stages have no symptoms because they do not affect the amount of hemoglobin in red blood cells, but levels of iron in the blood plasma and in body stores are low (see *Thinking It Through*). Iron deficiency anemia is the most common nutritional deficiency; cy anemia is the most common nutritional deficiency;

more than 2 billion people, or over 30% of the world's population, suffer from anemia, many due to iron deficiency.[43]

Iron also causes health problems if too much is consumed. Acute iron toxicity caused by excessive consumption of iron-containing supplements is one of the most common forms of poisoning among children under age 6. Iron poisoning may cause damage to the lining of the intestine, abnormalities in body acidity, shock, and liver failure. Even a single large dose can be fatal

Iron toxicity • Figure 8.26

To protect children, the labels on iron-containing drugs and supplements are required to display this warning.[44] Iron-containing products should be stored out of the reach of children or other individuals who might consume them in excess.

WARNING: CLOSE TIGHTLY AND KEEP OUT OF REACH OF CHILDREN. CONTAINS IRON, WHICH CAN BE HARMFUL OR FATAL TO CHILDREN IN LARGE DOSES. IN CASE OF ACCIDENTAL OVERDOSE, SEEK PROFESSIONAL ASSISTANCE OR CONTACT A POISON CONTROL CENTER IMMEDIATELY.

(**Figure 8.26**). A UL has been set at 45 mg/day from all sources.[41]

Accumulation of iron in the body over time, referred to as **iron overload**, is most commonly due to an inherited condition called **hemochromatosis**. Hemochromatosis occurs when genes involved in regulating iron uptake are defective, so excess iron is allowed to enter the circulation.[45] It is the most common genetic disorder in the Caucasian population, affecting more than 1 million people in the United States.[46] It has no symptoms early in life, but in middle age, nonspecific symptoms such as weight loss, fatigue, weakness, and abdominal pain develop. If allowed to progress, the accumulation of excess iron can damage the heart and liver and increase the individual's risks for diabetes and cancer. The treatment for hemochromatosis is simple: regular blood withdrawal. Iron loss through blood withdrawal will prevent the complications of iron overload, but to be effective, the treatment must be initiated before organs have been damaged. Therefore, genetic screening is essential to identify and treat individuals before any damage occurs.

hemochromatosis An inherited disorder that results in increased iron absorption.

Copper

It is logical that consuming too little iron will cause iron deficiency anemia, but consuming too little copper can also cause this problem. Iron status and copper status are interrelated because a copper-containing protein is needed for iron to be transported from the intestinal cells. Even if iron intake is adequate, iron can't get to cells throughout the body if copper is not present. Thus copper deficiency results in a secondary iron deficiency that may lead to anemia. Copper also functions as a component of a number of important proteins and enzymes that are involved in connective tissue synthesis, lipid metabolism, maintenance of heart muscle, and immune and central nervous system function.[41]

We consume copper in seafood, nuts and seeds, whole-grain breads and cereals, and chocolate; the richest dietary sources of copper are organ meats such as liver and kidney. As with many other trace minerals, soil content affects the amount of copper in plant foods. The RDA for copper for adults is 900 micrograms (µg)/day.[41]

When there is too little copper in the body, the protein collagen does not form normally, resulting in skeletal changes similar to those seen in vitamin C deficiency. Copper deficiency also causes elevated blood cholesterol, reflecting copper's role in cholesterol metabolism. Copper deficiency has been associated with impaired growth, degeneration of the heart muscle and the nervous system, and changes in hair color and structure. Because copper is needed to maintain the immune system, a diet that is low in copper increases the incidence of infections. Also, because copper is an essential component of one form of the antioxidant enzyme superoxide dismutase, a copper deficiency will weaken antioxidant defenses.

Severe copper deficiency is relatively rare, although it may occur in premature infants. It can also occur if zinc intake is high because high dietary zinc interferes with the absorption of copper. Copper toxicity from dietary sources is also rare but has occurred as a result of drinking from contaminated water supplies or consuming acidic foods or beverages that have been stored in copper containers. Toxicity is more likely to occur from supplements containing copper. Excessive copper intake causes abdominal pain, vomiting, and diarrhea. The UL has been set at 10 mg/day of copper.[41]

Zinc

Zinc, the most abundant intracellular trace mineral, helps regulate protein synthesis and is important in many other aspects of cellular metabolism. It is involved in the functioning of approximately 100 different enzymes, including a form of superoxide dismutase that is vital for protecting cells from free-radical damage. Zinc is needed to maintain adequate levels of metal-binding proteins, which also

Zinc and gene expression • Figure 8.27

One of zinc's most important roles is in gene expression. Zinc-containing DNA-binding proteins allow vitamin A, vitamin D, and a number of hormones to interact with DNA. The zinc forms "fingers" in the protein structure. When the vitamins or hormones bind to the protein, the zinc fingers bind to regulatory regions of DNA, increasing or decreasing the expression of specific genes and thus the synthesis of the proteins for which they code. Without zinc, these vitamins and hormones cannot function properly.

Ask Yourself

How could a zinc deficiency lead to a secondary vitamin A deficiency?

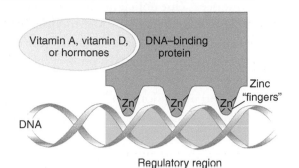

scavenge free radicals. Zinc is needed by enzymes that function in the synthesis of DNA and RNA, in carbohydrate metabolism, in acid–base balance, and in a reaction that is necessary for the absorption of folate from food. Zinc plays a role in the storage and release of insulin, the mobilization of vitamin A from the liver, and the stabilization of cell membranes. It influences hormonal regulation of cell division and is therefore needed for the growth and repair of tissues, the activity of the immune system, and the development of sex organs and bone. Some of the functions of zinc can be traced to its role in gene expression (**Figure 8.27**).[47]

Zinc transport from the mucosal cells of the intestine into the blood is regulated. When zinc intake is high, more zinc is held in the mucosal cells and lost in the feces when these cells die. When zinc intake is low, more dietary zinc passes into the blood for delivery to tissues.

Meeting zinc needs We consume zinc in red meat, liver, eggs, dairy products, vegetables, and seafood. Zinc from animal sources is better absorbed than that from plant sources because zinc in plant foods is often bound by phytates (**Figure 8.28**).

Zinc in health and disease Severe zinc deficiency is relatively uncommon in North America, but in developing

Food sources of zinc • Figure 8.28

Meat, seafood, dairy products, legumes, and seeds are good sources of zinc. Refined grains are not good sources because zinc is lost in milling and not added back. Yeast-leavened grain products are better sources of zinc than are unleavened products because yeast leavening reduces phytate content. The dashed lines represent the RDAs for adult men and women, which are 11 and 8 mg/day, respectively.

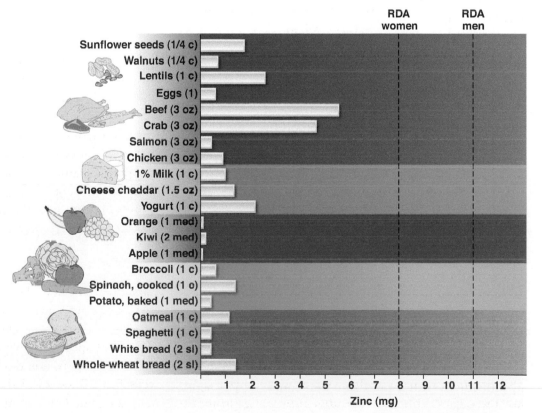

countries, it has important health and developmental consequences. Zinc deficiency interferes with growth and development, impairs immune function, and causes skin rashes and diarrhea. Mild zinc deficiency is a concern in the United States, particularly among the elderly who are at risk due to low dietary intake as well as decreases in absorption and utilization.[48] It is estimated that 40% of men and 45% of women over 50 consume less than the EAR for zinc.[41] Mild zinc deficiency results in diminished immune function and an increase in inflammation.[48] It has been hypothesized to play a role in the development of age-related diseases such as cardiovascular disease, type 2 diabetes, cancer, and autoimmune diseases.[49]

The risk of zinc deficiency is greater in areas where the diet is high in phytate, fiber, tannins, and oxalates, which limit zinc absorption. In the 1960s, a syndrome of growth depression and delayed sexual development was observed in Iranian and Egyptian men consuming a diet based on plant protein. The diet was not low in zinc, but it was high in grains containing phytates, which interfered with zinc absorption, thus causing the deficiency.

It is difficult to consume a toxic amount of zinc from food. However, high doses from supplements can cause toxicity symptoms. A single dose of 1 to 2 g can cause gastrointestinal irritation, vomiting, loss of appetite, diarrhea, abdominal cramps, and headaches. High intakes have been shown to decrease immune function, reduce concentrations of HDL cholesterol in the blood, and interfere with the absorption of copper. High doses of zinc can also interfere with iron absorption because iron and zinc are transported through the blood by the same protein. The converse is also true: Too much iron can limit the transport of zinc. Zinc and iron are often found together in foods, but food sources do not contain large enough amounts of either to cause imbalances.

Zinc supplements are marketed to improve immune function, enhance fertility and sexual performance, and cure the common cold. For individuals consuming adequate zinc, there is no evidence that extra zinc enhances immune function, fertility, or sexual performance. However, in individuals with a mild zinc deficiency,

supplementation can have beneficial immune, antioxidant, and anti-inflammatory effects that can help in the treatment of a variety of diseases, including diarrhea, pneumonia, and tuberculosis. In older adults, improving zinc status with supplements can decrease the incidence of infections and a type of age-associated blindness; in children, it can reduce the incidence of respiratory infections and improve growth.[50,51] Zinc supplements are most often taken to treat colds. When administered within 24 hours of the onset of cold symptoms, zinc supplements have been found to reduce the duration and severity of the common cold in healthy people; the mechanism by which they work is unclear.[52] A UL has been set at 40 mg/day from all sources.[41]

Selenium

The amount of selenium in food varies greatly, depending on the concentration of selenium in the soil where the food is produced (**Figure 8.29**). In regions of China with low soil selenium levels, a form of heart disease called

Soil selenium and health • Figure 8.29

As this map of China shows, the amount of selenium in the soil varies widely from one region to another. When the diet consists primarily of locally grown food, these differences affect selenium intake and, therefore, health. When the diet includes foods from many different locations, the low selenium content of foods grown in one geographic region is offset by the high selenium content of foods from other regions.

Hair and nail brittleness and loss occur in people living in regions of China with high levels of selenium in the soil. Other toxicity symptoms include nausea, diarrhea, abdominal pain, nervous system abnormalities, fatigue, and irritability.

Selenium deficiency causes muscular discomfort, weakness, and in some cases Keshan disease. However, Keshan disease is not caused entirely by selenium deficiency. It is believed to be due to a combination of selenium deficiency and a viral infection.[53]

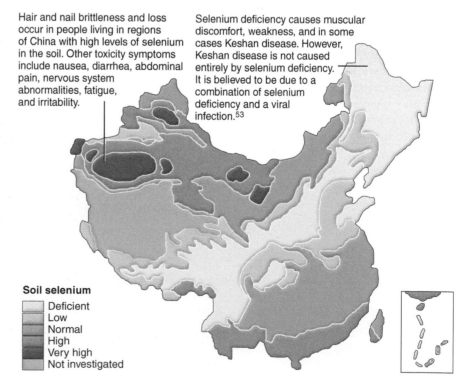

Soil selenium
- Deficient
- Low
- Normal
- High
- Very high
- Not investigated

Keshan disease occurs in children and young women. This disease can be prevented and cured with selenium supplements. In contrast, people living in regions of China with very high selenium in the soil may develop symptoms of selenium toxicity.

Selenium is incorporated into the structure of certain proteins. One of these proteins is the antioxidant enzyme **glutathione peroxidase**. Glutathione peroxidase neutralizes peroxides before they can form free radicals, which cause oxidative damage (**Figure 8.30**). In addition to its antioxidant role in glutathione peroxidase, selenium is part of a protein needed for the synthesis of the **thyroid hormones**, which regulate metabolic rate.

> **glutathione peroxidase** A selenium-containing enzyme that protects cells from oxidative damage by neutralizing peroxides.

Meeting selenium needs Selenium deficiencies and excesses are not a concern in the United States because the foods we consume come from many different locations around the country and around the world. The RDA for selenium for adults is 55 µg/day.[54] The average intake in the United States meets, or nearly meets, this recommendation for all age groups. Seafood, kidney, liver, and eggs are excellent sources of selenium. Grains, nuts, and seeds can be good sources, depending on the selenium content of the soil in which they were grown. Fruits, vegetables, and drinking water are generally poor sources. The UL for adults is 400 µg/day from food and supplements.[54]

Selenium and cancer An increased incidence of cancer has been observed in regions where selenium intake is low, suggesting that selenium plays a role in preventing cancer. In 1996, a study investigating the effect of selenium supplements on people with a history of skin cancer found that the supplement had no effect on the recurrence of skin cancer but that the incidence of lung, prostate, and colon cancer decreased in the selenium-supplemented group.[55] This result caused speculation that selenium supplements could reduce the risk of cancer. Continued study, however, has led to the conclusion that the reduction in the incidence of cancer seen in the 1996 study occurred primarily in people who began the study with low levels of selenium. It appears that an adequate level of selenium is necessary to prevent cancer, but the role of supplemental selenium in preventing cancer is still under investigation.[56]

Glutathione peroxidase • Figure 8.30 _____

Glutathione peroxidase is a selenium-containing enzyme that neutralizes peroxides before they can form free radicals. Selenium therefore can reduce the body's need for vitamin E, which neutralizes free radicals.

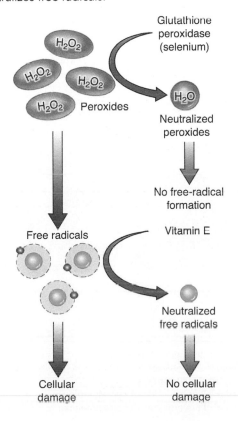

Iodine

About three-fourths of the iodine in the body is found in a small gland in the neck called the **thyroid gland**. Iodine is concentrated in this gland because it is an essential component of the thyroid hormones, which are produced here. Thyroid hormones regulate metabolic rate, growth, and development, and they promote protein synthesis.

Iodine in health and disease Thyroid hormone levels are carefully regulated. If blood levels drop, **thyroid-stimulating hormone** is released. This hormone signals the thyroid gland to take up iodine and synthesize more thyroid hormones. When the supply of iodine is adequate, thyroid hormones can be produced, and the return of thyroid hormones to normal levels turns off the synthesis of thyroid-stimulating hormone. If iodine is deficient, thyroid hormones cannot be synthesized (**Figure 8.31**). Without sufficient thyroid hormones, the metabolic rate slows, causing fatigue and weight gain.

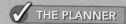
Iodine deficiency is a problem in developing countries around the world; this deficiency causes goiter and impairs cognitive development.

When thyroid hormone levels drop too low, thyroid-stimulating hormone (TSH) stimulates the thyroid gland to take up iodine and synthesize more hormones (blue arrows). If iodine is not available (purple arrows), thyroid hormones cannot be made, and the stimulation continues, causing the thyroid gland to enlarge.

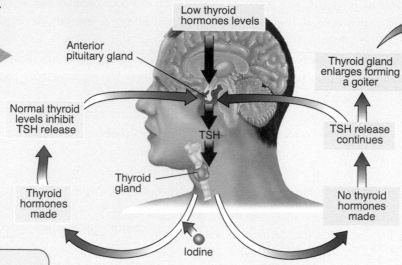

Low thyroid hormones levels

Anterior pituitary gland

Normal thyroid levels inhibit TSH release

TSH

Thyroid gland

Thyroid hormones made

Iodine

Iodine available

Thyroid gland enlarges forming a goiter

TSH release continues

No thyroid hormones made

Iodine deficient

© Mike Goldwater/Alamy Limited

Ask Yourself

Why does the thyroid gland enlarge when iodine is deficient?

Iodine deficiency impairs cognitive and motor development, which impairs school performance. Iodine deficient individuals my forfeit 15 IQ points.[57]

© Stefano Montesi/Demotix/ Corbis

A goiter, which is an enlarged thyroid gland, can be seen as a swelling in the neck. In milder cases of goiter, treatment with iodine causes the thyroid gland to return to its normal size, but it may remain enlarged in more severe cases.

Although iodine deficiency remains a global health issue, its incidence has declined dramatically since universal salt iodization was adopted in 1993. An estimated 70% of households worldwide now have access to iodized salt.[58] Excessive iodine intake can occur if the level of iodine added to salt is too high.

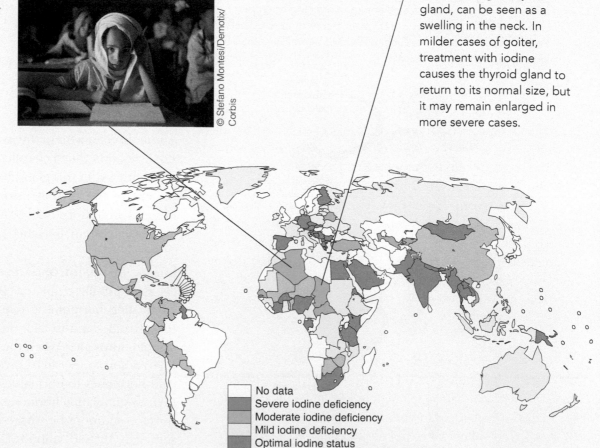

No data
Severe iodine deficiency
Moderate iodine deficiency
Mild iodine deficiency
Optimal iodine status
Risk of iodine-induced hyperthyroidism
Risk of adverse health consequences

The most obvious outward sign of iodine deficiency is an enlarged thyroid gland, called a **goiter** (see Figure 8.31), but because of the importance of the thyroid hormones for growth and development, other iodine deficiency disorders are also prevalent. If iodine is deficient during pregnancy, the risk of stillbirth and spontaneous abortion increases; insufficient iodine during pregnancy can cause a condition called **cretinism** in the child. Cretinism is characterized by symptoms that include impaired mental development, deaf mutism, and growth failure. In children and adolescents, iodine deficiency impairs mental function and reduces intellectual capacity. Though easily prevented, it is the world's most prevalent cause of brain damage.[58]

> **goiter** An enlargement of the thyroid gland caused by a deficiency of iodine.
>
> **cretinism** A condition resulting from poor maternal iodine intake during pregnancy that impairs mental development and growth in the offspring.

Iodine deficiency is most common in regions where the soil is low in iodine and there is little access to fish and seafood. The risk of iodine deficiency is also increased by the consumption of foods that contain **goitrogens**, substances that interfere with iodine utilization or with thyroid function. Goitrogens are found in turnips, rutabaga, cabbage, millet, and cassava. When these foods are boiled, the goitrogen content is reduced because some of these compounds leach into the cooking water. Goitrogens are primarily a problem in African countries where cassava is a dietary staple. Goitrogens are not a problem in the United States because the typical diet does not include large amounts of goitrogen-containing foods.

Chronically high intakes or a sudden increase in iodine intake can also cause an enlargement of the thyroid gland. For example, in a person with a marginal intake, a large dose from supplements could cause thyroid enlargement, even at levels that would not be toxic in a healthy person. The UL for adults is 1100 μg/day of iodine from all sources.[41]

Meeting iodine needs The iodine content of food varies, depending on the soil in which plants are grown or where animals graze. When the Earth was formed, all soils were high in iodine, but today mountainous areas and river valleys have little iodine left in the soil because it has been washed out by glaciers, snow, rain, and floodwaters. The iodine washed from the soil has accumulated in the oceans. Therefore, foods from the sea, such as fish, shellfish, and seaweed, are the best sources of iodine.

Today most of the iodine in the North American diet comes from **iodized salt** (**Figure 8.32**), but we also obtain iodine from contaminants and other additives in foods. Iodine-containing additives used in cattle feed and disinfectants used on milking machines and milk storage tanks increase the iodine content of dairy products. Iodine-containing sterilizing agents are also used in restaurants, and iodine is used in dough conditioners and some food colorings. The RDA for iodine for adults is 150 μg/day. Iodine deficiency is rare in the United States, but iodine intakes have been declining due to recommendations to reduce salt intake and the increasing use of noniodized salt in processed foods.[59] Recent surveys indicate that pregnant women in the United States have less than adequate iodine status during their first and second trimester.[60] Adequate iodine is particularly important during pregnancy because it is essential for normal brain development.

> **iodized salt** Table salt to which a small amount of sodium iodide or potassium iodide has been added in order to supplement the iodine content of the diet.

Iodized salt • Figure 8.32

Iodized salt was first introduced in Switzerland in the 1920s as a way to combat iodine deficiency. Salt was chosen because it is readily available, inexpensive, and consumed in regular amounts throughout the year. It takes only about half a teaspoon of iodized salt to provide the recommended amount of iodine. Iodized salt should not be confused with sea salt, which is a poor source of iodine because its iodine is lost in the drying process.

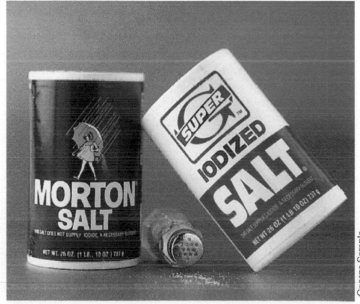

George Sample

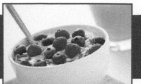
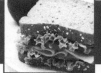
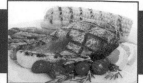

Chromium

Chromium is required to maintain normal blood glucose levels. It is believed to act by enhancing the effects of insulin.[61] Insulin facilitates the entry of glucose into cells and stimulates the synthesis of proteins, lipids, and glycogen. When chromium is deficient, more insulin is required to produce the same effect. A deficiency of chromium therefore affects the body's ability to regulate blood glucose, causing diabetes-like symptoms such as elevated blood glucose levels and increased insulin levels.

Dietary sources of chromium include liver, brewer's yeast, nuts, and whole grains. Milk, vegetables, and fruits are poor sources. Refined carbohydrates such as white breads, pasta, and white rice are also poor sources because chromium is lost in milling and is not added back in the enrichment process. Chromium intake can be increased by cooking in stainless-steel cookware because chromium leaches from the steel into the food. The recommended intake for chromium is 35 μg/day for men ages 19 to 50 and 25 μg/day for women ages 19 to 50.[41]

Overt chromium deficiency is not a problem in the United States; nevertheless, chromium, in the form of chromium picolinate, is a common dietary supplement. Because chromium is needed for insulin action and insulin promotes protein synthesis, chromium picolinate is popular with athletes and dieters who take it to reduce body fat and increase muscle mass. However, studies of chromium picolinate and other chromium supplements in healthy human subjects have not found them to have beneficial effects on muscle strength, body composition, or weight loss.[62] Toxicity is always a concern with nutrient supplements, but in the case of chromium, there is little evidence of dietary toxicity in humans. The DRI committee concluded that there was insufficient data to establish a UL for chromium.

Fluoride

Fluoride helps prevent **dental caries** (cavities) in both children and adults. During tooth formation (up until about age 13), ingested fluoride is incorporated into the crystals that make up tooth enamel. These fluoride-containing crystals are more resistant to acid than are crystals formed when fluoride is not present. Ingested fluoride, whether it is from the diet, the water supply, or supplements, is also secreted in saliva, which continually bathes the teeth. Fluoride in saliva prevents cavities in children and adults by reducing the amount of acid produced by bacteria, inhibiting the dissolution of tooth enamel by acid, and increasing enamel re-mineralization after acid exposure. Therefore ingested fluoride benefits dental health throughout life.[63] Fluoride in toothpaste and mouth rinses has the same topical effect but only remains in the mouth for a few hours after use.

Fluoride is also incorporated into the mineral crystals in bone. There is evidence that fluoride supplements stimulate bone formation and increase bone density, but there is no clear evidence that fluoride therapy reduces fractures and it may have side effects.[63] The amount of fluoride in drinking water does not affect bone health.[64]

Meeting fluoride needs Fluoride is present in small amounts in almost all soil, water, plants, and animals. The richest dietary sources of fluoride are toothpaste, tea, marine fish consumed with their bones, and fluoridated water (see *What Should I Eat?*). Because food readily absorbs the fluoride in cooking water, the fluoride content of food can be significantly increased when it is handled and prepared using water that contains fluoride. Cooking utensils also affect the fluoride content of foods. Foods cooked with Teflon utensils can pick up fluoride from the Teflon, whereas aluminum cookware can decrease the fluoride content of foods. Bottled water usually does not contain fluoride, so people who habitually drink bottled water need to obtain fluoride from other sources.

The recommended intake for fluoride for people 6 months of age and older is 0.05 mg/kg/day. This is equivalent to about 3.8 mg/day for a 76-kg man and 3.1 mg/day for a 61-kg woman. Fluoridated water provides about 0.7 to 1.2 mg fluoride /L of water. The American Academy of Pediatrics suggests a fluoride supplement of 0.25 mg/day for children 6 months to 3 years of age, 0.5 mg/day for children ages 3 to 6 years, and 1.0 mg/day for those ages 6 to 16 years who are receiving less than 0.3 mg/L of fluoride in the water supply. These supplements are available by prescription for children living in areas with low fluoride concentrations in the water supply.

Fluoridation of water To promote dental health, fluoride is added to public water supplies in many communities. Currently, about 75% of people served by public water systems receive fluoridated water.[65] When fluoride intake is low, tooth decay is more frequent (**Figure 8.33**). Water fluoridation is a safe, inexpensive way to prevent dental caries, but some people still believe that the added fluoride increases the risk of cancer and other diseases. These beliefs are not supported by scientific facts; the small amounts of fluoride consumed in drinking water promote dental health and do not pose a risk for health problems such as cancer, kidney failure, or bone disease.[65]

Although the levels of fluoride included in public water supplies are safe, too much fluoride can be toxic. In children, too much fluoride causes **fluorosis** (see Figure 8.33). Recently, there has been an

> **fluorosis** A condition caused by chronic overconsumption of fluoride, characterized by black and brown stains and cracking and pitting of the teeth.

Just the right amount of fluoride • Figure 8.33

This graph illustrates that the incidence of dental caries in children increases when the concentration of fluoride in the water supply is lower. If the fluoride concentration of the water is too high, it increases the risk of fluorosis.

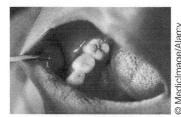

Too little fluoride makes teeth more susceptible to dental caries.

The optimal amount of fluoride makes teeth resistant to decay and does not cause fluorosis.

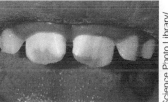

Too much fluoride (intakes of 2 to 8 mg/day or greater in children) causes teeth to appear mottled, a condition called fluorosis.

Caries per child (y-axis, 0–8) vs *Water fluoride (mg/liter)* (x-axis, 0–3)

Interpret the Data

Based on this graph, what concentration of water fluoride will protect against dental caries but not cause fluorosis?
a. 2.5 mg/L
b. 2 mg/L
c. 1 mg/l
d. 0.5 mg/l

increase in fluorosis in the United States due to chronic ingestion of fluoride-containing toothpaste.[66] The fluoride in toothpaste is good for your teeth, but swallowing it can increase fluoride intake to dangerous levels. Swallowed toothpaste is estimated to contribute about 0.6 mg/day of fluoride in young children. Due to concern over excess fluoride intake, the following warning is now required on all fluoride-containing toothpastes: "If you accidentally swallow more than used for brushing, seek professional help or contact a poison control center immediately."

In adults, doses of 20 to 80 mg/day of fluoride can result in changes in bone health that may be crippling, as well as changes in kidney function and possibly nerve and muscle function. Death has been reported in cases involving an intake of 5 to 10 g/day. The UL for fluoride is set at 0.1 mg/kg/day for infants and children younger than 9 years of age and at 10 mg/day for those 9 years and older.[37]

Manganese, Molybdenum, and Other Trace Minerals

In addition to the seven we have just examined, there are many other trace minerals in the human body. DRI recommendations have been set for two of them: manganese and molybdenum.[41]

Manganese is a constituent of some enzymes and an activator of others. Enzymes that require manganese are involved in carbohydrate and cholesterol metabolism, bone formation, synthesis of urea, and prevention of oxidative damage because manganese is a component of a form of superoxide dismutase. The recommended intake for manganese is 2.3 mg/day for adult men and 1.8 mg/day for adult women. The best dietary sources of manganese are whole grains, nuts, legumes, and leafy green vegetables.

Molybdenum is also needed to activate enzymes. It functions in the metabolism of sulfur-containing amino acids and nitrogen-containing compounds that are present in DNA and RNA, in the production of a waste product called uric acid, and in the oxidation and detoxification of various other compounds. The recommended intake for molybdenum is 45 µg/day for adult men and women. The molybdenum content of food varies with the molybdenum content of the soil in the regions where the food is produced. The most reliable sources include milk

A summary of the trace minerals   Table 8.4

Mineral	Sources	Recommended intake for adults	Major functions	Deficiency diseases and symptoms	Groups at risk of deficiency	Toxicity	UL
Iron	Red meats, leafy greens, dried fruit, legumes, whole and enriched grains	8–18 mg/day	Part of hemoglobin (which delivers oxygen to cells), myoglobin (which holds oxygen in muscle), and proteins needed for ATP production; needed for immune function	Iron deficiency anemia: fatigue; weakness; small, pale red blood cells; low hemoglobin levels; inability to maintain normal body temperature	Infants and preschool children, adolescents, women of childbearing age, pregnant women, athletes, vegetarians	Acute: Gastrointestinal upset, liver damage Chronic: fatigue, heart and liver damage, increased risk of diabetes and cancer	45 mg/day
Copper	Organ meats, nuts, seeds, whole grains, seafood, cocoa	900 µg/day	A component of proteins needed for iron transport, lipid metabolism, collagen synthesis, nerve and immune function, protection against oxidative damage	Anemia, poor growth, skeletal abnormalities	People who consume excessive amounts of zinc in supplements	Vomiting, abdominal pain, diarrhea, liver damage	10 mg/day
Zinc	Meat, seafood, whole grains, dairy products, legumes, nuts	8–11 mg/day	Regulates protein synthesis; functions in growth, development, wound healing, immunity, and antioxidant enzymes	Poor growth and development, skin rashes, decreased immune function	Vegetarians, low-income children, elderly people	Decreased copper absorption, depressed immune function	40 mg/day

Mineral	Sources	Recommended intake for adults	Major functions	Deficiency diseases and symptoms	Groups at risk of deficiency	Toxicity	UL
Selenium	Meats, seafood, eggs, whole grains, nuts, seeds	55 µg/day	Antioxidant as part of glutathione peroxidase, synthesis of thyroid hormones, spares vitamin E	Muscle pain, weakness, Keshan disease	Populations in areas where the soil is low in selenium	Nausea, diarrhea, vomiting, fatigue, changes in hair and nails	400 µg/day
Iodine	Iodized salt, seafood, seaweed, dairy products	150 µg/day	Needed for synthesis of thyroid hormones	Goiter, cretinism, impaired brain function, growth and developmental abnormalities	Populations in areas where the soil is low in iodine and iodized salt is not used	Enlarged thyroid	1110 µg/day
Chromium	Brewer's yeast, nuts, whole grains, meat, mushrooms	25–35 µg/day	Enhances insulin action	High blood glucose	Malnourished children	None reported	ND
Fluoride	Fluoridated water, tea, fish, toothpaste	3–4 mg/day	Strengthens tooth enamel, enhances remineralization of tooth enamel, reduces acid production by bacteria in the mouth	Increased risk of dental caries	Populations in areas with unfluoridated water, those who drink mostly bottled water	Fluorosis: mottled teeth, kidney damage, bone abnormalities	10 mg/day
Manganese	Nuts, legumes, whole grains, tea, leafy vegetables	1.8–2.3 mg/day	Functions in carbohydrate and cholesterol metabolism and antioxidant enzymes	Growth retardation	None	Nerve damage	11 mg/day
Molybdenum	Milk, organ meats, grains, legumes	45 µg/day	Cofactor for a number of enzymes	Unknown in humans	None	Arthritis, joint inflammation	2 mg/day

Note: UL, Tolerable Upper Intake Level; ND, not determined.

and milk products, organ meats, breads, cereals, and legumes. Molybdenum is readily absorbed from foods; the amount in the body is regulated by varying the amount excreted in the urine and bile.

There is evidence that arsenic, boron, nickel, silicon, and vanadium play a role in human health. The DRI committee reviewed the need for and functions of these minerals, but there was insufficient data to establish a recommended intake for any of them. Other trace minerals that are believed to play a physiological role in human health include aluminum, bromine, cadmium, germanium, lead, lithium, rubidium, and tin. Their specific functions have not been defined, and the DRI committee has not evaluated them. All the minerals, both those that are known to be essential and those that are still being assessed for their role in human health, can be obtained by choosing a variety of foods from each of the MyPlate food groups.

Table 8.4 provides a summary of the trace minerals.

CONCEPT CHECK	STOP

1. Why does iron deficiency cause fatigue?
2. How does selenium reduce the body's need for vitamin E?
3. What is the function of iodine?
4. How does fluoride protect the teeth?

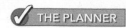
Summary

1 Water 240

- Water, which is found intracellularly and extracellularly, accounts for about 60% of adult body weight. The amount of water in the blood is a balance between the forces of **blood pressure** and osmosis.

- Because water isn't stored in the body, intake from fluids and foods, as shown in the illustration, must replace losses in urine, feces, sweat, and evaporation. Water intake is stimulated by the sensation of **thirst**. The kidneys regulate urinary water losses.

Water balance • Figure 8.2

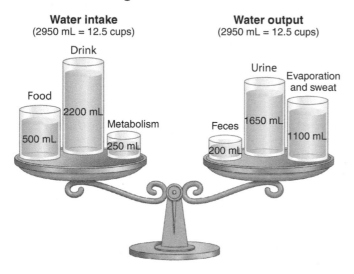

Water intake
(2950 mL = 12.5 cups)

Drink

Food

2200 mL

Metabolism

500 mL

250 mL

Water output
(2950 mL = 12.5 cups)

Urine

Evaporation and sweat

Feces

1650 mL

200 mL

1100 mL

- In the body, water is a **solvent** where chemical reactions occur; it also transports nutrients and wastes, provides protection, helps regulate temperature, and participates in chemical reactions and acid–base balance.

- **Dehydration** occurs when there is too little water in the body. **Water intoxication** causes **hyponatremia**, which can result in abnormal fluid accumulation in body tissues.

- The recommended intake of water is 2.7 L/day for women and 3.7 L/day for men; needs vary depending on environmental conditions and activity level.

2 An Overview of Minerals 247

- **Major minerals** and **trace minerals** are distinguished by the amounts needed in the diet and found in the body. Both plant and animal foods are good sources of minerals.

- Mineral bioavailability is affected by the food source of the mineral, the body's need, and interactions with other minerals, vitamins, and dietary components such as fiber, phytates, oxalates, and tannins, which are plentiful in the foods shown here.

Compounds that interfere with mineral absorption • Figure 8.9

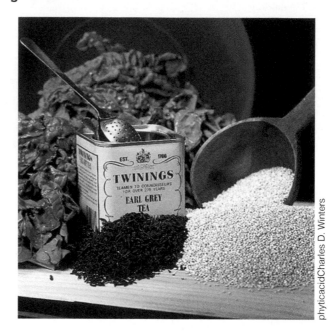

phyticacidCharles D. Winters

- Minerals are needed to provide structure and to regulate biochemical reactions, often as **cofactors**.

3 Electrolytes: Sodium, Potassium, and Chloride 251

- The minerals sodium, potassium, and chloride are **electrolytes** that are important in the maintenance of fluid balance and the functioning of nerves and muscles. The kidneys are the primary regulator of electrolyte and fluid balance.

- Sodium, potassium, and chloride depletion can occur when losses are increased by heavy and persistent sweating, chronic diarrhea, or vomiting. Diets high in sodium and low in potassium are associated with an increased risk of **hypertension**. The **DASH Eating Plan**—a dietary pattern moderate in sodium; high in potassium, magnesium, calcium, and fiber; and low in fat, saturated fat, and cholesterol—lowers blood pressure.

- As shown in the graph, processed foods add sodium to the diet. Potassium is highest in unprocessed foods such as fresh fruits and vegetables. Recommendations for health suggest that we increase our intake of potassium and consume less sodium.

Processing adds sodium • Figure 8.15

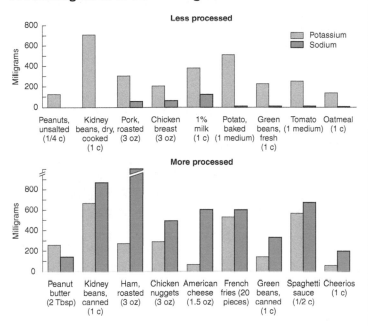

Restoring blood calcium levels • Figure 8.18

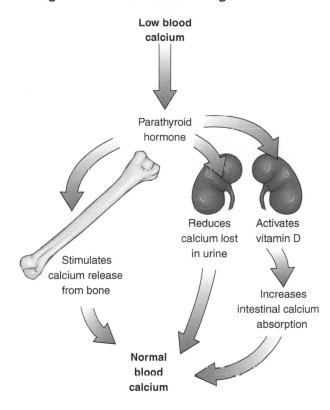

4 **Major Minerals and Bone Health 259**

- Bone is a living tissue that is constantly remodeled. **Peak bone mass** occurs in young adulthood. **Age-related bone loss** occurs in adults when more bone is broken down than is made. Bone loss is accelerated in women after **menopause**. **Osteoporosis** occurs when bone mass is so low that it increases the risk of bone fractures.

- Most of the calcium in the body is found in bone, but calcium is also needed for essential functions such as nerve transmission, muscle contraction, blood clotting, and blood pressure regulation. Good sources of calcium in the U.S. diet include dairy products, fish consumed with bones, and leafy green vegetables. As shown in the illustration, low blood calcium causes the release of parathyroid hormone (PTH), which affects the amount of calcium excreted in the urine, absorbed from the diet, and released from bone. When blood calcium is high, **calcitonin** blocks calcium release from bone.

- Phosphorus is widely distributed in foods. It plays an important structural role in bones and teeth. Phosphorus helps prevent changes in acidity and is an essential component of phospholipids, ATP, DNA, and RNA.

- Magnesium is important for bone health and blood pressure regulation, and it is needed as a cofactor and to stabilize ATP. The best dietary sources are whole grains and green vegetables.

- Sulfur is found in protein and is part of the structure of certain vitamins and of glutathione, which protects cells from oxidative damage.

5 **Trace Minerals 269**

- Iron functions as part of **hemoglobin**, **myoglobin**, and proteins involved in energy metabolism. The amount of iron absorbed depends on the form of iron and other dietary components. **Heme iron**, found in meats, is more absorbable than nonheme iron, which is the only form found in plant foods. **Iron deficiency anemia** is characterized by small, pale red blood cells such as those in the right-hand photo. It causes fatigue and decreased work capacity. The amount of iron transported from the intestinal cells to body cells depends on the amount needed. If too much iron is absorbed, as in **hemochromatosis**, the heart and liver can be damaged, and diabetes and cancer are more likely. A single large dose of iron is toxic and can be fatal.

Iron deficiency • Figure 8.25

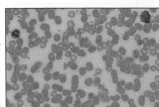
Normal red blood cells

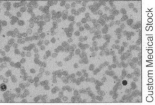
Iron deficiency anemia

B&B Photos/Custom Medical StockPhoto, Inc.

Custom Medical Stock Photo, Inc.

- Copper functions in proteins that affect iron and lipid metabolism, synthesis of connective tissue, antioxidant capacity, and iron transport. High levels of zinc can cause copper deficiency. A copper deficiency can result in anemia and skeletal abnormalities. Seafood, nuts, seeds, and whole-grain breads and cereals are good sources of copper.

- Zinc is needed for the activity of many enzymes, and zinc-containing proteins are needed for gene expression. Good sources of zinc include red meats, eggs, dairy products, and whole grains. The amount of zinc in the body is regulated primarily by the amount absorbed and lost through the small intestine. Zinc deficiency depresses immunity. Too much zinc depresses immune function and contributes to copper and iron deficiency.

- Selenium is part of the antioxidant enzyme **glutathione peroxidase** and is needed for the synthesis of **thyroid hormones**. Dietary sources include seafood, eggs, organ meats, and plant foods grown in selenium-rich soils. Selenium deficiency causes muscle discomfort and weakness and is associated with **Keshan disease**. Low selenium intake has been linked to increased cancer risk.

- Iodine is an essential component of thyroid hormones. The best sources of iodine are seafood, foods grown near the sea, and **iodized salt**. When iodine is deficient, the **thyroid gland** enlarges, forming a **goiter**. Iodine deficiency also affects growth and development. The use of iodized salt has reduced the incidence of iodine deficiency worldwide.

- Chromium is needed for normal insulin action and glucose utilization. It is found in liver, brewer's yeast, nuts, and whole grains.

- Fluoride is necessary for the maintenance of bones and teeth and the prevention of **dental caries**. Dietary sources of fluoride include fluoridated drinking water, toothpaste, tea, and marine fish consumed with bones. Too much fluoride causes **fluorosis** in children.

Key Terms

- age-related bone loss 261
- aldosterone 253
- antidiuretic hormone (ADH) 242
- blood pressure 241
- bone remodeling 261
- bone resorption 264
- calcitonin 263
- cofactor 251
- cretinism 279
- DASH (Dietary Approaches to Stop Hypertension) Eating Plan 256

- dehydration 244
- dental caries 280
- diuretic 247
- electrolyte 251
- fluorosis 281
- glutathione peroxidase 277
- goiter 279
- goitrogen 279
- heme iron 270
- hemochromatosis 274
- hemoglobin 269
- hypertension 253
- hyponatremia 245

- iodized salt 279
- ion 249
- iron deficiency anemia 271
- iron overload 274
- Keshan disease 277
- major mineral 247
- menopause 261
- mineral 247
- myoglobin 269
- osteopenia 260
- osteoporosis 261
- peak bone mass 261

- postmenopausal bone loss 261
- prehypertension 255
- sodium chloride 251
- solute 240
- solvent 243
- thirst 242
- thyroid gland 277
- thyroid hormone 277
- thyroid-stimulating hormone 277
- trace mineral 247
- water intoxication 245

What is happening in this picture?

This photo shows astronaut Pete Conrad riding a stationary bike during his 28-day stay aboard Skylab in 1973. Weight-bearing exercise and adequate nutrient intake are important for the maintenance of bone.

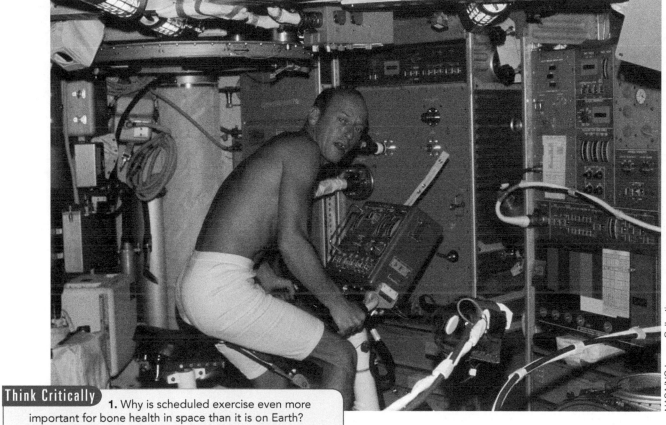

NASA/NG Image Collection

Think Critically

1. Why is scheduled exercise even more important for bone health in space than it is on Earth?
2. What nutrient other than calcium might be of particular concern for bone health in an astronaut? Why?

THE PLANNER ✓

Review your Chapter Planner on the chapter opener and check off your completed work.

Energy Balance and Weight Management

9

Wallis Simpson, the woman whose love affair with Edward VIII led him to abdicate the throne of England in 1936, famously said, "You can never be too rich or too thin." In much of the developed world, being too rich seems a hindrance to being too thin: The United Nations reports that the United States, with its high standard of living, has one of the highest obesity rates of all populous nations. The nation with the highest obesity rate? The tiny South Pacific island republic of Nauru, whose obesity rate began to climb in the 1970s when it boasted the highest per capita income in the world; today almost three out of four Nauruans are obese.

So does being rich make you too fat? There is certainly a connection between economic advances and energy expenditure. As people's income increases, their jobs become less physically demanding; they have greater leisure time; and their food supply becomes more available and varied. Being able to eat better and work less may seem advantageous, but there are consequences: The American Medical Association is so concerned about the health risks associated with obesity that it has declared it a disease, emphasizing its costs to the United States not only in dollars but also in productivity as a nation.

As developing nations strive for Western standards of consumption, weight problems manifest themselves in their populations as well. Obesity is a global problem with no easy solution. Clearly, getting richer doesn't keep you thin.

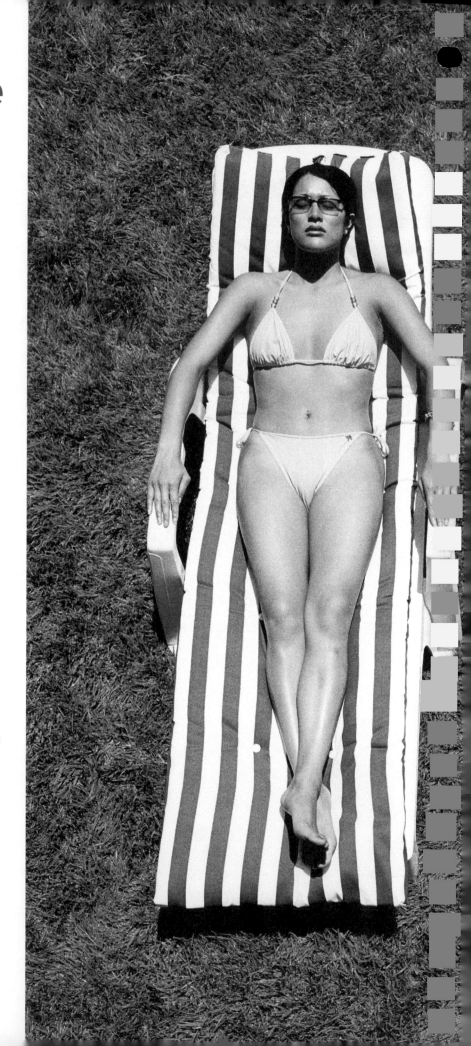

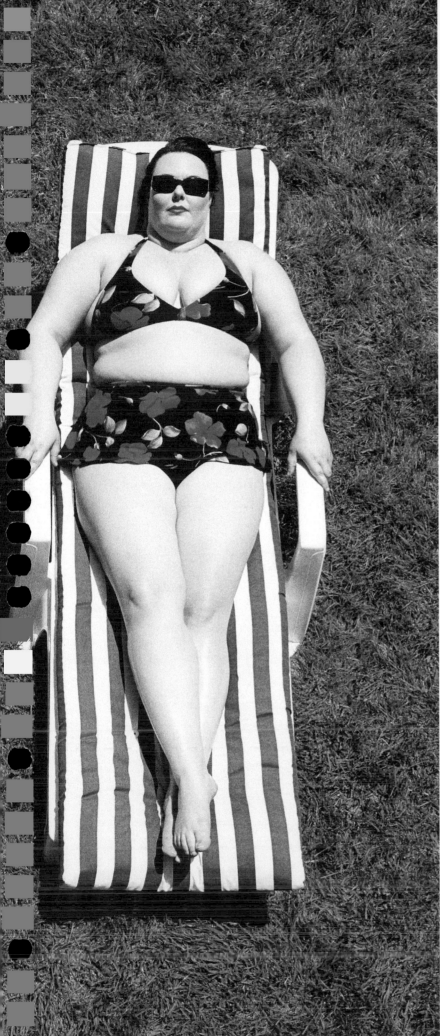

CHAPTER PLANNER ✓

Robert Daly/Stone/Getty Images

9.1 Body Weight and Health

LEARNING OBJECTIVES

1. **Discuss** the obesity epidemic.
2. **Describe** the health consequences of excess body fat.
3. **Calculate** your BMI and determine whether it indicates you are at a healthy weight.
4. **Discuss** how the amount and location of body fat affect the health risks associated with being overweight.

> **overweight** Being too heavy for one's height, usually due to an excess of body fat. Overweight is defined as having a body mass index (ratio of weight to height squared) of 25 to 29.9 kilograms/meter² (kg/m²).
>
> **obese** Having excess body fat. Obesity is defined as having a body mass index (ratio of weight to height squared) of 30 kg/m² or greater.

In the United States today, almost 69% of adults are either **overweight** or **obese**.[1] Carrying excess body weight usually involves excess body fat, which increases the risk of a host of chronic diseases. The number of people who carry excess fat has increased dramatically over the past five decades. In 1960, only 13.4% of American adults were obese. By 1990, about 23% were obese, and today almost 35% are obese (**Figure 9.1**). Excess body weight and fat are a major public health concern that affects both men and women of all ages and all racial and ethnic groups. Obesity rates for minorities often exceed those in the general population: Almost 48% of African Americans and over 42% of Hispanic Americans are obese.[1]

Obesity is not just an American problem but also a growing concern worldwide. It is such an important trend that the term *globesity* has been coined to reflect the escalation of global obesity and overweight. Around the world, approximately 1.4 billion adults are overweight, and of these, 500 million are obese; more than 10% of the world's adult population.[2] Once considered a problem only in high-income countries, overweight and obesity are now on the rise in low- and middle-income countries, particularly in urban settings.

Obesity across America • Figure 9.1

This map shows the percentage of the adult population classified as obese in each state in 2013.[14] The dramatic rise in overweight and obesity in the United States over the past few decades has led medical and public health officials to label the situation an epidemic.

> **Interpret the Data**
>
> How many states have an obesity rate of less than 20% of their population?

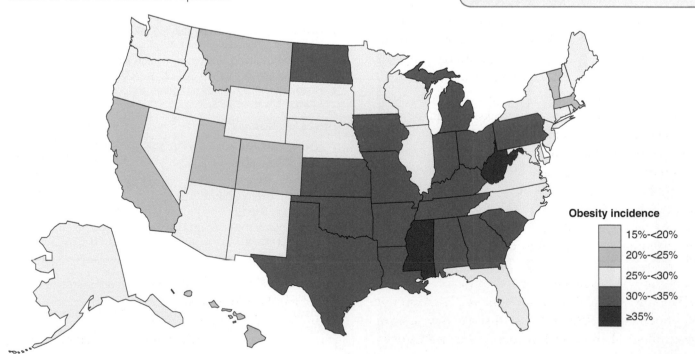

Obesity incidence
- 15%-<20%
- 20%-<25%
- 25%-<30%
- 30%-<35%
- ≥35%

Obesity-related health complications such as those highlighted here have reached epidemic proportions in the United States and around the world.

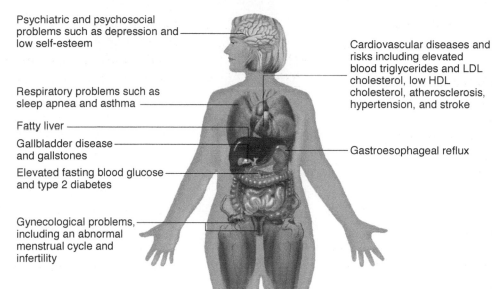

Psychiatric and psychosocial problems such as depression and low self-esteem

Respiratory problems such as sleep apnea and asthma

Fatty liver

Gallbladder disease and gallstones

Elevated fasting blood glucose and type 2 diabetes

Gynecological problems, including an abnormal menstrual cycle and infertility

Cardiovascular diseases and risks including elevated blood triglycerides and LDL cholesterol, low HDL cholesterol, atherosclerosis, hypertension, and stroke

Gastroesophageal reflux

Increased risk for cancers of the breast, colon, uterus, esophagus, pancreas, kidney, thyroid, and gallbladder

Arthritis and gout

What's Wrong with Having Too Much Body Fat?

Having too much body fat increases the risk of developing a host of chronic health problems, including high blood pressure, heart disease, high blood cholesterol, diabetes, gallbladder disease, liver disease, arthritis, sleep disorders, respiratory problems, menstrual irregularities, and cancers of the breast, uterus, prostate, and colon (**Figure 9.2**). Obesity also increases the incidence and severity of infectious disease and has been linked to poor wound healing and surgical complications. The more excess body fat you have, the greater your health risks. The longer you carry excess fat, the greater the risks; individuals who gain excess weight at a young age and remain overweight throughout life face the greatest health risks.

Being overweight also has psychological and social consequences. Overweight and obese individuals of any age are at increased risk of experiencing depression, negative self-image, and feelings of inadequacy.[3] They may also be discriminated against in college admissions, in the workplace, and even on public transportation. The physical health consequences of excess body fat may not manifest themselves as disease for years, but the psychological and social problems are experienced every day.

Because obesity increases health problems, it increases health care costs. Estimates suggest that obesity "costs" about $147 billion per year.[4] The greater the number of obese people, the higher the nation's health care expenses and the higher the cost to society as a whole in terms of lost wages and productivity.

What Is a Healthy Weight?

A healthy weight is a weight that minimizes the health risks associated with too much or too little body fat. Your body weight is the sum of the weight of your fat and your **lean body mass**. Some body fat is essential for health; too much or too little increases health risks (see Figure 9.2). How much weight and fat is too much or too little depends on your age, gender, and lifestyle and where your fat is located.

Body mass index (BMI) The current standard for assessing the healthfulness of body weight is **body mass index (BMI)**, which is determined by dividing body weight (in kilograms) by height (in meters) squared.

lean body mass Body mass attributed to nonfat body components such as bone, muscle, and internal organs; also called *fat-free mass*.

body mass index (BMI) A measure of body weight relative to height that is used to compare body size with a standard.

What's your BMI? • Figure 9.3

BMI is easily calculated from height and weight. It can be a useful tool, but other information is also needed to assess the health risks that are associated with high or low body weight.

To find your BMI, locate your height in the leftmost column and read across to your weight. Follow the column containing your weight up to the top line to find your BMI. A BMI < 18.5 kg/m² is classified as **underweight**, a BMI ≥ 25 and < 30 kg/m² is classified as overweight, and a BMI of ≥ 30 kg/m² is classified as obese. A BMI ≥ 40 kg/m² is considered **extreme obesity** or **morbid obesity**.[5]

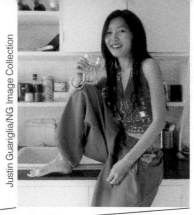

Justin Guariglia/NG Image Collection

◄ Being underweight is associated with increased risk of early death, but this does not mean that all thin people are at risk.[6] People who are naturally lean have a lower incidence of certain chronic diseases and do not face increased health risks due to their low body weight. However, low body fat due to starvation, eating disorders, or a disease process decreases energy reserves and the ability of the immune system to fight disease.

	UNDER-WEIGHT		NORMAL						OVERWEIGHT					OBESE										EXTREME OBESITY		
BMI	17	18	19	20	21	22	23	24	25	26	27	28	29	30	31	32	33	34	35	36	37	38	39	40	41	42
Height (feet/inches)	**Body Weight** (pounds)																									
4'10"	81	86	91	96	100	105	110	115	119	124	129	134	138	143	148	153	158	162	167	172	177	181	186	191	196	201
4'11"	84	89	94	99	104	109	114	119	124	128	133	138	143	148	153	158	163	168	173	178	183	188	193	198	203	208
5'0"	87	92	97	102	107	112	118	123	128	133	138	143	148	153	158	163	168	174	179	184	189	194	199	204	209	215
5'1"	90	95	100	106	111	116	122	127	132	137	143	148	153	158	164	169	174	180	185	190	195	201	206	211	217	222
5'2"	93	98	104	109	115	120	126	131	136	142	147	153	158	164	169	175	180	186	191	196	202	207	213	218	224	229
5'3"	96	102	107	113	118	124	130	135	141	146	152	158	163	169	175	180	186	191	197	203	208	214	220	225	231	237
5'4"	99	105	110	116	122	128	134	140	145	151	157	163	169	174	180	186	192	197	204	209	215	221	227	232	238	244
5'5"	102	108	114	120	126	132	138	144	150	156	162	168	174	180	186	192	198	204	210	216	222	228	234	240	246	252
5'6"	105	112	118	124	130	136	142	148	155	161	167	173	179	186	192	198	204	210	216	223	229	235	241	247	253	260
5'7"	108	115	121	127	134	140	146	153	159	166	172	178	185	191	198	204	211	217	223	230	236	242	249	255	261	268
5'8"	112	119	125	131	138	144	151	158	164	171	177	184	190	197	203	210	216	223	230	236	243	249	256	262	269	276
5'9"	115	122	128	135	142	149	155	162	169	176	182	189	196	203	209	216	223	230	236	243	250	257	263	270	277	284
5'10"	119	126	132	139	146	153	160	167	174	181	188	195	202	209	216	222	229	236	243	250	257	264	271	278	285	292
5'11"	122	129	136	143	150	157	165	172	179	186	193	200	208	215	222	229	236	243	250	257	265	272	279	286	293	301
6'0"	125	133	140	147	154	162	169	177	184	191	199	206	213	221	228	235	242	250	258	265	272	279	287	294	302	309
6'1"	129	137	144	151	159	166	174	182	189	197	204	212	219	227	235	242	250	257	265	272	280	288	295	302	310	318
6'2"	132	140	148	155	163	171	179	186	194	202	210	218	225	233	241	249	256	264	272	280	287	295	303	311	319	326
6'3"	136	144	152	160	168	176	184	192	200	208	216	224	232	240	248	256	264	272	279	287	295	303	311	319	327	335
6'4"	140	148	156	164	172	180	189	197	205	213	221	230	238	246	254	263	271	279	287	295	304	312	320	328	336	344

Someone who is overweight based on BMI but consumes a healthy diet and exercises regularly may be more fit and at lower risk for chronic diseases than someone with a BMI in the healthy range who is sedentary and eats a poor diet. ▶

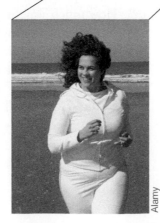

Alamy

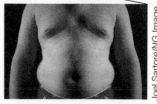

Jodi Cobb/NG Image Collection

Joel Sartore/NG Image Collection

▲ A high BMI may be caused by either too much body fat or a large amount of muscle. Therefore, in muscular athletes, BMI does not provide an accurate estimate of health risk. Both of these individuals have a BMI of 33, but only the man on the right has excess body fat. The high body weight of the man on the left is due to his large muscle mass. His body fat, and hence his risk of obesity-related health problems, is low.

A healthy BMI for adults is between 18.5 and 24.9 kg/m². People with a BMI in this range have the lowest health risks. Although BMI is not actually a measure of body fat, it is recommended as a way to assess body fatness that is better than measuring weight alone.[5] You can use **Figure 9.3** to determine your BMI or calculate it according to either of these equations:

$$\text{BMI} = \text{Weight in kilograms}/(\text{Height in meters})^2$$
or
$$\text{BMI} = [\text{Weight in pounds}/(\text{Height in inches})^2] \times 703$$

Body composition **Body composition**, which refers to the relative proportions of fat and lean tissue that make up the body, affects the risks associated with excess body weight. Having more than the recommended percentage of body fat increases health risks, whereas having more lean body mass does not. In general, women store more body fat than men do, so the level that is healthy for women is somewhat higher than the level that is healthy for men. A healthy level of body fat for young adult females is between 21 and 32% of total weight; for young adult males, it is between 8 and 19%.[7] With aging, lean body mass decreases and body fat increases, even if body weight remains the same. Some of this change may be prevented through exercise. Body composition can be measured using a variety of techniques (**Figure 9.4**).

Techniques for measuring body composition • Figure 9.4

The techniques available for assessing body composition differ in ease, availability, cost, and accuracy.

Underwater weighing relies on the fact that lean tissue is denser than fat tissue. The difference between a person's weight on land and his or her weight underwater is used to calculate body density; the higher a person's body density, the less fat he or she has. Underwater weighing is accurate but can't be used for small children or for ill or frail adults.

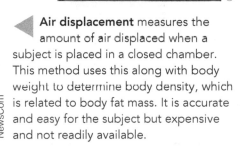

Skinfold thickness uses calipers to measure the thickness of the fat layer under the skin at several locations. This technique assumes that the amount of fat under the skin is representative of total body fat. It is fast, easy, and inexpensive but can be inaccurate if not performed by a trained professional.

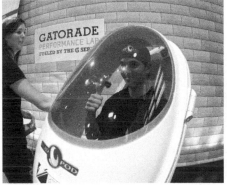
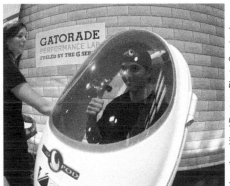

Air displacement measures the amount of air displaced when a subject is placed in a closed chamber. This method uses this along with body weight to determine body density, which is related to body fat mass. It is accurate and easy for the subject but expensive and not readily available.

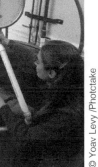

Bioelectric impedance analysis measures an electric current traveling through the body. It is based on the fact that current moves easily through lean tissue, which is high in water but is slowed by fat, which resists current flow. Bioelectric impedance measurements are fast, easy, and painless but can be inaccurate if the amount of body water is higher or lower than typical. For example, in someone who has been sweating heavily, the estimate of percentage body fat obtained using bioelectric impedance will be artificially high.

Dual-energy X-ray absorptiometry (DXA) distinguishes among various body tissues by measuring differences in levels of X-ray absorption. A single investigation can accurately determine total body mass, bone mineral mass, and body fat percentage, but the apparatus is expensive and not readily available.

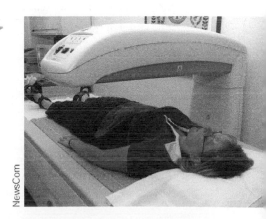

Excess fat in the visceral region increases health risks. Waist circumference measurements can help assess risk.

a. People who carry their excess fat around and above the waist have more visceral fat. Those who carry their extra fat below the waist, in the hips and thighs, have more subcutaneous fat. In the popular literature, these body types have been dubbed "apples" and "pears," respectively.

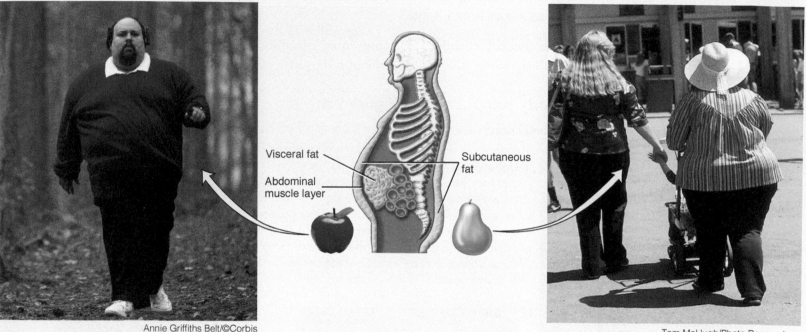

Visceral fat

Abdominal muscle layer

Subcutaneous fat

Annie Griffiths Belt/©Corbis

Tom McHugh/Photo Researchers

b. Waist circumference is indicative of the amount of visceral fat, the type of fat that is associated with increased health risk. Waist measurements along with BMI are used to estimate the health risk associated with excess body fat. These waist circumference "cutpoints" are not useful in patients with a BMI of 35 kg/m² or greater.

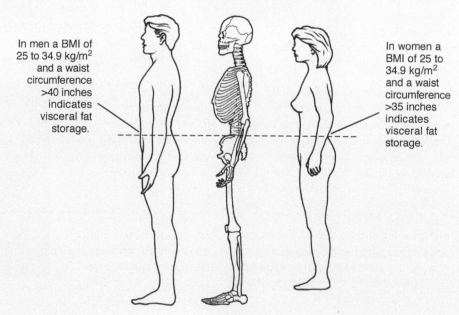

In men a BMI of 25 to 34.9 kg/m² and a waist circumference >40 inches indicates visceral fat storage.

In women a BMI of 25 to 34.9 kg/m² and a waist circumference >35 inches indicates visceral fat storage.

Location of body fat The location of body fat stores affects the risks associated with having too much fat (**Figure 9.5**). Excess **subcutaneous fat**, which is adipose tissue located under the skin, does not increase health risk as much as does excess **visceral fat**, which is adipose tissue located around the organs in the abdomen. Generally, fat in the hips and lower body is subcutaneous, whereas fat in the abdominal region is primarily visceral. An increase in visceral fat is associated with a higher incidence of heart disease, high blood cholesterol, high blood pressure, stroke, type 2 diabetes, and some types of cancer.[8]

Where your extra fat is deposited is determined primarily by your genes. Age, gender, ethnicity, and lifestyle also influence where fat is stored.[8] Visceral fat storage increases with age. Excess visceral fat is more common in men than in women, but after menopause, the amount of visceral fat in women increases. Caucasians and Asians have more visceral fat than African Americans with similar amounts of body fat.[8] Stress, tobacco use, and alcohol consumption predispose people to visceral fat deposition, and weight loss and exercise reduce the amount of visceral fat.

CONCEPT CHECK

1. **How** has the incidence of overweight and obesity changed in the United States over the past five decades?
2. **What** are two chronic disorders that are more common in obese individuals than in lean individuals?
3. **When** is a high BMI not associated with an increased health risk?
4. **What** pattern of fat distribution increases health risks?

9.2 Energy Balance

LEARNING OBJECTIVES

1. **Identify** lifestyle factors that have led to weight gain among Americans.
2. **Explain** the principle of energy balance.
3. **Describe** the components of energy expenditure.
4. **Calculate** your EER at various levels of activity.

The high rate of overweight and obesity in virtually every population group in the United States demonstrates that many Americans have been in energy imbalance.[9] According to the principle of **energy balance**, if you consume the same amount of energy—or calories—as you expend, your body weight will remain the same. If you consume more energy than you expend, you will gain weight, and if you expend more energy than you consume, you will lose weight. For many in the United States today, energy intake is exceeding energy expenditure.[9] Bringing it back into balance requires an understanding of how many calories we need and how we use energy.

> **energy balance**
> The amount of energy consumed in the diet compared with the amount expended by the body over a given period.

America's Energy Imbalance

Over the past several decades, changes in our food supply and lifestyle have affected what we eat, how much we eat, and how much exercise we get. Simply put, more Americans are overweight than ever before because we are eating more and burning fewer calories than we did 40 or 50 years ago.[9] Food is plentiful and continuously available, and little activity is required in our daily lives.

Eating more In America today, supermarkets, fast-food restaurants, and convenience marts make palatable, affordable food readily available to the majority of the population 24 hours a day. We are constantly bombarded with cues to eat: Advertisements entice us with tasty, inexpensive foods, and convenience stores, food courts, and vending machines tempt us with the sights and smells of fatty, sweet, high-calorie snacks. As a result, since 1970 the amount of energy available to us has increased by about 600 Calories per day, with the greatest increases in added fats, grains, dairy products, and sweeteners.[9] The accessibility of tempting treats stimulates **appetite**. Because appetite is

> **appetite** A desire to consume specific foods that is independent of hunger.

Portion distortion • Figure 9.6

The burger and French fry portions served in fast-food restaurants today are two to five times larger than they were when fast food first appeared about 50 years ago. Soft-drink portion sizes have also escalated. A large fast-food soft drink today contains 32 ounces, providing about 300 Calories, and 20-oz bottles have replaced 12-oz cans in many vending machines.

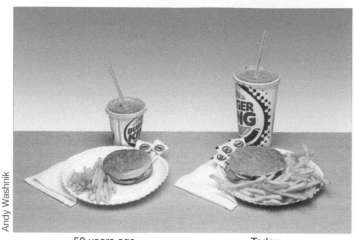

Andy Washnik

50 years ago　　　　　Today

Soft drinks
62%

French fries
57%

Cheeseburgers
24%

Percentage increase in portion size

triggered by external cues such as the sight or smell of food, it is usually appetite, and not **hunger**, that makes us stop for

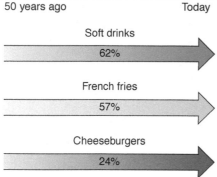

hunger A desire to consume food that is triggered by internal physiological signals.

an ice cream cone on a summer afternoon or give in to the smell of freshly baked chocolate chip cookies while strolling through the mall. Studies examining the relationship between the food environment and BMI have found that people in communities with more fast-food or quick-service restaurants tend to have higher BMIs.[9]

In addition to having more enticing choices available to us, we consume more calories today because portion sizes have increased (**Figure 9.6**). The more food that is put in front of people, the more they eat.[9] Portion size is associated with body weight; being served and consuming larger portions is associated with weight gain, whereas small portions are associated with weight loss.[9]

Social changes over the past few decades have also contributed to the increase in the number of calories Americans consume. Busy schedules and an increase in the number of single-parent households and households with two working parents mean that families are often too rushed to cook meals at home. As a result, prepackaged, convenience, and fast-food meals have become mainstays. These foods are typically higher in fat and energy than foods prepared at home.

Moving less Along with America's rising energy intake, there has been a decline in the amount of energy Americans expend, both at work and at play. Fewer American adults today work in jobs that require physical labor. People drive to work rather than walk or bike, take elevators instead of stairs, use dryers rather than hang clothes outside, and cut the lawn with riding mowers rather than with push mowers. All these modern conveniences reduce the amount of energy expended daily (**Figure 9.7**). Americans are also less active during their leisure time because busy schedules and long days at work and commuting leave little time for active recreation. Instead, at the end of the day, people tend to sit in front of television sets, video games, tablets, and computers.

Inactivity is also contributing to excess body weight among children. In the 1960s, schools provided daily physical education classes, and children spent their after-school hours playing outdoors; today, they are more

Activity reduces the risk of obesity • Figure 9.7

A typical office worker today walks only about 3000 to 5000 steps per day (2000 steps = approximately 1 mile). In contrast, in the Amish community—where automobiles and other modern conveniences are not allowed—a typical adult takes 14,000 to 18,000 steps a day. The overall incidence of obesity among the Amish is only 4%.[10]

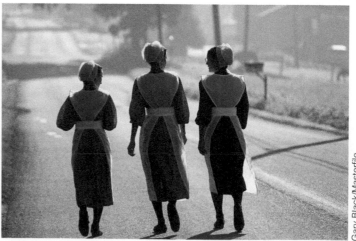

Gary Black/Masterfile

likely to spend their afternoons indoors watching television, texting with friends, and playing video games. As a result, they burn fewer calories, snack more, and consequently gain weight. In the United States, about 17% of children and adolescents ages 2 through 19 are obese.[1]

Balancing Energy Intake and Expenditure

The energy needed to fuel your body comes from the food you eat and the energy stored in your body. You use this energy to stay alive, process your food, move, and grow.

Energy intake The amount of energy you consume depends on what and how much you eat and drink. The carbohydrate, fat, protein, and alcohol consumed in food and drink all contribute energy: 4, 9, 4, and 7 Calories/gram, respectively (**Figure 9.8a**). Vitamins, minerals, and water, though essential nutrients, do not provide energy. You can determine your calorie intake by using food labels or looking up values in a food composition table or database (**Figure 9.8b**).

Energy expenditure The total amount of energy used by the body each day is called **total energy expenditure**. It includes the energy needed to maintain basic body functions as well as that needed to fuel physical activity and process food. In individuals who are growing or pregnant, total energy expenditure also includes the energy used to deposit new tissues. In women who are lactating, it includes the energy used to produce milk. A small amount of energy is also used to maintain body temperature in a cold environment.

For most people, about 60 to 75% of total energy expenditure is used for **basal metabolism**. Basal metabolism includes all the essential metabolic reactions and life-sustaining functions needed to keep you alive, such as breathing, circulating blood, regulating body temperature, synthesizing tissues, removing waste products, and sending nerve signals. The rate at which energy is used for these basic functions is the **basal metabolic rate (BMR)**. The energy expended for basal metabolism does *not* include the energy needed for physical activity or for the digestion of food and absorption of nutrients (**Figure 9.8c**).

> **basal metabolism** The energy expended to maintain an awake, resting body that is not digesting food.
>
> **basal metabolic rate (BMR)** The rate of energy expenditure under resting conditions. It is measured after 12 hours without food or exercise.

BMR increases with increasing body weight and is affected by body composition because it takes more energy to maintain lean tissue than to maintain body fat. BMR is generally higher in men than in women because men have a greater amount of lean body mass. BMR decreases with age, partly because of the decrease in lean body mass that occurs as we get older. BMR is also lower when calorie intake is consistently below the body's needs (see Figure 9.8c).[11] This drop in BMR reduces the amount of energy needed to maintain body weight. It is a beneficial adaptation in someone who is starving, but in someone who is trying to lose weight, it is frustrating because it makes weight loss more difficult.

Physical activity is the second major component of total energy expenditure. In most people, physical activity accounts for a smaller proportion of total energy expenditure than basal metabolism does—about 15 to 30% of energy requirements (**Figure 9.8d**). The energy we expend in physical activity includes both planned exercise and daily activities such as walking to work, typing, performing yard work, work-related activities, and even fidgeting. This **non-exercise activity thermogenesis (NEAT)** includes the energy expended for everything that is not sleeping, eating, or sports-like exercise. In most people it accounts for the majority of the energy expended for activity and varies enormously, depending on an individual's occupation and daily movements.

The amount of energy used for activity depends on the size of the person, how strenuous the activity is, and the length of time it is performed. Because it takes more energy to move a heavier object, the amount of energy expended for many activities increases as body weight increases. More strenuous activities, such as jogging, use more energy than do less strenuous activities, such as walking, but if you walk for an hour, you will probably burn as many calories as you would by jogging for 30 minutes (Appendix D).

We also use energy to digest food and to absorb, metabolize, and store the nutrients from this food. The energy used for these processes is called either the **thermic effect of food (TEF)** or **diet-induced thermogenesis**. This energy expenditure causes body temperature to rise slightly for several hours after a person has eaten. The energy required for TEF is estimated to be about 10% of energy intake but can vary, depending on the amounts and types of nutrients consumed (**Figure 9.8e**).

> **thermic effect of food (TEF)** or **diet-induced thermogenesis** The energy required for the digestion of food and absorption, metabolism, and storage of nutrients.

Nutrition InSight

What you weigh is determined by the balance between how much energy you take in and how much energy you expend.

a. The number of calories in a food depends on how much carbohydrate, fat, and protein it contains. Each of these tacos contains 9 g of protein, 16 g of carbohydrate, and 13 g of fat. The energy content of each is:

(9 g × 4 Cal/g protein)
+ (16 g × 4 Cal/g carbohydrate)
+ (13 g × 9 Cal/g fat)
= 217 Cal

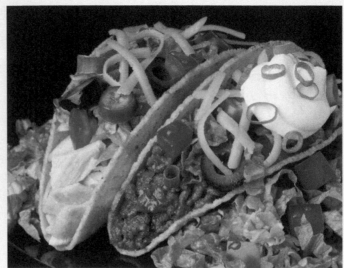

PhotoDisc, Inc./Getty Images

Current food label

Nutrition Facts

Serving Size 8 fl oz (240 mL)
Servings Per Container 2.5

Amount Per Serving

Calories 100

% Daily Value*

Total Fat 0 g   **0%**

Proposed food label

Nutrition Facts

1 Serving per container

Servings Size   1 bottle (20 fl oz)

Amount Per 20 fl oz

Calories   250

% DV*

0% | **Total Fat 0 g**

b. The Nutrition Facts panel shows the Calories per serving, but to know how many Calories your portion contains, you need to check the serving size. On the current food label (left) a serving is listed as 8 fl oz, so if you drink the whole bottle you will have had 2.5 servings, and thus 2.5 times the Calories per serving. The label on the right shows the proposed changes to the food label, which would make the Calories per serving more prominent and increase the serving size to one bottle, the amount most people typically consume.

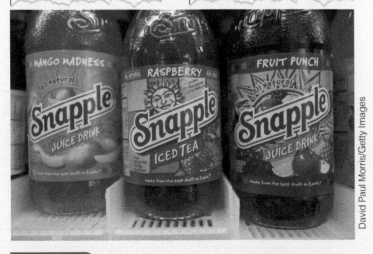

David Paul Morris/Getty Images

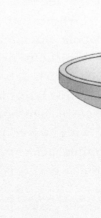

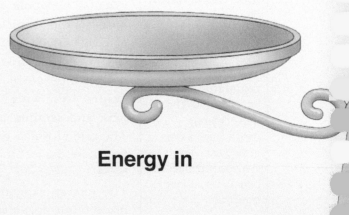

Energy in

Ask Yourself

Would the proposed changes to the Nutrition Facts label make you more aware of the number of calories you are consuming?

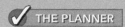

c. A person's BMR can be measured by collecting expired gases in a metabolic hood as shown. Measuring the oxygen consumed and carbon dioxide produced by aerobic metabolism can be used to estimate the amount of energy that is being expended. BMR is measured in the morning, in a warm room, before rising, and at least 12 hours after food intake or activity. **Resting metabolic rate (RMR)** is measured after 5 to 6 hours without food or exercise and yields values about 10 to 20% higher than BMR.[12]

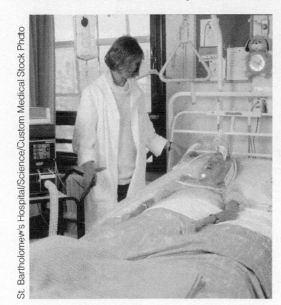

St. Bartholomew's Hospital/Science/Custom Medical Stock Photo

Factors that affect basal metabolism	
Factor	Effect
Higher lean body mass	↑
Greater height and weight	↑
Pregnancy	↑
Lactation	↑
Growth	↑
Low-calorie diet	↓
Starvation	↓
Fever	↑
Low thyroid hormone levels	↓
Stimulant drugs such as caffeine and tobacco	↑
Exercise	↑

Energy needs

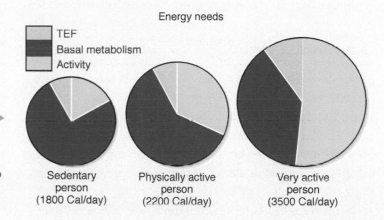

- TEF
- Basal metabolism
- Activity

d. Sedentary people must plan their intake carefully so it does not exceed energy expenditure. More active people burn more calories for activity so they can eat more and still maintain their weight. Very active people, such as professional athletes, can actually burn more calories for activity than they do for basal metabolism.

Sedentary person (1800 Cal/day)

Physically active person (2200 Cal/day)

Very active person (3500 Cal/day)

© swilmor/iStockphoto

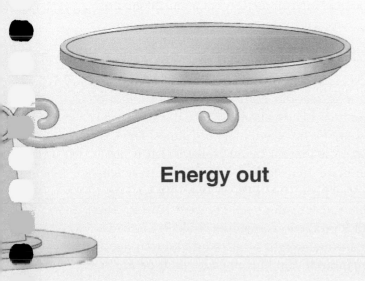

Energy out

e. The amount of energy used to process the food we eat varies with the size and composition of the meal. A bigger meal, such as the one on the left, requires more energy to process so has a higher TEF. A high-fat meal yields a lower TEF than one of similar size that is high in carbohydrate or protein because dietary fat is used and stored more efficiently.[13]

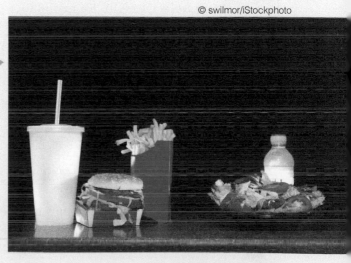

Energy balance: Storing and retrieving energy • Figure 9.9

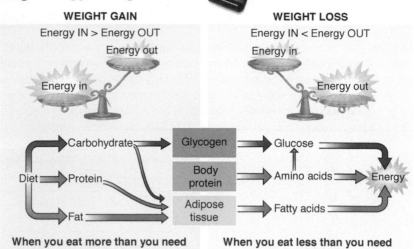

When calories are consumed in excess of needs, they are stored, mostly as fat. If the excess calories are consumed as fat, they are easily stored as body fat. If the excess calories are consumed as carbohydrate, they are stored as glycogen or converted into fat. If excess calories are consumed as protein, they are converted into body fat. When calorie intake is less than needs, energy can be retrieved from stores. Glycogen and body proteins can be broken down to supply glucose, and triglycerides in adipose tissue can be broken down to supply fatty acids.

WEIGHT GAIN
Energy IN > Energy OUT

WEIGHT LOSS
Energy IN < Energy OUT

When you eat more than you need

When you eat less than you need

The basics of weight gain and weight loss

If you consume more energy than you expend, the excess energy is stored for later use (**Figure 9.9**). A small amount of energy is stored as glycogen in liver and muscle, but most is stored as triglycerides in **adipocytes**, which make up adipose tis-

adipocyte A cell that stores fat.

sue. Adipocytes contain large fat droplets (see Figure 5.12b in Chapter 5). The cells increase in size as they accumulate more fat, and they shrink as fat is removed. If intake exceeds needs over the long term, adipocytes enlarge, and the amount of body fat increases, causing weight gain. The larger the number of adipocytes, the greater the body's ability to store fat. Most adipocytes are formed during infancy and adolescence, but excessive weight gain can cause the formation of new adipocytes at any time of life.

Stored energy is used when energy intake is reduced, both in the short term, such as when you haven't eaten a meal for a few hours, and in the long term, such as when you are trying to lose weight. To maintain a steady supply of blood glucose, liver glycogen is broken down (see Figure 9.9). Although protein is not considered a form of stored energy (see Chapter 6), when energy needs are not met, body protein, primarily muscle protein, can be broken down to yield amino acids, which can then be used to make glucose or produce ATP. Energy for tissues that don't require glucose is provided by the breakdown of stored fat (triglycerides). Nutrients consumed in the next meal replenish these stores, but with prolonged energy restriction, fat and protein are lost, and body weight is reduced. It is estimated that an energy deficit of about 3500 Calories results in the loss of a pound of adipose tissue.

Estimated Energy Requirements

The current recommendations for energy intake in the United States are the Estimated Energy Requirements (EER; see Chapter 2), the number of calories needed for a healthy individual to maintain his or her weight.[12] They are calculated using equations that take into account gender, age, height, weight, activity level, and life stage, all of which affect calorie needs.

To calculate your EER, you must first determine your physical activity level.[12] You can do this by keeping a daily log of your activities and recording the amount of time spent at each. Use **Figure 9.10** to help translate the amount of time you spend engaged in moderate-intensity or vigorous activity into an activity level (sedentary, low active, active, or very active). Each activity level corresponds to a numerical physical activity (PA) value that can be used to calculate your EER. For example, if you spend about an hour a day walking (a moderate-intensity activity) or about 30 minutes jogging (a vigorous activity), you are in the active category and should use the active PA value corresponding to your age and gender when calculating your EER.

Activity level has a significant effect on calorie needs. For example, a 22-year-old man who is 6 feet tall and weighs 185 pounds needs about 2770 Calories/day to maintain his weight if he is sedentary but almost 600 Calories/day more if he is at the active physical activity level.

Once you have determined your physical activity level, you can calculate your EER by entering your age, weight, height, and PA value (see Figure 9.10) into the appropriate EER prediction equation. **Table 9.1** provides equations for normal-weight adults and children age 9 and older. Equations for other groups are in Appendix A.

Physical activity level and PA value • Figure 9.10

Physical activity level, which is used to calculate EER, is categorized as sedentary, low active, active, or very active.[12] A sedentary person spends about 2.5 hours per day engaged in the activities of daily living, such as housework, homework, and yard work. Adding activity moves the person into the low-active, active, or very-active category. Activity can be moderate or vigorous or a combination of the two; compared to moderate-intensity activity, vigorous activity will burn the same number of calories in less time.

An adult in the very-active category spends at least 2.5 hours per day in moderate-intensity activity or at least 1.25 hours in vigorous activity.

An active adult spends at least 60 minutes per day engaged in moderate-intensity activity or at least 30 minutes in vigorous activity.

An adult in the low-active category spends at least 30 minutes per day engaged in moderate-intensity activity or at least 15 minutes in vigorous activity.

An adult in the sedentary category engages only in activities of daily living and not in moderate-intensity or vigorous activities.

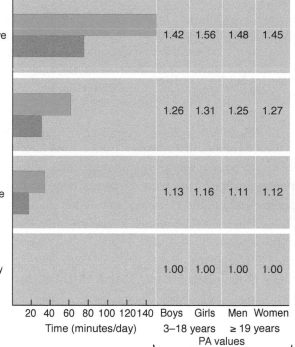

Ask Yourself

What are your activity level and corresponding PA value?

Each physical activity level is assigned a numerical physical activity (PA) value that can then be used in the EER calculation.

EER prediction equations   Table 9.1

Life stage	EER prediction equation*
Boys 9–18 years	EER = 88.5 − (61.9 × Age in yrs) + PA [(26.7 × Weight in kg) + (903 × Height in m)] + 25
Girls 9–18 years	EER = 135.3 − (30.8 × Age in yrs) + PA [(10.0 × Weight in kg) + (934 × Height in m)] + 25
Men ≥ 19 years	EER = 662 − (9.53 × Age in yrs) + PA [(15.91 × Weight in kg) + (539.6 × Height in m)]
Women ≥ 19 years	EER = 354 − (6.91 × Age in yrs) + PA [(9.36 × Weight in kg) + (726 × Height in m)]

For example, if you are an active 19-year-old male who weighs 72.7 kg and is 1.75 m tall, EER = 662 − (9.53 × 19 yrs) + 1.25 [(15.91 × 72.7 kg) + (539.6 × 1.75 m)] = 3107 Cal/day

*These equations are appropriate for determining EER in normal-weight individuals. Equations that predict the amount of energy needed for weight maintenance in overweight and obese individuals are also available (see Appendix A).

CONCEPT CHECK

1. Why are more Americans obese today compared to 50 years ago?

2. What happens to energy stores when energy intake exceeds expenditure?

3. Which component of energy expenditure is easiest to modify?

4. What is your EER?

9.3 What Determines Body Size and Shape?

LEARNING OBJECTIVES

1. **Discuss** genetic and environmental factors that affect body weight.
2. **List** four physiological signals that determine whether you feel hungry or full.
3. **Describe** how hormones regulate body fat levels.
4. **Discuss** factors that cause some people to gain weight more easily than others.

Y ou are probably shaped like your mother or your father. This is because much of the information that determines body size and shape is contained in the genes you inherit from your parents. Some of us inherit long, lean bodies, and others inherit huskier builds and the tendency to put on pounds (**Figure 9.11**). The genes involved in regulating body weight have been called **obesity genes**. Numerous obesity genes have been identified. They are responsible for the production of proteins that affect how much food you eat, how much energy you expend, and the way fat is stored in your body. Despite our growing knowledge, scientists still do not understand how these genes interact with each other and with your environment and the lifestyle choices you make to determine body weight and size.[15]

Genes versus Environment

The genes you inherit play a major role in determining your body weight. If one or both of your parents is obese, your risk of becoming obese is increased by a factor of 2 or 3, and the risk increases with the magnitude of the obesity. By studying identical twins, who have the same genetic makeup, researchers have been able to determine that about 75% of the variation in BMI can be attributed to genes.[16,17] This means that the remaining 25% is determined by the environment in which you live and the lifestyle choices you make.

Genes and body shape • Figure 9.11

The genes we inherit from our parents are important determinants of our body size and shape. The boy on the left inherited his father's long, lean body, whereas the boy on the right has his father's huskier build and will likely have a tendency to be overweight throughout his life.

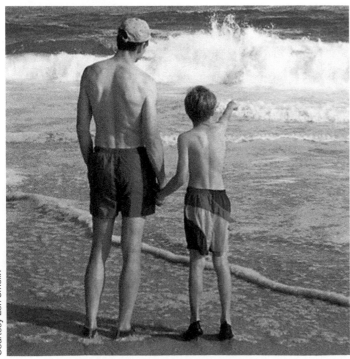

Courtesy Lori Smolin

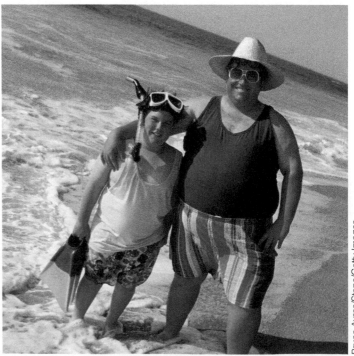

Bruce Ayres/Stone/Getty Images

When individuals who are genetically susceptible to weight gain find themselves in an environment where food is appealing and plentiful and physical activity is easily avoided, obesity is a likely outcome but not the only possible one. If you inherit genes that predispose you to being overweight but carefully monitor your diet and exercise regularly, you can maintain a healthy weight. It is also possible for individuals with no genetic tendency toward obesity to end up overweight if they consume a high-calorie diet and get little exercise. The interplay between genetics and lifestyle is illustrated by the higher incidence of obesity in Pima Indians living in Arizona than in a genetically similar group of Pima Indians living in Mexico (**Figure 9.12**).[18]

Regulation of Food Intake and Body Weight

What we eat and how much we exercise vary from day to day, but body weight tends to stay relatively constant for long periods. The body compensates for variations in diet and exercise by adjusting energy intake and expenditure to keep weight at a particular level, or **set point**. This set point, which is believed to be determined in part by genes, explains why your weight remains fairly constant, despite the added activity of a weekend hiking trip, or why most people gain back the weight they lose when they follow a weight-loss diet.[19]

To regulate weight and fatness at a constant level, the body must be able to respond both to short-term changes in food intake and to long-term changes in the amount of stored body fat. Signals related to food intake affect hunger and **satiety** over a short period—from meal to meal—whereas signals from adipose tissue trigger the brain to adjust both food intake and energy expenditure for long-term weight regulation.

> **satiety** The feeling of fullness and satisfaction caused by food consumption that eliminates the desire to eat.

Genes versus lifestyle • Figure 9.12

All Pima Indians carry genes that increase their risk of obesity but differences in lifestyle between different Pima populations cause their obesity rates to diverge.

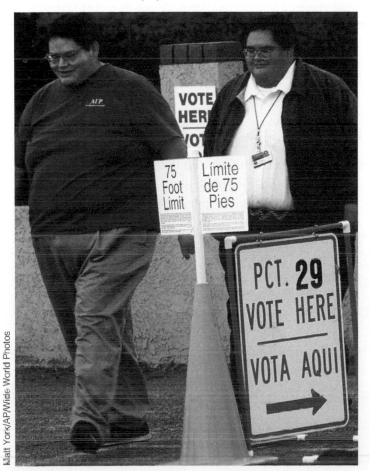

Matt York/AP/Wide World Photos

a. Genetic analysis of the Pima Indian population living in Arizona has identified a number of genes that may be responsible for this group's tendency to store excess body fat.[20] This, combined with an environment that fosters a sedentary lifestyle and consumption of high-calorie, high-fat processed foods, has resulted in a strikingly high incidence of obesity.

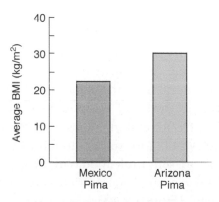

b. The Pima Indians of Mexico have the same genetic susceptibility to obesity as the Arizona Pimas but are farmers who work in the fields and consume the food they grow.[21] They still have higher rates of obesity than would be predicted from their diet and exercise patterns, suggesting that they possess genes that favor fat storage, but they are significantly less obese than the Arizona Pimas.[18]

Hunger is affected by sensations from the environment, signals from the gastrointestinal tract, and levels of nutrients and hormones circulating in the blood.

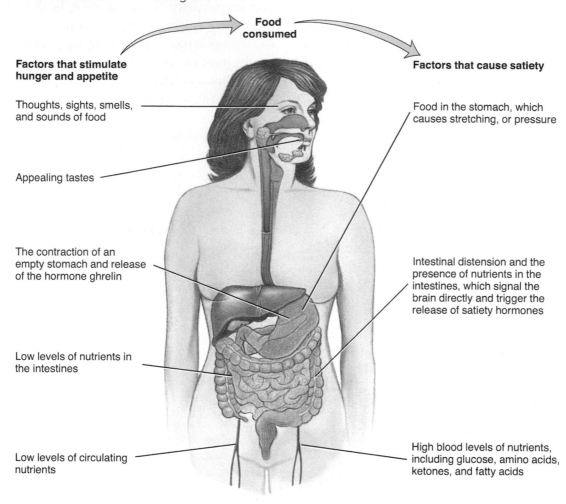

Food consumed

Factors that stimulate hunger and appetite

Thoughts, sights, smells, and sounds of food

Appealing tastes

The contraction of an empty stomach and release of the hormone ghrelin

Low levels of nutrients in the intestines

Low levels of circulating nutrients

Factors that cause satiety

Food in the stomach, which causes stretching, or pressure

Intestinal distension and the presence of nutrients in the intestines, which signal the brain directly and trigger the release of satiety hormones

High blood levels of nutrients, including glucose, amino acids, ketones, and fatty acids

Regulating how much we eat at each meal How do you know how much to eat for breakfast or when it is time to eat lunch? The physical sensations of hunger and satiety that determine how much you eat at each meal are triggered by neural and hormonal signals from the gastrointestinal tract, levels of nutrients and hormones circulating in the blood, and messages from the brain.[22] Some signals are sent before you eat to tell you that you are hungry, some are sent while food is in the gastrointestinal tract, and some occur when nutrients are circulating in the bloodstream (**Figure 9.13**).

The gastrointestinal tract releases hormones that are involved in the control of food intake. The hormone **ghrelin**, which is secreted by the stomach, is believed to stimulate the desire to eat at usual mealtimes. Blood levels of ghrelin rise an hour or two before a meal and drop very low after a meal. Peptide YY is one of a number of hormones that causes a reduction in appetite. It is released from the gastrointestinal tract after a meal, and the amount released is proportional to the number of calories in the meal.[22]

Psychological factors can also affect hunger and satiety. Some people eat for comfort and to relieve stress. Others lose their appetite when they experience these emotions. Psychological distress can alter the mechanisms that regulate food intake.

Regulating how much we weigh over the long term Sometimes we don't pay attention to how full we are after a meal, and we make room for dessert anyway. If this happens often enough, it can cause an increase in body weight and fatness. To return fatness to a set level, the body must be able to monitor how much fat is present. Some of this information comes from hormones.

Leptin is a good example of a hormone that can regulate body fatness in the long term. Leptin is produced by the adipocytes. The amount produced is proportional to the size of the adipocytes, and the effect of leptin on energy intake and expenditure depends on the amount released (see *What a Scientist Sees*). Unfortunately, leptin regulation, like other regulatory mechanisms, is much better at preventing weight loss than at preventing weight gain. Obese individuals generally have high levels of leptin, but these levels are not effective at reducing calorie intake and increasing energy expenditure.[23]

Despite regulatory mechanisms that act to keep our weight stable, changes in physiological, psychological, and environmental circumstances cause the level at which body weight is maintained to change, usually increasing it over time. This supports the hypothesis that the mechanisms that defend against weight loss are stronger than those that prevent weight gain.[24]

WHAT A SCIENTIST SEES
Leptin and Body Fat

The average person looking at the photo on the right sees a normal mouse and a very fat mouse. A scientist sees a clue to how body weight is regulated. The hormone leptin acts in a part of the brain called the hypothalamus to help maintain body fat at a normal level. As shown in the diagram, the effect of leptin depends on how much of it is present. If the mouse loses weight, fat is lost from adipocytes, and less leptin is released, causing an increase in food intake and a decrease in energy expenditure. If the mouse gains weight, the adipocytes accumulate fat, and more leptin is released, triggering events that decrease food intake and increase energy expenditure.

The mouse on the left inherited a defective leptin gene, so it produces no leptin. Even when the adipocytes enlarge, leptin levels do not increase. The lack of leptin continues to signal the mouse to eat more and expend less energy. The mouse on the right also inherited a defective leptin gene, but treatment with leptin injections returned its weight to normal.

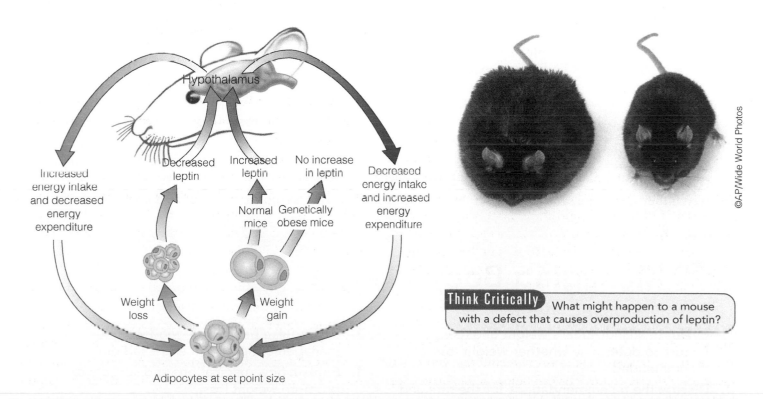

©AP/Wide World Photos

Think Critically What might happen to a mouse with a defect that causes overproduction of leptin?

Differences in NEAT can affect body weight • Figure 9.14

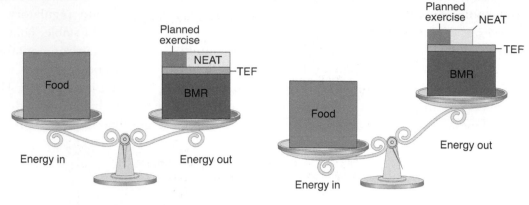

The number of calories a person expends in NEAT can affect their body weight. Person 1 (illustrated by the scale on the left) is weight stable. She eats the same number of calories as she burns per day. Person 2 (illustrated by the scale on the right) is gaining weight. She eats the same number of calories as person 1 and burns the same number of calories for BMR, TEF, and planned exercise, but her total energy expenditure is lower because she burns fewer calories through NEAT.

Person 1: Energy balance

Person 2: Weight gain

Why Do Some People Gain Weight More Easily?

A few cases of human obesity have been linked directly to defects in specific genes,[20] but mutations in single genes are not responsible for most human obesity.[15] Rather, variations in many genes interact with one another and affect metabolic rate, food intake, fat storage, and activity level. These in turn affect body weight, determining why some of us stay lean and others put on pounds.

Some people, such as the Pima Indians discussed earlier, may gain weight more easily because they inherited genes that make them more efficient at using energy and storing fat. Throughout human history, starvation has threatened survival. Over time, the human body has evolved ways to conserve body fat stores and prevent weight loss. Individuals with the "thriftiest" metabolism would have been more likely to survive. In the United States today, however, food is abundant, so people who inherited these "thrifty genes" are more likely to be obese.

Some people may gain weight more easily because they inherit a tendency to expend less energy on activity. Even if they spend the same amount of time engaged

in planned exercise as a lean person, a heavier person's total energy expenditure may be lower because he or she expends less energy for NEAT activities, such as housework, walking between classes, fidgeting, and moving to maintain posture (**Figure 9.14**). One of the factors hypothesized to contribute to obesity is the inability of susceptible individuals to compensate for increases in energy intake by increasing energy expenditure through NEAT. When obese and lean individuals who were overfed by 1000 Cal/day were compared, the lean study subjects walked more and sat less than the obese study subjects, thus burning off more of the extra calories.[25]

CONCEPT CHECK

1. **What** is the role of genes in regulating body weight?

2. **Why** do we feel hungry at about the same times every day?

3. **What** happens to leptin levels when you lose weight?

4. **Why** are some of us fat and some of us lean?

9.4 Managing Body Weight

LEARNING OBJECTIVES

1. **Evaluate** an individual's weight and risk factors to determine whether weight loss is recommended.

2. **Discuss** the recommendations for the rate and amount of weight loss.

3. **Distinguish** between a good weight management program and a fad diet.

4. **Explain** how medications and surgery can promote weight loss.

Weight-loss decisions • Figure 9.15

This decision tree can be used to determine whether someone would benefit from weight loss.[5]

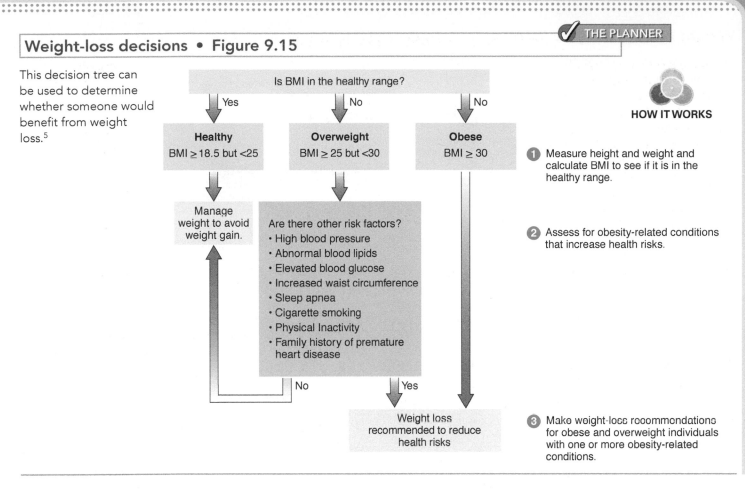

HOW IT WORKS

1 Measure height and weight and calculate BMI to see if it is in the healthy range.

2 Assess for obesity-related conditions that increase health risks.

3 Make weight-loss recommendations for obese and overweight individuals with one or more obesity-related conditions.

anaging your body weight to keep it in the healthy range requires maintaining a balance between energy intake and energy expenditure. For some people, weight management may mean avoiding weight gain as they age by making healthy food choices, controlling portion size, and maintaining an active lifestyle. For others, it may mean making major lifestyle changes in order to reduce their weight into the healthy range and keep it there.

Who Would Benefit from Weight Loss?

These days, just about everybody wants to lose a few pounds or more, but not everyone who is concerned about weight needs to lose weight in order to be healthy. The risks associated with carrying excess weight are related to the degree of the excess, the location of the excess fat, and the presence of other diseases or risk factors that often accompany excess body fat (**Figure 9.15**).

Weight-Loss Goals and Guidelines

The medical goal for weight loss is for overweight or obese people to reduce the health risks associated with their

excess body fat. The general recommendation is to lose 5 to 10% of body weight within 6 months. This amount of weight loss can lower blood pressure, reduce the risk of developing type 2 diabetes, improve blood cholesterol profiles, and reduce the need for medications to control blood pressure, blood glucose, and blood lipid levels.[5] After 6 months, risk factors can be assessed to determine the need for additional weight loss.

Because a pound of adipose tissue provides about 3500 Calories, losing a pound of fat requires decreasing intake and/or increasing expenditure by this amount. The approach that is best for an individual depends on personal preferences and his or her readiness to make lifestyle changes. Whatever the approach, losing weight slowly, at a rate of 1/2 to 2 pounds per week, helps ensure that most of what is lost is fat and not lean tissue. The more severe energy restriction needed for rapid weight loss leads to greater losses of water and protein and causes a more significant drop in BMR.

Successful long-term weight management requires changing the behavior patterns that led to weight gain in the first place. People who cut calories to lose weight generally achieve a maximal weight loss at about 6 months,

Weight cycling • Figure 9.16

Managing weight is an ongoing process that requires long-term changes in lifestyle. Often, weight loss leads to a pattern of repeated cycles of weight loss and gain, referred to as *weight cycling* or *yo-yo dieting*. Although this cycle was once thought to increase visceral fat storage and make future weight loss more difficult, current research shows that the benefits of weight loss outweigh any risk associated with weight cycling. [26]

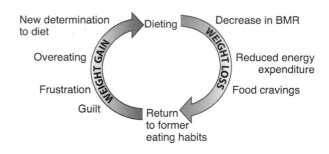

after which they regain some or all of the weight. This weight gain often leads to repeated cycles of weight loss and regain (**Figure 9.16**). Compared to diet alone, combining diet, activity, and **behavior modification** results in greater short-term weight loss and better weight maintenance in the long term (see *What Should I Eat?*).[5]

> **behavior modification** A process that is used to gradually and permanently change habitual behaviors.

Decreasing energy intake For healthy weight loss, intake must be low in energy but high in nutrients in order to provide for all the body's nutrient needs (see *Thinking it Through*). Even when choosing nutrient-dense foods, it is difficult to meet nutrient needs with an intake of fewer than 1200 Calories/day; therefore, dieters consuming less than this amount should take a multivitamin/multi-mineral supplement. Medical supervision is recommended if intake is below 800 Calories/day.

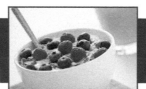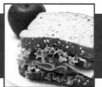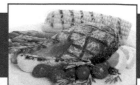

© Sara Winter/iStockphoto   © Jill Chen/iStockphoto   © Steve Mcsweeny/iStockphoto

WHAT SHOULD I EAT?

Weight Management

✔ THE PLANNER

Balance your intake and output
- Know your calorie needs and monitor what you eat.
- Weigh yourself frequently; if the number goes up, cut down your calories.
- When you add dessert, add extra exercise.
- Watch your alcohol consumption and count the calories in alcoholic beverages.

Cut down on calories
- Replace your sugar-sweetened soft drink with a glass of water with lemon.
- Put less dressing on your salad, less mayonnaise on your sandwich, and less butter on your toast
- Control your snacks—pour chips or crackers into a one-serving bowl rather than eating right from the bag or box.
- Choose a small drink and a small order of fries if you have fast food.

- Fill up on veggies—add less cheese and more vegetables to your pizza or omelet to fill you up with fewer calories
- When you eat out, share an entrée with a friend or take some home for lunch the next day.

Increase activity
- Go for a bike ride.
- Try bowling or miniature golf instead of watching TV on Friday nights.
- Take a walk during your lunch break or after dinner.
- Play tennis; you don't have to be good to get plenty of exercise.
- Boost your NEAT calories—small changes such as getting off the bus one stop early or parking at the back of the lot all add up.

 Use iProfile to calculate the number of calories you consume as between-meal snacks.

A Case Study on Food Choices and Body Weight

Leticia gained 15 pounds in her freshman year of college. She couldn't figure out why. She didn't think she was eating any differently than she did at home. She is a healthy 18-year-old who is 5 feet 4 inches tall and now weighs 155 lb.

 1 What is her BMI? Is it in the healthy range? Does she need to lose weight? (Hint: Use the decision tree in Figure 9.15.)

Your answer:

Leticia decides to keep a diary of what and when she eats. The diary shows that she eats a lot at night while studying. She tends to keep an open bag of chips or a package of cookies and bottle of cola at her desk. She estimates that she eats enough to add about 600 Calories to her daily intake.

 2 Suggest some behavioral strategies to reduce the number of calories she consumes while studying.

Your answer:

 3 Use iProfile to suggest some satisfying snacks with 200 Calories or less that Leticia could keep in her dorm room to replace the high-calorie ones she has been eating.

Your answer:

Leticia's food diary shows that her highest caloric meals are the ones she eats when she leaves campus to have lunch with friends at fast-food restaurants. Meal A, shown below, is her typical lunch, and Meal B is the lower-calorie lunch that she plans to replace it with.

 4 How can Meal B have fewer calories even though it looks like more food?

Your answer:

 5 Why might Meal B satisfy hunger just as well as or better than Meal A?

Your answer:

(Check your answers in online appendix L)

Meal A

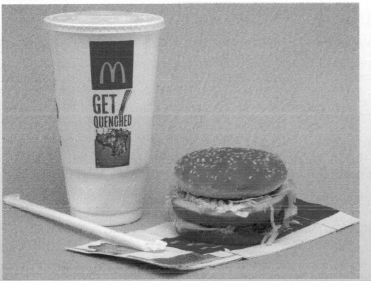

Andy Washnik

Meal B

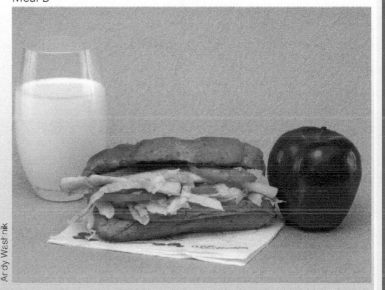

Andy Washnik

Increasing physical activity Exercise increases energy expenditure and therefore makes weight loss easier. If food intake stays the same, adding enough exercise to expend 200 Calories 5 days a week will result in the loss of a pound in about 3½ weeks. Exercise also promotes muscle development, and because muscle is metabolically active tissue, increased muscle mass increases energy expenditure. In addition, physical activity improves overall fitness and relieves boredom and stress. Weight loss is maintained better when physical activity is included. The benefits of exercise are discussed more fully in Chapter 10.

To achieve and maintain a healthy body weight, the 2010 *Dietary Guidelines for Americans* recommend that adults engage in the equivalent of 150 minutes of moderate-intensity aerobic activity per week.[9] Those who are overweight or obese may need to gradually increase their weekly minutes of aerobic physical activity over time and decrease calorie intake to achieve a negative energy balance and reach a healthy weight. The amount of activity needed to achieve and maintain a healthy body weight varies; some may need more than the equivalent of 300 minutes per week of moderate-intensity activity.

Modifying behavior To successfully lose weight and keep it off, the food consumption and exercise patterns that led to weight gain need to be identified and replaced with new ones that promote and maintain weight loss (**Figure 9.17**). Successful behavior modification includes regular self-monitoring of food intake, physical activity, and weight. Behavior modification can help you to establish patterns of food intake and exercise that you can maintain throughout your life without gaining weight.

Managing America's weight To become a thinner nation, we need strategies that can help all Americans improve their food choices, reduce portion sizes, and increase their physical activity.[27] Although successful weight management ultimately depends on an individual's choices, food manufacturers and restaurants can help us cut calories by offering healthier foods and by packaging or serving foods in smaller portions. Communities can help increase activity by providing parks, bike paths, and other recreational facilities for people of all ages. Businesses and schools can contribute by offering more opportunities for physical activity at the workplace and during the school day.

Even small changes, if they are consistent, can arrest the increase in obesity in the population. It has been estimated that a population-wide shift in energy balance of only 100 Calories/day, the equivalent of walking a mile or cutting out a scoop of ice cream, would prevent further weight gain in 90% of the population.[24]

Suggestions for Weight Gain

As difficult as weight loss is for some people, weight gain can be equally elusive for underweight individuals. The first step toward weight gain is to rule out medical reasons for low body weight. This is particularly important when weight loss occurs unexpectedly. If low body weight is due to low-energy intake or high-energy expenditure, gradually increasing consumption of energy-dense foods is suggested. Energy intake can be increased by eating meals more frequently; adding healthy high-calorie snacks, such as nuts, peanut butter, or milkshakes, between meals; and replacing low-calorie drinks such as water and diet beverages with 100% fruit juices and milk.

To encourage a gain in muscle rather than fat, muscle-strengthening exercise should be a component of any weight-gain program. This approach requires extra calories to fuel the activity needed to build muscles. These weight-gain recommendations apply to individuals who are naturally thin and have trouble gaining weight on the recommended energy intake. However, this dietary approach may not promote weight gain for those who limit intake because of an eating disorder.

Diets and Fad Diets

Want to lose 10 lb in just 5 days? What dieter wouldn't? People who are desperate to lose weight are prey to all sorts of diets that promise quick fixes. They willingly eat a single food for days at a time, select foods on the basis of special fat-burning qualities, and consume odd combinations at specific times of the day. Most diets, no matter how outlandish, will promote weight loss because they reduce energy intake. Even diets that focus on modifying fat or carbohydrate intake or promise to allow unlimited amounts of certain foods work because intake is reduced. The true test of the effectiveness of a weight-loss plan is whether it promotes weight loss that can be maintained over the long term.

People often don't recognize that if you lose weight, you need to eat less to stay at the lower weight. For example, an inactive 30-year-old, 5'4" woman who weighs 170 lb needs to consume about 2100 Calories/day to maintain her weight. If she loses 40 lb but does not change her activity

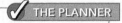
ABCs of behavior modification • Figure 9.17

Behavior modification is based on the theory that behaviors involve three factors: antecedents or cues that lead to a behavior, the behavior itself, and the consequences of the behavior. These are referred to as the ABCs of behavior modification. The example shown here illustrates how changing the antecendent can change behavior and help reduce food intake to manage weight.

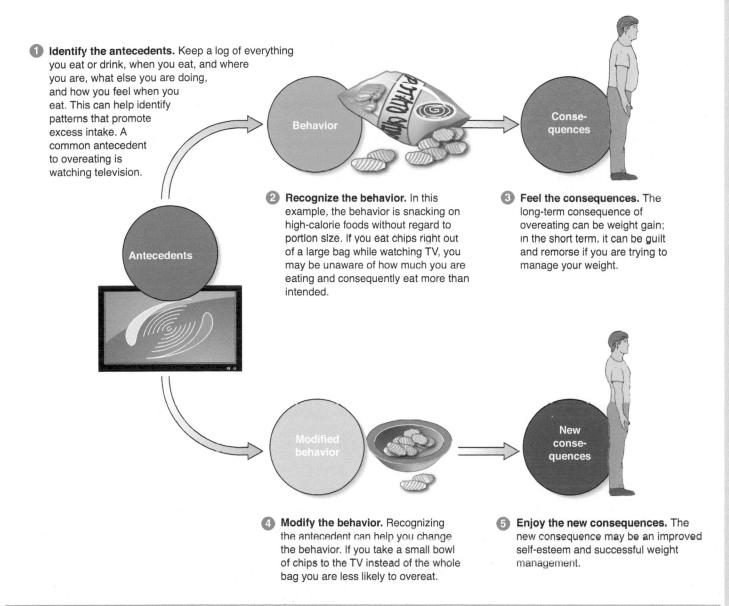

1 **Identify the antecedents.** Keep a log of everything you eat or drink, when you eat, and where you are, what else you are doing, and how you feel when you eat. This can help identify patterns that promote excess intake. A common antecedent to overeating is watching television.

2 **Recognize the behavior.** In this example, the behavior is snacking on high-calorie foods without regard to portion size. If you eat chips right out of a large bag while watching TV, you may be unaware of how much you are eating and consequently eat more than intended.

3 **Feel the consequences.** The long-term consequence of overeating can be weight gain; in the short term, it can be guilt and remorse if you are trying to manage your weight.

4 **Modify the behavior.** Recognizing the antecedent can help you change the behavior. If you take a small bowl of chips to the TV instead of the whole bag you are less likely to overeat.

5 **Enjoy the new consequences.** The new consequence may be an improved self-esteem and successful weight management.

level, she will need to consume only about 1880 Calories to maintain her healthier reduced weight. If, once the weight is lost, she resumes her pre-weight-loss dietary pattern, eating 2100 Calories/day, she will regain all the lost weight.

Effective weight-management programs promote healthy weight-loss diets and encourage changes in the lifestyle patterns that led to weight gain. When selecting a program, look for one that is based on sound nutrition

Distinguishing between healthy diets and fad diets   Table 9.2

A healthy diet . . .	A fad diet . . .
Promotes a healthy dietary pattern that meets nutrient needs, includes a variety of foods, suits food preferences, and can be maintained throughout life.	Limits food selections to a few food groups or promotes rituals such as eating only specific food combinations. As a result, it may be limited in certain nutrients and in variety.
Promotes a reasonable weight loss of 0.5 to 2 lb/week and does not restrict energy to under 1200 Cal/day.	Promotes rapid weight loss of much more than 2 lb/week.
Promotes or includes physical activity.	Advertises weight loss without the need to exercise.
Is flexible enough to be followed when eating out and includes foods that are easily obtained.	May require a rigid menu or avoidance of certain foods or may include "magic" foods that promise to burn fat or speed up metabolism.
Does not require costly supplements.	May require the purchase of special foods, weight-loss patches, expensive supplements, creams, or other products.
Promotes a change in behavior. Teaches new eating habits. Provides social support.	Does not recommend changes in activity and eating habits, recommends an eating pattern that is difficult to follow for life, or provides no support other than a book that must be purchased.
Is based on sound scientific principles and may include monitoring by qualified health professionals.	Makes outlandish and unscientific claims, does not support claims that it is clinically tested or scientifically proven, claims that it is new and improved or based on some new scientific discovery, or relies on testimonials from celebrities or connects the diet to trendy places such as Beverly Hills.

and exercise principles, suits your individual preferences in terms of food choices as well as time and costs, and promotes long-term lifestyle changes. Quick fixes are tempting, but if the program's approach is not one that can be followed for a lifetime, it is unlikely to promote successful weight management (**Table 9.2**).

Some of the most common methods for reducing calorie intake include using food guides such as My-Plate for diet planning, eating a moderate to high protein diet, choosing preportioned meals or liquid meals, and reducing the fat or carbohydrate content of the diet (**Figure 9.18**). All these methods cause weight loss by limiting, in one way or another, the number of calories consumed.

Weight-Loss Medications and Supplements

Prescription medications for the treatment of obesity include those that reduce appetite by affecting the activity of brain neurotransmitters (for example, phentermine, trade name Adipex) and those that decrease the absorption of fat in the intestine (for example, orlistat, brand name Xenical). Medications such as these are recommended along with diet and exercise for individuals with a BMI $\geq$ 30 kg/m^2 or a BMI $\geq$ 27 kg/m^2 with one or more obesity-related risk factors. Weight-loss medication may also be considered for anyone who would benefit from weight loss but who has not been able to lose enough weight through lifestyle modification to improve health.[5] As with any treatment, the risks should be weighed against the benefits before starting a medication for weight loss. One of the major disadvantages of drug treatment is that even if the drug promotes weight loss, the weight is usually regained when the drug is discontinued.

Like prescription drugs, over-the-counter weight-loss medications are regulated by the FDA and must adhere to strict guidelines regarding the dose per pill and the effectiveness of the ingredients. The FDA has approved

Common dieting methods • Figure 9.18

Weight-loss diets take a variety of forms, but all cause weight loss by promoting a reduction in energy intake.

a. Food guides

The MyPlate My Weight Manager recommends amounts from various food groups to meet the dieter's goals. Diets based on food guides are varied and are likely to meet nutrient needs. They teach meal-planning skills that are easy to apply away from home and can be used over the long term. ▼

Daily Calorie Limit			Daily Food Group Targets		More Info▸		
			Grains	**Vegetables**	**Fruits**	**Dairy**	**Protein Foods**
Allowance	2000	Target	6 oz.	2½ cup(s)	2 cup(s)	3 cup(s)	5½ oz.
Eaten	0	Eaten	0 oz.	0 cup(s)	0 cup(s)	0 cup(s)	0 oz.
Remaining	2000	Status	-	-	-	-	-

High protein menu

Breakfast

8 oz. nonfat yogurt

Ham slices

Vanilla oatbran porridge

Snack

4 oz. nonfat cottage cheese

Lunch

Hard-boiled egg with herb mayonnaise

5 oz. steak

8 oz. nonfat yogurt

Snack

4 oz. nonfat yogurt

Dinner

1 lb. shrimp sauteed in herbs

8 oz. tandoori chicken cutlets

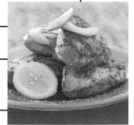

Images of Africa/Getty

b. Moderate to high protein diets

Many popular weight-loss diets promote a protein intake of 25% or more of calories. These high-protein diets rely ▲ on meat and eggs as the primary source of calories. The high protein content promotes satiety and preserves muscle mass, but this approach has not been shown to be more effective for weight loss than other calorie-restricted diets.[5,28] These diets are difficult to stick with in the long term, and low intakes of fruits, vegetables, and grains reduce nutritional adequacy.

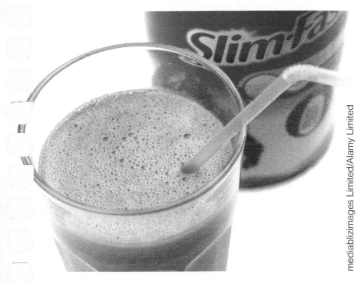

medialblizimages Limited/Alamy Limited

c. Liquid and prepackaged meals
▲ Liquid formulas and preportioned meals make portion control easy, but they are not practical when traveling or eating out, and they do not teach the food-selection skills needed to make a long-term lifestyle change. Programs that rely exclusively on liquid formulas are not recommended without medical supervision.

d. Reduced fat diets

Low-fat diets typically reduce calorie intake ▶ because fat is high in calories. Low-fat diets can include large quantities of fresh fruits and vegetables, which are low in fat and calories and high in nutrients. But just because a food is low in fat does not mean it is low in calories. In the 1990s, low-fat cookies, crackers, and cakes flooded the market. These foods were low in fat but not in calories. When eaten in excess, they contributed to weight gain.

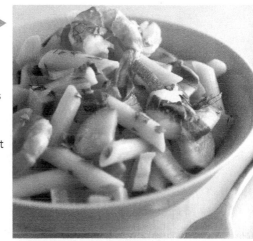

Think Critically Which of these diet plans will promote weight loss? Which are best for long-term weight management?

food and drink photos/Masterfile

Branislav Senic/iStockphoto

e. Carbohydrate-restricted diets

Carbohydrate-restricted diets limit total carbohydrate or allow only low glycemic index carbs, such as legumes and vegetables. Low-carb diets promote weight loss because people eat less. This may be due to metabolic changes that suppress appetite, but intake is also reduced because of the monotony of the food choices.[29] Low-carb diets that restrict choices from entire food groups are not nutritionally adequate and are rarely adhered to in the long term. ▶

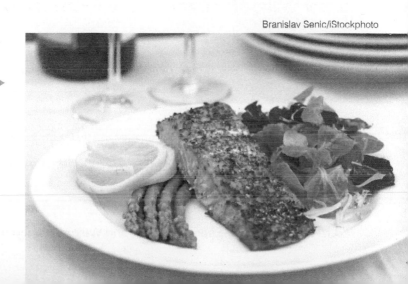

only a limited number of substances for sale as nonprescription weight-loss medications. One of these is a nonprescription version of orlistat (**Figure 9.19**). As with prescription drugs, any weight loss that occurs with over-the-counter weight-loss medications is usually regained when the product is no longer consumed.

In addition to weight-loss medications, hundreds of dietary supplements claim to promote weight loss. As with other dietary supplements, weight-loss supplements are not strictly regulated by the FDA, so their safety and effectiveness may not have been carefully tested. Some products claiming to be weight-loss supplements have been found to contain hidden prescription drugs or compounds that have not been adequately studied in humans.[30] It cannot be assumed that a product is safe simply because it is labeled a dietary supplement or as "herbal" or "all natural."

Weight-loss supplements that contain soluble fiber promise to reduce the amount you eat by filling up your stomach. Although they are safe, their use may contribute to only small amounts of weight loss.[31] Hydroxycitric acid, conjugated linoleic acid, and chromium picolinate are weight-loss supplements that promise to enhance fat loss by altering metabolism so as to prevent the synthesis and deposition of fat. None of these supplements has been shown to be effective for promoting weight loss in humans.[31] Supplements that boost energy expenditure, often called "fat burners," can be effective but have serious and potentially life-threatening side effects. One of the most popular and controversial herbal fat burners is ephedra, a stimulant that increases blood pressure and heart rate and constricts blood vessels. Due to safety concerns, the FDA banned it in 2004. After the ban was instituted, supplement manufacturers began substituting other herbal products, such as bitter orange, that contain similar stimulants and therefore may have similar side effects.[31] Fat burners also typically contain guarana, an herbal source of caffeine. Green tea extract is another

Alli: Blocking fat absorption • Figure 9.19

Alli is an over-the-counter version of the prescription drug orlistat. It acts by disabling the enzyme lipase, which breaks triglycerides into fatty acids and monoglycerides. When Alli is present, the triglycerides are not broken down, so they cannot be absorbed. The undigested fat is eliminated in the feces. This cuts the number of calories from fat that get into your body, but it is not without side effects. Fat in the colon may cause gas, diarrhea, and more frequent and hard-to-control bowel movements.

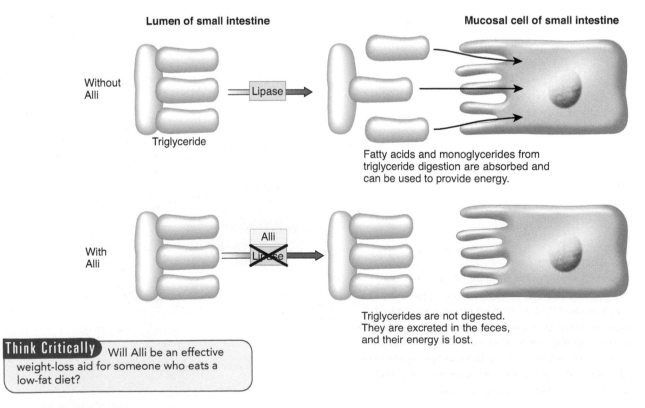

Lumen of small intestine   **Mucosal cell of small intestine**

Without Alli

Lipase

Triglyceride

Fatty acids and monoglycerides from triglyceride digestion are absorbed and can be used to provide energy.

With Alli

Alli

Lipase

Triglycerides are not digested. They are excreted in the feces, and their energy is lost.

Think Critically Will Alli be an effective weight-loss aid for someone who eats a low-fat diet?

popular supplement used to boost metabolism and aid weight loss. It is also a source of caffeine as well as phytochemicals call catechins. Studies have shown it to have only a small effect on weight loss in certain populations Consuming green tea is safe, but green tea extract has been associated with liver damage.[31]

Taking some dietary supplements results in weight loss through water loss—either because these supplements are diuretics or because they cause diarrhea. Water loss decreases body weight but does not cause a decrease in body fat. Herbal laxatives found in weight-loss teas and supplements include senna, aloe, buckthorn, rhubarb root, cascara, and castor oil. Overuse of these substances can have serious side effects, including diarrhea, electrolyte imbalances, and liver and kidney toxicity.[32]

Weight-Loss Surgery

For individuals who have a BMI ≥ 40 or a BMI ≥ 35 with one or more obesity-related risk factors and who have failed to lose sufficient weight to improve their health using lifestyle interventions, there are a number of surgical weight loss options. **Adjustable gastric banding** and **gastric sleeve surgery** both restrict the amount of food that can be consumed (**Figure 9.20**).

Weight-loss surgery • Figure 9.20

Gastric banding, gastric sleeve surgery, and gastric bypass are three common surgical approaches to treating obesity.

a. Gastric banding involves surgically placing an adjustable band around the upper part of the stomach, creating a small pouch. The narrow opening between the stomach pouch and the rest of the stomach slows the rate at which food leaves the pouch. This promotes weight loss by reducing the amount of food that can be consumed at one time and slowing digestion. Gastric banding entails less surgical risk and is more easily reversible than other types of weight-loss surgery.

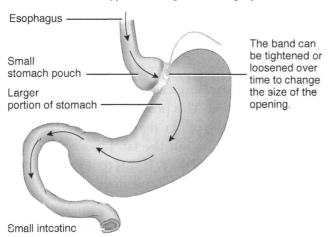

b. Gastric sleeve surgery involves surgically removing a large part of the stomach. This reduces the amount of food that can be consumed at one time. The procedure is not reversible, and since it is relatively new, the long-term risks and effectiveness are not known.

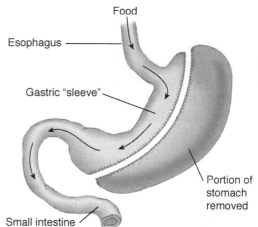

c. The type of gastric bypass surgery shown here involves bypassing part of the stomach and small intestine by connecting the intestine to the upper portion of the stomach. Food intake is reduced because the stomach is smaller, and absorption is reduced because the small intestine is shortened. Gastric bypass entails short-term surgical risks and a long-term risk of nutrient deficiencies, particularly of vitamin B_{12}, folate, calcium, and iron, because absorption of these nutrients is reduced.

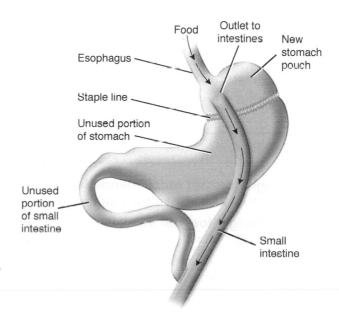

eating disorder A psychological illness characterized by specific abnormal eating behaviors, often intended to control weight.

anorexia nervosa An eating disorder characterized by self-starvation, a distorted body image, abnormally low body weight, and a pathological fear of becoming fat.

bulimia nervosa An eating disorder characterized by the consumption of a large amount of food at one time (binge eating) followed by purging behaviors such as self-induced vomiting to prevent weight gain.

aspects of food and eating overpower the role of food as nourishment, an **eating disorder** may develop. Eating disorders affect physical and nutritional health and psychosocial functioning. If untreated, they can be fatal.

Types of Eating Disorders

Mental health guidelines define a number of eating disorders including **anorexia nervosa**, **bulimia nervosa**, and **binge-eating disorder** (**Table 9.3**).[40]

What Causes Eating Disorders?

We do not completely understand what causes eating disorders, but we do know that genetic, psychological, and sociocultural factors contribute to their development

(**Figure 9.21**). Eating disorders can be triggered by traumatic events such as sexual abuse or by day-to-day occurrences such as teasing or judgmental comments by a friend or a coach. Eating disorders occur in people of all ages, races, and socioeconomic backgrounds, but some groups are at greater risk than others. Women are more likely than men to develop eating disorders. Professional dancers, models, and others who are concerned about maintaining a low body weight are most likely to develop eating disorders. Eating disorders commonly begin in adolescence, when physical, psychological, and social development is occurring rapidly.

Psychological issues People with eating disorders often have low self-esteem. *Self-esteem* refers to the judgments people make and maintain about themselves—a general attitude of approval or disapproval about worth and capability. A poor **body image** contributes to low self-esteem. Eating disorders are characterized not only by dissatisfaction with one's body but

binge-eating disorder An eating disorder characterized by recurrent episodes of binge eating accompanied by a loss of control over eating in the absence of purging behavior.

body image The way a person perceives and imagines his or her body.

Distinguishing among eating disorders Table 9.3

Characteristic	Eating disorder		
	Anorexia nervosa	**Bulimia nervosa**	**Binge-eating disorder**
Body weight	Below normal	Usually normal	Above normal
Binge eating	Possibly	Yes, at least once a week for 3 months	Yes, at least once a week for 3 or more months
Purging	Possibly	Yes, at least once a week for 3 months	No
Restricts food intake	Yes	Yes	Yes
Body image	Dissatisfaction with body and distorted image of body size	Dissatisfaction with body and distorted image of body size	Dissatisfaction with body
Fear of being fat	Yes	Yes	Not excessive
Self-esteem	Low	Low	Low
Typical age of onset	Preadolescence/adolescence	Adolescence/young adults	Adults of all ages

Eating disorders are caused by a combination of genetic, psychological, and sociocultural factors. Although these disorders are not necessarily passed from parent to child, the genes that a person inherits contribute to psychological and biological characteristics that can predispose him or her to developing an eating disorder. When placed in the right sociocultural environment, an individual who carries such genes will be more likely than others to develop an eating disorder.

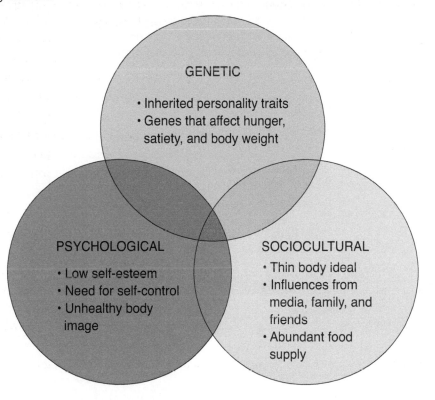

GENETIC
- Inherited personality traits
- Genes that affect hunger, satiety, and body weight

PSYCHOLOGICAL
- Low self-esteem
- Need for self-control
- Unhealthy body image

SOCIOCULTURAL
- Thin body ideal
- Influences from media, family, and friends
- Abundant food supply

also with distorted body image. Someone with a distorted body image is unable to judge the size of his or her own body. Thus, even if a young woman achieves a body weight comparable to that of a fashion model, she may continue to see herself as fat and strive to lose more weight.

People with eating disorders are often perfectionists who set very high standards for themselves and strive to be in control of their bodies and their lives. Despite their many achievements, they feel inadequate, defective, and worthless. They may use their relationship with food to gain control over their lives and boost their self-esteem. Controlling their food intake and weight demonstrates their ability to control other aspects of their lives and they can associate this control with success.

Sociocultural issues What is viewed as an "ideal" body differs across cultures and has changed throughout history (**Figure 9.22**). Cultural ideals about body size are linked to body image and the incidence of eating disorders.[43] Eating disorders occur in societies where food is abundant and the body ideal is thin. They do not occur in societies where food is scarce and people must worry about where their next meal is coming from.

U.S. culture today is a culture of thinness. Messages about what society views as a perfect body—the ideal that we should strive for—are constantly delivered by television, movies, magazines, advertisements, and even toys. Tall, lean fashion models adorn billboards and magazine covers. Thinness is associated with beauty, success, intelligence, and vitality. A young woman facing a future in which she must be independent, have a prestigious job, maintain a successful love relationship, bear and nurture children, manage a household, and keep up with fashion trends can become overwhelmed. Unable to master all these roles, she may look for some aspect of her life that she can control. Food intake and body weight are natural choices because thinness is associated with success. These messages about how we should look are hard to ignore and can create

What is viewed as a desirable body size and shape is influenced by society and culture.

a. A fuller figure is still desirable in many cultures. Young women in these cultures, such as the Zulu of South Africa, may struggle to gain weight in order to achieve what is viewed as the ideal female body. As television images of very thin Western women become more accessible, the Zulu cultural view of plumpness as desirable may be changing.[41]

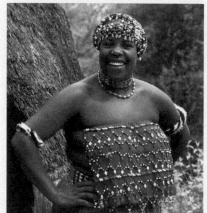

SC Photos/Alamy

b. Thinness has not always been the beauty standard in the United States. This time line shows how the female body ideal has changed over the years. As female models, actresses, and other cultural icons have become thinner over the past several decades, the incidence of eating disorders has increased.

Lillian Russell

Actress Lillian Russell **1900** is considered a beauty at about 200 pounds

Bettmann/© Corbis

Marilyn Monroe

The thinner flapper **1920s** look becomes popular

© Bettmann/© Corbis

The curvy figure of **1950s** Marilyn Monroe becomes the beauty standard

Twiggy

Twiggy, who weighs **1960s** less than 100 pounds, is the leading model

© Bettmann/© Corbis

Jane Fonda's workout **1980s** book is a best seller

The fashion ideal today is thin but well muscled **Today**

Masterfile

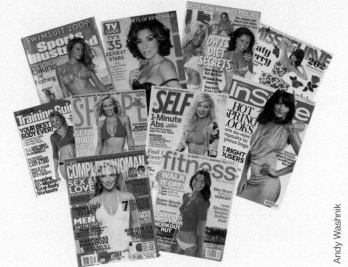

Andy Washnik

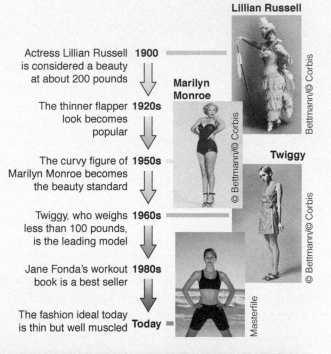

Michael Nichols/NG Image Collection

c. Magazine covers and advertisements emphasize thinness as a standard for female beauty. These "ideal" bodies are frequently atypical of normal, healthy women. Fashion models today weigh 23% less than the average female. Although many women strive for this thin ideal, only 1% of young women have a chance of being as thin as a supermodel.[42]

d. The toys that children play with set a cultural standard for body ideal. Little girls playing with Barbie dolls want to be like Barbie when they grow up, and boys playing with Superman, Batman, or GI Joe action figures want to be like them. This includes looking like them. Unfortunately, Barbie's measurements would be virtually unachievable if Barbie were life-sized. The same is true of the big chest, muscular arms and legs, and flat stomach with "six-pack" abs seen on male action figures.

pressure to achieve this ideal body. But it is a standard that is very difficult to meet—a standard that is contributing to disturbances in body image and eating behavior.

Although men currently represent a small percentage of people with eating disorders, the numbers are increasing.[44] This is likely due to increasing pressure to achieve an ideal male body. Advertisements directed at men are showing more and more exposed skin, with a focus on well-defined abdominal and chest muscles.

Anorexia Nervosa

Anorexia means lack of appetite, but in the case of the eating disorder anorexia nervosa, it is a desire to be thin, rather than a lack of appetite, that causes individuals to decrease their food intake. Anorexia nervosa is characterized by a distorted body image, excessive dieting that leads to severe weight loss, and a pathological fear of being fat. It typically begins in adolescence and affects 0.5 to 3.7% of women in their lifetime. There is a 5% death rate in the first 2 years, and the death rate can reach 20% in untreated individuals.[45]

The psychological component of anorexia nervosa revolves around an overwhelming fear of gaining weight, even in individuals who are already underweight. It is not uncommon for individuals with anorexia to feel that they would rather be dead than fat. Anorexia is also characterized by disturbances in body image or perception of body size that prevent those with this disorder from seeing themselves as underweight even when they

are dangerously thin. People with this disorder may use body weight and shape as a means of self-evaluation: "If I weren't so fat, everyone would like and respect me, and I wouldn't have other problems." However, no matter how much weight they lose, they do not gain self-respect, inner assurance, or the happiness they seek. Therefore, they continue to restrict their intake and use other behaviors to lose weight.

The most obvious behaviors associated with anorexia are those that contribute to the maintenance of a body weight that is less than minimally normal. These behaviors include restriction of food intake, binge-eating and purging episodes in some patients, strange eating rituals, and excessive activity (**Figure 9.23**). For some individuals with anorexia, the increase in activity is surreptitious, such as going up and down stairs repeatedly or getting off the bus a few stops too early. For others, the activity takes the form of strenuous physical exercise. They may become fanatical athletes and feel guilty if they cannot exercise. They link exercise and eating, so a certain amount of exercise earns them the right to eat, and if they eat too much, they must pay the price by adding extra exercise. They do not stop when they are tired; instead, they train compulsively beyond reasonable endurance.

The first obvious physical manifestation of anorexia is weight loss. As weight loss becomes severe, symptoms of starvation begin to appear. Starvation affects mental function, causing the person to become apathetic, dull, exhausted, and depressed. Fat stores are depleted. Other symptoms that appear include muscle wasting,

A day in the life of a person with anorexia • Figure 9.23

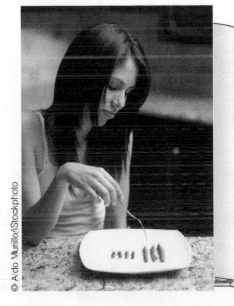

For individuals with anorexia, food and eating become an obsession. In addition to restricting the total amount of food they consume, people with anorexia develop personal diet rituals, limiting certain foods and eating them in specific ways. Although they do not consume very much food, they are preoccupied with food and spend an enormous amount of time thinking about it, talking about it, and preparing meals for others. Instead of eating, they move the food around the plate and cut it into tiny pieces.

© Aldo Murillo/iStockphoto

Dear Diary,
    For breakfast today I had a cup of tea. For lunch I ate some lettuce and a slice of tomato, but no dressing. I cooked dinner for my family. I love to cook, but it is hard not to taste. I tried a new chicken recipe and served it with rice and asparagus. I even made a chocolate cake for dessert but I didn't even lick the bowl from the frosting. When it came time to eat, I only took a little. I told my mom I nibbled while cooking. I pushed the food around on my plate so no one would notice that I only ate a few bites. I was good today - I kept my food intake under control. The scale says I have lost 20 pounds but I still look fat.

inflammation and swelling of the lips, flaking and peeling of the skin, growth of fine hair (lanugo hair) on the body, and dry, thin, brittle hair on the head. In females, estrogen levels drop, and in some women menstruation becomes irregular or stops. In males, testosterone levels decrease. In the final stages of starvation, the person experiences abnormalities in electrolyte and fluid balance and cardiac irregularities. Suppression of immune function leads to infection, which further increases nutritional needs.

The goal of treatment for anorexia nervosa is to help resolve the underlying psychological and behavioral problems while providing for physical and nutritional rehabilitation. Treatment requires an interdisciplinary team of nutritional, psychological, and medical specialists and typically requires years of therapy. The goal of nutrition intervention is to promote weight gain by increasing energy intake and expanding dietary choices.[46] In more severe cases of anorexia, hospitalization is required so that food intake and exercise behaviors can be controlled. Intravenous nutrition may be necessary to keep a patient with anorexia alive. Some people with anorexia make full recoveries, but about half have poor long-term outcomes—remaining irrationally concerned about weight gain and never achieving normal body weight. Some patients with anorexia also transition to bulimia nervosa.[47]

Bulimia Nervosa

The word *bulimia* comes from the Greek *bous* ("ox") and *limos* ("hunger"), denoting hunger of such intensity that a person could eat an entire ox. The term *bulimia nervosa* was coined in 1979 by a British psychiatrist who suggested that bulimia consists of powerful urges to overeat in combination with a morbid fear of becoming fat and avoidance of the fattening effects of food by inducing vomiting and/or abusing purgatives.[48]

Bulimia is characterized by frequent episodes of binge eating followed by inappropriate behaviors such as self-induced vomiting to avoid weight gain. Like individuals with anorexia, those with bulimia have an intense fear of becoming fat and a negative body image, accompanied by a distorted perception of body size. Because self-esteem is highly tied to impressions of body shape and weight, people with bulimia may blame all their problems on their appearance. They are preoccupied with the fear that once they start eating, they will not be able to stop. They may engage in continuous dieting, which leads to a preoccupation with food. They are often socially isolated and may avoid situations that will expose them to food, such as going to parties or out to dinner; thus they become further isolated.

Bulimia typically begins with food restriction motivated by the desire to be thin. Overwhelming hunger may finally cause the dieting to be interrupted by a period of overeating. Eventually a pattern develops that consists of semistarvation interrupted by periods of gorging. During a binge-eating episode, a person with bulimia experiences a sense of lack of control. Binges usually last less than 2 hours and occur in secrecy. Eating stops when the food runs out or when pain, fatigue, or an interruption intervenes. The amount of food consumed in a binge may not always be enormous, but the individual perceives it as a binge episode (**Figure 9.24**).

A day in the life of a person with bulimia • Figure 9.24

The amount of food consumed during a binge varies but is typically on the order of 3400 Calories, while a normal young woman may consume only about 2000 Calories in an entire day. Self-induced vomiting is the most common purging behavior. At first, a physical maneuver such as sticking a finger down the throat is needed to induce vomiting, but patients eventually learn to vomit at will. Bingeing and purging are followed by intense feelings of guilt and shame.

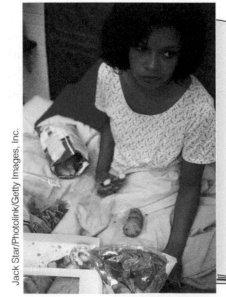

Jack Star/Photolink/Getty Images, Inc.

Dear Diary,
    Today started well. I stuck to my diet through breakfast, lunch, and dinner, but by 8 PM I was feeling depressed and bored. I thought food would make me feel better. Before I knew it I was at the convenience store buying two pints of ice cream, a large bag of chips, a one pound package of cookies, a half dozen candy bars, and a quart of milk. I told the clerk I was having a party. But it was a party of one. Alone in my dorm room I started by eating the chips, then polished off the cookies and the candy bars, washing them down with milk and finishing with the ice cream. Luckily no one was around so I was able to vomit without anyone hearing. I feel weak and guilty but also relieved that I got rid of all those calories. Tomorrow, I will start a new diet.

A day in the life of a person with binge-eating disorder • Figure 9.25

People with binge-eating disorder often seek help for their weight rather than for their disordered eating pattern. It is estimated that about 5 million women and 3 million men in the United States suffer from binge-eating disorder.[50]

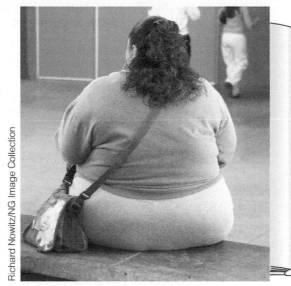

Richard Nowitz/NG Image Collection

Dear Diary,

I got on the scale today. What a mistake! My weight is up to 250 pounds. I hate myself for being so fat. Just seeing that I gained more weight made me feel ashamed – all I wanted to do was bury my feelings in a box of cookies or a carton of ice cream. Why do I always think the food will help? Once I started eating I couldn't stop. When I finally did I felt even more disgusted, depressed, and guilty. I am always on a diet but it is never long before I lose control and pig out. I know my eating and my weight are not healthy but I just can't seem to stop.

After binge episodes, individuals with bulimia use various behaviors to eliminate the extra calories and prevent weight gain. Some use behaviors such as fasting or excessive exercise, but most use purging behaviors such as vomiting or taking laxatives, diuretics, or other medications. Self-induced vomiting does eliminate some of the food before the nutrients have been absorbed, preventing weight gain, but laxatives and diuretics cause only water loss. Nutrient absorption is almost complete before food enters the colon, where laxatives have their effect. The weight loss associated with laxative abuse is due to dehydration. Diuretics also cause water loss, but via the kidney rather than the GI tract. They do not cause fat loss.

It is the purging portion of the binge/purge cycle that is most hazardous to health. Vomiting brings stomach acid into the mouth. Frequent vomiting can cause tooth decay, sores in the mouth and on the lips, swelling of the jaw and salivary glands, irritation of the throat and esophagus, and changes in stomach capacity and the rate of stomach emptying.[46] It also causes broken blood vessels in the face due to the force of vomiting, as well as electrolyte imbalance, dehydration, muscle weakness, and menstrual irregularities. Laxative and diuretic abuse can also lead to dehydration and electrolyte imbalance.

The overall goal of therapy for people with bulimia nervosa is to reduce or eliminate bingeing and purging behavior by separating the patients' eating behavior from their emotions and their perceptions of success and promoting eating in response to hunger and satiety. Psychological issues related to body image and a sense of lack of control over eating must be resolved. Nutritional therapy must address physiological imbalances caused by purging episodes as well as provide education on nutrient needs and how to meet them. Treatment has been found to speed recovery, especially if it is provided soon after symptoms begin, but for some women, this disorder may remain a chronic problem throughout life.[49]

Binge-Eating Disorder

Binge-eating disorder is the most common eating disorder. Unlike anorexia and bulimia, binge-eating disorder is not uncommon in men, who account for about 40% of cases.[50] It is most common in overweight individuals (**Figure 9.25**). Individuals with binge-eating disorder engage in recurrent episodes of binge eating and experience a loss of control over eating but do not regularly engage in purging behaviors.

The major complications of binge-eating disorder are the health problems associated with obesity, which include diabetes, high blood pressure, high blood cholesterol levels, gallbladder disease, heart disease, and certain types of cancer. Treatment of binge-eating disorder involves counseling to improve body image and self-acceptance, a nutritious reduced-calorie diet and increased exercise to promote weight loss, and behavior therapy to reduce bingeing.

Eating disorder	Who is affected	Characteristics and consequences
Anorexia athletica	Athletes in weight-dependent sports such as dance, figure skating, gymnastics, track and field, cycling, wrestling, and horse racing	Engaging in compulsive exercise to lose weight or maintain a very low body weight. Can lead to more serious eating disorders and serious health problems, including kidney failure, heart attack, and death.
Female athlete triad	Female athletes in weight-dependent sports	A syndrome involving energy restriction, along with high levels of exercise, that causes low estrogen levels. Low estrogen levels lead to amenorrhea and interfere with calcium balance, eventually causing reductions in bone mass and an increased risk of bone fractures (discussed further in Chapter 10).
Bigorexia (muscle dysmorphia or reverse anorexia)	Bodybuilders and avid gym-goers; more common in men than in women	An obsession with being small and underdeveloped. Those affected believe that their muscles are inadequate, even when they have good muscle mass. They become avid weightlifters and may experiment with steroids or other muscle-enhancing drugs.
Avoidant/restrictive food intake disorder	Infants/children/adults	Similar to anorexia nervosa in that the individual avoids eating and experiences weight loss and the other physical symptoms of anorexia. However, there is no distorted body image or fear of weight gain.
Selective eating disorder	Children	Children with this disorder will eat only a few foods, mostly those high in carbohydrate. If the disorder continues for long periods, it increases the risk of malnutrition.
Night-eating syndrome	Obese adults and those experiencing stress	A disorder that involves consuming most of the day's calories late in the day or at night. People with this disorder—which contributes to weight gain—are tense, anxious, upset, or guilty while eating. A similar disorder, in which a person may eat while asleep and have no memory of the events, is called nocturnal sleep-related eating disorder (NS-RED) and is considered a sleep disorder, not an eating disorder.
Pica	Pregnant women, children, people with psychiatric disturbances and developmental disabilities, people whose family or ethnic customs include eating certain nonfood substances, people who are hungry and try to ease hunger and cravings with nonfood substances	Craving and eating nonfood items such as dirt, clay, paint chips, plaster, chalk, laundry starch, coffee grounds, and ashes. Depending on the items consumed, pica can cause perforated intestines and contribute to mineral deficiencies or intestinal infections (discussed further in Chapter 11).
Diabulimia (insulin misuse)	People taking insulin to control diabetes	Without insulin glucose cannot enter cells to provide fuel, blood levels rise, and weight drops. Manipulating insulin doses can be used to control weight. However, the consequences of uncontrolled blood sugar include blindness, kidney disease, heart disease, nerve damage, and amputations.

Eating Disorders in Special Groups

Although anorexia and bulimia are most common in women in their teens and 20s, eating disorders occur in both genders and all age groups. Both male and female athletes are at high risk for eating disorders, with an incidence that exceeds that seen in nonathletes.[51] Eating disorders occur during pregnancy and are becoming more frequent among younger children due to social values about food and body weight. They also occur in individuals with diabetes. A number of less common eating disorders appear in special groups in the general population (**Table 9.4**).

Preventing and Getting Treatment for Eating Disorders

Because eating disorders are often triggered by weight-related criticism, elimination of this type of behavior can help prevent them. Another important target for reducing the incidence of eating disorders is the media. If the unrealistically thin body ideal presented by the media could be altered, the incidence of eating disorders would likely decrease. Even with these interventions, however, eating disorders are unlikely to go away entirely. Education through schools and communities about the symptoms and complications of eating disorders can help people identify friends and family members who are at risk and persuade those with early symptoms to seek help.

The first step in preventing individuals from developing eating disorders is to recognize those who are at risk. Early intervention can help prevent at-risk individuals from developing serious eating disorders. Excessive concerns about body weight, having friends who are preoccupied with weight, being teased by peers about weight, and family problems all predispose a person to developing an eating disorder.

Once an eating disorder has developed, the person usually does not get better on his or her own. The actions of family members and friends can help people suffering from eating disorders get help before their health is impaired. But it is not always easy to persuade a friend or relative with an eating disorder to agree to seek help. People with eating disorders are good at hiding their behaviors and denying the problem, and often they do not want help. When confronted, one person might be relieved that you are concerned and willing to help, whereas another might be angry and defensive. When approaching someone about an eating disorder, it is important to make it clear that you are not forcing the person to do anything he or she doesn't want to do. Continued encouragement can help some people agree to seek professional help.

CONCEPT CHECK STOP

1. **Which** eating disorder is characterized by extreme weight loss? Which is characterized by excess weight?

2. **What** factors contribute to the higher incidence of eating disorders among women than among men?

3. **What** is meant by body image?

4. **How** does a food binge differ from "normal" overeating?

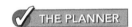 THE PLANNER

Summary

1 Body Weight and Health 290

- The number of Americans who are **overweight** and **obese** has reached epidemic proportions, as seen in this obesity map. Excess body fat increases the risk of chronic diseases such as diabetes, heart disease, high blood pressure, and certain types of cancer.

Obesity across America • Figure 9.1

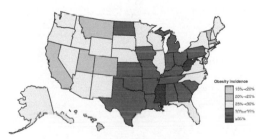

Obesity incidence
15%–<20%
20%–<25%
25%–<30%
30%–<35%
≥35%

- **Body mass index (BMI)** can be used to evaluate the health risks of a particular body weight and height. Measures of **body composition** can be used to determine the proportion of a person's weight that is due to fat. Excess **visceral fat** is a greater health risk than excess **subcutaneous fat**.

---

2 Energy Balance 295

- Americans have gotten fatter because they are consuming more calories due to poor food choices and larger portion sizes, as illustrated in the photo, and moving less due to modern lifestyles in which computers, cars, and other conveniences reduce the amount of energy expended in work and play.

Portion distortion • Figure 9.6

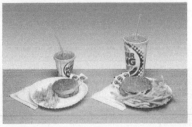

Andy Washnik

- The principle of **energy balance** states that if energy intake equals energy expenditure, body weight will remain constant. Energy is provided to the body by the carbohydrate, fat, and protein in the food we eat. This energy is used to maintain **basal metabolic rate (BMR)**, to support activity, and to digest food and to absorb, metabolize, and store the nutrients (**thermic effect of food (TEF)**). When excess energy is consumed, it is stored, primarily as fat in **adipocytes**, causing weight gain. When energy in the diet does not meet needs, energy stores in the body are used, and weight is lost.

- The energy needs of healthy people can be predicted by calculating their Estimated Energy Requirements (EERs). A person's EER depends on gender, age, life stage, height, weight, and level of physical activity.

3 What Determines Body Size and Shape? 302

- The genes people inherit affect their body size and shape, as illustrated by the father and son shown here, but environmental factors and personal choices concerning the amount and type of food consumed and the amount and intensity of exercise performed also affect body weight.

Genes and body shape • Figure 9.11

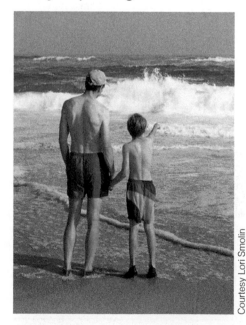

Courtesy Lori Smolin

- **Hunger** and **satiety** from meal to meal are regulated by signals from the gastrointestinal tract, hormones, and levels of circulating nutrients. Signals from fat cells, such as the release of **leptin**, regulate long-term energy intake and expenditure.

- Inheriting an efficient metabolism or expending less energy through **nonexercise activity thermogenesis (NEAT)** may contribute to obesity.

4 Managing Body Weight 306

- Weight loss is recommended for those with a BMI above the healthy range who have excess body fat and risk factors associated with obesity, such as diabetes, hypertension, abnormal lipid levels, and an increased waist circumference. The goal of weight loss should be 5 to 10% of body weight within the first 6 months.

- Successful weight loss involves a reduction in energy intake, an increase in energy expenditure, and **behavior modification** to change behaviors that led to weight gain and help keep weight in a healthy range over the long term. To lose a pound of adipose tissue, energy expenditure must be increased or intake decreased by approximately 3500 Calories. Slow, steady weight loss of 1/2 to 2 lb/week is more likely to be maintained than rapid weight loss.

- If being **underweight** is not due to a medical condition, weight gain can be accomplished by increasing energy intake and lifting weights to increase muscle mass.

- A good weight-loss program is one that promotes physical activity and a wide variety of nutrient-dense food choices, does not require the purchase and consumption of special foods or combinations of foods, and can be followed for life.

- Weight-loss medications are recommended when conventional weight-loss methods fail. Weight-loss surgery is recommended for those whose health is seriously compromised by their body weight and conventional weight-loss methods have failed. Some common surgical approaches to treating obesity are **gastric bypass**, shown here, **gastric sleeve surgery**, and **adjustable gastric banding**.

Gastric bypass • Figure 9.20b

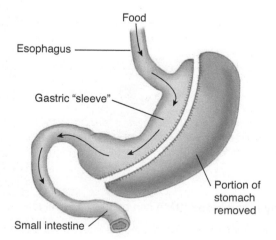

Food

Esophagus

Gastric "sleeve"

Portion of stomach removed

Small intestine

5 Eating Disorders 317

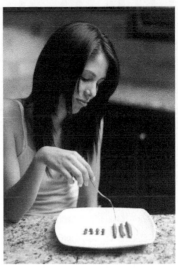
© Aldo Murillo/iStockphoto

- **Eating disorders** are psychological disorders that involve dissatisfaction with body weight. **Anorexia nervosa** involves self-starvation, as shown here, resulting in an abnormally low body weight. **Bulimia nervosa** is characterized by repeated cycles of binge eating followed by purging and other behaviors to prevent weight gain. **Binge-eating disorder** is characterized by bingeing without purging. People with this disorder are typically overweight.

- Eating disorders are caused by a combination of genetic, psychological, and sociocultural factors. The lean body ideal in the United States is believed to contribute to disturbances in **body image** that lead to eating disorders. Treatment involves medical, psychological, and nutritional intervention to stabilize health, change attitudes about body size, and improve eating habits while supplying an adequate diet.

Key Terms

- adipocyte 300
- adjustable gastric banding 315
- anorexia nervosa 318
- appetite 295
- basal metabolic rate (BMR) 297
- basal metabolism 297
- behavior modification 308
- binge-eating disorder 318
- body composition 293

- body image 318
- body mass index (BMI) 291
- bulimia nervosa 318
- eating disorder 318
- energy balance 295
- extreme obesity or morbid obesity 292
- gastric bypass 316
- gastric sleeve surgery 315
- ghrelin 304

- hunger 296
- lean body mass 291
- leptin 305
- liposuction 316
- nonexercise activity thermogenesis (NEAT) 297
- obese 290
- obesity genes 302
- overweight 290
- resting metabolic rate (RMR) 299

- satiety 303
- set point 303
- subcutaneous fat 295
- thermic effect of food (TEF) or diet-induced thermogenesis 297
- total energy expenditure 297
- underweight 292
- visceral fat 295

What is happening in this picture?

Sumo wrestlers train for many hours each day and eat huge amounts of food. The result is a high BMI and a large waist but surprisingly little visceral fat.

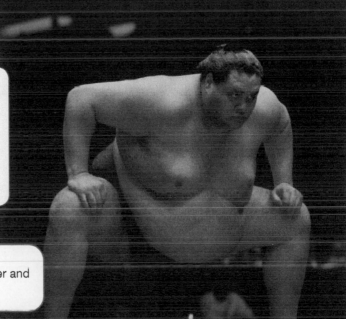
Cusp and Flirt/Masterfile

Think Critically

1. Why do these individuals have a low level of visceral fat?
2. Do you think they are at risk for diabetes and heart disease?
3. What type of fat is hanging over the belt of this wrestler?
4. What may happen if this wrestler retires and stops exercising but keeps eating large amounts of food?

THE PLANNER ✔

Review your Chapter Planner on the chapter opener and check off your completed work.

Nutrition, Fitness, and Physical Activity

Lance Armstrong seemed a phenomenal athlete: cancer survivor, seven-time winner of the Tour de France bicycle race, a philanthropist and role model for millions with his Livestrong organization. Yet by his own admission he was a cheat who rode to his many victories aided by a blood-doping regimen he justified by saying it was impossible to win the Tour de France without doping.

Few people face the challenges of athletes like Armstrong, but many of us struggle with the challenge of getting enough physical activity in a world that demands less and less physical exertion.

Advances in technology have introduced consumers to more and more "labor-saving" devices, so to stay fit people have had to allot time for physical exertion. Physical fitness has always been a priority for a society's military and athletes, and idleness an indulgence of the elites, or "leisure class," but as jobs have become less labor-intensive for most people, we have had to seek

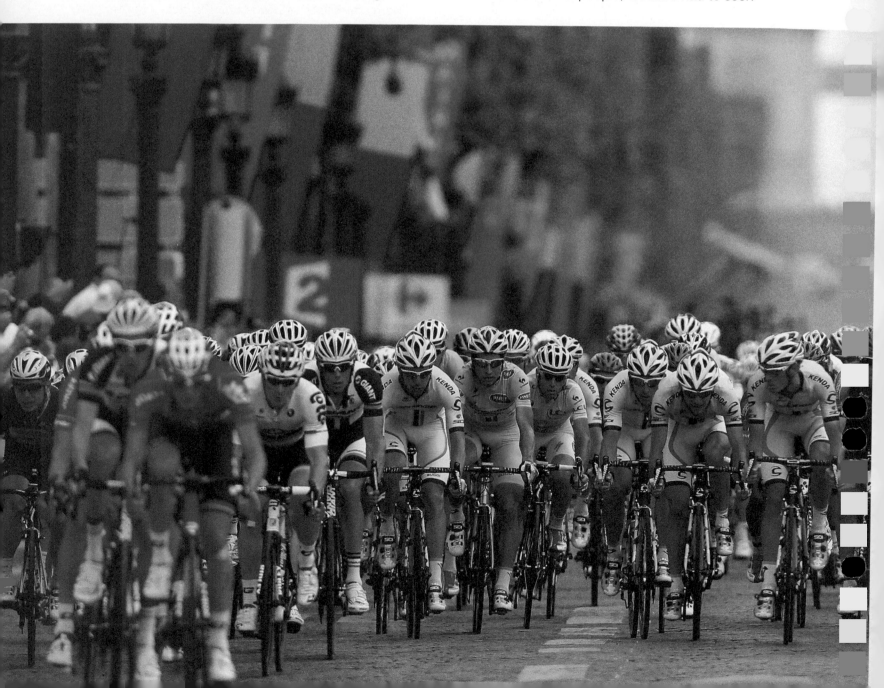

out ways of staying fit. Fitness crazes and fad diets litter our recent history—from jogging and kickboxing to spin classes and Zumba; from eating your Wheaties to a high-carb diet to an all-meat diet.

As technological innovation continues to ease the daily physical challenges and exertions we face, like the *honest* mega athlete we have to pay a lot more attention to what we eat and how much activity we need to remain healthy.

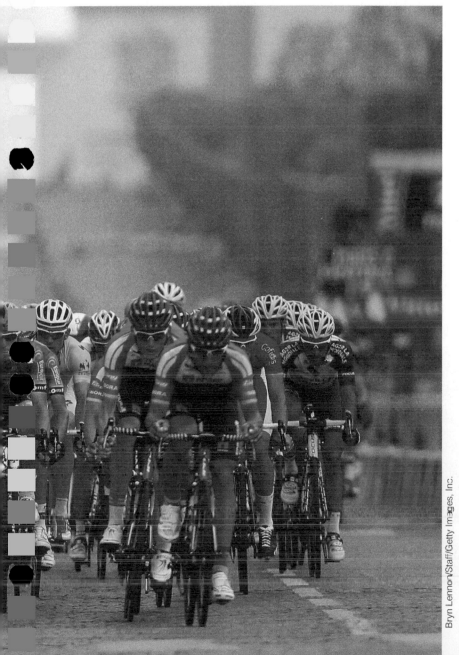

Bryn Lennon/Staff/Getty Images, Inc.

CHAPTER PLANNER ✓

❏ Stimulate your interest by reading the introduction and looking at the visual.
❏ Scan the Learning Objectives in each section:
   p. 330 ❏ p. 332 ❏ p. 335 ❏ p. 339 ❏ p. 345 ❏ p. 355 ❏
❏ Read the text and study all figures and visuals. Answer any questions.

Analyze key features:

❏ Nutrition InSight, p. 333 ❏   p. 344 ❏
❏ Process Diagram, p. 340 ❏
❏ What a Scientist Sees, p. 342 ❏   p. 356 ❏
❏ Thinking it Through, p. 353 ❏
❏ Debate, p. 358 ❏
❏ Stop: Answer the Concept Checks before you go on:
   p. 332 ❏ p. 334 ❏ p. 338 ❏ p. 344 ❏ p. 354 ❏ p. 359 ❏

End of chapter and online review:

❏ Review the Summary, online links to Additional Resources, and Key Terms.
❏ Answer the online Critical and Creative Thinking Questions.
❏ Answer What is happening in this picture?
❏ Complete the online Self-Test and check your answers.

10.1 Food, Physical Activity, and Health

LEARNING OBJECTIVES

1. **Discuss** how food and physical activity interact to promote health.
2. **Explain** the impact of physical activity on chronic disease.
3. **Discuss** the role of physical activity in weight management.

ood and physical activity are both necessary to achieve optimal health. The right foods provide the nutrients needed to promote health and reduce disease risk. Adequate physical activity improves your **fitness** and overall health. However, the link between food and physical activity goes beyond the fact that both promote health and reduce disease risk. Physical activity burns calories and utilizes nutrients, which must be supplied by the diet. Therefore, the foods you eat are necessary to fuel your activity and optimize athletic performance (**Figure 10.1**). The connection between diet and physical activity holds true whether your fitness goal is to keep your weight in the healthy range, to reduce your risk of chronic disease, to be able to complete your daily activities, or to perform optimally in athletic competitions.

fitness A set of attributes related to the ability to perform routine physical activities without undue fatigue.

Physical Activity Reduces the Risk of Chronic Disease

Physical activity includes both planned exercise and daily activities such as cleaning, cooking, yard work, and recreation. Adequate amounts of regular physical activity not only make everyday tasks easier but can also prevent or delay the onset of chronic conditions such as cardiovascular disease, hypertension, type 2 diabetes, breast and colon cancer, and bone and joint disorders (**Figure 10.2**).[1] The health benefits of physical activity are so great that they can even overcome some of the health risks of carrying excess body fat. Adequate physical activity reduces overall mortality, regardless of whether the person is lean, normal weight, or obese.[1] So even if you can't take off the pounds, you'll still benefit from being active. If you are in a profession that requires high levels of activity, such as construction worker or ski instructor, your everyday activities may be enough to optimize your health and prevent weight gain, but for most of us to achieve these benefits we must add exercise to our days.

In addition to decreasing the risk of disease, adequate physical activity improves mood and self-esteem and increases vigor and overall well-being. Physical activity has also been shown to reduce depression and anxiety, as well as to improve the quality of life.[2] The mechanisms involved are not clear, but one hypothesis has to do with

Food and physical activity benefit health • Figure 10.1

The energy and nutrients in food fuel our activity, and physical activity in turn affects our energy and nutrient needs. Both food and physical activity are necessary for optimal health.

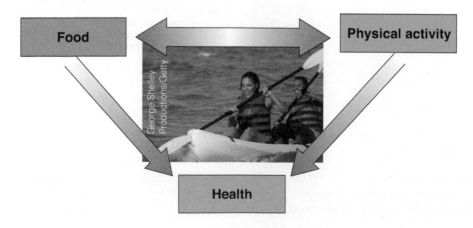

endorphins
Compounds that cause a natural euphoria and reduce the perception of pain under certain stressful conditions.

the production of **endorphins**. Certain types of activity stimulate the release of these chemicals, which are thought to be natural mood enhancers that play a role in triggering what athletes describe as an "exercise high." In addition to causing this state of exercise euphoria, endorphins are thought to aid in relaxation, pain tolerance, and appetite control.

Physical Activity Makes Weight Management Easier

Physical activity makes weight management easier because it increases both energy needs and lean body mass. During moderate to

strenuous physical activity, energy expenditure can rise well above the resting rate, and some of this increase persists for many hours after activity slows.[3] Over time, regular exercise increases lean body mass. Even at rest, lean tissue uses more energy than fat tissue; therefore, the increase in lean body mass increases basal metabolism. The combination of increased energy output during physical activity, the rise in energy expenditure that persists for a period after activity, and the increase in basal needs over the long term can have a major impact on total energy

Regular physical activity reduces the risk of cardiovascular disease because it strengthens the heart muscle, lowers blood pressure, and increases HDL (good) cholesterol levels in the blood.

Regular physical activity reduces the risk of colon cancer and breast cancer.

Physical activity improves flexibility and balance.

Physical activity increases the sensitivity of tissues to insulin and decreases the risk of developing type 2 diabetes.

Regular physical activity increases muscle mass, strength, and endurance.

The strength and flexibility promoted by exercise can help improve joint function.

Weight-bearing activity stimulates bones to become denser and stronger and therefore reduces the risk of osteoporosis.

Cameron Lawcn/NG Image Collection

Health benefits of physical activity • Figure 10.2

Engaging in enough of the right types of activity improves strength and endurance, reduces the risk of chronic disease, aids weight management, reduces sleeplessness, improves self-image, and helps relieve stress, anxiety, and depression.

Physical activity increases energy expenditure • Figure 10.3

The total amount of energy we expend each day is the sum of the energy used for basal metabolism, physical activity, and the thermic effect of food (TEF). Adding 30 minutes of moderate activity to a sedentary lifestyle can increase energy expenditure by as much as 300 Calories. A program of regular exercise increases muscle mass, which increases basal metabolism, further increasing total energy expenditure.

Ask Yourself

Why does regular exercise cause an increase in basal metabolism?

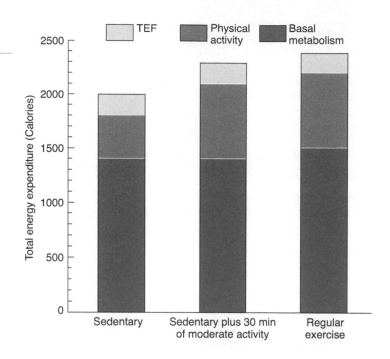

expenditure (**Figure 10.3**). The more energy you expend, the more food you can consume while maintaining a healthy weight. As discussed in Chapter 9, exercise is an essential component of any weight-reduction program: It increases energy needs, promotes loss of body fat, and slows the loss of lean tissue that occurs with energy restriction.[4]

CONCEPT CHECK STOP

1. **What** is the relationship between food, physical activity, and health?
2. **How** does physical activity affect heart health?
3. **Why** does physical activity help manage weight?

10.2 The Four Components of Fitness

LEARNING OBJECTIVES

1. **Describe** the overload principle.
2. **List** the characteristics of a fit individual.
3. **Explain** how aerobic exercise affects heart rate and aerobic capacity.
4. **Compare** the amount of muscle in a fit and unfit individual.

When you exercise, changes occur in your body: You breathe harder, your heart beats faster, and your muscles stretch and strain. If you exercise regularly, you adapt to the exercise you perform and as a result can continue for a few minutes longer, lift a heavier weight, or stretch a millimeter farther. This is known as the **overload principle**: The more you do, the more you are capable of doing. For example, if you run a given distance three times a week, in a few weeks you can run farther; if you lift heavy books for a few days, by the next week you have more muscle and can lift more books more easily. These adaptations improve your overall fitness.

A person's fitness is defined by his or her endurance, strength, flexibility, and body composition (**Figure 10.4**). A fit person can continue an activity for a longer period than an unfit person can before fatigue forces him or her to stop.

> **overload principle** The concept that the body adapts to the stresses placed on it.

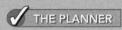

Your fitness depends on your cardiorespiratory endurance, muscle strength and endurance, flexibility, and the proportion of your body that is lean tissue versus fat.

a. Aerobic activity such as jogging, bicycling, or swimming strengthens the cardiovascular and respiratory systems. A quick way to keep your activity in the aerobic range is to proceed at a pace that is slow enough to allow you to carry on a conversation but fast enough that you cannot sing while exercising.

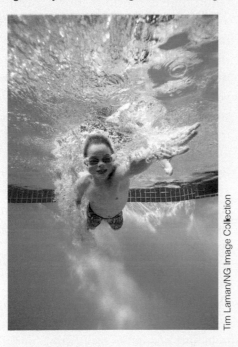

Tim Laman/NG Image Collection

b. Weightlifting stresses the muscles, causing them to adapt by increasing in size and strength—a process called **hypertrophy**. The larger, stronger muscles can lift the same weight more easily. Muscles that are not used due to a lapse in weight training, injury, or illness become smaller and weaker. This process is called **atrophy**. Thus, there is truth to the saying, "Use it or lose it."

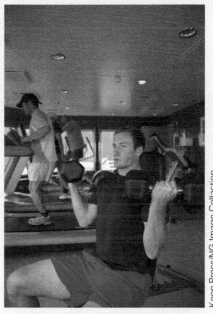

Keen Press/NG Image Collection

c. Flexibility exercises can be static or dynamic. In a static stretch, such as that shown here, a position that stretches a muscle or group of muscles to its farthest point is held for about 30 seconds. Dynamic stretching involves motion. It uses controlled leg and arm swings, torso twists, and side lunges to extend muscles gently to the limits of their range of motion. The combination of static and dynamic stretching that is best depends on the person and their sport.[5]

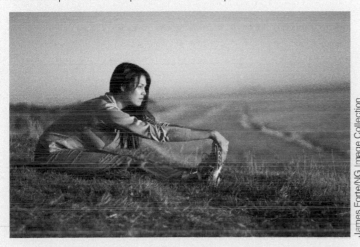

James Forte/NG Image Collection

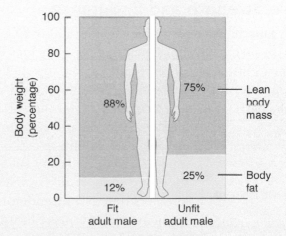

d. A fit person has more muscle mass than an unfit person of the same height and weight. Becoming fit by engaging in aerobic activity and muscle-strengthening exercise has a positive impact on body composition, reducing body fat, and increasing the proportion of lean tissue.

Cardiorespiratory Endurance

How long you can jog or ride your bike depends on the ability of your cardiovascular and respiratory systems, referred to jointly as the cardiorespiratory system, to deliver oxygen and nutrients to your tissues and remove wastes. **Cardiorespiratory endurance** is enhanced by regular **aerobic activity** (**Figure 10.4a**).

Regular aerobic activity strengthens the heart muscle and increases the amount of blood pumped with each heartbeat. This in turn decreases **resting heart rate**, the rate at which the heart beats when the body is at rest to supply blood to the tissues. The more fit you are, the lower your resting heart rate and the more blood your heart can pump to your muscles during exercise. In addition to increasing the amount of oxygen-rich blood that is pumped to your muscles, regular aerobic activity increases the ability of your muscles to use oxygen to produce ATP. Your body's maximum ability to generate ATP using aerobic metabolism is called your **aerobic capacity**, or VO_2 max. Aerobic capacity is a function of the ability of the cardiorespiratory system to deliver oxygen to the cells and the ability of the cells to use oxygen to produce ATP. The greater your aerobic capacity, the more intense activity you can perform before lack of oxygen affects your performance.

Muscle Strength and Endurance

Greater **muscle strength** enhances the ability to perform tasks such as pushing or lifting. In daily life, this could mean lifting a gallon of milk off the top shelf of the refrigerator with one hand, carrying a full trash can out to the curb, or moving a couch into your new apartment. Greater **muscle endurance** enhances your ability to continue repetitive muscle activity, such as shoveling snow or raking leaves. Muscle strength and endurance are increased by repeatedly using muscles in activities that require moving against a resisting force. This type of exercise is called **muscle-strengthening exercise**, strength-training exercise, or resistance-training exercise and includes activities such as weightlifting and calisthenics (**Figure 10.4b**).

cardiorespiratory endurance The efficiency with which the body delivers to cells the oxygen and nutrients needed for muscular activity and transports waste products from cells.

aerobic activity Endurance activity that increases heart rate and uses oxygen to provide energy as ATP.

aerobic capacity The maximum amount of oxygen that can be consumed by the tissues during exercise. Also called maximal oxygen consumption, or VO_2 max.

muscle-strengthening exercise Activities that are specifically designed to increase muscle strength, endurance, and size; also called strength-training exercise or resistance-training exercise.

Flexibility

When you think of fitness, you may picture someone with bulging muscles, but fitness also involves flexibility. Flexibility determines your range of motion—how far you can bend and stretch muscles and ligaments. Regularly moving your limbs, neck, and torso through their full range of motion helps increase and maintain flexibility. If your flexibility is poor, you cannot easily bend to tie your shoes or stretch to remove packages from the car. Being flexible can enhance postural stability and balance.[6] Stretching improves flexibility but has not been shown to reduce injury (**Figure 10.4c**). However, an exercise warm-up that includes both cardiorespiratory activities and stretching has benefits for certain types of sports such as dancing.

Body Composition

Individuals who are physically fit have a greater proportion of muscle and a smaller proportion of fat than do unfit individuals of the same weight (**Figure 10.4d**). The amount of body fat a person has is also affected by gender and age. In general, women have more stored body fat than men. For young adult women, a healthy amount of body fat is 21 to 32% of total weight; in adult men, a healthy amount is 8 to 19%.[7]

CONCEPT CHECK	

1. **Why** do your muscles get bigger when you lift weights?
2. **What** distinguishes a fit person from an unfit one?
3. **How** does aerobic activity affect heart rate?
4. **Why** do fit individuals have more lean tissue?

10.3 Physical Activity Recommendations

LEARNING OBJECTIVES

1. **Describe** the amounts and types of activity recommended to improve health.
2. **Classify** activities as aerobic or anaerobic.
3. **Plan** a fitness program that can be integrated into your daily routine.
4. **Explain** overtraining syndrome.

To reduce the risk of chronic disease, public health guidelines, including the 2010 Dietary Guidelines, advise at least 150 minutes of moderate-intensity or 75 minutes of vigorous-intensity aerobic physical activity each week or an equivalent combination of both (**Figure 10.5**).[6,8,9] Even a small amount of exercise is better than none, and greater

Physical activity recommendations • Figure 10.5

A healthy lifestyle minimizes sedentary activities and includes some planned exercise and a variety of everyday activities. At least 150 minutes of aerobic activity is recommended as well as activities that improve muscle strength and flexibility. Achieving the recommended amounts and types of activity will help improve and maintain fitness and health.[6,8] In general, more exercise is better than less.

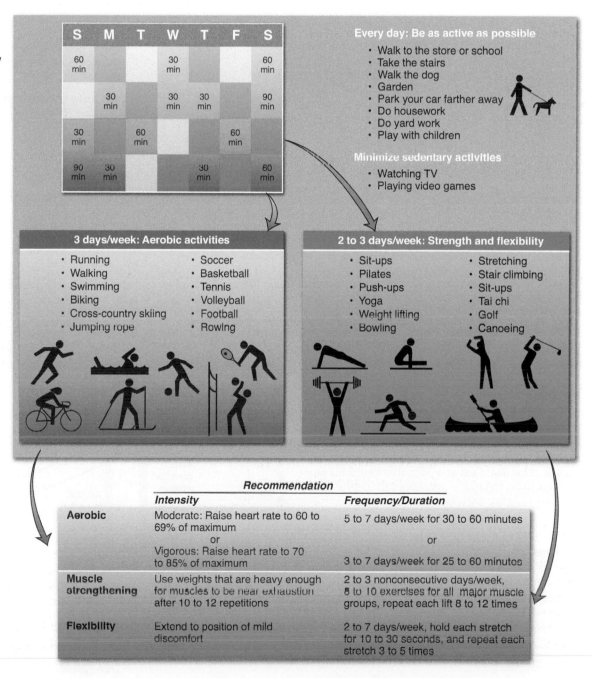

	Recommendation	
	Intensity	*Frequency/Duration*
Aerobic	Moderate: Raise heart rate to 60 to 69% of maximum or Vigorous: Raise heart rate to 70 to 85% of maximum	5 to 7 days/week for 30 to 60 minutes or 3 to 7 days/week for 25 to 60 minutes
Muscle strengthening	Use weights that are heavy enough for muscles to be near exhaustion after 10 to 12 repetitions	2 to 3 nonconsecutive days/week, 8 to 10 exercises for all major muscle groups, repeat each lift 8 to 12 times
Flexibility	Extend to position of mild discomfort	2 to 7 days/week, hold each stretch for 10 to 30 seconds, and repeat each stretch 3 to 5 times

health benefits can be obtained by exercising more vigorously or for a longer duration. Moderate-intensity exercise is the equivalent of walking 3 miles in about an hour or bicycling 8 miles in about an hour. Vigorous-intensity exercise is equivalent to jogging at a rate of 5 miles per hour or faster or bicycling at 10 miles per hour or faster.[9] Adults should also include muscle-strengthening activities on two or more days per week, but time spent in muscle-strengthening activities does not count toward meeting the aerobic activity guidelines. Only about 21% of U.S. adults 18 years and older currently meet the physical activity guidelines for both aerobic and muscle-strengthening physical activity.[10]

What to Look for in a Fitness Program

A complete fitness program includes aerobic activity for cardiovascular conditioning, stretching exercises for flexibility, and muscle-strengthening exercises to increase muscle strength and endurance and maintain or increase muscle mass.[9,11] The program should be integrated into an active lifestyle that includes a variety of everyday activities, enjoyable recreational activities, and a minimum amount of time spent in sedentary activities (see Figure 10.5).

Moderate or vigorous aerobic activity should be performed most days of the week. An activity is aerobic if

Finding your aerobic zone • Figure 10.6

Checking your heart rate during your exercise session can help you determine if you are exercising in your aerobic zone.

a. You can check your heart rate by feeling the pulse at the side of your neck, just below the jawbone. A pulse is caused by the heart beating and forcing blood through the arteries. The number of pulses per minute equals heart rate.

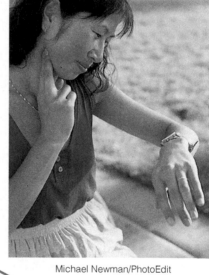

Michael Newman/PhotoEdit

b. You can calculate your aerobic zone by multiplying your maximum heart rate by 0.6 and 0.85. Maximum heart rate is dependent on age and can be estimated in men by subtracting age from 220 and in women by subtracting 88% of age from 206, according to the following equations.[13]

Men: Maximum heart rate = 220 − age
Women: Maximum heart rate = 206 − (0.88 × age)
For example, a 20-year-old man would have a maximum heart rate of 200 (220 − 20) beats per minute. If he exercises at a pace that keeps his heart rate between 120 (0.6 × 200) and 170 (0.85 × 200) beats per minute, he is in his aerobic zone.

Interpret the Data

What is the aerobic zone for a 30-year-old woman? What happens to this range when she turns 40?

Maximum heart rate

85% of maximum

Aerobic zone for women

60% of maximum

Aerobic zone for men

Heart rate (beats/min)

—— Female
—— Male

Age (years)

maximum heart rate The maximum number of beats per minute that the heart can attain.

it raises your heart rate to 60 to 85% of your **maximum heart rate**; when you are exercising at an intensity in this range, you are said to be in your **aerobic zone** (**Figure 10.6**). For a sedentary individual who is beginning a fitness program, mild exercise such as walking can raise the heart rate into the aerobic zone. As fitness improves, an exerciser must perform more intense activity to raise the heart rate to this level.

Aerobic activities of different intensities can be combined to meet recommendations and achieve health benefits. The total amount of energy expended in physical activity depends on the intensity, duration, and frequency of the activity. Vigorous physical activity, such as jogging, that raises heart rate to the high end of the aerobic zone (70 to 85%) improves fitness more and burns more calories per unit of time than does moderate-intensity activity, such as walking, which raises heart rate only to the low end of the zone (60 to 69%).

Individuals should structure their fitness program based on their needs, goals, and abilities. For example, some people might prefer a short, intense workout such as a 30-minute run, while others would rather work out for a longer time, at a lower intensity, such as a 1-hour walk. Some may choose to complete all their exercise during the same session, while others may spread their exercise throughout the day, in shorter bouts. Three short bouts of 10-minute duration can be as effective as a continuous bout of 30 minutes for reducing the risk of chronic disease.[11] It is preferable to spread your aerobic activity throughout the week rather than cram it all into the weekend. Exercising at least 3 days produces health benefits and reduces the risk of injury and fatigue. A combination of intensities, such as a brisk 30-minute walk twice during the week in addition to a 20-minute jog on 2 other days, can meet recommendations.

Muscle strengthening and stretching can be performed less often than aerobic activities (see Figure 10.5). Muscle strengthening is needed only 2 to 3 days a week at the start of a fitness program and 2 days a week after the desired strength has been achieved. Muscle strengthening should not be done on consecutive days. The rest between sessions gives the muscles time to respond to the stress by getting stronger. Increasing the amount of weight lifted increases muscle strength, whereas increasing the number of repetitions improves muscle endurance. Flexibility exercises can be performed 2 to 7 days

per week. Time spent stretching does not count toward meeting aerobic or strength-training guidelines.

In addition to following these physical activity recommendations, it is important to minimize sedentary time. A few hours of planned exercise cannot compensate for extended periods of time spent in sedentary pastimes. Therefore, even people who exercise enough to meet physical activity guidelines may be at increased risk of cardiovascular disease, depression, increased waist circumference, and other adverse effects if they spend long periods sitting in a car, at a desk, or in front of the television.[6,12] Reducing total time spent in sedentary pursuits and breaking up periods of sedentary activity with short bouts of physical activity and standing, which can attenuate the adverse effects of sedentary behavior, should be a goal for all adults, regardless of their exercise habits.

Creating an Active Lifestyle

Incorporating activity into your day-to-day life may require a change in lifestyle, which is not always easy (**Table 10.1**).

Suggestions for starting and maintaining an exercise program   Table 10.1

Start slowly. Set specific, attainable goals. Once you have met them, add more.

- Walk around the block after dinner.
- Get off the bus or subway one stop early.
- Use half of your lunch break to exercise.
- Do a few biceps curls each time you take the milk out of the refrigerator.

Make your exercise fun and convenient

- Opt for activities you enjoy: Bowling and dancing may be more fun for you than using a treadmill at the gym.
- Find a partner to exercise with you.
- Choose times that fit your schedule.

Stay motivated

- Vary your routine: Swim one day and mountain bike the next.
- Challenge your strength or endurance once or twice a week and do moderate workouts on other days.
- Track your progress by recording your activity.
- Reward your success with a new book, movie, or workout clothes.

Keep your exercise safe

- Warm up before you start and cool down when you are done.
- Wear light-colored or reflective clothing that is appropriate for the environmental conditions.
- Don't overdo it: Alternate hard days with easy days and take a day off when you need it.
- Listen to your body and stop before an injury occurs.

Many people avoid exercise because they do not enjoy it, think it requires them to join an expensive health club, have little motivation to do it alone, or find it inconvenient or uncomfortable. Finding an activity you enjoy, setting aside a time that is realistic and convenient, and finding a place that is appropriate and safe are important steps in starting and maintaining a fitness program. Riding your bike to class or work rather than driving, taking a walk during your lunch break, and enjoying a game of catch or tag with your friends or family are all effective ways to increase your everyday activity level. The goal is to gradually make lifestyle changes that increase physical activity.

Before beginning a fitness program, check with your physician to be sure that the activities are appropriate for you, considering your medical history (**Figure 10.7**). If you choose to exercise outdoors rather than in a gym, reduce or curtail exercise in hot, humid weather in order to avoid heat-related illness. In cold weather, wear clothing that allows for evaporation of sweat while providing protection from the cold. Start each exercise session with a warm-up, such as mild stretching or easy jogging, to increase blood flow to the muscles. End with a cool-down period, such as walking or stretching, to prevent muscle cramps and slowly reduce heart rate.

Don't overdo it. If you don't rest enough between exercise sessions, fitness and performance will not improve. During rest, the body replenishes energy stores, repairs damaged tissues, and builds and strengthens muscles. In athletes, excessive training without sufficient rest to allow for recovery can lead to **overtraining syndrome**. The most common symptoms of this condition are fatigue, performance decline, and mood disturbances.[14] Athletes may become moody, easily irritated, or depressed; experience altered sleep patterns; or lose their competitive desire and enthusiasm. It may take weeks or months to recover. In addition to the physical demands of training, psychological factors such as excessive expectations from a coach or family members, competitive stress, personal or emotional problems, and school- or work-related demands contribute to the

> **overtraining syndrome**
> A collection of emotional, behavioral, and physical symptoms that occurs when the amount and intensity of exercise exceeds an athlete's capacity to recover.

Physical activity is for everyone • Figure 10.7

Almost anyone of any age can be active, no matter where they live, how old they are, or what physical limitations they have.

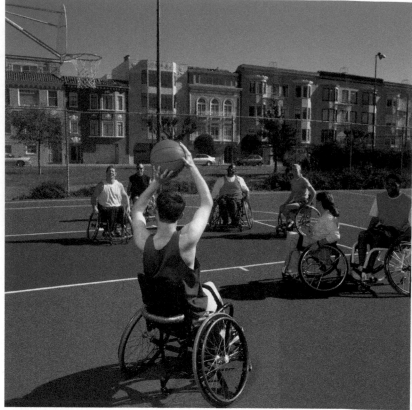

David Papas/Getty Images

development of overtraining syndrome. Overtraining syndrome occurs only in serious athletes who are training extensively, but rest is essential for anyone who is working to increase fitness.

CONCEPT CHECK

1. **How** much aerobic activity is recommended to reduce the risk of chronic disease?
2. **What** is your aerobic zone?
3. **What** types of activities should be part of a fitness program?
4. **Who** is at risk for overtraining syndrome?

10.4 Fueling Activity

LEARNING OBJECTIVES

1. **Compare** the fuels used to generate ATP by anaerobic and aerobic metabolism.
2. **Discuss** the effect of exercise duration and intensity on the type of fuel used.
3. **Describe** the physiological changes that occur in response to exercise training.

The body runs on energy from the carbohydrate, fat, and protein in food and body stores. These fuels are needed whether you are writing a term paper, riding your bike to class, or running a marathon. Before they can be used to fuel activity, their energy must be transferred to the high-energy compound ATP, the immediate source of energy for body functions. ATP can be generated both in the absence of oxygen, by **anaerobic metabolism**, and in the presence of oxygen, by **aerobic metabolism** (**Figure 10.8**). The type of metabolism that predominates during an activity determines how much carbohydrate, fat, and protein are used to fuel the activity.

The availability of oxygen determines whether ATP is produced predominantly by anaerobic versus aerobic

Anaerobic versus aerobic metabolism • Figure 10.8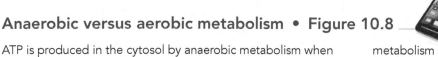

ATP is produced in the cytosol by anaerobic metabolism when no oxygen is available. Anaerobic metabolism produces ATP very rapidly but uses only glucose as a fuel. The **lactic acid** that is produced can be used as a fuel for aerobic metabolism. Aerobic metabolism requires oxygen, takes place in the mitochondria, and can use carbohydrate, fat, or protein to produce ATP. Aerobic metabolism produces the majority of ATP; it is slower but more efficient at generating ATP than anaerobic metabolism.

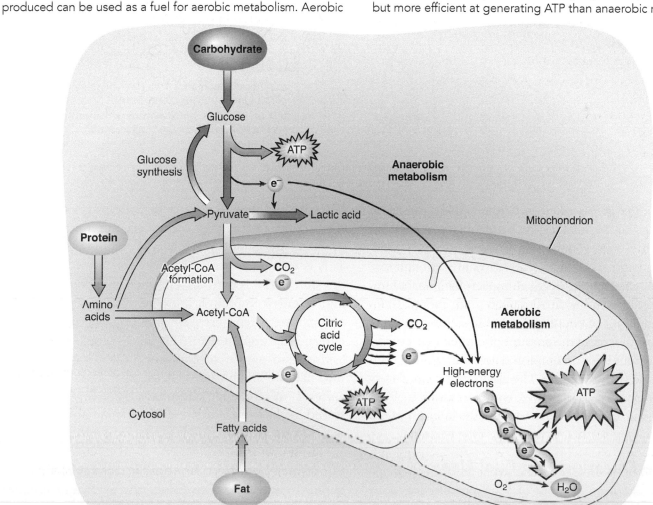

Getting oxygen to muscle cells • Figure 10.9

When you exercise, your muscles need more oxygen. Your body responds to this need by breathing faster and deeper in order to take in more oxygen through the lungs and by increasing heart rate in order to deliver the additional oxygen to your muscles.

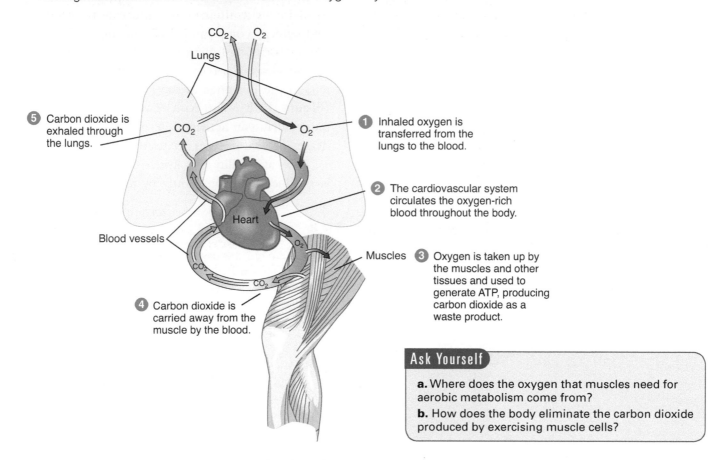

5 Carbon dioxide is exhaled through the lungs.

1 Inhaled oxygen is transferred from the lungs to the blood.

2 The cardiovascular system circulates the oxygen-rich blood throughout the body.

3 Oxygen is taken up by the muscles and other tissues and used to generate ATP, producing carbon dioxide as a waste product.

4 Carbon dioxide is carried away from the muscle by the blood.

Ask Yourself

a. Where does the oxygen that muscles need for aerobic metabolism come from?

b. How does the body eliminate the carbon dioxide produced by exercising muscle cells?

metabolism. Oxygen is taken in by the respiratory system and delivered to the muscles by the blood (**Figure 10.9**). When you are at rest, your muscles do not need much energy, and your heart and lungs are able to deliver enough oxygen to meet your energy needs using aerobic metabolism. When you exercise, your muscles need more energy. To increase the amount of energy provided by aerobic metabolism, you must increase the amount of oxygen delivered to the muscles. Your body accomplishes this by increasing both heart rate and breathing rate. The ability of the circulatory and respiratory systems to deliver oxygen to tissues is affected by how long an activity is performed, the intensity of the activity, and the physical conditioning of the exerciser.

Exercise Duration and Fuel Use

When you take the first steps of your morning jog, your muscles increase their activity, but your heart and lungs have not had time to step up their delivery of oxygen to them. To get the energy they need, the muscles rely on the small amount of ATP that is stored in resting muscle. This is enough to sustain activity for a few seconds. As the stored ATP is used up, enzymes break down another high-energy compound, **creatine phosphate**, to convert ADP (adenosine diphosphate) to ATP, allowing your activity to continue. But, like the amount of ATP, the amount of creatine phosphate stored in the muscle at any time is small and soon runs out (**Figure 10.10**).

creatine phosphate A compound stored in muscle that can be broken down quickly to make ATP.

Short-term energy: Anaerobic metabolism After about 15 seconds of exercise, the ATP and creatine phosphate in your muscles are used up, but your heart

Changes in the source of ATP over time • Figure 10.10

The source of the ATP that fuels muscle contraction changes over the first few minutes of exercise. If the intensity of activity remains moderate, aerobic metabolism will predominate after about 5 minutes.

Instant energy
During the first few seconds of exercise, the muscles get energy from stored ATP. Then, for the next 10 seconds or so, creatine phosphate stored in the muscles is broken down to form more ATP.

Short-term energy
Anaerobic metabolism of glucose, obtained either from the blood or from muscle glycogen, becomes the predominant source of ATP when creatine phosphate stores have been depleted. Thirty seconds into the activity, anaerobic pathways are operating at full capacity.

Long-term energy
After about 2 to 3 minutes, oxygen delivery to the muscles has increased enough to support aerobic metabolism, which uses fatty acids and glucose to produce ATP.

Interpret the Data

After about 10 minutes of moderate exercise, which ATP-producing system is operating at highest capacity?

Graph: Activity of energy systems (percent) vs. Exercise duration (10 sec, 30 sec, 2 min, 10 min)

— ATP-creatine phosphate
— Anaerobic metabolism of glucose
— Aerobic metabolism of glucose and fatty acids

rate and breathing have not increased enough to deliver more oxygen to the muscles. To get more energy at this point, your muscles must produce the additional ATP without oxygen (see Figure 10.8). This anaerobic metabolism can produce ATP very rapidly but can use only glucose as a fuel (**Figure 10.11**). The amount of glucose is limited, so anaerobic metabolism cannot continue indefinitely.

Fuels for anaerobic and aerobic metabolism • Figure 10.11

The glucose used to fuel muscle contraction comes from muscle glycogen breakdown or blood glucose. Blood glucose is supplied by the breakdown of liver glycogen, glucose synthesis by the liver, and carbohydrate consumed in the diet. Some of the fatty acids used as fuel come from triglycerides stored in the muscle, but most come from those in adipose tissue. The amino acids available to the body come from the digestion of dietary proteins and from the breakdown of body proteins.

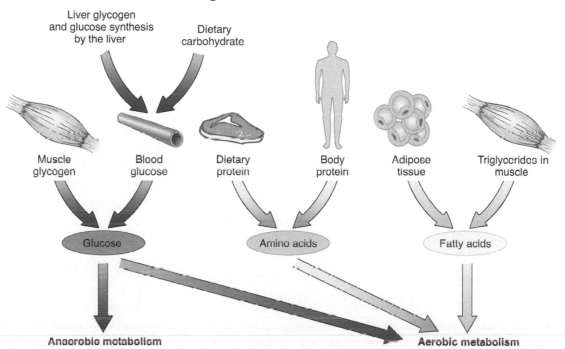

Liver glycogen and glucose synthesis by the liver — Dietary carbohydrate

Muscle glycogen — Blood glucose — Dietary protein — Body protein — Adipose tissue — Triglycerides in muscle

Glucose — Amino acids — Fatty acids

Anaerobic metabolism   **Aerobic metabolism**

WHAT A SCIENTIST SEES
The Fat-Burning Zone

Have you ever jumped onto a treadmill and chosen the workout that puts you in the "fat-burning zone" rather than the one that puts you in the "cardio zone" because your goal was to lose weight? The fat-burning zone is a lower-intensity aerobic workout that keeps your heart rate between about 60 and 69% of maximum. The cardio zone is a higher-intensity aerobic workout that keeps the heart rate between about 70 and 85% of maximum.

However, do you really burn more fat during a slow 30-minute jog in the fat-burning zone than during a vigorous 30-minute run in the cardio zone? A scientist sees that you do burn a higher percentage of calories from fat during a lower-intensity aerobic workout, but that's not the whole story. When you pick up the pace and exercise in what the treadmill calls the cardio zone, you continue to burn fat. The graph shows that 50% of the calories burned come from fat during the lower-intensity workout (that is, in the fat-burning zone) and only 40% come from fat during the higher-intensity workout. Looking at the actual numbers of calories burned, however, the scientist sees that at the higher intensity, you burn just as much fat (about 150 Calories/hour) but a much greater number of calories overall.

Think Critically Which workout will help you lose the most weight: 30 minutes in the cardio zone or 30 minutes in the fat-burning zone? Why?

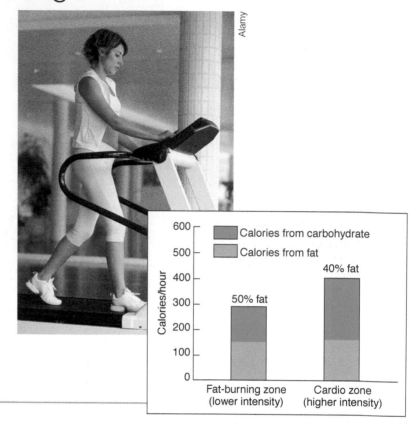

Long-term energy: Aerobic metabolism After you have been exercising for 2 to 3 minutes, your breathing and heart rate have increased to supply more oxygen to your muscles. This allows aerobic metabolism to predominate. Aerobic metabolism produces ATP at a slower rate than does anaerobic metabolism, but it is much more efficient, producing about 18 times more ATP for each molecule of glucose. As a result, glucose is used more slowly than in anaerobic metabolism. In addition, aerobic metabolism can use fatty acids, and amino acids from protein, to generate ATP (see Figure 10.11).

In a typical adult, about 90% of stored energy is found in adipose tissue; this provides an ample supply of fatty acids. When you continue to exercise at a low to moderate intensity, aerobic metabolism predominates, and fatty acids become the primary fuel source for your exercising muscles (see *What a Scientist Sees*). When you pick up the pace, the relative amount of ATP generated by anaerobic versus aerobic metabolism and the fuels you burn will change.

Protein as a fuel for exercise Although protein is not considered a major energy source for the body, even

at rest, small amounts of amino acids are used for energy. The amount increases if your diet does not provide enough total energy to meet needs, if you consume more protein than you need, or if you are involved in endurance exercise (see Chapter 6).

When the nitrogen-containing amino group is removed from an amino acid, the remaining carbon compound can be broken down to produce ATP by aerobic metabolism or, in some cases, used to make glucose (see Figure 10.8). Exercise that continues for many hours increases the use of amino acids both as an energy source and as a raw material for glucose synthesis. Strength training does not increase the use of protein for energy, but it does increase the demand for amino acids for muscle building and repair.

Exercise Intensity and Fuel Use

The energy contributions made by anaerobic and aerobic metabolism combine to ensure that your muscles get enough ATP to meet the demands you place on them. The relative contribution of each type of metabolism

The effect of exercise intensity on fuel use • Figure 10.12

Exercise intensity determines the contributions of carbohydrate, fat, and protein as fuels for ATP production. At rest and during low- to moderate-intensity exercise, aerobic metabolism predominates, so fatty acids are an important fuel source. As exercise intensity increases, the proportion of energy supplied by anaerobic metabolism increases, so glucose becomes the predominant fuel. Keep in mind, however, that during exercise, the total amount of energy expended is greater than the amount expended at rest.

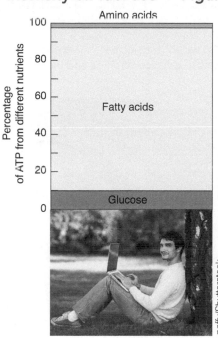

Rest

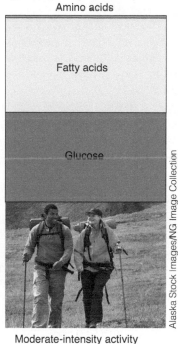

Moderate-intensity activity

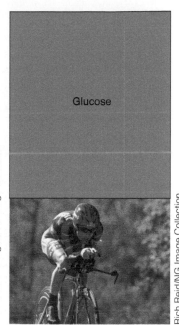

High-intensity activity

depends on the intensity of your activity. With low-intensity activity, sufficient ATP can be produced by aerobic metabolism. With intense exercise, more ATP is needed, but oxygen delivery to and use by the muscles becomes limited, so the muscles must get the additional ATP they need by using anaerobic metabolism (**Figure 10.12**).

Lower-intensity exercise relies on aerobic metabolism, which is more efficient than anaerobic metabolism and uses both glucose and fatty acids to produce ATP. The body's fat reserves are almost unlimited, so if fat is the fuel, exercise can theoretically continue for a very long time. For example, it is estimated that a 130-pound woman has enough energy stored as body fat to run 1000 miles. However, even aerobic activity uses some glucose, which means that if exercise continues long enough, glycogen stores are eventually depleted, causing fatigue.

Fatigue has many causes, including glycogen depletion, increased muscle acidity, and other changes in the muscle cells and the concentrations of molecules involved in muscle metabolism.[15] Fatigue occurs much more quickly with high-intensity exercise than with lower-intensity exercise because more intense exercise relies more on anaerobic metabolism, which can use only glucose for fuel. Glycogen stores thus are rapidly depleted (**Figure 10.13**). Anaerobic metabolism also produces lactic acid. With low-intensity exercise, the small amounts of lactic acid produced are carried

Fatigue: "Hitting the wall" • Figure 10.13

Glycogen depletion is a concern for athletes because the amount of stored glycogen available to produce glucose during exercise is limited. When athletes run out of glycogen, they experience a feeling of overwhelming fatigue that is sometimes referred to as "hitting the wall" or "bonking."

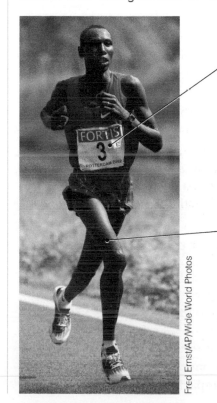

Between 60 and 120 grams of glycogen are stored in the liver; glycogen stores are highest just after a meal. Liver glycogen is used to maintain blood glucose between meals and during the night. Eating a high-carbohydrate breakfast will replenish the liver glycogen you used while you slept.

There are about 200 to 500 g of glycogen in the muscles of a 70-kg (154-lb) person. The glycogen in a muscle is used to fuel that muscle's activity.

Aerobic training causes physiological changes in the cardiovascular system that increase the delivery of oxygen to cells. It also causes changes in the muscle cells that increase glycogen storage and the ability to use oxygen to generate ATP.[17]

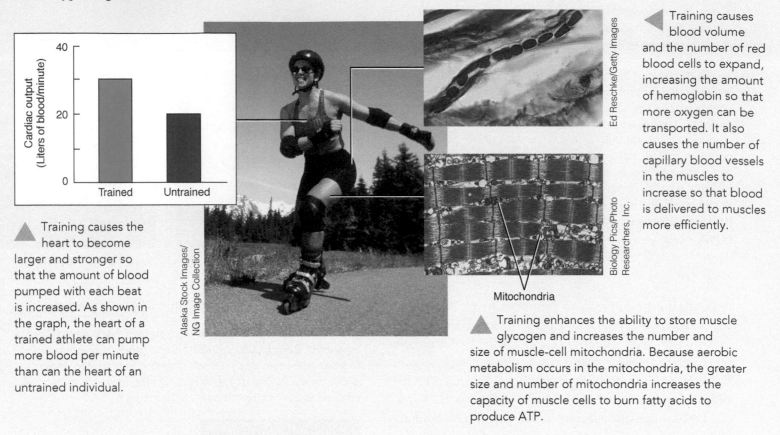

Training causes the heart to become larger and stronger so that the amount of blood pumped with each beat is increased. As shown in the graph, the heart of a trained athlete can pump more blood per minute than can the heart of an untrained individual.

Alaska Stock Images/NG Image Collection

Ed Reschke/Getty Images

Training causes blood volume and the number of red blood cells to expand, increasing the amount of hemoglobin so that more oxygen can be transported. It also causes the number of capillary blood vessels in the muscles to increase so that blood is delivered to muscles more efficiently.

Biology Pics/Photo Researchers, Inc.

Mitochondria

Training enhances the ability to store muscle glycogen and increases the number and size of muscle-cell mitochondria. Because aerobic metabolism occurs in the mitochondria, the greater size and number of mitochondria increases the capacity of muscle cells to burn fatty acids to produce ATP.

---

away from the muscles and used by other tissues as an energy source or converted back into glucose by the liver. During high-intensity exercise, the amount of lactic acid produced exceeds the amount that can be used, and the lactic acid builds up in the muscle and subsequently in the blood. Lactic acid buildup accompanies exercise-associated muscle fatigue, but it is still not known to what extent lactic acid causes fatigue.[15,16]

Fitness Training and Fuel Use

When you exercise regularly to improve your fitness, the training causes physiological changes in your body. The changes caused by repeated bouts of aerobic exercise increase the amount of oxygen that can be delivered to the muscles and the ability of the muscles to use oxygen to generate ATP by aerobic metabolism (**Figure 10.14**).[17] This increased aerobic capacity allows fatty acids to be used for fuel during higher intensity activity so that glycogen is spared and the onset of fatigue is delayed. Training aerobically also increases the amount of glycogen stored in the muscles. Because trained athletes store more glycogen and use it more slowly, they can sustain aerobic exercise for longer periods at higher intensities than can untrained individuals.

CONCEPT CHECK   STOP

1. **What** fuels are used in anaerobic metabolism?

2. **What** type of metabolism does a marathon runner rely on?

3. **Why** is a trained athlete able to perform at a higher intensity for a longer time than an untrained person?

10.5 Energy and Nutrient Needs for Physical Activity

LEARNING OBJECTIVES

1. **Compare** the energy and nutrient needs of athletes and nonathletes.
2. **Explain** why athletes are at risk for dehydration and hyponatremia.
3. **Discuss** the recommendations for food and drink during extended exercise.
4. **Plan** pre- and postcompetition meals for a marathon runner.

Good nutrition is essential to performance, whether you are a marathon runner or a mall walker. Your diet must provide enough energy to fuel activity, enough protein to maintain muscle mass, sufficient micronutrients to metabolize the energy-yielding nutrients, and enough water to transport nutrients and cool your body. The major difference between the nutritional needs of a serious athlete and those of a casual exerciser is the amount of energy and water required.

Energy Needs

The amount of energy expended for any activity depends on the intensity, duration, and frequency of the activity and the weight of the exerciser (**Figure 10.15**). Whereas casual exercise may burn only 100 additional Calories/day, the training required for an endurance athlete, such as a marathon runner, may increase energy expenditure

Factors affecting energy expenditure • Figure 10.15

This graph illustrates the impact of running pace and body weight on energy expenditure per hour. The longer an individual continues to run, the greater the amount of energy expended. Body weight affects energy needs because moving a heavier body requires more energy than moving a lighter one. Therefore, if the pace is the same, a 170-lb woman requires more energy to run for an hour than does a 125-lb woman.

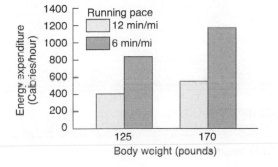

by 2000 to 3000 Calories/day. Some athletes require 6000 Calories/day to maintain their body weight. In general, the more intense the activity, the more energy it requires, and the more time spent exercising, the more energy is expended (see Appendix D). Running for 60 minutes, for instance, involves more work than walking for the same amount of time and therefore requires more energy.

Gaining or losing weight Body weight and composition can affect exercise performance. In sports such as football and weightlifting, having a large amount of muscle is advantageous, and athletes may try to build muscle and increase body weight. Healthy weight gain can be achieved through a combination of increased energy intake, adequate protein intake, and muscle-strengthening exercise to promote an increase in lean tissue rather than fat.

In sports such as ballet, gymnastics, and certain running events, small, light bodies offer an advantage, so athletes may restrict energy intake in order to maintain a low body weight. While a slightly leaner physique may be beneficial in these sports, dieting to maintain an unrealistically low weight may threaten health and performance. An athlete who needs to lose weight should do so in advance of the competitive season to prevent the calorie restriction from affecting performance. The general guidelines for healthy weight loss should be followed: Reduce energy intake by 200 to 500 Calories/day, increase activity, and change the behaviors that led to weight gain (see Chapter 9).

Unhealthy weight-loss practices Athletes who participate in sports that require weight restriction to optimize performance are vulnerable to eating disorders. The motivation and self-discipline characteristic of successful athletes contribute to their increased risk of anorexia and bulimia (see Chapter 9).[18] In athletes who develop anorexia, the restricted food intake can affect growth and maturation and impair exercise performance. In athletes who

Female athlete triad • Figure 10.16

Women with female athlete triad typically have low body fat, do not menstruate regularly (amenorrhea), and may experience multiple or recurrent stress fractures.[20] Neither adequate dietary calcium nor the increase in bone mass caused by weight-bearing exercise can compensate for the bone loss caused by low estrogen levels. Treatment involves increasing energy intake and reducing activity so that menstrual cycles resume.

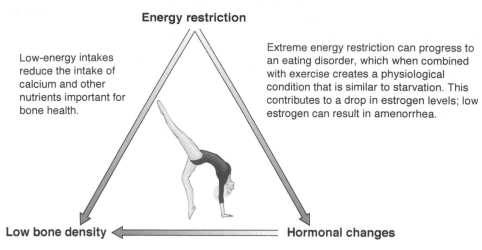

Energy restriction

Low-energy intakes reduce the intake of calcium and other nutrients important for bone health.

Extreme energy restriction can progress to an eating disorder, which when combined with exercise creates a physiological condition that is similar to starvation. This contributes to a drop in estrogen levels; low estrogen can result in amenorrhea.

Low bone density ← **Hormonal changes**

Estrogen is needed for calcium homeostasis in the bone and for calcium absorption in the intestines. Low levels lead to low peak bone mass, premature bone loss, and increased risk of stress fractures and osteoporosis.

Think Critically Why is bone loss accelerated in young girls who are not menstruating?

---

develop bulimia, purging can cause dehydration and electrolyte imbalance, which affect performance and endanger overall health.[19] In addition to using restricted food intake or purging to keep body weight low, athletes are more likely than nonathletes to engage in compulsive exercise behaviors in order to increase energy expenditure.

In female athletes, the pressure to reduce body weight and fat in order to improve performance, achieve an ideal body image, and meet goals set by coaches, trainers, or parents may lead to a combination of symptoms referred to as the **female athlete triad.** This syndrome includes energy restriction, changes in hormone levels that affect the menstrual cycle, and low bone mineral density; these symptoms can progress to more serious conditions including eating disorders, amenorrhea, and osteoporosis (**Figure 10.16**).[20]

Athletes involved in sports that have weight classes, such as wrestling and boxing, are at particular risk for unhealthy weight-loss practices because they are under pressure to lose weight before a competition so that they can compete in a lower-weight class. Competing at the high end of a weight class is thought to offer an advantage over smaller opponents. To lose weight rapidly, these athletes may use sporadic diets that severely restrict energy intake or dehydrate themselves through such practices as vigorous exercise, fluid restriction, wearing of vapor-impermeable suits, or use of hot environments, such as saunas and steam rooms, to increase sweat loss. They may also resort to even more extreme measures, such as vomiting and the use of

diuretics and laxatives. These practices can be dangerous and even fatal (**Figure 10.17**). They may impair performance and can adversely affect heart and kidney function, temperature regulation, and electrolyte balance.

Making weight • Figure 10.17

After three young wrestlers died while exercising in plastic suits in order to sweat off water, wrestling guidelines were changed to improve safety.[21] Weight classes were altered to eliminate the lightest class, plastic sweat suits were banned, weigh-ins were moved to 1 hour before competition, and mandatory weight-loss rules were instituted. The percentage of body fat can be no less than 5% for college wrestlers and 7% for high school wrestlers.

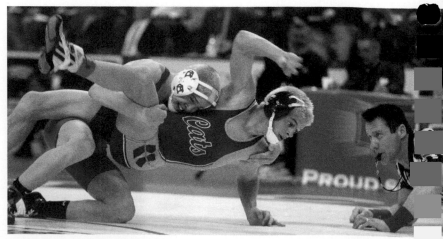

Carolyn Kaster/©AP/Wide World Photos

Carbohydrate, Fat, and Protein Needs

The source of energy in an athlete's diet can be as important as the amount. To maximize glycogen stores and optimize performance, a diet providing about 6 to 10 g of carbohydrate/kg of body weight per day is recommended for athletes in training (**Figure 10.18**).[22] The recommended amount of fat is the same as that for the general population—between 20 and 35% of energy. To allow for enough carbohydrate, fat intakes at the lower end of this range may be needed for some athletes. Diets that are very low in fat (less than 20% of calories) do not benefit performance. Protein is not a significant energy source, accounting for only about 5% of energy expended, but dietary protein is needed to maintain and repair lean tissues, including muscle. A diet in which 15 to 20% of calories come from protein will meet the needs of most athletes.

As discussed in Chapter 6, competitive athletes participating in endurance or strength sports may require extra protein. In endurance events, such as marathons, protein is used for energy and to maintain blood glucose. Athletes participating in these events may benefit from 1.2 to 1.4 g of protein/kg of body weight per day. Athletes participating in strength events require amino acids to synthesize new muscle proteins and may benefit from 1.2 to 1.7 g/kg per day.[22] While this amount is greater than the RDA (0.8 g/kg per day), it is not greater than the amount of protein habitually consumed by athletes.[23] For example, an 85-kg man consuming 3000 Calories, of which 15 to 20% is from protein, would be consuming 1.6 g of protein/kg of body weight.

Vitamin and Mineral Needs

An adequate intake of vitamins and minerals is essential for optimal performance. These micronutrients are needed for energy production, oxygen delivery, protection against oxidative damage, and repair and maintenance of body structures.

Exercise increases the amounts of many vitamins and minerals used both in metabolism during exercise and in repairing tissues after exercise. In addition, exercise may increase losses of some micronutrients. Nevertheless, special micronutrient recommendations have not been made for athletes, and most athletes can meet their needs by consuming a balanced diet that meets their energy needs.[22] Because athletes must eat more food to satisfy their higher energy needs, they consume extra vitamins and minerals with these foods, particularly if they choose nutrient-dense foods. Athletes who restrict their intake in order to maintain a low body weight may be at risk for vitamin and mineral deficiencies.

Antioxidants and oxidative damage Exercise increases the amount of oxygen used by the muscles and the rate of ATP-producing metabolic reactions. This increased oxygen use increases the production of free radicals, which can lead to oxidative damage and contribute to muscle fatigue.[24] To protect the body from oxidative damage, muscle cells contain antioxidant defenses, some of which may interact with dietary antioxidants such as vitamin C, vitamin E, β-carotene, and selenium. Despite the importance of antioxidants for health and performance, there is little evidence that supplementation with antioxidants improves human performance.[25]

Iron and anemia Iron is a component of hemoglobin, which is needed for the delivery of oxygen to cells; myoglobin, which stores oxygen within muscle cells; and other iron-containing proteins that are essential for the production of ATP by aerobic metabolism. Exercise increases the need for

Proportions of energy-yielding nutrients in an athlete's diet • Figure 10.18

The proportions of carbohydrate, fat, and protein recommended in the diets of athletes, shown in the pie chart to the right, are within the ranges recommended for the general population: 45 to 65% of total energy from carbohydrate, 20 to 35% of energy from fat, and 10 to 35% of energy from protein.

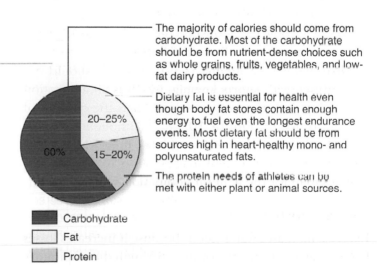

The majority of calories should come from carbohydrate. Most of the carbohydrate should be from nutrient-dense choices such as whole grains, fruits, vegetables, and low-fat dairy products.

Dietary fat is essential for health even though body fat stores contain enough energy to fuel even the longest endurance events. Most dietary fat should be from sources high in heart-healthy mono- and polyunsaturated fats.

The protein needs of athletes can be met with either plant or animal sources.

■ Carbohydrate
□ Fat
■ Protein

20–25%
60%
15–20%

Diluting blood sodium • Figure 10.22

Water and sodium are lost in sweat. Drinking plain water during extended periods of excessive sweating can dilute the sodium remaining in the blood. Hyponatremia occurs in about 6% of male ultra-endurance athletes.[29]

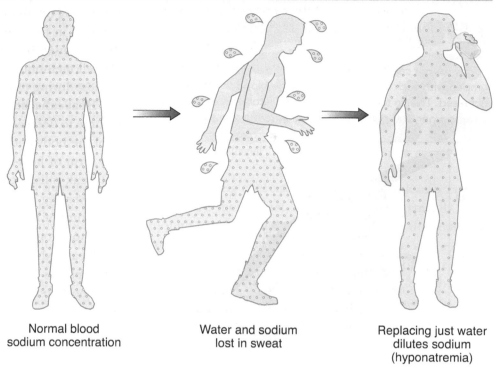

Normal blood sodium concentration

Water and sodium lost in sweat

Replacing just water dilutes sodium (hyponatremia)

Hyponatremia Sweating helps us stay cool. But if the water and sodium lost in sweat are not replaced in the right proportions, low blood sodium, or hyponatremia, may result (see Chapter 8). For most activities, sweat losses can be replaced with plain water, and lost electrolytes can be replaced during the meals following exercise. However, during endurance events such as marathons and triathalons, when sweating continues for many hours, both water and sodium need to be replenished. If an athlete replaces the lost fluid with plain water, the sodium that remains in the blood is diluted, causing hyponatremia (**Figure 10.22**). As sodium concentrations in the blood decrease, water moves into body tissues by osmosis, causing swelling. Fluid accumulation in the lungs interferes with gas exchange, and fluid accumulation in the brain causes disorientation, seizure, coma, and death.

The risk of hyponatremia can be reduced by consuming a sodium-containing sports drink during long-distance events, increasing sodium intake several days prior to a competition, and avoiding acetaminophen, aspirin, ibuprofen, and other nonsteroidal anti-inflammatory drugs, which may contribute to the development of hyponatremia by interfering with kidney function. The early symptoms of hyponatremia may be similar to those of dehydration: nausea, muscle cramps, disorientation, slurred speech, and confusion. A proper diagnosis is important because drinking water alone will make the problem worse. Mild symptoms of hyponatremia can be treated by eating salty foods or drinking a sodium-containing beverage, such as a sports drink. More severe symptoms require medical attention.

Fluid recommendations for exercise Anyone who is exercising should consume extra fluids. Because thirst is not a reliable short-term indicator of the body's water needs, it is important to schedule regular fluid breaks. To ensure hydration, adequate amounts of fluid should be consumed before, during, and after exercise.

Exercisers should drink generous amounts of fluid in the 24 hours before an exercise session and about 2 cups of fluid 4 hours before exercise. During exercise, whether casual or competitive, exercisers should try to drink enough fluid to prevent weight loss.[22] Drinking 6 to 12 ounces (oz) of fluid every 15 to 20 minutes for the duration of the exercise should maintain adequate hydration. To restore lost water after exercise, each pound of weight lost should be replaced with 16 to 24 oz (2 to 3 cups) of fluid.[22]

The best type of beverage to consume during exercise depends on the duration of the exercise. For exercise lasting an hour or less, water is the only fluid needed, particularly if one of your exercise goals is weight management.

A typical 16-oz sports drink provides about 100 Calories, so it will replace about half of the calories expended during a 40-minute ride on a stationary bicycle.

For exercise lasting more than 60 minutes, sports drinks or other beverages containing a small amount of carbohydrate (about 10 to 20 g of carbohydrate/cup) and electrolytes (around 150 milligrams of sodium/cup) are recommended.[22] The carbohydrate is a source of glucose for the muscle and thus delays fatigue. Commercial sports drinks contain rapidly absorbed sources of carbohydrate, such as glucose, sucrose, or glucose polymers (chains of glucose molecules). The right proportion of carbohydrate to water is important. If the concentration of carbohydrate is too low, it will not help performance; if it is too high, it will delay stomach emptying. Water and carbohydrate trapped in the stomach do not benefit the athlete and may cause stomach cramps. Because fruit juices and soft drinks contain twice as much sugar as sports drinks, they are not recommended unless they are diluted with an equal volume of water. The sodium in sports drinks helps prevent hyponatremia and also enhances intestinal absorption of water and glucose and stimulates thirst. Flavored beverages also tempt athletes to drink more, helping to ensure adequate hydration.

Food and Drink to Optimize Performance

For most of us, a trip to the gym requires no special nutritional planning, but for competitive athletes, when and what they eat before, during, and after competition are as important as a balanced overall diet. The type and amount of food eaten at these times may give or take away the extra seconds that can mean victory or defeat.

Maximizing glycogen stores Glycogen stores are a source of glucose, and larger glycogen stores allow exercise to continue for longer periods. Glycogen stores and hence endurance are increased by increasing carbohydrate intake (**Figure 10.23**).

Serious endurance athletes who want to substantially increase their muscle glycogen stores before a competition may choose to follow a dietary regimen referred to as **glycogen supercompensation** or **carbohydrate loading**. Such a regimen involves resting for one to three days before competition while consuming a very high-carbohydrate diet.[30] The diet should provide 10 to 12 g of carbohydrate/kg of body weight per day. For a 150-lb person, this is equivalent to about 700 g of carbohydrate per day. Having a stack of pancakes with syrup and a glass of milk or a plate of pasta with garlic bread and a glass of juice provides more than 200 g of carbohydrate. A number of commercial high-carbohydrate beverages (50 to 60 g of carbohydrate in 8 fluid oz) are available to help athletes consume the amount of carbohydrate recommended to maximize glycogen stores. (These should not be confused with sports drinks designed to be consumed during competition, which contain only about 10 to 20 g of carbohydrate in 8 fluid oz.) Trained athletes who follow a carbohydrate-loading regimen can double their muscle glycogen content.[30]

Although glycogen supercompensation is beneficial to endurance athletes, it provides no benefit, and even has some disadvantages, for those exercising for less than 90 minutes. For every gram of glycogen in the muscle, about 3 g of water is also deposited. This water will cause

> **glycogen supercompensation** or **carbohydrate loading** A regimen designed to increase muscle glycogen stores beyond their usual level.

Dietary carbohydrate and endurance • Figure 10.23

The amount of carbohydrate consumed in the diet affects the level of muscle glycogen and hence an athlete's endurance. This graph shows endurance capacity during cycling exercise after three days of a low-carbohydrate diet (less than 5% of energy from carbohydrate), a normal diet (about 55% of energy from carbohydrate), and a high-carbohydrate diet (82% of energy from carbohydrate).[31]

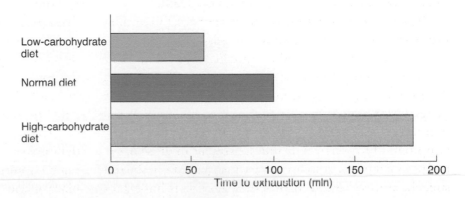

weight gain and may cause some muscle stiffness. As glycogen is used, the water is released. This can be an advantage when exercising in hot weather, but the extra weight is a disadvantage for individuals competing in short-duration events.

What to eat before exercise A pre-exercise meal should be consumed two to four hours before exercise, provide enough fluid to maintain hydration, and be high in carbohydrate (60 to 70% of calories). The carbohydrate will help maintain blood glucose and maximize glycogen stores. Muscle glycogen is depleted by activity, but liver glycogen is used to supply blood glucose and is depleted even during rest if no food is ingested. The meal should contain about 300 Calories and be moderate in protein (10 to 20%) and low in fat (10 to 25%) and fiber in order to minimize gastrointestinal distress and bloating during competition (**Figure 10.24**). Spicy foods, which can cause heartburn, and large amounts of simple sugars, which can cause diarrhea, should also be avoided unless the athlete is accustomed to eating these foods.

What to eat during exercise Most people don't need to eat while they exercise. If the activity lasts longer than an hour, however, it is important to consume carbohydrate during exercise in order to maintain glucose supplies. Carbohydrate consumption during exercise is particularly important for athletes who exercise in the morning before eating breakfast.

For exercise that lasts longer than an hour, carbohydrate intake should begin shortly after exercise begins, and regular amounts should be consumed every 15 to 20 minutes during exercise. The carbohydrate should provide a combination of glucose and fructose. (Fructose alone is not as effective as the combination and may cause diarrhea.) This carbohydrate can be obtained from a sports drink, but consuming a solid-food snack or a carbohydrate gel with water is also appropriate. About 30 to 60 g of carbohydrate (the amount in a large banana or an energy bar) each hour is recommended (see *Thinking It Through*).[22]

Snacks and sports drinks also provide sodium. Although the amount of sodium lost in sweat during exercise lasting less than three to four hours is usually not enough to affect health or performance, a snack or beverage containing sodium is recommended for exercise lasting more than an hour. This will reduce the risk of hyponatremia, improve glucose and water absorption, and stimulate thirst.

What to eat after exercise When you stop exercising, your body must shift from the task of breaking down glycogen, triglycerides, and muscle proteins for fuel to the job of restoring muscle and liver glycogen, depositing lipids, and synthesizing muscle proteins. Meals eaten after exercise should replenish lost fluid, electrolytes, and glycogen and provide protein for building and repairing muscle tissue.

The precompetition meal • Figure 10.24

When we don't eat overnight, liver glycogen stores are reduced, so replenishing glycogen by eating is particularly important first thing on the morning of a competition. A high-carbohydrate meal—such as cereal, milk, and juice—2 to 4 hours before competition can restore liver glycogen. The effects of different foods should be tested during training, not during competition. In addition to providing nutritional clout, a meal that includes "lucky" foods may provide an added psychological advantage.

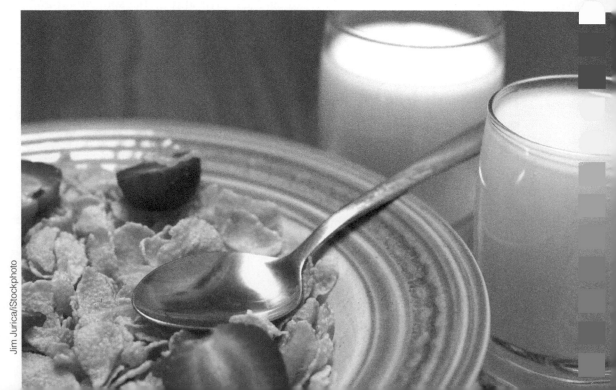

Jim Jurica/iStockphoto

A Case Study on Snacks for Exercise 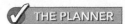 THE PLANNER

Mark enjoys long-distance cycling. On weekends, he often goes on a 40 or 50-mile ride, which takes him 3–4 hours. Despite the sports drink in his bike bottle, after about 2 hours, he gets hungry and fatigued, so he is looking for a snack that's easy to carry.

 1 Should Mark choose a high-carbohydrate, high-protein, or high-fat snack to provide the energy he needs to continue his ride? Why?

Answer: Mark should choose a snack that is high in carbohydrate and low in fat because carbohydrate is the fuel that is depleted during prolonged exercise and too much fat can delay stomach emptying and cause stomach upset.

One option for Mark is half of a turkey sandwich and a cup of grapes. This provides about 300 Calories with 50 g of carbohydrate, 5 g of fat, and 10 g of protein.

 2 Suggest another snack, with similar amounts of calories, carbohydrate, fat, and protein that Mark could put together using items he might have in his kitchen.

Your answer:

The bike shop sells a variety of energy or endurance bars that claim to prevent hunger and maintain blood glucose during extended activity. These provide about 50 g of carbohydrate and no more than 10 g of fat. Mark wonders if he should just bring a candy bar instead.

 3 Compare the amounts of carbohydrate and fat in the sandwich and grapes with the amounts in the endurance bars and the candy bars shown here. Which of the three is a better option for Mark? Why?

Your answer:

 4 Portability and cost are also important in choosing a snack for exercise. How do the sandwich and grapes, the snack you suggested, the endurance bars, and the candy bars compare in terms of these?

Your answer:

(Check your answers in online appendix L)

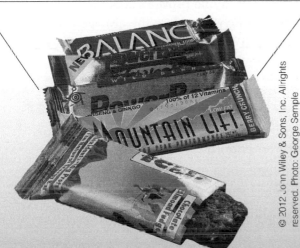

Nutrition Facts	Amount/Serving	% DV*	Amount/Serving	% DV*
Serving Size 1 bar (65g)	Total Fat 2g	3%	Total Carb 45g	15%
	Saturated Fat 0.5g	3%	Dietary Fiber 3g	12%
Calories 230	Trans Fat 0g		Sugars 14g	
Calories from Fat 20	Cholesterol 0mg	0%	Other Carb 28g	
Calories from Sat Fat 5	Sodium 90mg	4%		
*Percent Daily Values (DV) are based on a 2,000 calorie diet.	Potassium 145mg	4%	Protein 10g	

Vitamin A 0% • Vitamin C 100% • Calcium 30% • Iron 35% • Vitamin E 100%
Thiamin 100% • Riboflavin 100% • Niacin 100% • Vitamin B₆ 100%
Folate 100% • Vitamin B₁₂ 100% • Biotin 100% • Pantothenic Acid 100%
Phosphorus 35% • Magnesium 35% • Zinc 35% • Copper 35% • Chromium 20%

Nutrition Facts
Serving Size 1 bar (2 oz.) (57g)

Amount Per Serving		
Calories 271	Calories from Fat 122	
		% Daily Value*
Total Fat 14g		21%
Saturated Fat 5g		26%
Trans Fat 0g		
Cholesterol 5mg		2%
Sodium 140mg		6%
Total Carbohydrates 35g		12%
Dietary Fiber 1g		5%
Sugars 30g		
Protein 4g		

Vitamin A 2%	•	Vitamin C 0%
Calcium 5%	•	Iron 2%

*Based on a 2,000 calorie diet

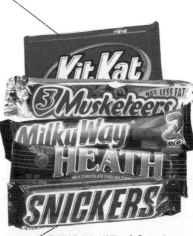

WHAT SHOULD I EAT?

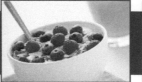
© Sara Winter/iStockphoto

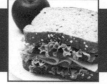
© Jill Chen/iStockphoto

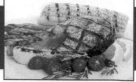
© Steve Mcsweeny/iStockphoto

Before, During, and After Exercise

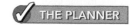
✓ THE PLANNER

A few hours before you exercise
- Fill a water bottle 4 hours before exercise and finish it before you start.
- Plan to have a high-carb meal like pasta but pass on the high-fat cream sauce.
- Have a pancake breakfast.
- Fix a bowl of cereal with low-fat milk.

During your short workouts (≤ 60 min)
- Fill your water bottle with water.
- Take a swallow of water every 15 min.

During your long workouts (>60 min)
- Fill your water bottle with a sports drink.
- Take a sip of fluid at every sign or intersection to make sure you consume at least 6 oz every 15 min.
- Carry a piece of fruit and a bagel to snack on.
- Bring a bar that's high in carbohydrates.

When you are finished
- Drink 16 to 24 oz for each pound of weight lost.
- Refuel with a sandwich or a plate of pasta and a glass of chocolate milk.

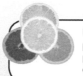
Use iProfile to plan a precompetition meal that provides at least 50 g of carbohydrate.

After exercise, the first priority for all exercisers is to replace fluid losses. For serious athletes competing on consecutive days, glycogen replacement is also a priority. To maximize glycogen replacement, a snack or beverage providing about 1.0 to 1.5 g of easily absorbed carbohydrate per kilogram of body weight should be consumed within 30 minutes after the competition and again every 2 hours for about 6 hours.[22] This is about 50 to 100 g of carbohydrate for a 70-kg (154-lb) person—the equivalent of 2 cups of pasta or 2 cups of low-fat chocolate milk. Consuming foods such as these that contain both carbohydrate and protein may enhance glycogen synthesis even more than does consuming carbohydrate alone.[32,33] Including protein with carbohydrate in postexercise foods or beverages also stimulates muscle protein synthesis and provides the amino acids needed for muscle protein synthesis and repair (see *What Should I Eat?*).[34]

The glycogen-restoring regimen just described can replenish muscle and liver glycogen within 24 hours of an athletic event and is critical for optimizing performance on the following day. Athletes who aren't competing again the next day can replenish their glycogen stores more slowly by consuming high-carbohydrate foods for the next day or so. A diet providing about 65% of calories

from carbohydrate, or about 400 g of carbohydrate in a 2500-Calorie diet, should provide sufficient carbohydrate during the recovery period.[22] If this carbohydrate comes from whole foods, it also provides protein to allow for maintenance and repair.

Most of us are not competitive athletes, so we don't need a special glycogen replacement strategy to ensure that our glycogen stores are replenished before our next visit to the gym. If your routine includes 30 to 60 minutes at the gym, a typical diet that provides about 55% of calories from carbohydrate will replace the glycogen used so that you will be ready for a workout again the next day.

CONCEPT CHECK STOP

1. **Why** might a low-carbohydrate diet be a poor choice for an endurance athlete?

2. **Why** is dehydration more likely when it is hot and humid?

3. **How** much of what fluid should you drink during a 2-hour bike ride?

4. **What** should an athlete eat as a precompetition meal and why?

10.6 Ergogenic Aids

LEARNING OBJECTIVES

1. **Assess** the health risks associated with using anabolic steroids.

2. **Explain** how supplements might enhance performance in short, intense activities.

3. **Describe** one way in which a supplement might improve endurance.

itius, altius, fortius—faster, higher, stronger—is the motto of the Olympic Games. For as long as there have been competitions, athletes have yearned for anything that would give them a competitive edge. Everything from bee pollen and high-dose vitamins to ancient herbs and hormones has been used as an **ergogenic aid**.

> **ergogenic aid**
> A substance, an appliance, or a procedure that improves athletic performance.

Athletes are willing to go to great lengths to improve performance and are therefore susceptible to the lures of ergogenic supplements. Many of the vitamins, minerals, and other substances in these supplements are involved in providing energy for exercise or promoting recovery from exercise. Most supplements do not improve athletic performance, and the few that do have a small effect compared to the benefits of an overall healthy diet (**Figure 10.25**). When considering whether to use an ergogenic supplement or any other type of supplement, an individual risk–benefit analysis should be used to determine whether the supplement is appropriate for you.

Vitamin and Mineral Supplements

Many of the promises made to athletes about the benefits of vitamin and mineral supplements are extrapolated from the biochemical functions of these micronutrients. For example, B vitamins are promoted to enhance ATP production because of their roles in muscle energy metabolism. Vitamin B_6, vitamin B_{12}, and folic acid are promoted for aerobic exercise because they are involved in the transport of oxygen to exercising muscles. These vitamins are indeed needed for energy metabolism, and a deficiency of one or more of them will interfere with ATP production and impair athletic performance. But providing more than the recommended amount does not deliver more oxygen to the muscles, cause more ATP to be produced, or enhance athletic performance.

Supplements of vitamin E, vitamin C, and selenium are promoted to athletes because of their antioxidant functions. As discussed earlier, exercise increases oxidative processes and therefore increases the production of free radicals, which cause cellular damage and have been associated with fatigue. However, antioxidant supplements have not been found to improve performance.[25]

Supplements of chromium (chromium picolinate) and vanadium (vanadyl sulfate) are marketed to increase lean body mass and decrease body fat. Chromium is needed for insulin action, and insulin promotes protein

The impact of diet and supplements on performance • Figure 10.25

This figure illustrates the relative importance of various nutrition strategies for exercise performance. Along with talent and training, eating a healthy overall diet provides the most significant benefit. Sports foods and beverages can supply energy and ensure hydration during an athletic event; most ergogenic supplements provide little or no performance boost.

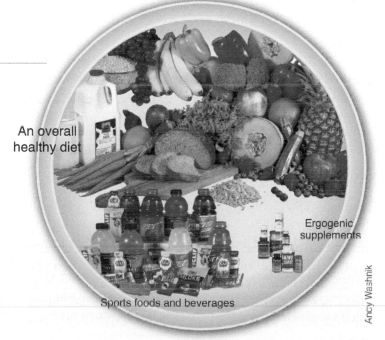

An overall healthy diet

Ergogenic supplements

Sports foods and beverages

Ancy Washnik

WHAT A SCIENTIST SEES
Anabolic Steroids

Athletes looking at this photograph see the bulging muscles and enhanced performance that can be achieved with anabolic steroid use. A scientist sees that these are not the only effects that anabolic steroids have. These drugs make the body think natural testosterone is being produced, and therefore, as shown in the diagram, the body shuts down its own testosterone production. Natural testosterone stimulates and maintains the male sexual organs and promotes the development of bones and muscles and the growth of skin and hair. The synthetic testosterone in anabolic steroids has a greater effect on muscle, bone, skin, and hair than it does on sexual organs. Without natural testosterone, the sexual organs are not maintained; this leads to shrinkage of the testicles and a decrease in sperm production.[37,38]

In adolescents, the use of anabolic steroids causes cessation of bone growth and stunted height. Anabolic steroid use may also cause oily skin and acne, water retention in the tissues, yellowing of the eyes and skin, coronary artery disease, liver disease, and sometimes death. Users may experience psychological and behavioral side effects such as violent outbursts, insomnia, and depression, possibly leading to suicide.[37,38]

When testosterone levels are low, the hypothalamus releases a hormone that stimulates the anterior pituitary to secrete a hormone that increases the production of testosterone by the testes. High levels of either natural or synthetic testosterone inhibit the release of the stimulatory hormone from the hypothalamus, shutting down the synthesis of natural testosterone.

Think Critically Why does anabolic steroid use promote muscle development while causing the testes to shrink?

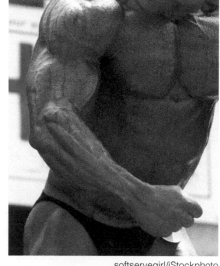
softservegirl/iStockphoto

Despite the risks, between 1 million and 3 million athletes in the United States have used anabolic steroids.[39] Anabolic steroids are controlled substances and are banned by the International Olympic Committee, the National Collegiate Athletic Association (NCAA), and most other sporting organizations.

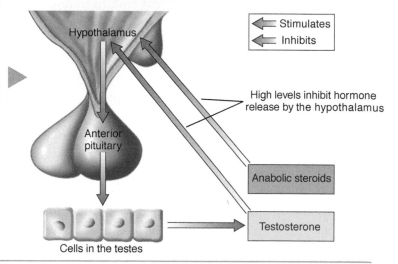

Stimulates
Inhibits

Hypothalamus

High levels inhibit hormone release by the hypothalamus

Anterior pituitary

Anabolic steroids

Cells in the testes

Testosterone

---

synthesis. However, studies have not consistently demonstrated that supplemental chromium has any effect on muscle strength, body composition, or other aspects of health (see Chapter 8).[35] Vanadium is also believed to assist the action of insulin, but there is no evidence that supplemental vanadium increases lean body mass.[36]

Supplements to Build Muscle

Protein supplements are often marketed to athletes with the promise of enhancing muscle growth or improving performance. Adequate protein is necessary for muscle growth, but consuming extra protein, either as food or as supplements, does not increase muscle growth or strength. Muscles enlarge in response to exercise stress. The protein provided by expensive supplements will not meet an athlete's

needs any better than the protein found in a balanced diet. If an athlete's diet provides enough energy, it usually provides enough protein, without a supplement.

Anabolic steroids accelerate protein synthesis. When taken in conjunction with exercise and an adequate diet, they cause increases in muscle size and strength. However, they have extremely dangerous side effects (see *What a Scientist Sees*). The Anabolic Steroid Control Act of 1990 made possession of anabolic steroids without a prescription illegal. The act was amended in 2004 to include **steroid precursors**, which are compounds that can be converted into steroid hormones in the body. The best known of these

anabolic steroids Synthetic fat-soluble hormones that mimic testosterone and are used to increase muscle strength and mass.

is androstenedione, often referred to as "andro." It was launched to public prominence when professional baseball player Mark McGwire announced his use of it during the 1998 major league baseball season, when he hit 70 home runs, breaking the league's single-season home-run record. Contrary to marketing claims, the use of andro or other steroid precursors has not been found to increase testosterone levels or produce any ergogenic effects, and they may cause some of the same side effects as anabolic steroids.[40]

Growth hormone is another hormone used to increase muscle protein synthesis. Despite this physiological effect, however, it has not been shown to enhance muscle strength, power, or aerobic exercise capacity, but there is evidence that it improves anaerobic exercise capacity.[41] Prolonged use of growth hormone can cause heart dysfunction, high blood pressure, and excessive growth of some body parts, such as hands, feet, and facial features.[41] Growth hormone is on the World Anti-Doping Agency's list of banned substances.

Supplements of the amino acids ornithine, arginine, and lysine are marketed with the promise that they will stimulate the release of growth hormone and, in turn, enhance the growth of muscles. Large doses of these amino acids have been shown to stimulate the release of growth hormone. However, growth hormone levels in the blood of athletes taking these amino acids are no greater than levels typically resulting from exercise alone. Also, supplements of these amino acids have not been found to cause greater increases in muscle mass and strength than those achieved through strength-training exercise alone.[42,43]

Supplements to Enhance Performance in Short, Intense Activities

A number of supplements are marketed to athletes who seek to improve performance in sports that depend on quick bursts of intense activity. Supplements of β-hydroxy-β-methylbutyrate, known as HMB, claim to increase strength and muscle growth and improve muscle recovery; however, the outcome of research studies has been variable. Overall, studies have found a small increase in strength in previously untrained men, but the effects in trained weightlifters are trivial, as is the effect of HMB on body composition.[44]

Bicarbonate is a supplement that may enhance performance in high-intensity activities. Because bicarbonate acts as a buffer in the body, supplementing it is thought to neutralize acid and thus delay fatigue and allow improved performance. Taking sodium bicarbonate, which is just baking soda from the kitchen cupboard, before exercise has been found to have a moderately positive effect on performance in sports, such as sprint cycling and sprint swimming, which entail intense exercise lasting only 1 to 7 minutes, as well as to enhance endurance in longer continuous and intermittent exercise, such as running and cycling.[45] However, just because baking soda is an ingredient in your cookies does not mean that it is risk free. Many people experience abdominal cramps and diarrhea after taking sodium bicarbonate, and other possible side effects have not been carefully researched.

One of the most popular ergogenic supplements is **creatine**. This nitrogen-containing compound is found primarily in muscle, where it is used to make creatine phosphate (**Figure 10.26**). Higher levels of creatine and creatine phosphate provide more quick energy for short-term muscular activity. Creatine supplementation has been shown to increase muscle creatine phosphate levels and improve performance in high-intensity exercise lasting 30 seconds or less. It is therefore beneficial for exercise that requires explosive bursts of energy, such as sprinting and weightlifting, but not for long-term endurance activities, such as

Creatine boosts creatine phosphate • Figure 10.26

Creatine can be synthesized in the liver and kidneys and is consumed in the diet in meat and milk. The more creatine consumed, the greater the amount of creatine stored in the muscles. Increasing creatine intake with supplement use has been shown to increase levels of muscle creatine and creatine phosphate, which is made from it.[46] During short bursts of intense activity, the creatine phosphate can transfer a phosphate group to ADP, forming creatine, and ATP that can be used for muscle contraction.

Ask Yourself

Why might creatine supplements have a greater ergogenic effect in someone who consumes a vegetarian diet than in someone who consumes a diet high in meat and dairy products?

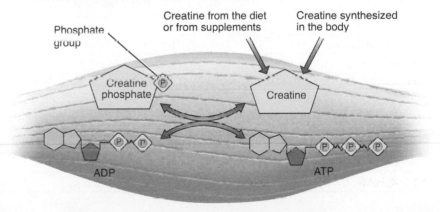

Debate | Energy Drinks for Athletic Performance?

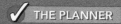

The Issue: Energy drinks are sold alongside sports drinks, and manufacturers of these beverages often sponsor athletes and athletic events. Should they be used as ergogenic aids? Is drinking them a safe way to improve your game?

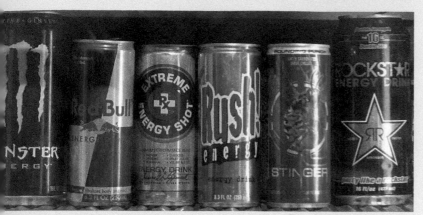

Tony Cenicola/Redux Pictures

The popularity of energy drinks with names like Red Bull, Monster, and Full Throttle has soared over the past decade. They promise to keep you alert to study, work, drive, party all night, and perhaps excel at your next athletic competition. The main ingredients in these drinks are sugar and caffeine. Glucose is an important fuel for exercise, and caffeine is known to enhance endurance, so these drinks may seem like an ideal ergogenic aid.

A traditional sports drink, like Gatorade, contains about 28 g of sugar in 16 oz; a typical energy drink provides twice this much (55 to 60 g, or about 14 teaspoons). Since carbohydrate fuels activity, it may seem that the additional sugar would provide energy for prolonged exercise. But more is not always better during activity. The double load of sugar cannot be absorbed quickly, and unabsorbed sugar in the stomach can cause GI distress and also slow fluid absorption.

The caffeine content of energy drinks ranges from 50 to about 500 mg per can or bottle. Caffeine is an effective ergogenic aid that enhances endurance when consumed before or during exercise.[48] But too much caffeine, referred to as *caffeine toxicity*, causes nervousness, anxiety, restlessness, insomnia, gastrointestinal upset, tremors, increased blood pressure, and rapid heartbeat. A number of cases of caffeine-associated death, seizure, and cardiac arrest have occurred after consumption of energy drinks.[49–51] Even if the caffeine in an energy drink increases endurance, depending on when it is consumed, it can affect timing and coordination and hurt overall performance. Caffeine is also a diuretic; at the levels contained in these drinks, it may contribute to dehydration, particularly in first-time users.[52] The FDA limits the amount of caffeine in soft drinks to 0.02% (about 71 mg in 12 oz), but energy drinks are considered dietary supplements, so the caffeine content is not regulated.

Energy drinks often also contain other ingredients that promise to improve performance, such as B vitamins, taurine, guarana, and ginseng. B vitamins are needed to produce ATP, so they are marketed to enhance energy production from sugar. But unless you are deficient in these vitamins, drinking them in an energy drink will not enhance your ATP production. Taurine is an amino acid that may reduce the amount of muscle damage and improve exercise performance and capacity, but not all research supports these claims.[51] Guarana is an herbal ingredient that contains caffeine as well as small amounts of the stimulants theobromine and theophylline. The extra caffeine from guarana (not included in the caffeine listed for these beverages) may contribute to caffeine toxicity. Ginseng is also claimed to have performance-enhancing effects, but these effects have not been demonstrated scientifically.[50,53] In general, the amounts of these ingredients are too small to have much effect, and the safety of consuming them in combination with caffeine prior to or during exercise has yet to be established.[50]

So should you down an energy drink before your next competition? They do provide a caffeine boost, but is it so much caffeine that you risk dehydration, high blood pressure, and heart problems? Energy drinks provide sugar to fuel activity, but will they upset your stomach? What about the herbal ingredients—do they offer a benefit you are looking for?

Think Critically: Use the table below to assess the advantages and disadvantages of consuming an 8-oz can of Red Bull versus a 12-oz can of Coca-Cola Classic before your 30-minute run.

How much caffeine is in your beverage?

Beverage	Serving (fluid ounces)	Caffeine (mg)	Sugar (g)	Energy (Calories)
Coffee	8	100–200	0	0
Coca-Cola Classic	8	23	26	93
Mountain Dew	8	36	31	113
Monster	8	80	27	100
Jolt Cola	8	80	30	120
Arizona Caution Extreme Energy Shot	8	100	33	130
Red Bull	8	80	28	110
Rockstar	8	80	31	140
Full Throttle	8	80	28	110

marathons.[46] Athletes also take creatine supplements to increase muscle mass and strength. Creatine in combination with resistance training has been found to increase muscle strength and size more than resistance training alone.[47]

There is little evidence of any adverse effects of creatine supplementation in healthy people; however, high-dose (3–5 g/day) creatine supplementation should not be used by individuals with renal disease or those at risk for renal dysfunction such as those with diabetes or hypertension.[54] The FDA has advised consumers to consult a physician before using creatine.

Supplements to Enhance Endurance

Sprinters and weightlifters can benefit from increases in creatine phosphate levels, but endurance athletes are more concerned about running out of glycogen. Glycogen is spared when fat is used as an energy source, allowing exercise to continue for a longer time before glycogen is depleted and fatigue sets in. Supplements that increase the amount of fat or oxygen available to the muscle cells are used to increase endurance.

Carnitine supplements are marketed as fat burners—substances that increase the utilization of fat during exercise. Carnitine is needed to transport fatty acids into the mitochondria, where they are used to produce ATP by aerobic metabolism. We ingest carnitine in red meats and dairy products, and it is synthesized in the body. Even when dietary carnitine is low, enough carnitine is made in the body to ensure efficient use of fatty acids. Carnitine supplements have not been shown to increase endurance.[55]

Medium-chain triglycerides (MCT) are composed of fatty acids with medium-length carbon chains (8 to 10 carbons). These fatty acids can be absorbed directly into the blood without first being incorporated into chylomicrons. They are therefore absorbed quickly, causing blood fatty acids levels to rise and thereby increasing the availability of fat as a fuel for exercise. Nevertheless, research has not found that supplementation with MCT increases endurance, spares glycogen, or enhances performance.[56]

Caffeine is a stimulant found in coffee, tea, soft drinks, and energy drinks (see *Debate: Energy Drinks for Athletic Performance?*). Consuming 3 to 6 mg of caffeine per kilogram of body weight, an amount equivalent to about 2.5 cups of percolated coffee, up to an hour before exercising as well as consuming smaller doses of caffeine during exercise (1 to 2 mg/kg) have been shown to improve endurance.[46] Caffeine enhances the release of fatty acids. When fatty acids are used as a fuel source, less glycogen is used, and the onset of fatigue is delayed. Athletes who are unaccustomed to caffeine respond better to it than do those who consume caffeine routinely. Caffeine also improves concentration and enhances alertness, but in some athletes, it may impair performance by causing gastrointestinal upset or caffeine toxicity symptoms.

Athletes also use the hormone erythropoietin, known as EPO, to enhance endurance. Natural erythropoietin is produced by the kidneys and stimulates cells in the bone marrow to differentiate into red blood cells. EPO can enhance endurance by increasing the number of red blood cells and hence the ability to transport oxygen to the muscles. It therefore increases aerobic capacity and spares glycogen. However, too much EPO can cause production of too many red blood cells, which can lead to excessive blood clotting, heart attacks, and strokes. EPO was banned in 1990, after it was linked to the deaths of more than a dozen cyclists.[57]

Other Supplements

In addition to the supplements discussed thus far, hundreds of other products are marketed to athletes. Most have no effect on performance. For example, brewer's yeast is a source of B vitamins and some minerals but has not been found to have any ergogenic properties. Likewise, there is no evidence to support claims that bee pollen or wheat germ oil enhances performance. Royal jelly is a substance that worker bees produce to help the queen bee grow larger and live longer, but it does not appear to enhance athletic capacity in humans. Supplements of DNA and RNA are marketed to aid in tissue regeneration. DNA and RNA are needed to synthesize proteins, but they are not required in the diet, and supplements do not help replace damaged cells.

Herbal products are also marketed to athletes. Most have not been studied extensively for their ergogenic effects, so the only evidence of their benefits is anecdotal. Many can harm health as well as performance, so athletes should consider the risks before using these products.

CONCEPT CHECK	

1. How do anabolic steroids affect the production of testosterone?
2. Why are creatine supplements beneficial for sprint and strength athletes?
3. How does caffeine increase endurance?

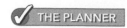
Summary

1 Food, Physical Activity, and Health 330

- Food fuels physical activity, and physical activity in turn affects energy and nutrient needs. As shown in the illustration, both food and physical activity promote health. Regular physical activity can reduce the risk of chronic diseases such as obesity, heart disease, diabetes, and osteoporosis. It can reduce overall mortality even in obese individuals.

Food and physical activity benefit health • Figure 10.1

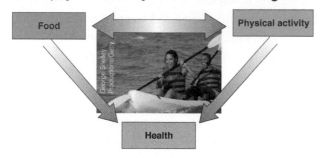

- Physical activity helps manage body weight by increasing energy expenditure, and by increasing the proportion of body weight that is lean tissue.

2 The Four Components of Fitness 332

- How fit an individual is depends on his or her **cardiorespiratory endurance**, **muscle strength**, **muscle endurance**, flexibility, and body composition. Regular **aerobic activity**, such as the swimming shown here, improves **aerobic capacity**. **Muscle-strengthening exercise** increases muscle strength and endurance. Stretching improves flexibility. Fit individuals have a higher percentage of lean tissue than unfit individuals of the same body weight.

The components of fitness • Figure 10.4a

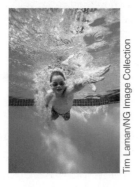

3 Physical Activity Recommendations 335

- To reduce the risk of chronic disease, a minimum of 30 minutes of moderate-intensity aerobic activity on most days is recommended, as indicated by the calendar. A well-designed fitness program involves aerobic activity, stretching, and muscle-strengthening exercises.

Physical activity recommendations • Figure 10.5

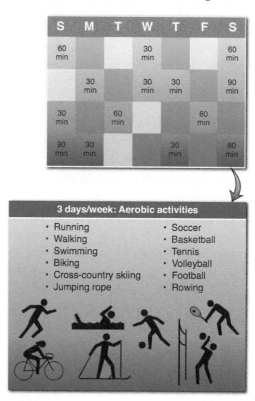

- A fitness program should include activities that are enjoyable, convenient, and safe. Rest is important to allow the body to recover and rebuild. In serious athletes, inadequate rest relative to training can lead to **overtraining syndrome**.

4 Fueling Activity 339

- The graph illustrates that during the first 10 to 15 seconds of exercise, ATP and **creatine phosphate** stored in the muscle provide energy to fuel activity. During the next 2 to 3 minutes, the amount of oxygen at the muscle remains limited, so ATP is generated by the **anaerobic metabolism** of glucose. After a few minutes, the delivery of oxygen at the muscle increases, and ATP can be generated by **aerobic metabolism**. Aerobic metabolism is more efficient than anaerobic metabolism and can utilize glucose, fatty acids, and amino acids as energy sources. The use of protein as an energy source increases when exercise continues for many hours.

Changes in the source of ATP over time • Figure 10.10

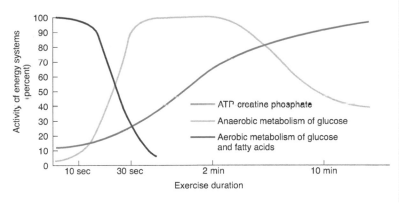

- For short-term, high-intensity activity, ATP is generated primarily from the anaerobic metabolism of glucose from glycogen stores. Anaerobic metabolism uses glucose rapidly and produces **lactic acid**. Both of these factors are associated with the onset of fatigue. For lower-intensity exercise of longer duration, aerobic metabolism predominates, and both glucose and fatty acids are important fuel sources.

- Fitness training causes changes in the cardiovascular system and muscles that improve oxygen delivery and utilization, allowing aerobic activity to be sustained for longer periods at higher intensity.

5 Energy and Nutrient Needs for Physical Activity 345

- The diet of an active individual should provide sufficient energy to fuel activity. The pressure to compete and maintain a body weight that is optimal for their sport puts some athletes at risk for eating disorders. A combination of excessive exercise and energy restriction puts female athletes at risk for the **female athlete triad**, shown here.

Female athlete triad • Figure 10.16

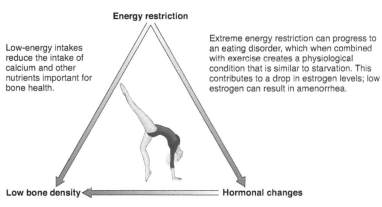

- To maximize glycogen stores, optimize performance, and maintain and repair lean tissue, a diet providing about 60% of energy from carbohydrate, 20 to 25% of energy from fat, and about 15 to 20% of energy from protein is recommended.

- Sufficient vitamins and minerals are needed to generate ATP from macronutrients, to maintain and repair tissues, and to transport oxygen and wastes to and from the cells. Most athletes who consume a varied diet that meets their energy needs also meet their vitamin and mineral needs from their diet alone. Those who restrict their food intake may be at risk for deficiencies. Increased iron needs and greater iron losses due to fitness training put athletes, particularly female athletes, at risk for iron deficiency.

- Water is needed to ensure that the body can be cooled and that nutrients and oxygen can be delivered to body tissues. If water intake is inadequate, dehydration can lead to a decline in exercise performance and increase the risk of **heat-related illness**. Adequate fluid intake before exercise ensures that athletes begin exercise well hydrated. Fluid intake during and after exercise must replace water lost in sweat and from evaporation through the lungs. Plain water is an appropriate fluid to consume for most exercise. Beverages containing carbohydrate and sodium are recommended for exercise lasting more than an hour. Drinking plain water during extended exercise increases the risk of hyponatremia.

- Competitive endurance athletes may benefit from **glycogen supercompensation** (**carbohydrate loading**), which maximizes glycogen stores before an event. Meals eaten before competition should help ensure adequate hydration, provide moderate amounts of protein, be high enough in carbohydrate to maximize glycogen stores, be low in fat and fiber to speed gastric emptying, and satisfy the psychological needs of the athlete. During exercise, athletes need beverages and food to replace lost fluid and provide carbohydrate and sodium. Postcompetition meals should replace lost fluids and electrolytes, provide carbohydrate to restore muscle and liver glycogen, and provide protein for muscle protein synthesis and repair.

6   Ergogenic Aids 355

- Many types of **ergogenic aids** are marketed to improve athletic performance. Some are beneficial for certain types of activity, but many offer little or no benefit. An individual risk–benefit analysis should be used to determine whether a supplement is appropriate for you.

- Athletes may take protein supplements or use hormones to build muscle. **Anabolic steroids** are hormones that when combined with muscle-strengthening exercise increase muscle size and strength, but these supplements are illegal and have dangerous side effects.

- **Creatine** supplementation increases muscle creatine phosphate levels, as illustrated here, and has been shown to increase muscle mass and improve performance in short-duration, high-intensity exercise.

Creatine boosts creatine phosphate • Figure 10.26

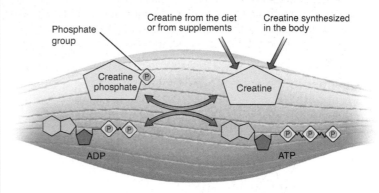

- Caffeine use can improve performance in endurance activities, but high doses can cause caffeine toxicity and contribute to dehydration in some athletes. EPO can enhance endurance by increasing the number of red blood cells, but it is dangerous and is a banned substance.

Key Terms

- aerobic capacity 334
- aerobic activity 334
- aerobic metabolism 339
- aerobic zone 337
- anabolic steroids 356
- anaerobic metabolism 339
- atrophy 333
- cardiorespiratory endurance 334

- creatine 357
- creatine phosphate 340
- endorphins 331
- ergogenic aid 355
- female athlete triad 346
- fitness 330
- glycogen supercompensation or carbohydrate loading 351

- heat cramps 349
- heat exhaustion 349
- heat stroke 349
- heat-related illnesses 348
- hypertrophy 333
- lactic acid 339
- maximum heart rate 337
- muscle endurance 334

- muscle strength 334
- muscle-strengthening exercise 334
- overload principle 332
- overtraining syndrome 338
- resting heart rate 334
- sports anemia 348
- steroid precursors 356

What is happening in this picture?

During competitive events, cyclists often spend 6 or more hours a day riding their bikes. This rider is picking up a musette bag, which contains water bottles and snacks. He will carry the bottles on his bike and the food in his jersey pockets to have water and fuel available during his ride.

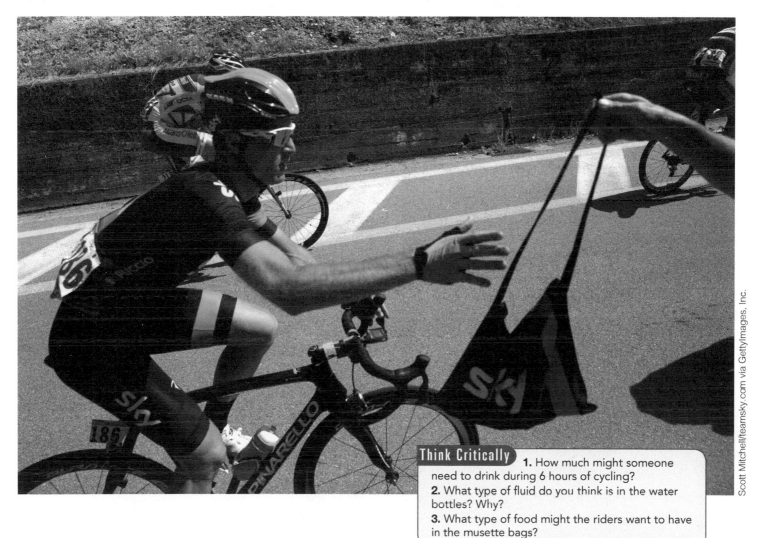

Scott Mitchell/teamsky.com via GettyImages, Inc.

Think Critically
1. How much might someone need to drink during 6 hours of cycling?
2. What type of fluid do you think is in the water bottles? Why?
3. What type of food might the riders want to have in the musette bags?

THE PLANNER ✔

Review your Chapter Planner on the chapter opener and check off your completed work.

LEARNING OBJECTIVES

1. **Describe** how the embryo and fetus are nourished.

2. **Discuss** why appropriate weight gain is important during pregnancy.

3. **Explain** why morning sickness, heartburn, and constipation are common during pregnancy.

4. **Review** the risks associated with the hypertensive disorders of pregnancy and gestational diabetes.

Whether you end up 6 feet 4 inches or 5 feet 3 inches tall, you begin as a single cell that arises from the union of a sperm and an egg. Over the course of 40 weeks, this cell grows and develops into a fully formed human baby. Prenatal growth and development are carefully orchestrated processes that require adequate supplies of calories and all the essential nutrients in order to progress normally.

In the days after **fertilization**, the single cell divides rapidly to form a ball of cells (**Figure 11.1**). The cells then begin to differentiate

> **fertilization** The union of a sperm and an egg.

PROCESS DIAGRAM

Prenatal development • Figure 11.1

✓ THE PLANNER

This cross section shows the path of the egg and developing embryo from the ovary, where the egg is produced, through the oviduct to the uterus, where most prenatal development occurs.

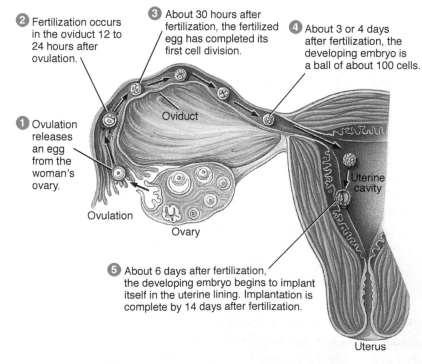

1 Ovulation releases an egg from the woman's ovary.

2 Fertilization occurs in the oviduct 12 to 24 hours after ovulation.

3 About 30 hours after fertilization, the fertilized egg has completed its first cell division.

4 About 3 or 4 days after fertilization, the developing embryo is a ball of about 100 cells.

5 About 6 days after fertilization, the developing embryo begins to implant itself in the uterine lining. Implantation is complete by 14 days after fertilization.

Oviduct

Ovulation

Ovary

Uterine cavity

Uterus

6 During the embryonic stage of development, from 2 to 8 weeks after fertilization, cells differentiate and arrange themselves in the proper locations to form the major organ systems. The embryo shown here is about 5 to 6 weeks old and less than 3 cm long. The organ systems and external body structures are not fully developed.

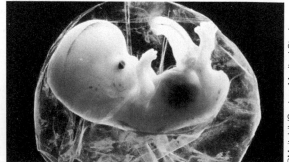

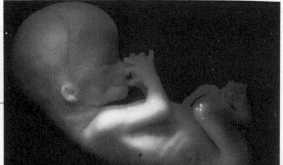

HOW IT WORKS

7 The fetal stage of development begins at 9 weeks after fertilization and continues until birth. During this time, the fetus grows, and internal and external body structures continue to develop. This fetus is about 16 weeks old and about 16 cm long.

©Meitchik/Custom Medical Stock Photo, Inc.

Biophoto Associates/PhotoResearchers

The placenta • Figure 11.2

The placenta is made up of branchlike projections that extend from the embryo into the uterine lining, placing maternal and fetal blood in close proximity. The placenta allows nutrients and oxygen to pass from maternal blood to fetal blood and waste products to be transferred from fetal blood to maternal blood. Fetal blood travels to and from the placenta via the umbilical cord.

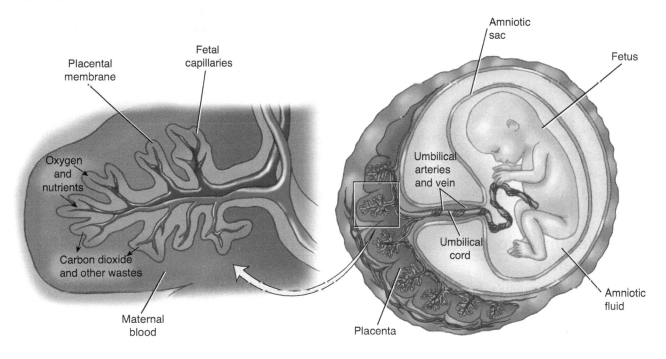

Nourishing the Embryo and Fetus

The embryonic stage of development lasts until the eighth week after fertilization. During this time, the cells differentiate to form the multitude of specialized cell types that make up the human body. At the end of this stage, the embryo is about 3 centimeters (cm) long and has a beating heart. The rudiments of all major external and internal body structures have been formed.

and move to form body structures. During these early steps in development, this ball of cells obtains the nutrients it needs from the fluids around it. About a week after fertilization, the developing embryo begins burrowing into the lining of the uterus; and by two weeks, **implantation** is complete, and the cluster of cells has become an **embryo**.

implantation The process through which a developing embryo embeds itself in the uterine lining.

embryo A developing human from 2 through 8 weeks after fertilization.

The early embryo gets its nourishment by breaking down the lining of the uterus, but soon this source is inadequate to meet its growing needs. After about five weeks, the **placenta** takes over the role of nourishing the embryo (**Figure 11.2**). The placenta also secretes hormones that are necessary to maintain pregnancy.

From the ninth week on, the developing offspring is a **fetus**. During the fetal period, structures formed during the embryonic period grow and mature. The placenta continues to nourish the fetus until birth. During this time, the length of the fetus increases from about 3 cm to around 50 cm. The fetal period usually ends after 40 weeks, with the birth of an infant weighing 3 to 4 kilograms (6.5 to 9 pounds).[1]

Infants who are born on time but have failed to grow well in the uterus are said to be **small for gestational age**.

placenta An organ produced from maternal and embryonic tissues. It secretes hormones, transfers nutrients and oxygen from the mother's blood to the fetus, and removes metabolic wastes.

fetus A developing human from the ninth week after fertilization to birth.

Discomforts of Pregnancy

The physiological changes that occur during pregnancy can cause uncomfortable side effects. For example, the expansion in blood volume necessary to nourish the fetus often causes an accumulation of extracellular fluid in the tissues, a condition known as **edema**. Edema can be uncomfortable but does not increase medical risks unless it is accompanied by a rise in blood pressure.

Almost 70% of women experience nausea and vomiting during the first trimester of pregnancy.[9] This is referred to as **morning sickness**, but symptoms can occur at any time during the day or night. Morning sickness is thought to be related to hormones that are released early in pregnancy. The symptoms may be alleviated by eating small, frequent snacks of dry, starchy foods, such as plain crackers or bread. In most women, the symptoms of morning sickness decrease significantly after the first trimester, but in some they last for the entire pregnancy and, in severe cases, may require intravenous nutrition.[10]

The hormones produced during pregnancy to relax uterine muscles also relax the muscles of the gastrointestinal tract. This relaxation, along with crowding of the organs by the growing baby, can cause heartburn and constipation (**Figure 11.5**). Heartburn can be reduced by limiting high-fat foods, which leave the stomach slowly; avoiding substances, such as caffeine and chocolate, that are known to cause heartburn; eating small, frequent meals; and remaining upright after eating. Constipation can be prevented by maintaining a moderate level of physical activity and consuming plenty of fluids and high-fiber foods. Hemorrhoids are common during pregnancy as a result of both constipation and changes in blood flow.

Crowding of the gastrointestinal tract • Figure 11.5

During pregnancy, the uterus enlarges and pushes higher into the abdominal cavity, exerting pressure on the stomach and intestines.

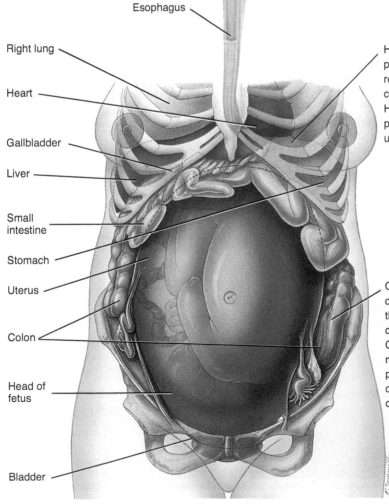

Esophagus

Right lung

Heart

Gallbladder

Liver

Small intestine

Stomach

Uterus

Colon

Head of fetus

Bladder

Heartburn is common during pregnancy because the sphincter relaxes, allowing acidic stomach contents to leak into the esophagus. Heartburn increases as pregnancy progresses because the enlarging uterus crowds the stomach.

Constipation is common during pregnancy because the relaxed muscles of the colon are less efficient. Constipation becomes more of a problem late in pregnancy, when the weight of the uterus puts pressure on the colon.

Ask Yourself

Why is heartburn common during pregnancy?

Complications of Pregnancy

Most of the 3.95 million women who give birth every year in the United States have healthy pregnancies. However, about 12% of babies are born too soon, 8% have low or very low birth weights, and about 6 out of 1000 of those born alive die in their first year of life.[11] In the United States, about 21 out of every 100,000 women die as a result of childbirth.[12] If complications that occur during pregnancy are caught early, they can usually be managed, resulting in the delivery of a healthy baby.

High blood pressure About 5 to 10% of pregnant women in the United States experience high blood pressure during pregnancy.[13] **Hypertensive disorders of pregnancy** refers to a spectrum of conditions involving elevated blood pressure during pregnancy. It accounts for more than 12% of pregnancy-related maternal deaths in the United States.[14]

High blood pressure that is present before the pregnancy or diagnosed before 20 weeks of gestation is referred to as chronic hypertension; it complicates about 3% of pregnancies.[15,16] **Gestational hypertension** is an abnormal rise in blood pressure that occurs after the 20th week of pregnancy and resolves within 12 weeks of birth; it complicates about 6% of pregnancies and may signal the potential for a more serious condition called preeclampsia.[15,16] Preeclampsia is characterized by high blood pressure, severe headaches, changes in vision, rapid weight gain, abdominal pain, and swelling of the hands and feet. It is dangerous to the baby because blood flow to the placenta is reduced, and it is dangerous to the mother because it can progress to a more severe condition called **eclampsia**, in which life-threatening seizures occur. Preeclampsia can often be managed with bed rest and careful medical monitoring, but if symptoms are severe it may necessitate early delivery of the baby. The condition usually resolves after delivery. Preeclampsia and eclampsia are more common in mothers under 18 and over 35 years of age, low-income mothers, obese mothers, and mothers with chronic hypertension or kidney disease.

The causes of hypertension during pregnancy are not fully understood. At one time, low-sodium diets were

> **preeclampsia** A condition characterized by elevated blood pressure, a rapid increase in body weight, protein in the urine, and edema. Also called *toxemia*.
>
> **eclampsia** Convulsions or seizures during or immediately after pregnancy. Untreated, it can lead to coma or death.

prescribed to prevent preeclampsia, but studies have not found such diets to be beneficial in lowering blood pressure or preventing this condition.[17] Calcium may play a role in preventing hypertensive disorders of pregnancy. Women with a high intake of calcium have a low incidence of these disorders, and calcium supplements have been found to reduce the risk of preeclampsia in high-risk women.[18] Calcium supplements are not routinely recommended for healthy pregnant women; however, pregnant teens, individuals with inadequate calcium intake, and women who are known to be at risk of developing preeclampsia may benefit from additional dietary calcium.[18]

Gestational diabetes Diabetes that develops in a pregnant woman is known as **gestational diabetes**. Glucose passes freely across the placenta, so when the mother's blood glucose levels are high the growing fetus receives extra glucose and hence extra calories. The baby grows rapidly and is at risk for being large for gestational age and consequently at increased risk for difficult delivery and abnormal blood glucose levels at birth. Controlling the mother's blood glucose through changes in diet and activity, and in some cases medication, reduces the risks to the baby. Gestational diabetes is common in obese women and those with a family history of type 2 diabetes and occurs more frequently among Asian, African American, Hispanic/Latino, and Native American women than among Caucasian women.[19] It usually resolves after the birth, but up to half of women who have had gestational diabetes develop type 2 diabetes within the next 5 to 10 years.[20] Babies born to mothers with gestational diabetes are at increased risk of developing diabetes as adults.[20]

> **gestational diabetes** A condition characterized by high blood glucose levels that develop during pregnancy.

CONCEPT CHECK

1. **How** are nutrients and oxygen transferred from mother to fetus?

2. **How** does a mother's weight gain during pregnancy affect the health of her child?

3. **Why** do heartburn and constipation tend to increase later in pregnancy?

4. **How** does gestational diabetes in a mother affect the baby?

11.2 Nutritional Needs During Pregnancy

LEARNING OBJECTIVES

1. **Compare** the energy and protein needs of pregnant and nonpregnant women.
2. **Explain** why pregnancy increases the need for many vitamins and minerals.
3. **Discuss** the need for dietary supplements during pregnancy.

During pregnancy, the mother's diet must provide all of her nutrients as well as those needed for the baby's growth and development. Because the increase in nutrient needs is greater than the increase in energy needs, a nutrient-dense diet is essential.

Energy and Macronutrient Needs

Although pregnant women are eating for two, they don't need to eat twice as much as they normally do. During the first trimester, energy needs are not increased above levels for nonpregnant women. During the second and third trimesters, an additional 340 and 452 Calories/day, respectively, is recommended (**Figure 11.6**).[21]

Protein needs are increased during pregnancy because protein is needed for the synthesis of new blood cells, formation of the placenta, enlargement of the uterus and breasts, and growth of the baby (see Figure 11.6). An additional 25 grams (g) of protein above the RDA for nonpregnant women, or 1.1 g/kg/day, is recommended for the second and third trimesters of pregnancy.

To ensure sufficient glucose to fuel the fetal and maternal brains during pregnancy, the RDA for carbohydrate is increased by 45 g, to 175 g/day. If this carbohydrate comes from whole grains, fruits, and vegetables, it will also provide the additional 3 g/day of fiber recommended during pregnancy.

Although it is not necessary to increase total fat intake during pregnancy, additional amounts of the essential fatty acids linoleic and α-linolenic acid are recommended because they are incorporated into the placenta and fetal tissues. The long-chain polyunsaturated fatty acids docosahexaenoic acid (DHA) and arachidonic acid (ARA) are important because they not only support maternal health but are essential for development of the eyes and nervous system in the fetus.[22]

Despite increases in the recommended intakes of protein, carbohydrate, and specific fatty acids during pregnancy, the distribution of calories from protein, carbohydrate, and fat should be about the same as that recommended for the general population.

Energy and macronutrient recommendations • Figure 11.6

This graph illustrates the difference between the recommended daily intake of energy, protein, carbohydrate, fiber, essential fatty acids, and water for 25-year-old nonpregnant women and 25-year-old pregnant women during the third trimester.

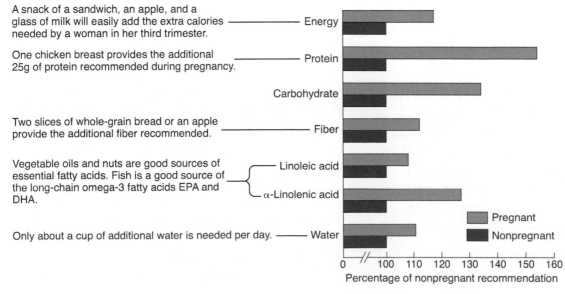

A snack of a sandwich, an apple, and a glass of milk will easily add the extra calories needed by a woman in her third trimester. — Energy

One chicken breast provides the additional 25g of protein recommended during pregnancy. — Protein

Carbohydrate

Two slices of whole-grain bread or an apple provide the additional fiber recommended. — Fiber

Vegetable oils and nuts are good sources of essential fatty acids. Fish is a good source of the long-chain omega-3 fatty acids EPA and DHA. — Linoleic acid / α-Linolenic acid

Only about a cup of additional water is needed per day. — Water

Pregnant
Nonpregnant

0   100 110 120 130 140 150 160
Percentage of nonpregnant recommendation

Micronutrient needs during pregnancy • Figure 11.7

The graph compares the recommended micronutrient intakes for 25-year-old nonpregnant women and 25-year-old women during the third trimester of pregnancy.

The need for B vitamins increases as energy needs increase.

The need for folate, vitamin B$_{12}$, iron, and zinc increases to support the formation of new maternal and fetal cells.

The requirements for zinc and vitamin B$_6$ rise to meet the need for increased protein synthesis.

Calcium, phosphorus, magnesium, vitamin D, and vitamin C are needed to provide for the growth and development of bone and connective tissue.

Vitamin A is needed for cell differentiation and development. Low intake can cause low birth weight and premature birth, but too much can increase the risk of heart defects, cleft palate, and other developmental defects.

Iodine and selenium are needed for the synthesis of thyroid hormones. Iodine deficiency causes developmental disorders.

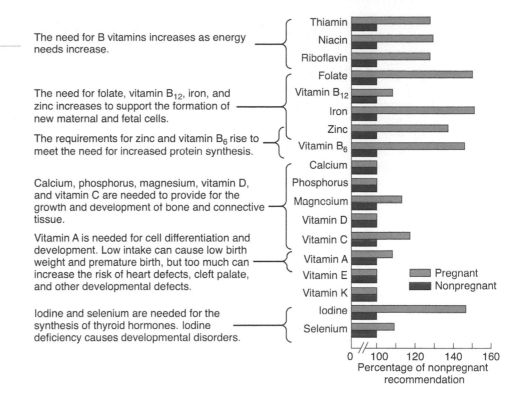

Fluid and Electrolyte Needs

During pregnancy, a woman will accumulate 6 to 9 liters (L) of water. Some of this water is intracellular, resulting from the growth of tissues, but most is due to increases in the volume of blood and the fluid between cells. The need for water increases from 2.7 L/day in nonpregnant women to 3 L/day during pregnancy.[23] Despite changes in the amount and distribution of body water during pregnancy, there is no evidence that the requirements for potassium, sodium, and chloride are different for pregnant women than for nonpregnant women.

Vitamin and Mineral Needs

Many vitamins and minerals are needed for the growth of new tissues in both mother and child (**Figure 11.7**). For many of these nutrients, the increased need is easily met with the extra food the mother consumes. For others, the increased need is met because their absorption is increased during pregnancy. For a few, including calcium, vitamin D, folate, vitamin B$_{12}$, iron, and zinc, there is a risk that the woman will not consume adequate amounts without supplementation.

Calcium and vitamin D During gestation, the fetus accumulates about 30 g of calcium, mostly during the third trimester, when the bones are growing rapidly and the teeth are forming. However, the RDA is not increased during pregnancy because calcium absorption doubles.[24] The RDA for calcium can be met by consuming three to four servings of dairy products daily. Women who are lactose intolerant can meet their calcium needs with yogurt, cheese, reduced-lactose milk, calcium-rich vegetables, calcium-fortified foods and beverages, and calcium supplements. Many pregnant women fail to consume adequate amounts of calcium. Low calcium intake increases the risk that the mother will develop preeclampsia.[18]

Adequate vitamin D is essential to ensure efficient calcium absorption. The RDA for vitamin D during pregnancy is 600 IU (15 µg)/day, the same as it is for nonpregnant women.[24] This is based on the assumption of minimal sun exposure.

Folate and vitamin B$_{12}$ Folate is needed for the synthesis of DNA and hence for cell division. Adequate folate intake before conception and during early pregnancy is crucial because rapid cell division occurs in the first days and weeks of pregnancy.

Low folate levels increase the risk of abnormalities in the formation of the *neural tube*, which forms the baby's brain and spinal cord (see Chapter 7, Figure 7.17). Neural tube closure, a critical step in neural tube development, occurs between 21 and 28 days after conception, often before a woman knows she is pregnant. Therefore,

WHAT A SCIENTIST SEES
Folate Fortification and Neural Tube Defects

Consumers reading the ingredient list on this box of pasta see that it is made from a coarse flour called semolina, with added niacin, thiamin, riboflavin, iron, and folic acid. In 1998, the United States and Canada began requiring the addition of folic acid to pasta and other enriched grain products in order to increase intake in women of childbearing age, with the goal of reducing the incidence of neural tube defects. Enriched grains were chosen for fortification because they are commonly consumed in regular amounts by this target population. Because high folic acid intake can mask the symptoms of vitamin B_{12} deficiency, the amount added to enriched grains was kept low enough to avoid this problem in any segment of the population but high enough to reduce the risk of neural tube defects. A scientist can see that this public health measure has succeeded. Since the initiation of folic acid fortification, the incidence of neural tube defects has been reduced by almost 50% in the United States and Canada (see graph).[25,26]

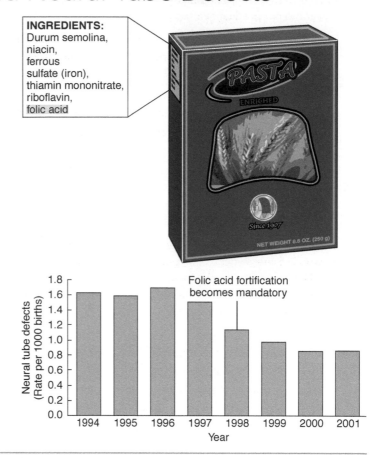

INGREDIENTS:
Durum semolina,
niacin,
ferrous
sulfate (iron),
thiamin mononitrate,
riboflavin,
folic acid

Think Critically Suggest some reasons why fortifying grains with folic acid has not completely eliminated neural tube defects.

it is recommended that all women capable of becoming pregnant is consume 400 μg daily of synthetic folic acid from fortified foods, supplements, or a combination of the two, in addition to a varied diet that is rich in natural sources of folate, such as leafy greens, legumes, and orange juice (see *What a Scientist Sees*).

Folate continues to be important even after the neural tube closes. Folate deficiency can cause macrocytic anemia in the mother, and inadequate folate intake is associated with prematurity, low birth weight, and birth defects.[27] During pregnancy, the RDA is 600 μg/day.[28]

Vitamin B_{12} is essential for the regeneration of active forms of folate. A deficiency of vitamin B_{12} can therefore result in macrocytic anemia in the mother and impaired growth and cognitive development in the fetus.[29] Based on the amount of vitamin B_{12} transferred from mother to fetus during pregnancy and on the increased efficiency of vitamin B_{12} absorption during pregnancy, the RDA for pregnancy is set at 2.6 μg/day.[28] This recommendation is easily met by consuming a diet containing even small amounts of animal products. Pregnant women who consume vegan diets must include vitamin B_{12} supplements or foods or beverages fortified with vitamin B_{12} to meet their needs as well as those of the fetus.

Iron and zinc Iron needs are high during pregnancy because iron is required for the synthesis of hemoglobin and other iron-containing proteins in both maternal and fetal tissues. The RDA for pregnant women is 27 mg/day, 50% higher than the recommended amount for nonpregnant women.[30] Many women start pregnancy with diminished iron stores and quickly become iron deficient. This occurs even though iron absorption is increased during pregnancy and iron losses decrease because menstruation ceases. Iron deficiency anemia during pregnancy is associated with low birth weight, preterm delivery, and impaired cognitive development.[31] Because most of the transfer of iron from mother to fetus occurs during the third trimester, babies who are born prematurely may not have time to accumulate sufficient iron.

Meeting iron needs during pregnancy requires a well-planned diet. Red meat is a good source of the more absorbable heme iron, and leafy green vegetables and fortified cereals are good sources of nonheme iron. Consuming citrus fruit, which is high in vitamin C, or meat, which contains heme iron, along with foods that are good sources of nonheme iron, can enhance iron absorption. Iron supplements are typically recommended and iron is included in prenatal supplements.

Zinc is involved in the synthesis and function of DNA and RNA and the synthesis of proteins. It is therefore extremely important for growth and development. Zinc deficiency during pregnancy is associated with increased risks of fetal malformations, premature birth, and low birth weight.[32] Because zinc absorption is inhibited by high iron intake, iron supplements may compromise zinc status if the mother's diet is low in zinc. The RDA for zinc is 13 mg/day for pregnant women age 18 and younger and 11 mg/day for pregnant women age 19 and older.[30] As is the case with iron, the zinc in red meat is more absorbable than the zinc from other sources.

Meeting Nutrient Needs with Food and Supplements

The energy and nutrient needs of pregnancy can be met by following the MyPlate Daily Food Plans for Moms (**Figure 11.8**).

Daily Food Plan for Moms • Figure 11.8

This Daily Food Plan for Moms (www.choosemyplate.gov) is for a 26-year-old woman who is 5 feet 4 inches tall, gets 30 to 60 minutes of exercise a day, and weighed 125 lb before she became pregnant. Energy needs are not increased during the first trimester, so the recommended amounts from each group for the first trimester are the same as for a nonpregnant woman.

Ask Yourself

Compared to a nonpregnant woman, how many more cups of milk should a woman in her third trimester be consuming?

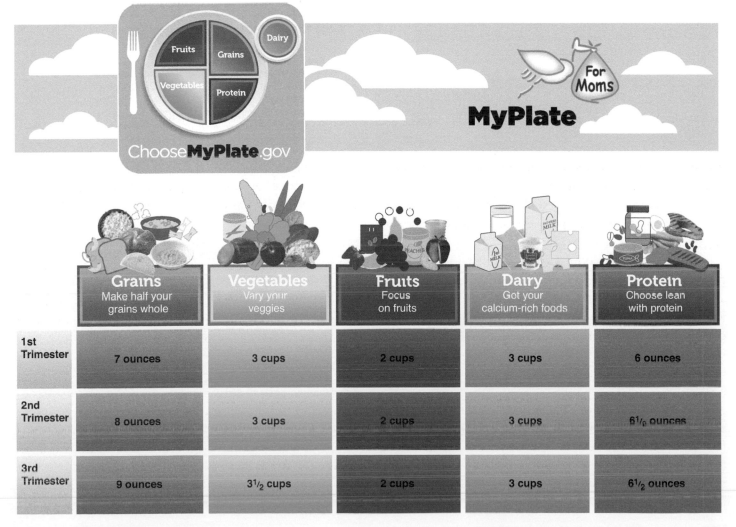

	Grains Make half your grains whole	Vegetables Vary your veggies	Fruits Focus on fruits	Dairy Got your calcium-rich foods	Protein Choose lean with protein
1st Trimester	7 ounces	3 cups	2 cups	3 cups	6 ounces
2nd Trimester	8 ounces	3 cups	2 cups	3 cups	6½ ounces
3rd Trimester	9 ounces	3½ cups	2 cups	3 cups	6½ ounces

Even when a healthy diet is consumed, it is difficult to meet all the vitamin and mineral needs of pregnancy. Therefore, prenatal supplements are generally prescribed for pregnant women. These supplements include the additional folic acid and iron discussed earlier.[1] Prenatal supplements, however, must be taken along with, not in place of, a carefully planned diet (**Figure 11.9**) (see *Thinking It Through*).

Food Cravings and Aversions

Most women experience some food cravings and aversions during pregnancy. The foods most commonly craved are ice cream, sweets, candy, fruit, and fish. Common aversions include coffee, highly seasoned foods, and fried foods. It is not known why women have these cravings and aversions. It has been suggested that hormonal or physiological changes during pregnancy—in particular, changes in taste and smell—may be the cause, but psychological and behavioral factors are also involved.

Usually, the foods that pregnant women crave are not harmful and can be safely included in the diet to meet not only nutritional needs but also emotional needs and

Prenatal supplements • Figure 11.9

Prenatal supplements cannot take the place of a well-planned diet. They typically do not provide enough calcium to meet the needs of pregnant women; to do so, the tablet would have to be very large. They also lack protein needed for tissue synthesis; complex carbohydrates needed for energy; essential fatty acids for brain and nerve tissue development; fiber and fluid to help prevent constipation; and the phytochemicals found in a healthy diet.

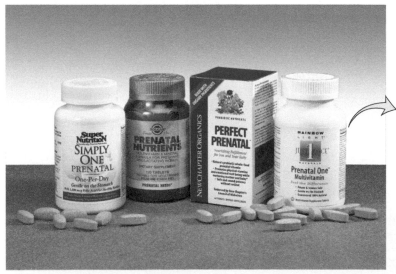

Supplement Facts

Serving Size 1 Tablet
Servings Per Container 60

Amount Per 1 Tablet	% Daily Value
Vitamin A (as beta carotene) 5000 IU	63%
Vitamin C (as ascorbic acid) 85 mg	100%
Vitamin D (as cholecalciferol) 400 IU	200%
Vitamin E (as d-alpha tocopheryl acetate) 22 IU	67%
Vitamin K 90 mcg	100%
Thiamin 1.4 mg	100%
Riboflavin 1.6 mg	100%
Niacin (as niacinamide) 17 mg	100%
Vitamin B_6 (as pyridoxine HCl) 2.6 mg	137%
Folic acid 1000 mcg	167%
Vitamin B_{12} (as cyanocobalamin) 2.6 mg	100%
Pantothenic Acid (as as d-calcium pantothenate) 6 mg	100%
Iron (as iron fumarate) 27 mg	100%
Iodine (kelp) 220 mcg	100%
Zinc (as monomethionine & gluconate) 11mg	100%
Selenium (as sodium selenate) 60 mcg	100%
Copper (as copper sulfate) 1000 mcg	100%
Calcium (as calcium carbonate) 200 mg	20%

* Daily Values based on RDAs for pregnant women ages 19-50
Other ingredients: stearic acid, vegetable stearate, silicon dioxide, croscarmellose sodium, microcrystalline cellulose, natural coating (contains hydroxypropyl methylcellulose, titanium dioxide, riboflavin, polyethylene glycol and polysorbate)

A Case Study on Nutrient Needs for a Successful Pregnancy

Tina is a moderately active 26-year-old at the end of her fourth month of pregnancy. She is 5 feet 4 inches tall and weighed 125 lb at the start of her pregnancy. She is concerned about gaining too much weight because her sister gained 50 lb during her pregnancy and has had difficulty losing the excess weight since her baby was born. Tina's obstetrician recommends that she gain 25 to 35 lb during her pregnancy, but she would like to keep her weight gain to only 15 lb.

 1 Based on the graph below, why would gaining only 15 lb put the baby at risk? Why would gaining 50 lb put the baby at risk?

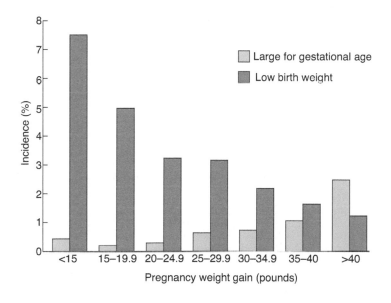

Your answer:

Tina's typical diet provides enough calories for a nonpregnant woman, but during her second and third trimesters, she needs additional calories and nutrients. To decide what to add to her diet, she compares her typical intake to the Daily Food Plan for Moms she finds at ChooseMyPlate.gov. Her current diet includes 8 ounces (oz) of grains, 1.5 cups of vegetables, 1 cup of fruit, 2 cups of dairy, and 6 oz of protein foods.

 2 Use Figure 11.8 to compare Tina's current intake to the MyPlate recommendations for the second trimester of pregnancy. How much from which groups does she need to add to her diet?

Your answer:

Tina is taking a prenatal supplement but is curious about whether her diet alone can meet her nutrient needs. She analyzes her diet and finds that she is meeting her needs for all nutrients except iron. Her current diet provides only 13.5 mg of iron—significantly less than the RDA of 27 mg for pregnant women.

3 Use iProfile to find foods that Tina could add to her diet to increase her iron intake by 13.5 mg/day. How many calories would your suggestions add?

Your answer:

4 Considering the foods you suggested to increase her iron intake, do you think it is reasonable for Tina to consume 27 mg of iron each day from her diet alone? Why or why not?

Your answer:

(Check your answers in online Appendix L)

WHAT SHOULD I EAT?

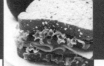
© Sara Winter/iStockphoto

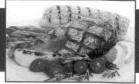
© Jill Chen/iStockphoto   © Steve Mcsweeny/iStockphoto

During Pregnancy

✓ **THE PLANNER**

Make nutrient-dense choices
- Have yogurt and granola for a midmorning snack.
- Put some peanut butter on your banana to add some protein to your snack.
- Have a cup of pasta Florentine (with spinach)—it provides both a natural and a fortified source of folate.

Drink plenty of fluids
- Have a glass of low-fat milk to boost fluid and calcium intake.
- Keep a bottle of water at your desk or in your car.
- Relax with a cup of tea.

Indulge your cravings, within reason
- Enjoy an ice cream cone—it provides calcium and protein.
- Enjoy oatmeal cookies with a glass of low-fat milk.

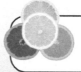
Use iProfile to plan a nutritious 300-Calorie snack for a pregnant woman.

Pica • Figure 11.10

This African American woman in Georgia is eating a white clay called kaolin, which some women crave during pregnancy. Eating kaolin is also a traditional remedy for morning sickness. This example of pica may be related to cultural beliefs and traditions, but pica is also believed to be triggered by nutrient deficiencies, stress, and anxiety. It is most common in African American women, women who live in rural areas, and in those with a childhood or family history of pica.[33]

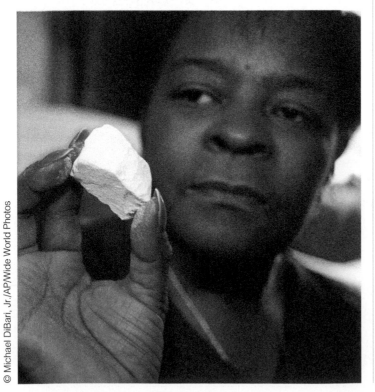
© Michael DiBari, Jr./AP/Wide World Photos

individual preferences (see *What Should I Eat?*). However, **pica** during pregnancy can have serious health consequences. Women with pica commonly consume nonfood substances such as clay, laundry starch, and ashes. Consuming large amounts of these substances can reduce intake of nutrient-dense foods, inhibit nutrient absorption, increase the risk of consuming toxins, and cause intestinal obstructions. Complications of pica include iron deficiency anemia, lead poisoning, and parasitic infestations.[33] Anemia and high blood pressure are more common in those with pica than among other pregnant women, but it is not clear whether pica is a result of these conditions or a cause. In newborns, anemia and low birth weight are often related to pica in the mother (**Figure 11.10**).

> **pica** An abnormal craving for and ingestion of nonfood substances that have little or no nutritional value.

CONCEPT CHECK 🛑 STOP

1. **What** snack could a pregnant woman add to her day to meet her increased energy and protein needs?

2. **Why** isn't the recommendation for dietary calcium increased during pregnancy?

3. **Why** are iron supplements recommended during pregnancy?

11.3 Factors That Increase the Risks Associated with Pregnancy

LEARNING OBJECTIVES

1. **Explain** what is meant by critical periods of prenatal development.

2. **Discuss** how nutritional status can influence the outcome of pregnancy.

3. **Explain** how a pregnant woman's age and health status affect the risks associated with pregnancy.

4. **Describe** the effects of alcohol, mercury, and cocaine on the outcome of pregnancy.

A nything that interferes with embryonic or fetal development can cause a baby to be born too soon or too small or result in birth defects. The embryo and fetus are particularly vulnerable to damage because their cells are dividing rapidly, differentiating, and moving to form organs and other structures. Developmental errors can be caused by deficiencies or excesses in the maternal diet and by harmful substances that are present in the environment, consumed in the diet, or taken as medications or recreational drugs. Any chemical, biological, or physical agent that causes a birth defect is called a **teratogen**. And because each organ system develops at a different time and rate, each has a **critical period** during which exposure to a teratogen is most likely to disrupt development and cause irreversible damage (**Figure 11.11**). Severe damage can result in miscarriage. Some women are at increased risk for complications during pregnancy because of their

Critical periods of development • Figure 11.11

The critical periods of development are different for different body systems. Because the majority of cell differentiation occurs during the embryonic period, this is the time when exposure to teratogens can do the most damage, but vital body organs can still be affected during the fetal period. One in every 33 babies born in the United States has a birth defect.[34]

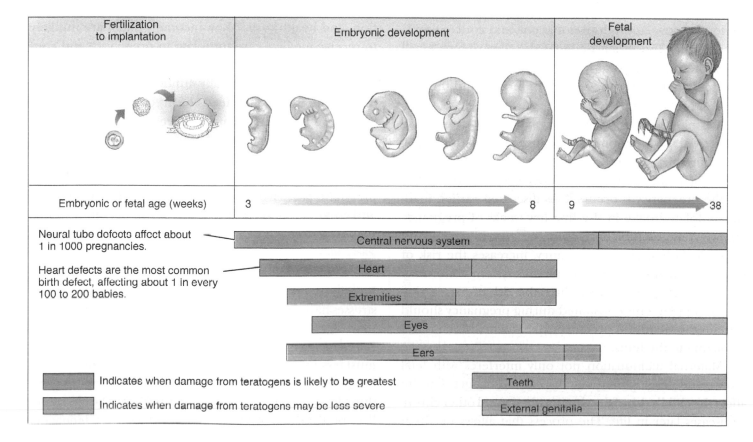

Fertilization to implantation	Embryonic development	Fetal development

Embryonic or fetal age (weeks) 3 ——————————→ 8   9 ——————————→ 38

Neural tube defects affect about 1 in 1000 pregnancies. — Central nervous system

Heart defects are the most common birth defect, affecting about 1 in every 100 to 200 babies. — Heart

Extremities

Eyes

Ears

▢ Indicates when damage from teratogens is likely to be greatest

▢ Indicates when damage from teratogens may be less severe

Teeth

External genitalia

Exposure to Toxic Substances

A pregnant woman's exposure to toxins in food, water, and the environment can affect the developing fetus. Even substances that seem innocuous can be dangerous. For example, herbal remedies, including herbal teas, should be avoided unless their consumption during pregnancy has been determined to be safe.[3]

Caffeine When consumed in excess, coffee and other caffeine-containing beverages have been associated with increased risks of miscarriage or low birth weight. However, moderate caffeine consumption, less than 200 mg/day, the amount in one or two cups of coffee or about two or three 20-oz caffeinated soft drinks, does not appear to increase the risk of miscarriage or low birth weight.[45]

Mercury in fish Fish has both benefits and risks for pregnant women. It is a source of lean protein for tissue growth and of omega-3 fatty acids and iodine needed for brain development, but if it is contaminated with mercury, consumption during pregnancy can cause developmental delays and brain damage. Rather than avoid fish, pregnant women should be informed consumers. The 2010 Dietary Guidelines recommend that pregnant women consume 8 to 12 oz/week of seafood from a variety of types of fish and shellfish.[46] Exposure to mercury from fish can be controlled by avoiding varieties that are high in mercury and limiting intake of fish that contain lower amounts of mercury (**Table 11.2**).

Food-borne illness The immune system is weakened during pregnancy, increasing susceptibility to and the severity of certain food-borne illnesses. *Listeria* infection is 18 times more common in pregnant women than in the general population. Infection during pregnancy is associated with an increased risk of miscarriage and stillbirth; the infection can be transmitted to the fetus, causing meningitis and serious blood infections.[48] About one-third of fetuses with *Listeria* infections do not survive.[49] The bacteria are commonly found in unpasteurized milk, soft cheeses, and uncooked hot dogs and lunch meats (see Table 11.2).

Toxoplasmosis is an infection caused by a parasite. If a pregnant woman becomes infected, there is about a 40% chance that she will pass the infection to her unborn baby.[50] Infected babies may develop vision and hearing loss, intellectual disability, and/or seizures, and some die within a few days of birth. The toxoplasmosis parasite is found in cat feces, soil, and undercooked infected meat (see Table 11.2). Pregnant women should follow the safe food-handling recommendations discussed in Chapter 13.

Alcohol Alcohol consumption during pregnancy is one of the leading causes of preventable birth defects. Alcohol is a teratogen that is particularly damaging to the developing nervous system.[51] It also indirectly affects fetal growth and development because it is a toxin that reduces blood flow to the placenta, thereby decreasing the delivery of oxygen and nutrients to the fetus. Use of

---

Food safety during pregnancy[47]   **Table 11.2**

Eat 8 to 12 oz of a variety of fish per week. Choose fish that are lower in mercury, such as salmon, shrimp, canned light tuna, pollock, catfish, and cod.

Don't eat swordfish, shark, king mackerel, or tilefish, which can be high in mercury.

Check local advisories about the safety of fish caught from streams, rivers, and lakes. If no advice is available, eat up to 6 oz per week but don't consume any other fish during that week.

Don't drink raw (unpasteurized) milk or consume products made with unpasteurized milk, such as certain Mexican-style soft cheeses.

Don't eat refrigerated smoked fish, cold deli salads, or refrigerated pâtés or meat spreads.

Don't eat hot dogs and luncheon meats unless they have been reheated to steaming hot.

Don't eat raw or undercooked meat, poultry, fish, shellfish, or eggs.

Don't eat unwashed fruits and vegetables, raw sprouts, or unpasteurized juice.

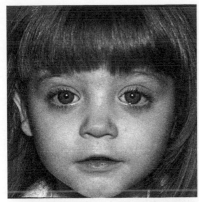
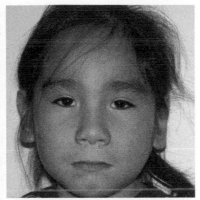
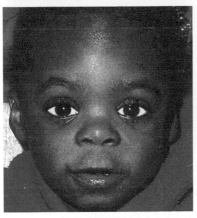
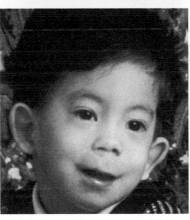

© 2012 Susan Astley PhD, University of Washington.

Dangers of alcohol use during pregnancy • Figure 11.15

The facial characteristics shared by children with fetal alcohol syndrome (FAS) include a low nasal bridge, short nose, distinct eyelids, and a thin upper lip. Newborns with FAS may be shaky and irritable, with poor muscle tone. Other problems associated with FAS include heart and urinary tract defects, impaired vision and hearing, and delayed language development. Below-average intellectual function is the most common and most serious effect.

Cigarette smoke If a woman smokes cigarettes during pregnancy, her baby will be affected before birth and throughout life. The carbon monoxide in cigarette smoke binds to hemoglobin in maternal and fetal blood, reducing the amount of oxygen delivered to fetal tissues. The nicotine absorbed from cigarette smoke is a teratogen that can affect brain development.[54,55] Nicotine also constricts arteries and limits blood flow, reducing the amounts of oxygen and nutrients delivered to the fetus.[56] Cigarette smoking during pregnancy reduces birth weight and increases the risks of stillbirth, preterm delivery, neurobehavioral problems, and early infant death.[3,54] In women who don't smoke, environmental exposure to cigarette smoke has been found to increase the risk of having a low-birthweight baby. The risks of **sudden infant death syndrome (SIDS)**, or **crib death**, and respiratory problems are also increased in children exposed to cigarette smoke both in the uterus and after birth.[57] The effects of maternal smoking follow children throughout life; these children are more likely to develop lung problems later in life.[58]

> **sudden infant death syndrome (SIDS) or crib death** The unexplained death of an infant, usually during sleep.

Drug use Certain drugs—whether over-the-counter, prescribed, or illegal—can affect fetal development. For example, the acne medications Accutane and Retin-A are derivatives of vitamin A that can cause birth defects if used during pregnancy. A woman who is considering becoming pregnant should discuss her plans with her physician in order to determine the risks associated with any medication she is taking.

Abuse of illegal substances during pregnancy is a national health issue. It is estimated that about 4.4% of pregnant women use illicit drugs.[59] The risk to the infant depends on the drug. Marijuana and cocaine can cross the placenta and enter the fetal blood. Prenatal marijuana exposure may cause subtle abnormalities in infant neurobehavior, such as increased irritability and muscle

alcohol can also impair maternal nutritional status, further increasing the risks to the fetus.

Prenatal exposure to alcohol can cause a spectrum of disorders, depending on the amount, timing, and duration of the exposure. One of the most severe outcomes of alcohol use during pregnancy is delivery of a baby with **fetal alcohol syndrome (FAS)** (**Figure 11.15**). Not all babies who are exposed to alcohol while in the uterus have FAS. The term **fetal alcohol spectrum disorders (FASDs)** is used to refer to all the physical and behavioral disorders or conditions and functional or mental impairments linked to prenatal alcohol exposure.[52] As many as 2 to 5% of young school children in the United States are affected by FASDs.[53] Because alcohol consumption in each trimester has been associated with fetal abnormalities, and there is no level of alcohol consumption that is known to be safe, complete abstinence from alcohol is recommended during pregnancy.

> **fetal alcohol syndrome (FAS)** A characteristic group of physical and mental abnormalities in an infant resulting from maternal alcohol consumption during pregnancy.

tremors, but it has not been shown to affect fetal growth or cause birth defects.[59] Cocaine use creates problems for both the mother and the infant before, during, and after delivery.[60] Cocaine is a teratogen that interferes with nervous system development and may cause permanent changes in brain structure and function.[59] Cocaine also constricts blood vessels, thereby reducing the delivery of oxygen and nutrients to the fetus. Cocaine use during pregnancy is associated with an increased risk of miscarriage, fetal growth retardation, premature labor and delivery, low birth weight, and birth defects.[61] Exposure to cocaine and other illegal drugs before birth has also been shown to affect infant behavior and influence learning and attention span during childhood.[59]

CONCEPT CHECK ⬛STOP

1. **Why** does the effect of a given teratogen vary, depending on when a pregnant woman is exposed to it?

2. **How** does malnutrition during pregnancy affect the health of the child at birth and later in life?

3. **Why** are the requirements for some nutrients different in pregnant teenage girls than in pregnant adult women?

4. **How** much alcohol can be safely consumed during pregnancy?

11.4 Lactation

LEARNING OBJECTIVES

1. **Describe** the events that trigger milk production and let-down.

2. **Discuss** the energy and water needs of lactating women.

3. **Compare** the micronutrient needs of lactating women with those of nonpregnant, nonlactating women.

T he need for many nutrients is even greater during lactation than during pregnancy. The milk produced by a breast-feeding mother must meet all the nutrient needs of her baby, who is bigger and more active than he or she was in the womb. To meet these needs, a lactating woman must choose a varied, nutrient-dense diet that follows the MyPlate Daily Food Plans for breast-feeding women.

Milk Production and Let-Down

let-down The release of milk from the milk-producing glands and its movement through the ducts and storage sinuses.

Lactation involves both the synthesis of milk components—proteins, lactose, and lipids—and the movement of these components through the milk ducts to the nipple (**Figure 11.16**). Milk production and **let-down** are triggered by hormones that are released in response to an infant's suckling. The pituitary hormone **prolactin** stimulates

Anatomy of milk production • Figure 11.16

Throughout pregnancy, hormones prepare the breasts for lactation by stimulating the enlargement and development of the milk ducts and milk-producing glands, called *alveoli* (singular *alveolus*). During lactation, milk travels from the alveoli through the ducts to the milk storage sinuses and then to the nipple.

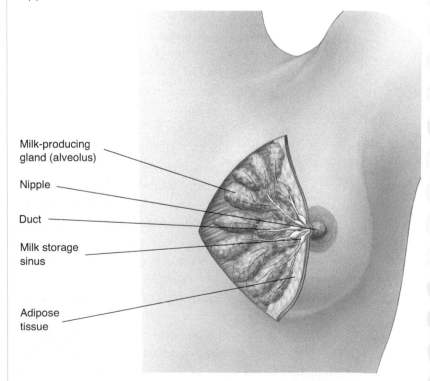

Milk-producing gland (alveolus)

Nipple

Duct

Milk storage sinus

Adipose tissue

This graph compares the energy and macronutrient recommendations for 25-year-old nonpregnant women and 25-year-old women during the third trimester of pregnancy and the first 6 months of lactation.

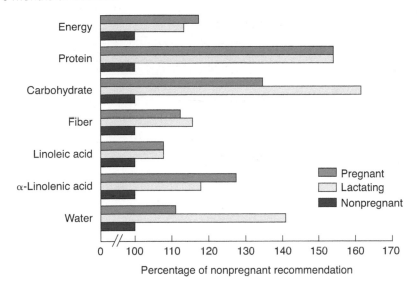

Ask Yourself

Why is the need for water greater during lactation than during pregnancy?

milk production; the more the infant suckles, the more milk is produced. Let-down is caused by **oxytocin**, another pituitary hormone. Oxytocin release is also stimulated by suckling, but as nursing becomes routine, oxytocin release and let-down may occur in response to just the sight or sound of an infant. Let-down can be inhibited by nervous tension, fatigue, or embarrassment. Because let-down is essential for breast-feeding and makes suckling easier for the child, slow let-down can make feeding difficult.

Energy and Nutrient Needs During Lactation

Human milk contains about 70 Calories/100 milliliters (160 Calories/cup). During the first 6 months of lactation, an average infant consumes 600 to 900 mL (about 2.5 to 4 cups)/day, so approximately 500 Calories are required from the mother each day. Much of this energy must come from the diet, but some can come from maternal fat stores. Because some of the energy for milk production comes from fat stores, the increase in recommended energy intake is lower during lactation than during pregnancy, even though total energy demands are greater (**Figure 11.17**). An additional 330 Calories/day above nonpregnant, nonlactating needs are recommended during the first 6 months of lactation, and an additional 400 Calories/day are recommended for the second 6 months. Beginning 1 month after birth, most lactating women lose 0.5 to 1 kg (1 to 2 lb)/month for 6 months. Rapid weight loss is not recommended during lactation because it can decrease milk production.

To ensure adequate protein for milk production, the RDA for lactation is increased by 25 g/day. The recommended intakes of total carbohydrate, fiber, and the essential fatty acids linoleic and α-linolenic acid are also higher during lactation (see Figure 11.17).[21] Since the fatty acid composition of the mother's diet determines the fatty acid composition of her breast milk, adequate intake of omega-3 and omega-6 fatty acids ensures a healthy balance of these essential fatty acids in her breast milk.[62]

To avoid dehydration and ensure adequate milk production, lactating women need to consume about 1 L/day of additional water.[23] Consuming an extra glass of milk, juice, or water at each meal and whenever the infant nurses can help ensure adequate fluid intake.

The recommended intakes for several vitamins and minerals are increased during lactation to meet the needs for synthesizing milk and to replace the nutrients

This graph compares the vitamin and mineral recommendations for 25-year-old nonpregnant women and 25-year-old women during the third trimester of pregnancy and the first 6 months of lactation.

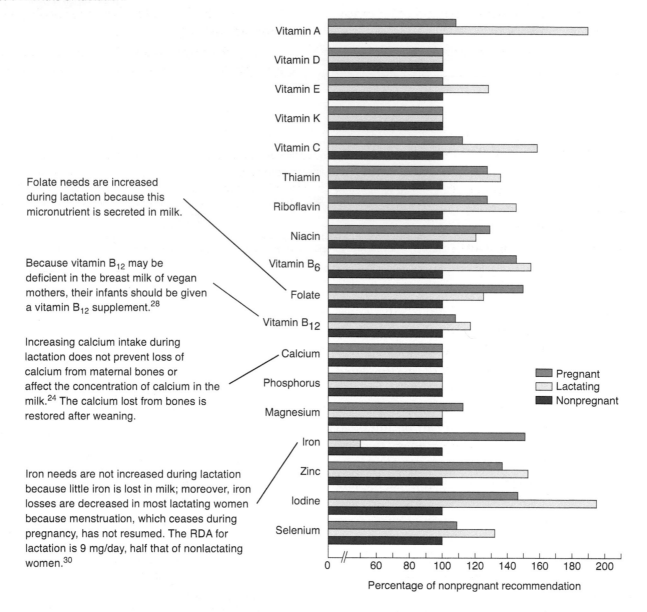

Folate needs are increased during lactation because this micronutrient is secreted in milk.

Because vitamin B_{12} may be deficient in the breast milk of vegan mothers, their infants should be given a vitamin B_{12} supplement.[28]

Increasing calcium intake during lactation does not prevent loss of calcium from maternal bones or affect the concentration of calcium in the milk.[24] The calcium lost from bones is restored after weaning.

Iron needs are not increased during lactation because little iron is lost in milk; moreover, iron losses are decreased in most lactating women because menstruation, which ceases during pregnancy, has not resumed. The RDA for lactation is 9 mg/day, half that of nonlactating women.[30]

secreted in the milk (**Figure 11.18**). For some nutrients, including thiamin, riboflavin, vitamin B_6, vitamin B_{12}, vitamin A, vitamin D, selenium, and iodine, low maternal intake reduces the amount secreted into the milk.[63,64] For example, low levels of vitamin B_{12} in a mother's diet can result in low levels of vitamin B_{12} in her milk. For other nutrients, including folate, calcium, iron, copper, and zinc, levels in the milk are maintained at the expense of maternal stores.[63,64]

CONCEPT CHECK STOP

1. **What** causes milk let-down?

2. **Where** does the energy for milk production come from?

3. **Why** is the recommended calcium intake for a new mother not increased while she is lactating?

LEARNING OBJECTIVES

1. **Explain** how growth charts are used to monitor the nutritional well-being of infants.

2. **Contrast** the energy and macronutrient needs of infants and adults.

3. **Compare** the benefits of breast-feeding and formula-feeding.

4. **Discuss** the importance of choosing foods that are appropriate for a child's developmental stage.

fter the umbilical cord is cut, a newborn must actively obtain nutrients rather than being passively fed through the placenta. The energy and nutrients an infant consumes must support his or her continuing growth and development, as well as his or her increasing activity level.

Infant Growth and Development

During **infancy**—the first year of life—growth and development are extremely rapid. Infants get bigger and develop physically, intellectually, and socially. Adequate nutrition is essential for achieving growth and developmental milestones.

Healthy infants follow standard patterns of growth—that is, whether a newborn weighs 6 lb or 8 lb at birth, the rate of growth should be approximately the same: rapid initially and slowing slightly as the infant approaches his or her first birthday. A rule of thumb is that an infant's birth weight should double by 4 months of age and triple by 1 year of age. In the first year of life, most infants increase their length by 50%. Growth is the best indicator of adequate nutrition in an infant.

Growth can be assessed in infants and children using growth charts (**Figure 11.19**). The growth charts used for infants were developed by the World Health Organization based on growth

Growth charts • Figure 11.19

This growth chart can be used to compare a boy's length and weight at a particular age to standards for optimal growth. A similar chart is available for girls. Growth charts for boys and girls from birth to 24 months of age are also available to monitor weight for length and head circumference.

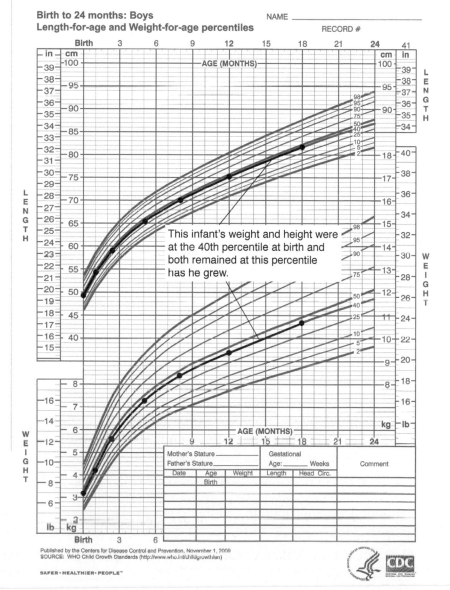

This infant's weight and height were at the 40th percentile at birth and both remained at this percentile has he grew.

Interpret the Data

A 23-month-old boy who weighs 13 kg is at the _____ percentile.

a. 25th   b. 50th

c. 75th   d. 90th

patterns of breast-fed infants living in optimal conditions. To use a growth chart, the infant's weight and/or height is plotted on the graph, and the resulting percentile indicates where the infant's growth falls in relation to optimal growth patterns for infants of the same age.[65] Children usually remain at the same percentile as they grow. For instance, a child who is at the 50th percentile for height and the 25th percentile for weight generally remains close to these percentiles throughout childhood. Small and premature infants often follow a pattern that is parallel to, but below, the growth curve for a period of time and then experience catch-up growth that brings them into the same range as children of the same age.

Slight variations in growth rate are normal, but a consistent pattern of not following the established growth curve or a sudden change in growth pattern is cause for concern and could indicate overnutrition or undernutrition. For example, a rapid increase in weight without an increase in height may indicate that the infant is being overfed. Just as there are critical periods in prenatal life, there are critical periods during infancy when nutrition can have permanent effects on growth and development and long-term health. Evidence suggests that accelerated weight gain in the first 2 years of life increases the risk of obesity, diabetes, high blood pressure, harmful blood lipid levels, and cardiovascular disease in adulthood.[66] A pattern of accelerated weight increase should be addressed early in life to reduce the likelihood of these chronic conditions later.

Growth that is slower than the predicted pattern indicates **failure to thrive**, a catchall term for any type of growth failure in a young child. The cause may be a congenital condition, disease, poor nutrition, neglect, abuse, or psychosocial problems. The treatment is usually an individualized plan that includes adequate nutrition and careful monitoring by physicians, dietitians, and other health-care professionals. Undernutrition during infancy can permanently affect growth and development as well as health later in life. Because the first year of life is a critical period for brain development, undernutrition interferes with learning and affects behavior. Undernutrition in childhood is a risk factor for diabetes, high blood pressure, and cardiovascular disease in adulthood, especially in undernourished children who experience rapid weight gain after infancy.[67]

failure to thrive Inability of a child's growth to keep up with normal growth curves.

Energy and Nutrient Needs of Infants

The rapid growth rate of infants increases their need for energy, protein, and vitamins and minerals that are important for growth. Human milk and commercially produced formula are designed to meet infants' nutrient needs. Nevertheless, infants may still be at risk for iron, vitamin D, and vitamin K deficiencies and for suboptimal levels of fluoride.

Energy and macronutrients Infants require more calories and protein per kilogram of body weight than do individuals at any other time of life (**Figure 11.20a**).[21] As infants grow older, their rate of growth slows, but they become more mobile, so the amount of energy they need for activity increases. Because infants change so much during the first year, energy recommendations are made for three age groups—0 to 3 months, 4 to 6 months, and 7 to 12 months—and nutrient recommendations are made for two age groups—0 to 6 months and 7 to 12 months (see inside cover).

The combination of high energy demands and a small stomach means that infants require an energy-dense diet. Healthy infants consume about 55% of their energy as fat during the first 6 months of life and 40% during the second 6 months. These percentages are far higher than the 20 to 35% of energy from fat recommended in the adult diet (**Figure 11.20b**). This high-fat diet allows the small volume of food that fits in an infant's stomach to provide enough energy to meet the infant's needs and provides essential fatty acids needed for growth and development.

Fluid needs Infants have a higher proportion of body water than do adults, and they lose proportionately more water in urine and through evaporation. Urine losses are high because the kidneys are not fully developed and hence are unable to reabsorb as much water as adult kidneys. Water losses through evaporation are proportionately higher in infants than in adults because infants have a larger surface area relative to body weight. As a result, they need to consume more water per unit of body weight than do adults. Nevertheless, healthy infants who are exclusively breast-fed do not require additional water.[23] In older infants, some water is obtained from food and from beverages other than milk. When water losses

Energy and macronutrient needs • Figure 11.20

The amount of energy and the distribution of energy-yielding nutrients required by infants are strikingly different from what is recommended in the adult diet.

a. The total amount of energy required by a newborn is less than the amount needed by an adult. When this amount is expressed as Calories/kg of body weight, however, we see that infants require about three times more energy than an adult male.

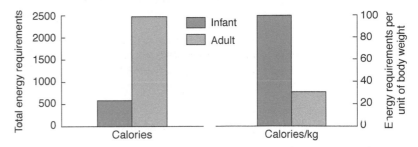

Carbohydrate is a major contributor to an infant's energy intake; most of this comes from lactose.

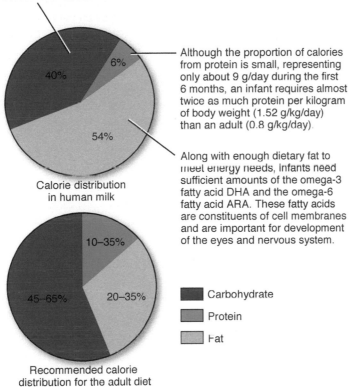

Calorie distribution in human milk

Recommended calorie distribution for the adult diet

Although the proportion of calories from protein is small, representing only about 9 g/day during the first 6 months, an infant requires almost twice as much protein per kilogram of body weight (1.52 g/kg/day) than an adult (0.8 g/kg/day).

Along with enough dietary fat to meet energy needs, infants need sufficient amounts of the omega-3 fatty acid DHA and the omega-6 fatty acid ARA. These fatty acids are constituents of cell membranes and are important for development of the eyes and nervous system.

b. Comparing the distribution of calories from carbohydrate, fat, and protein in human milk with that recommended for an adult illustrates proportionally how much more fat infants need. As an infant grows and solid foods are introduced into the diet, the percentage of calories from carbohydrate in the diet increases and the percentage from fat decreases.

- Carbohydrate
- Protein
- Fat

---

are increased by diarrhea or vomiting, additional fluids may be needed.

Micronutrients at risk Iron is the nutrient that is most commonly deficient in infants who are consuming adequate energy and protein. Iron deficiency usually is not a problem during the first 6 months of life because infants have iron stores at birth and the iron in human milk, though not abundant, is very well absorbed. The AI for iron from birth to 6 months is 0.27 mg/day. After 4 to 6 months, iron stores are depleted, but iron needs remain high. The RDA for infants 7 to 12 months old increases to 11 mg/day.[30] By this age, the diet of breast-fed infants

should contain other sources of iron. Formula-fed infants should be fed iron-fortified formula.

Breast milk is low in vitamin D. Therefore, it is recommended that breast-fed and partially breast-fed infants be supplemented with 400 IU (10 µg)/day of vitamin D beginning in the first few days of life and continuing until they are consuming about 1 L (4 cups) of vitamin D–fortified formula or milk daily.[24,68] Infant formulas contain at least 400 IU (10 µg)/L of vitamin D. Formula-fed infants who consume at least 1 L/day of formula can meet their vitamin D needs from the formula alone; those consuming less than 1 L/day should receive a vitamin D supplement of 400 IU (10 µg)/day. The amount of sun

The Issue: The fatty acids docosahexaenoic acid (DHA) and arachidonic acid (ARA) are essential for development of the retina and brain. Breast milk provides these fatty acids and some infant formulas in the United States are fortified with them. Advertisements suggest that these formulas provide an advantage for infant development. Will feeding babies formula fortified with DHA and ARA make them smarter and improve their vision?

DHA and ARA are polyunsaturated fatty acids that can be made in the body from the essential omega-3 fatty acid α-linolenic acid and the essential omega-6 fatty acid linoleic acid, respectively (see Figure 5.13). DHA and ARA are an integral structural part of cell membranes in the brain and retina and are essential for normal brain development and vision.[70] Accumulation of these fatty acids in the brain and retina occurs most rapidly in the third trimester of pregnancy and the first 24 months after birth, so adequate amounts are crucial during these developmental periods.

Many studies have suggested that babies who are breast-fed have higher IQs than those who are formula fed.[71] The high DHA and ARA content of breast milk compared to standard formula is hypothesized to be responsible for this difference and has led some companies to fortify their infant formula with DHA and ARA. Unlike most other nutrients, however, the amounts of DHA and ARA in breast milk are variable, depending on maternal diet, so it is unclear what constitutes optimal levels. The amounts of these fatty acids transferred to the fetus by the placenta during the third trimester may be enough to ensure adequate amounts for brain development.[70] Infants born at term are also capable of synthesizing DHA and ARA, so those fed unfortified formula may be able to meet their needs if they have enough α-linolenic acid and linoleic acid in their diet. But there is wide individual variation in the ability to convert α-linolenic acid to DHA, and in some infants conversion may be too low for optimal development of the brain and retina.[72] Infants born before term cannot synthesize enough of these fatty acids, so DHA and ARA must be included in formula for premature infants.[73]

So, will higher intakes of these fatty acids make children smarter or improve their vision? Numerous studies have explored the impact that postnatal intake of these fatty acids has on intelligence and vision. Some have found that higher intakes of DHA increase blood levels of DHA in infants and are associated with improvements in cognitive development or vision compared to infants with lower intakes.[70, 74, 75] But not all studies agree. Recent analyses that combine results from many studies have found that supplementing infant formula with DHA and ARA does not improve the IQ of infants or children.[76,77] The results of combined analyses on visual acuity are more mixed, with some analyses concluding that it improves vision in infants up to a year of age.[78]

There are a number of reasons studies on the effects of fortified formulas are inconsistent. Differences may be due to variations in the DHA content of the formulas, the duration of formula-feeding, and the methods used to assess visual acuity and cognitive development. Higher intelligence seen in breast-fed infants may be due more to factors such as maternal IQ, income level, and the amount of time mothers spend with their infants than to whether they are breast- or formula-fed.[79]

When it comes to brain and eye development, no one knows exactly how much DHA or ARA an infant needs. A direct link between use of fortified formula and better vision or higher IQ compared to use of unfortified formula has yet to be established, but fortified formulas are generally recommended.[72] They may not make your baby smarter, but published literature has not demonstrated these formulas to be harmful for infants.[80] Breast milk is always best, so the biggest downside to fortified formulas is that advertising may make new mothers believe that they are as good as or better for their babies than breast milk.

Think Critically: Why is breast milk still better than these fortified formulas?

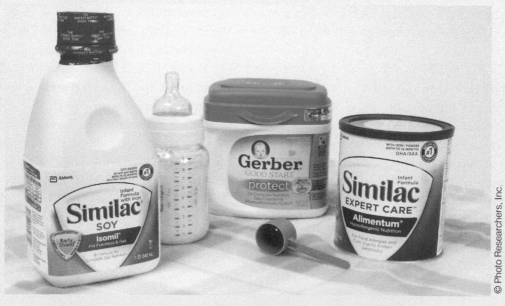

© Photo Researchers, Inc.

exposure necessary to maintain an adequate level of vitamin D in any given infant at any point in time is not easy to determine. Light-skinned infants are more likely than darker-skinned babies to meet their vitamin D needs from sunlight.[68]

Infants are at risk for vitamin K deficiency because little vitamin K crosses the placenta, and the infant's gut is sterile, so there are no bacteria to synthesize this vitamin. Because lack of vitamin K can cause bleeding, it is recommended that all newborns receive an intramuscular injection containing 0.5 to 1.0 mg of vitamin K, which provides enough of the vitamin to last until the intestines have been colonized with bacteria that synthesize it.[69]

Fluoride is important for tooth development, even before the teeth erupt. Breast milk is low in fluoride, and formula manufacturers use unfluoridated water in preparing liquid formula. Therefore, breast-fed infants, infants who are fed premixed formula, and those who are fed formula mixed with low-fluoride water at home are often given fluoride supplements beginning at 6 months of age. In areas where drinking water is fluoridated, infants who are fed formula reconstituted with tap water should not be given fluoride supplements.

Meeting Needs with Breast Milk or Formula

Because of its health and nutritional benefits, breast-feeding is the recommended choice for the newborn of a healthy, well-nourished mother (see *Debate: DHA/ARA-Fortified Infant Formulas*). Health professionals in the United States recommend exclusive breast-feeding for the first 6 months of life and breast-feeding with complementary foods for at least the first year and as long thereafter as mutually desired.[81] Breast-feeding after the first year continues to provide nutrition, comfort, and an emotional bond between mother and child. As infants begin consuming other foods, their demand for milk is reduced, and milk production decreases, but lactation can continue as long as suckling is maintained.

Whether they are breast-fed or formula-fed, young infants should be fed frequently, on demand. For breast-fed infants, a feeding should last approximately 10 to 15 minutes at each breast. Bottle-fed newborns may consume only a few ounces at each feeding; as the infant grows, the amount consumed will increase to 4 to 8 oz (**Figure 11.21**). A well-fed newborn, whether breast-fed or bottle-fed, should urinate enough to soak six to eight diapers a day and gain about 0.15 to 0.23 kg (0.33 to 0.5 lb)/week.

Dos and don'ts of bottle-feeding • Figure 11.21

Proper bottle-feeding technique supports the infant's nutritional and overall health.

a. During bottle feeding, the infant's head should be higher than his or her stomach, and the bottle should be tilted so that there is no air in the nipple. Just as breast-fed infants alternate breasts, bottle-fed infants should be held alternately on the left and right sides to promote equal development of the head and neck muscles.

b. Infants should never be put to bed with a bottle because saliva flow decreases during sleep, and the formula remains in contact with the teeth for many hours. This causes **nursing bottle syndrome**, rapid and serious decay of the upper teeth. Usually the lower teeth are protected by the tongue.

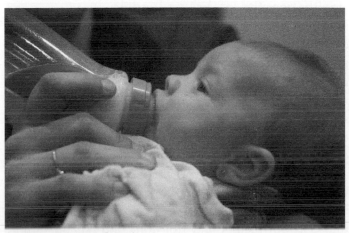

Joel Sartore/NG Image Collection

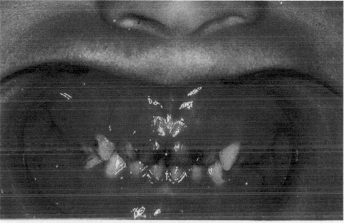

K.L. Boyd, D.D.S./Custom MedicalStock Photo, Inc.

Nutritional composition of breast milk and infant formula   Table 11.3

Nutrient	Amount in breast milk	Amount in formula	Comparisons
Protein	1.8 g/100 mL	1.4 g/100 mL	The relatively low protein content of human milk and formula protects the immature infant kidneys from a too-high load of nitrogen wastes. Alpha-lactalbumin, the predominant protein in human milk, forms a soft, easily digested curd in the infant's stomach. Most formula is made from cow's milk that is modified to mimic the protein concentration and amino acid composition of human milk.
Fat	4 g/100 mL	4.8 g/100 mL	The fat in human milk is easily digested. Human milk is high in cholesterol and the essential fatty acids linoleic acid and α-linolenic acid, as well as their long-chain derivatives ARA and DHA, which are essential for normal brain development, eyesight, and growth. The fat in formula is derived from vegetable oils and provides linoleic and α-linolenic acid. Some formulas are also supplemented with ARA and DHA.
Carbohydrate	7 g/100 mL	7.3 g/100 mL	Lactose, the primary carbohydrate in human milk and most formula, enhances calcium absorption. Because it is digested slowly, it stimulates the growth of beneficial acid-producing bacteria. Oligosaccharides in milk protect against respiratory and gastrointestinal disease.
Sodium	1.3 mg/100 mL	0.7 mg/100 mL	Because breast milk and formula are both low in sodium, the fluid needs of breast-fed and formula-fed infants can be met without an excessive load on the kidneys.
Calcium	22 mg/100 mL	53 mg/100 mL	The ratio of calcium to phosphorus in breast milk and formula enhances calcium absorption.
Phosphorus	14 mg/100 mL	38 mg/100 mL	
Iron	0.03 mg/100 mL	0.1 mg/100 mL	Iron and zinc are present in limited amounts in breast milk but are readily absorbed. Most infant formulas are fortified with iron and zinc because the forms present are less absorbable than those in breast milk.
Zinc	3.2 mg/100 mL	5.1 mg/100 mL	
Vitamin D	4 IU/100 mL	41 IU/100 mL	Formulas are fortified with vitamin D, which is present at low levels in breast milk.

Nutrients in breast milk and formula Human milk is tailored to meet the needs of human infants. The composition of milk changes continuously to suit the needs of a growing infant. The first milk, called **colostrum**, which is produced by the breast for up to a week after delivery, has beneficial effects on the gastrointestinal tract, acting as a laxative that helps the baby excrete the thick, mucusy stool produced during life in the womb. Colostrum looks watery, but the nutrients it supplies meet the infant's needs until mature milk production begins. Mature breast milk contains an appropriate balance of nutrients in forms that are easily digested and absorbed. Infant formulas try to replicate human milk as closely as possible in order to match the growth, nutrient absorption, and other benefits associated with breast-feeding (**Table 11.3**).

colostrum The first milk, produced by the breast late in pregnancy and for up to a week after delivery. Compared to mature milk, it contains more water, protein, immune factors, minerals, and vitamins and less fat.

Health benefits of breast-feeding Despite a nutritional profile that is similar, infant formulas can never exactly duplicate the composition of human milk.[64] Antibody proteins and immune-system cells pass from the mother to her child in the breast milk, providing immune protection for the infant. A number of enzymes and other proteins in breast milk prevent the growth of harmful microorganisms, and several of the carbohydrates in breast milk protect against viruses that cause diarrhea. One substance favors the growth of the beneficial bacterium *Lactobacillus bifidus* in the infant's colon; this bacterium inhibits the growth of disease-causing organisms. Growth factors and hormones present in human

The benefits of breast-feeding[81] • Figure 11.22

Breast-feeding benefits both infants and their mothers.

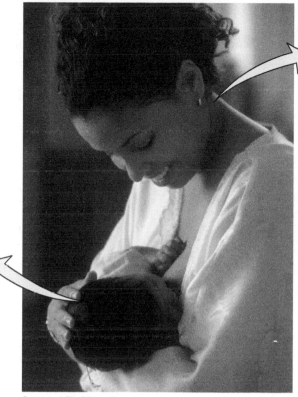

Cusp and Flirt/Masterfile

Benefits for infants

- Provides optimum nutrition
- Enables strong bonding with mother
- Enhances immune protection
- Reduces allergies
- Decreases ear infections, respiratory illnesses, and asthma
- Reduces the likelihood of constipation, diarrhea, or chronic digestive diseases
- Reduces risk for SIDS
- Lowers risk for obesity, type 1 and 2 diabetes, heart disease, hypertension, high cholesterol, and childhood leukemia
- Aids in the development of the facial muscles, speech development, and correct formation of the teeth
- Lessens the risk of overfeeding because the amount of milk consumed cannot be monitored visually

Benefits for mothers

- Provides relaxing, emotionally enjoyable interaction; strengthens bonding with infant
- Reduces financial costs
- Requires less preparation and clean-up time; always available
- Causes uterine contractions that help the uterus return to its normal size more quickly after delivery
- Increases energy expenditure, which may speed return to prepregnancy weight
- Lowers risk of developing type 2 diabetes and breast and ovarian cancers
- Improves bone density and decreases risk of fractures
- Inhibits ovulation, lengthening the time between pregnancies; however, breast-feeding cannot be relied on for birth control
- Decreases the risk of postpartum depression
- Enhances self-esteem in the maternal role

milk promote maturation of the infant's gastrointestinal, cardiovascular, nervous, and endocrine systems. In addition to the numerous health benefits that breast-feeding has for infants it has physical, emotional, and financial advantages for the mother (**Figure 11.22**).

When is formula-feeding better? Despite the benefits of breast milk, formula-feeding may be the best option in some cases. Common illnesses such as colds and skin infections are not passed to the infant in breast milk, but a few, such as tuberculosis and HIV infection, are.[81] Some drugs can also pass from the mother to the baby in breast milk, which means that women who are taking medications should check with their physician about whether they can safely breast-feed while taking their medication. Because alcohol and drugs such as cocaine and marijuana can be passed to a baby in breast milk, alcoholic and drug-addicted mothers are counseled not to breast-feed. Nicotine from cigarette smoke is also rapidly transferred from maternal blood to milk, and heavy smoking may decrease the supply of milk.

Although alcoholic mothers are counseled not to breast-feed, occasional limited alcohol consumption while breast-feeding is probably not harmful if alcohol intake is timed so as to minimize the amount present in milk when the infant is fed. Consuming a single alcoholic drink is safe if the mother then waits at least 4 hours before breast-feeding. Alternatively, milk can be expressed before consuming the drink and fed to the infant later.[46]

Feeding an infant with formula requires more preparation and washing than breast-feeding, but it can give the mother a break because other family members can share the responsibility. For preterm infants and those with genetic abnormalities, formula may be the best option because there are special formulas to meet these infants' unique needs. If an infant is too small or weak to take a bottle, pumped breast milk or formula can be fed through a tube.

Safe Feeding for the First Year

Whether infants are breast-fed or formula-fed, care must be taken to ensure that their needs are met and their food is safe. If proper measurements are not used in preparing formula, the infant can receive an excess or a deficiency of nutrients and an improper ratio of nutrients to fluid

(**Figure 11.23**). If the water and equipment used in preparing formula are not clean or if the prepared formula is left unrefrigerated, food-borne illness may result. Because sanitation is often lacking in developing nations, infections that lead to diarrhea and dehydration occur more frequently in formula-fed infants than in breast-fed infants.

Bacterial contamination is not a concern when a baby is breast-fed, but care must be taken to avoid contamination when milk is pumped from the breast and stored for later feedings. Hands, breast pumps, bottles, and nipples must be washed. Breast milk that is not immediately fed to the baby can be kept refrigerated for 24 to 48 hours. Warming breast milk in a microwave is not recommended because microwaving destroys some of its immune properties and

Safe infant feeding • Figure 11.23

To avoid bacterial contamination, wash hands before preparing formula. Clean bottles and nipples by washing them in a dishwasher or placing them in boiling water for five minutes. Boil water for one to two minutes and cool it before using it to mix powdered formula or dilute concentrates. Cover and refrigerate opened cans of ready-to-feed and liquid concentrate formula and use the formula within the period indicated on the can. Prepare formula immediately before a feeding and discard any excess.

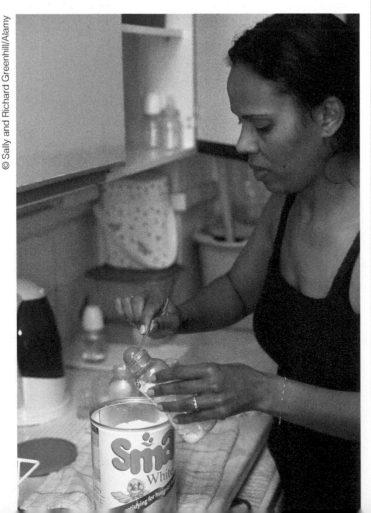

© Sally and Richard Greenhill/Alamy

may result in dangerously hot milk. The best way to warm milk is by running warm water over the bottle.

A concern that is unique to feeding breast milk is that substances in the maternal diet may pass into the milk and cause adverse reactions in the infant. For example, caffeine in the mother's diet can make the infant jittery and excitable, so a mother should avoid consuming large amounts of caffeine while breast-feeding. Most of these reactions seem to be unique to a particular mother and child, so as long as a food does not affect the infant's health or response to feeding, it can be included in the mother's diet.

Food allergies Food allergies are common in infants. Because infants' digestive tracts are immature, they allow the absorption of incompletely digested proteins, which triggers a response from the immune system (see Chapters 3 and 6). After about 3 months of age, the risk of developing food allergies is reduced because incompletely digested proteins are less likely to be absorbed. Many children who develop food allergies before age 3 years eventually outgrow them. Allergies that appear after 3 years of age are more likely to be problematic throughout the individual's life.

Exclusive breast-feeding for the first 4 to 6 months reduces an infant's risk of developing a food allergy.[82] If a formula-fed baby becomes allergic to the milk proteins used in the formula, soy formulas should be used. For infants who cannot tolerate milk or soy protein, formulas made from predigested proteins are an option.

Appropriate introduction of solid and semisolid foods can reduce the risk of an infant developing food allergies. The most commonly recommended first food is iron-fortified infant rice cereal mixed with formula or breast milk, because this cereal is easily digested and rarely causes allergic reactions. After rice has been successfully included in the diet, other grains can be introduced, with wheat cereal given last because it is more likely than other cereals to cause an allergic reaction. Each new food should be offered for a few days without the addition of any other new foods. If an allergic reaction occurs, it is then likely that the newly introduced food caused it. Foods that cause symptoms such as rashes, digestive upsets, or respiratory problems should be discontinued, and the symptoms should no longer be present before any other new foods are added.

Developmentally appropriate foods Although most of an infant's nutritional needs are met by breast milk or

Nourishing a developing infant • Figure 11.24

Foods that are offered to infants should be appropriate for their developmental and digestive abilities.

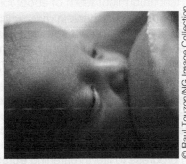
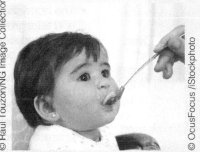
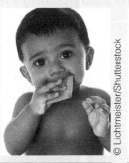
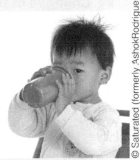

© Raul Touzon/NG Image Collection
© OcusFocus /iStockphoto
© Lichtmeister/Shutterstock
© Saturated (formerly AshokRodrigues)\ © Saturated/iStockphoto

Age	Birth to 4 months	4 to 6 months	6 to 9 months	9 to 12 months
Developmental milestones	The infant takes milk by means of a licking motion of the tongue called *suckling*, which strokes or milks the liquid from the nipple. Solid food placed in the mouth at an early age is usually pushed out as the tongue thrusts forward	The tongue is held farther back in the mouth, allowing solid food to be accepted without being expelled. The infant can hold his or her head up and is able to sit, with or without support.	The infant can sit without support, chew, hold food, and easily move hand to mouth.	The infant can drink from a cup and feed him/herself.
Foods	Breast milk or iron-fortified infant formula.	Breast milk or formula, iron-fortified infant cereal; Rice cereal is usually the first solid food introduced because it is easily digested and less likely than other grains to cause allergies. After cereals, puréed vegetables and fruits can be introduced.	Breast milk or formula, iron-fortified infant cereal, puréed or strained vegetables, fruits, meats and beans, limited finger foods.	Breast milk or formula, iron-fortified infant cereal, chopped vegetables, soft fruits, meats and beans, nonchoking finger foods such as dry cereal, cooked pasta, and well-cooked vegetables.

infant formula, solid and semisolid foods can be gradually introduced into the diet starting at 4 to 6 months of age. By this time, the infant's feeding abilities and gastrointestinal tract are mature enough to handle solid foods (**Figure 11.24**). Cow's milk should never be fed to infants because it is too high in protein and too low in iron.[83] At 1 year of age, whole cow's milk can be offered; it can be used until 2 years of age, after which reduced-fat or low-fat milk can be used. As a child becomes familiar with more variety, food choices should be made from each of the food groups. To avoid choking, foods that can easily lodge in the throat, such as raw carrots, grapes, and hot dogs, should not be offered to infants or toddlers.

The American Academy of Pediatrics and the Dietary Guidelines recommend that fruit juice not be introduced until after 6 months of age and then be limited to 4 to 6 oz per day. Only 100% fruit juice should be offered. Fruit juice should be offered only from a cup; juice consumed from a covered cup or bottle encourages consumption over a long period of time and may allow prolonged contact with the teeth.[84] Honey should not be fed to children less than 1 year old because it may contain spores of *Clostridium botulinum*, the bacterium that causes botulism poisoning (discussed in Chapter 13). Older children and adults are not at risk from botulism spores because the environment in a mature gastrointestinal tract prevents the bacteria from growing.

CONCEPT CHECK STOP

1. **What** does it mean if a child whose birth weight was in the 50th percentile is now in the 30th percentile for growth?

2. **Why** do infants need more fat than adults?

3. **Why** is breast milk the best choice for healthy mothers and babies?

4. **When** can solid food be introduced into an infant's diet?

5 Nutrition for Infants 387

- Growth is the best indicator of adequate nutrition in an infant. Healthy infants follow standard patterns of growth. Growth charts can be used to compare an infant's growth with optimal growth patterns. Slow growth indicates **failure to thrive**, whereas excess weight gain may predispose a child to obesity. Undernutrition and overnutrition during infancy can have permanent effects on growth and development and the risk of chronic disease later in life.

- Infants require more calories and protein per kilogram of body weight than do individuals at any other time of life. Fat and fluid needs are also proportionately higher than in adults. Infants are at risk for deficiencies of iron, vitamin D, and vitamin K, as well as low fluoride intake.

- Breast milk is the ideal food for infants. It meets nutrient needs; it is always available; it requires no special equipment, mixing, or sterilization; and it provides immune protection. There are many infant formulas on the market that are patterned after human milk and provide adequate nutrition to a baby. Formula-feeding is the best option when the mother has certain infections or is taking prescription or illicit drugs, or when the infant has special nutritional needs.

- Introducing solid foods between 4 and 6 months of age, as shown here, adds iron and other nutrients to the diet. Newly introduced foods should be appropriate to the child's stage of development and offered one at a time in order to monitor for food allergies.

Nourishing a developing infant: 4 to 6 months • Figure 11.24

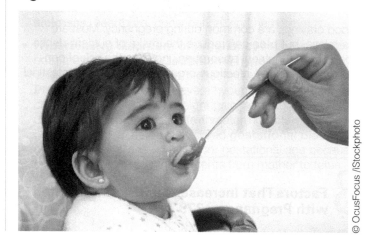

© OcusFocus /iStockphoto

Key Terms

- cesarean section 368
- colostrum 392
- critical period 379
- Down syndrome 381
- eclampsia 371
- edema 370
- embryo 367
- failure to thrive 387
- fertilization 366
- fetal alcohol spectrum disorders (FASDs) 383
- fetal alcohol syndrome (FAS) 383

- fetus 367
- gestational diabetes 371
- gestational hypertension 371
- hypertensive disorders of pregnancy 371
- implantation 367
- infancy 385
- lactation 368
- large for gestational age 368
- let-down 384
- low birth weight 368

- morning sickness 370
- nursing bottle syndrome 391
- nutritional programming 380
- oxytocin 385
- pica 378
- placenta 367
- preeclampsia 371
- preterm or premature 368
- prolactin 384
- small for gestational age 367

- Special Supplemental Nutrition Program for Women, Infants, and Children (WIC) 380
- sudden infant death syndrome (SIDS) or crib death 383
- teratogen 379
- trimester 368
- very low birth weight 368

What is happening in this picture?

Ultrasound imaging, shown here, uses sound waves to visualize the embryo or fetus in the uterus. It can be used to assess the progress of the pregnancy and identify fetal and maternal health problems.

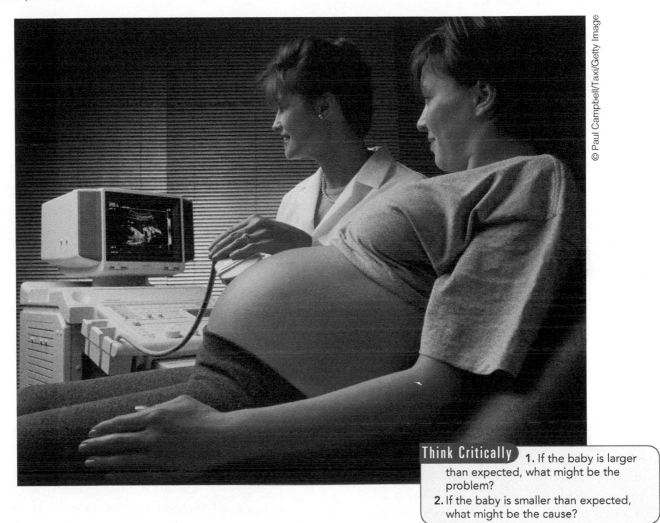

© Paul Campbell/Taxi/Getty Image

Think Critically

1. If the baby is larger than expected, what might be the problem?
2. If the baby is smaller than expected, what might be the cause?

THE PLANNER ✓

Review your Chapter Planner on the chapter opener and check off your completed work.

Nutrition from 1 to 100

12

In *As You Like It*, Shakespeare allotted a human lifetime seven acts to be played upon the world's stage, beginning with "the infant, mewling and puking in the nurse's arms" and ending in "second childishness . . . sans teeth, sans eyes, sans taste." While our senses and abilities do diminish as we age, with proper nutrition and health maintenance, we may not quite reach the state of helplessness described by the Bard.

For "the whining schoolboy"—and girl— "with . . . shining morning face," nutrition and healthy

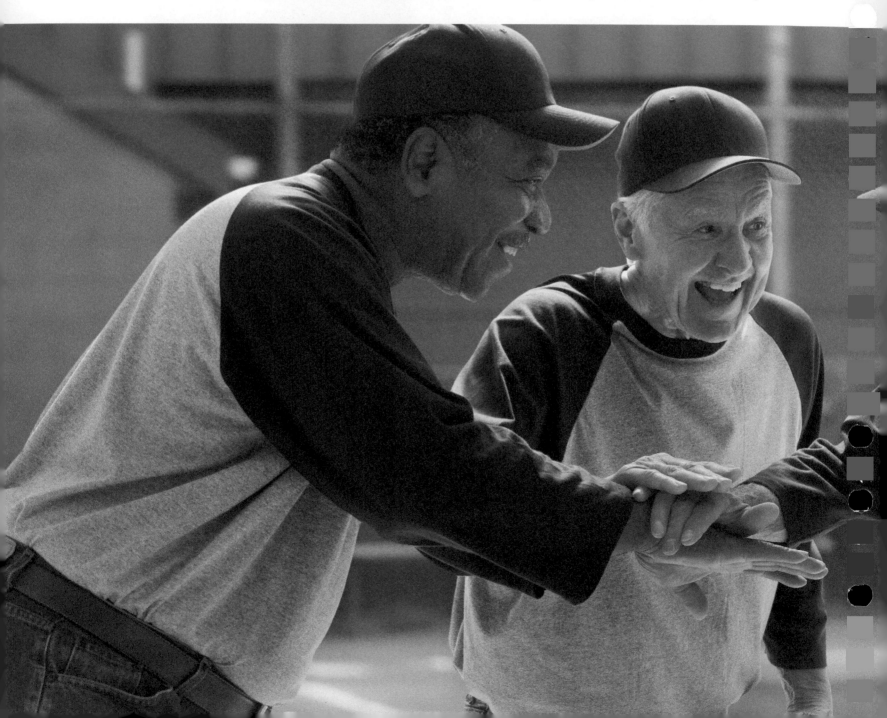

development go hand in hand. As the adolescent becomes "the lover," then "the soldier" of young adulthood, good nutrition is still necessary to maintain health and build a foundation of well-being for the mature "justice, in fair round belly with good capon lin'd"—Shakespeare's archetype of middle age. In his characterization of the closing years of life, "the lean and slipper'd pantaloon . . . a world too wide for his shrunk shank," Shakespeare highlights the muscle withering of old age that, along with other physical, social, and mental changes present a new set of challenges to maintaining nutritional health.

Good nutrition habits adopted in our early years will serve us well through the seven acts of our own "strange eventful history."

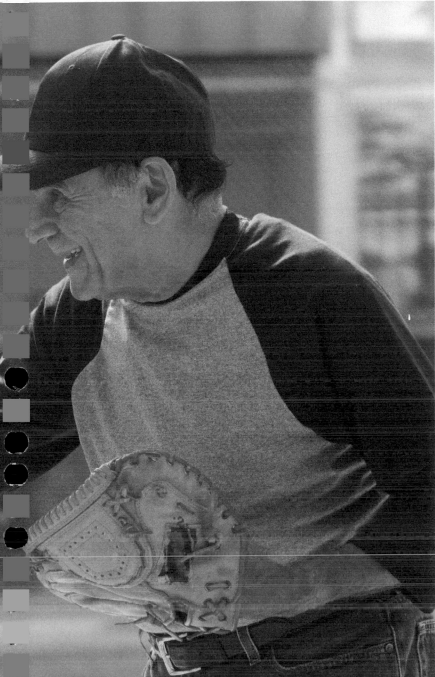

Jose Luis Pelaez Inc/Getty Images

CHAPTER OUTLINE

CHAPTER PLANNER ✔

- ❏ Stimulate your interest by reading the introduction and looking at the visual.
- ❏ Scan the Learning Objectives in each section:
  p. 402 ❏ p. 412 ❏ p. 417 ❏ p. 428 ❏
- ❏ Read the text and study all figures and visuals. Answer any questions.

Analyze key features

- ❏ What a Scientist Sees, p. 405 ❏
- ❏ Nutrition InSight, p. 408 ❏ p. 412 ❏ p. 422 ❏
- ❏ Thinking It Through, p. 410 ❏
- ❏ Debate, p. 418 ❏
- ❏ Process Diagram, p. 430 ❏
- ❏ Stop: Answer the Concept Checks before you go on:
  p. 411 ❏ p. 416 ❏ p. 427 ❏ p. 432 ❏

End of chapter and online review:

- ❏ Review the Summary, Key Terms, and online links to Additional Resources.
- ❏ Answer the online Critical and Creative Thinking Questions.
- ❏ Answer What is happening in this picture?
- ❏ Complete the online Self-Test and check your answers.

12.1 Nutrition for Children

LEARNING OBJECTIVES

1. **Describe** how children's nutrient needs change as they grow.
2. **Discuss** how children's eating habits develop.
3. **Explain** the impact of diet and lifestyle during childhood on the risk of chronic disease.

Nutrient intake during childhood affects health throughout life. The foods a child consumes must supply the energy and nutrients needed for growth and development as well as for maintenance and activity. Foods offered to children must also be appropriate for their stage of physical development and suit their developing tastes. A nutritious, well-balanced eating pattern and an active lifestyle allow children to grow to their potential and can prevent or delay the onset of the chronic diseases that plague adults. Therefore, learning healthy eating and exercise habits will benefit not only today's children but also tomorrow's adults.

Energy and Nutrient Needs of Children

As children grow and become more active, their requirements for energy and most nutrients increase. The average 2-year-old needs about 1000 Calories and 13 grams of protein per day. By age 6, that child needs about 1600 Calories and 19 g of protein per day.[1] The total amount of protein and energy needed continue to increase as children grow into adults; however, the amounts needed per kilogram of body weight decrease (**Figure 12.1**).

The recommended range of carbohydrate intake for children is the same as for adults: 45 to 65% of total energy intake. To provide enough energy to support rapid growth and development, the recommended range of fat intake is higher for children than for adults: 30 to 40% of total energy intake for 1- to 3-year-olds and 25 to 35% for 4- to 18-year-olds. As children grow, the recommended proportion of calories from fat decreases because a higher fat diet is no longer needed to meet energy and developmental needs.

Infants have high water needs, but by 1 year of age, their evaporative losses have decreased and their kidneys have matured, decreasing the loss of water in urine. Therefore, as with adults, in most situations, children can meet their water needs by drinking enough to satisfy thirst.[2] Water needs increase with illness, when the environmental temperature is high, and when activity increases losses from sweat.

Because children are smaller than adolescents and adults, the recommended amounts of most micronutrients are also smaller (see inside cover). Recommended intakes do not differ for boys and girls until about age 9, at which time sexual maturation causes differences in nutrient requirements. Like adults, children who consume a varied, nutrient-dense diet can meet all their vitamin and mineral requirements with food.

The majority of toddlers and preschoolers in the United States meet recommendations for micronutrient intakes.[3] However, children's dietary patterns are high in sugar-sweetened beverages, desserts, and salty snacks, and low in dairy foods, vegetables, fruits, seafood, and whole grains. This dietary pattern tends to be high in sodium, sugar, and saturated fat and low in nutrients of public health concern including calcium, vitamin D, potassium, and fiber.

Calcium, vitamin D, and bone health Calcium intake in school-age children has been declining, primarily due to a decrease in the consumption of dairy products. Adequate calcium intake during childhood is essential for achieving maximum peak bone mass, which is important for preventing osteoporosis later in life (see Chapter 8). The RDA for calcium is 700 mg/day for toddlers (ages 1 to 3) and 1000 mg/day for young children (ages 4 to 8).[6]

Energy needs • Figure 12.1

As children grow, their larger body size causes the total amount of energy they need to increase, but as growth slows, energy needs per kilogram of body weight decline.

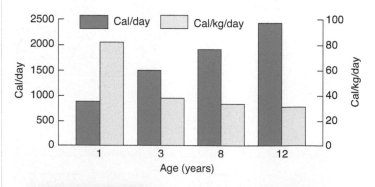

Interpret the Data

How many more Calories per day does a 12-year-old child need than an 8-year-old child?

Vitamin D, which is needed for calcium absorption, is also essential for bone health. Low intakes of milk combined with limited sun exposure contribute to low blood levels of vitamin D in many children in the United States.[7] The RDA is 600 IU (15 µg)/day for children and adolescents.[6]

Iron and anemia Children's iron needs are high because iron is required for growth. The RDA is 7 mg/day for toddlers and 10 mg/day for young children; the latter recommendation is higher than the RDA for adult men. The high needs and finicky eating habits of young children often lead to iron deficiency anemia, a condition that can impair learning ability and intellectual performance.[8] If anemia is diagnosed, iron supplements are usually prescribed until the child's iron stores have been replenished. These supplements should be kept out of the reach of children to prevent iron toxicity from supplement overdoses (see Chapter 8).

Developing Healthy Eating Habits

Much of what we choose to eat as adults depends on what we learned to eat as children. Caregivers are responsible for deciding what foods should be offered to a child and when and where they should be eaten. The child must then decide whether to eat, what foods to eat, and how much to consume. As children grow older, their choices are increasingly affected by social activities, what they see at school, and what their friends are eating.

What to offer? Children should be offered a balanced and varied diet that is adequate in energy and essential nutrients and is appropriate to their developmental needs. A healthy diet is based on whole grains, vegetables, and fruits; includes adequate dairy and other high-protein foods; is low in sodium and added sugars, and contains moderate amounts of fat. MyPlate can be used as a guide for meeting the dietary goals of preschoolers and older children (**Figure 12.2**).

MyPlate recommendations for children • Figure 12.2

MyPlate recommends amounts of food from each group that are appropriate for young children. The recommendations shown here are for a 3-year-old and an 8-year-old boy who engage in more than 60 minutes of activity daily. Food choices to meet these amounts should be spread throughout the meals and snacks served each day.

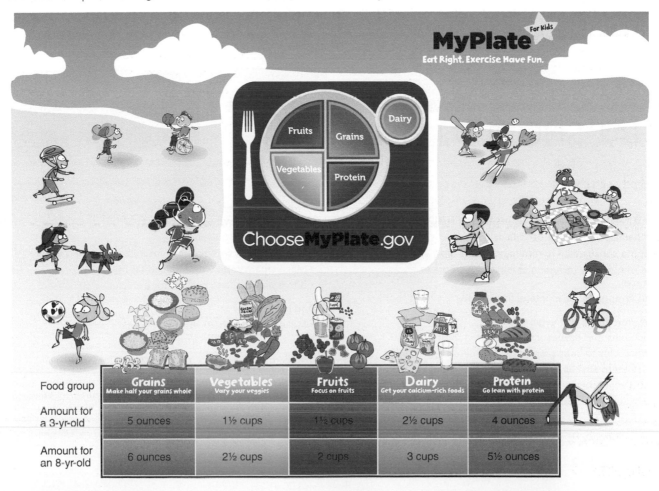

Food group	Grains Make half your grains whole	Vegetables Vary your veggies	Fruits Focus on fruits	Dairy Get your calcium-rich foods	Protein Go lean with protein
Amount for a 3-yr-old	5 ounces	1½ cups	1½ cups	2½ cups	4 ounces
Amount for an 8-yr-old	6 ounces	2½ cups	2 cups	3 cups	5½ ounces

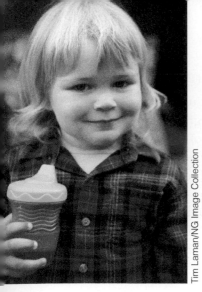

Tim Laman/NG Image Collection

**Limiting juice consumption •
Figure 12.3** _____

More than half the fruit children consume is as juice rather than whole fruit. Although 100% fruit juice can be part of a healthy diet, too much can cause diarrhea, over- or undernutrition, and dental caries. It is recommended that juice not be offered to children in containers that can be carried around, encouraging continuous sipping.[9,10]

It isn't always easy to persuade a child to eat a variety of foods from all the food groups, as recommended by MyPlate. To increase variety, new foods should be introduced into a child's diet regularly. Children's food preferences are learned through repeated exposure to foods; a new food may need to be offered 8 or 10 times before the child will accept it. Children are also more likely to eat a new food if it is introduced at the beginning of a meal, when the child is hungry, and if the child sees his or her parents or peers eating it. Incorporating healthy foods into familiar dishes can also increase the variety of the diet. Vegetables can be added to soups and casseroles, for example, and lean meats can be added to spaghetti sauce, stews, or pizza. Getting children to consume the recommended amount of fruit is usually not difficult, but most servings should come from fruit, with limited amounts from 100% juice, not fruit drinks or juice cocktails. The American Academy of Pediatrics recommends limiting juice to 4 to 6 ounces/day for children ages 1 to 6 and 8 to 12 oz/day for children age 7 and older (**Figure 12.3**).[10]

No matter how erratic children's food intake may be, caregivers should continue to offer a variety of healthy foods at each meal and let children select what and how much they will eat. Children, like adults, tend to eat greater quantities when larger portions are provided.[11] When children are allowed to serve themselves, they eat more appropriate portions than they do when a large portion is put in front of them.

The best indicator that a child is receiving adequate nourishment—neither too little nor too much—is a normal growth pattern. Growth is most rapid in the first year of life, when an infant's length increases by 50%, or about 10 inches. In the second year of life, children generally grow about 5 inches; in the third year, 4 inches; and thereafter, about 2 to 3 inches/year. Although growth often occurs in spurts, growth patterns are predictable and can be monitored by comparing a child's growth pattern with standard patterns shown on growth charts (online Appendix E).[12] The stature a child will eventually attain is affected by genetic, environmental, and lifestyle factors. A child whose parents are 5 feet tall may not have the genetic potential to grow to 6 feet.

WHAT SHOULD I EAT?

 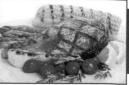

© Sara Winter/iStockphoto © Jill Chen/iStockphoto © Steve Mcsweeny/iStockphoto

Childhood

✓ THE PLANNER

Serve children frequent nutritious meals and snacks
- Smear peanut butter on a banana or an apple.
- Offer some carrots with hummus or yogurt dip.
- Make a rainbow by including at least four colors in every meal.
- Cut and arrange foods in interesting shapes.

Sneak in more fruits and vegetables
- Bake bananas and berries into breads and muffins.
- Add vegetables to soups, tacos, and casseroles.
- Blend fruit into shakes and smoothies.
- Mix extra vegetables into spaghetti sauce.

Include calcium where you can
- Have macaroni and cheese.
- Make oatmeal with reduced-fat milk rather than water.
- Make cream soup with reduced-fat milk.
- Serve pudding and custard for a calcium-rich dessert.

Add iron
- Make your spaghetti sauce with meat.
- Cook your stew in an iron pot.
- Beef up your tacos and burritos.
- Serve iron-fortified breakfast cereal.

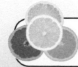

Use iProfile to find snacks that children would enjoy that are high in iron.

WHAT A SCIENTIST SEES
Breakfast and School Performance

This breakfast looks appealing, but regardless of what's on the plate, many children and teens do not make time for breakfast; they are more likely to skip breakfast than to skip any other meal.[13] What a scientist sees is the impact breakfast has on nutritional status and school performance. Skipping breakfast may result in a span of 15 or more hours without food. Because breakfast provides energy and nutrients to the brain, children who skip it are more likely to have academic, emotional, and behavioral problems than those who eat breakfast.[14] Studies have found that compared with nonbreakfast eaters, children who routinely eat breakfast have better nutrient intakes, and these improvements in nutrient intakes are associated with improvements in academic performance, reductions in hyperactivity, better psychosocial behaviors, and less absence and tardiness (see graph).[15,16]

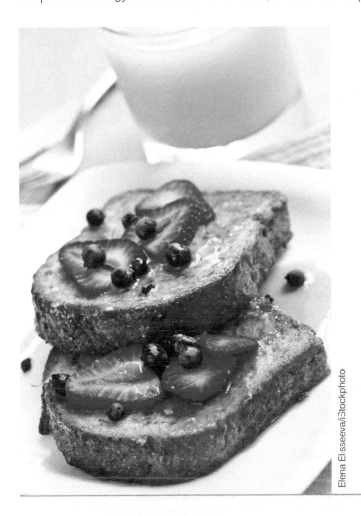

Elena Elisseeva/iStockphoto

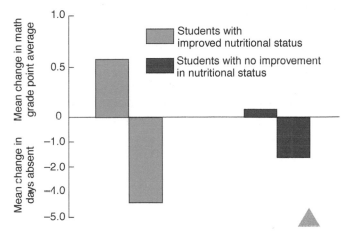

Implementation of a free school breakfast program in the Boston Public Schools improved the nutritional status of many students. Those whose nutritional status improved showed greater improvements in math grades and fewer school absences than students whose nutritional status was not improved.[15]

Think Critically In addition to enhancing learning by fueling the brain after the overnight fast, in what other ways might breakfast contribute to better school performance?

When a child does not get enough to eat, weight gain slows, and if the deficiency continues, growth in height slows. If food intake is excessive, a child is at risk for becoming obese and developing the chronic diseases that are increasingly common in U.S. adults (see *What Should I Eat?*).

When and where to offer meals and snacks Because children have small stomachs and high nutrient needs, they should consume small, nutrient-dense meals and snacks, ideally every two to three hours throughout the day. Establishing a consistent meal pattern is important because children thrive on routine and feel secure when they know what to expect. Starting the day with a good breakfast is particularly important; children who eat breakfast are more likely than those who do not to meet their daily nutrient needs and do better in school (see *What a Scientist Sees*).[15] Snacks should be as

Typical meal and snack patterns for 3- and 8-year-old children   Table 12.1

Food	Amount 3-year-old	Amount 8-year-old	Food	Amount 3-year-old	Amount 8-year-old
Breakfast			**Snack**		
Whole grain cereal	1/2 cup	1 cup	Broccoli crowns	4	6
Milk, 2%	1/2 cup	1/2 cup	Ranch salad dressing	1 tsp	2 tsp
Banana	1/2 medium	1 medium			
			Dinner		
Snack			Chicken drumsticks	1	2
Peanut butter	2 Tbsp	2 Tbsp	Baked sweet potato	1/2 cup	1 cup
Whole wheat crackers	5	5	Green beans	1/4 cup	1/2 cup
Milk, 2%	1/2 cup	1 cup	Milk, 2%	1/2 cup	1 cup
			Graham crackers	1	2
Lunch					
Vegetable soup	1/2 cup	1 cup	**Snack**		
Grilled tuna sandwich	1/2	1	Yogurt	1/2 cup	1 cup
Tomato	1/4 medium	1/2 medium	Berries	1/2 cup	3/4 cup
Orange	1/2 medium	1 medium			
Milk, 2%	1/2 cup	1 cup			

nutritious as meals to ensure that nutrient needs are met (**Table 12.1**).

The setting in which a meal is consumed is also important. Children need companionship, conversation, and a pleasant location at mealtimes. Eating meals together helps children connect with family and culture and is associated with better school performance and decreased risk of unhealthy weight-loss practices and substance abuse. Children learn by example; therefore, the eating patterns, attitudes, and feeding styles of their caregivers influence what they learn to eat. Children whose mothers' eat a healthy diet are more likely to have a healthy diet.[17] Children should be given plenty of time to finish eating. Slow eaters are unlikely to finish eating if they are abandoned by siblings who run off to play and adults who leave to wash dishes. Moreover, if mealtime is to be a nutritious, educational, and enjoyable experience, it should not be a battle zone. Food is not a reward or a punishment: It is simply nutrition.

Meals at day care or school   It is not easy to ensure that meals eaten away from home are nutritious because there is no guarantee that what is served at school or brought from home will be eaten. A packed lunch should contain foods that the child likes and that do not require refrigeration. For children who do not bring meals from home, federal school breakfast and lunch programs provide free or low-cost meals containing age-appropriate foods.

The **National School Lunch Program** provides free or reduced cost lunches to eligible children. In 2012, nearly 32 million children participated in the program.[18] While

How good are children's diets? • Figure 12.4

The Healthy Eating Index scores diets based on how well they meet the recommendations of the 2010 Dietary Guidelines and MyPlate. A score of 100% indicates that on average the recommendation was met or exceeded. Some recommendations target getting adequate amounts so higher scores mean a higher intake; others focus on moderation so higher scores indicate lower and hence more desirable intakes. For all, a higher percentage indicates a higher quality diet. In general, children do not eat enough vegetables or whole grains, and they consume too many empty calories as well as too much sodium.[21]

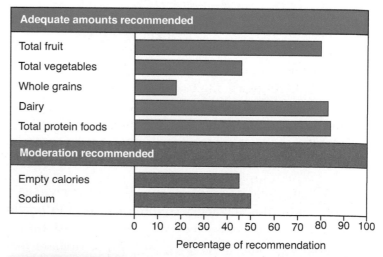

Interpret the Data

According to the graph, which of the following is consumed in an amount farthest from what is recommended?

a. sodium   c. total fruit
b. total vegetables   d. whole grains

the program has provided meals for over 50 years, the specific requirements for these meals have changed over the years. The Healthy Hunger-Free Kids Act of 2010 provided a new set of school lunch standards based on the 2010 Dietary Guidelines and designed to promote nutrition education by teaching children to make appropriate food choices. Each lunch must include fruits and vegetables, half of the grains offered must be whole, and only low-fat or fat-free milk can be offered. Meals must be low in saturated fat and include only ingredients with 0 *trans* fat. The sodium content of meals will be reduced gradually over a 10-year period.[19] In addition to lunches, federal guidelines regulate meals provided as part of the School Breakfast Program and foods sold in school vending machines. Vending machine snacks must have fewer than 200 Calories, less than 230 mg of sodium, less than 35% of calories from fat, and less than 35% of their weight from sugar. The only beverages that can be sold in vending machines are water, low-fat and fat-free milk, fruit and vegetable juices, and fruit and vegetable juices diluted with water but containing no sweeteners.[20]

Nutrition and Health Concerns in Children

The diets of U.S. children today are not as healthy as they could be, and as a result, children are not as healthy as they could be (**Figure 12.4**). Some of the nutrition and health concerns affecting children in the United States are related to their dietary and exercise patterns. The high-caloric, high-sugar, high-salt, high-saturated-fat diet and low-activity lifestyle that contribute to obesity and chronic disease in adults are having the same effects in children. Other nutrition-related health concerns in children include dental caries and lead poisoning.

The rising rate of childhood obesity A child's weight is assessed by determining his or her body mass index (BMI) and plotting it on a gender-specific BMI-for-age growth chart to determine his or her percentile. The BMI percentile is then used to classify the child as obese, overweight, healthy

weight, or underweight (**Figure 12.5**).[22] It is estimated that about 17% of U.S. children and adolescents ages 2 through 19 are obese.[23] Along with obesity come a number of other chronic conditions, including type 2 diabetes, high blood pressure, and elevated blood cholesterol, as well as social and psychological challenges (**Figure 12.6**).

Reducing the incidence of childhood overweight/obesity requires changes in eating and activity patterns, behavioral counseling, and the support of caregivers. The goal is to promote healthy body weight in all children and

BMI-for-age percentiles • Figure 12.5

This growth chart shows the BMI-for-age percentiles for boys 2 to 20 years of age. The colored areas represent BMI values associated with underweight, healthy weight, overweight, and obesity. A similar growth chart can be used to assess body weight in girls (see online Appendix E).

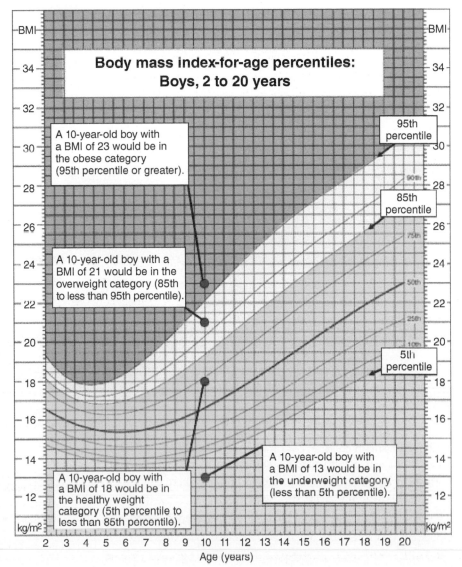

Body mass index-for-age percentiles: Boys, 2 to 20 years

A 10-year-old boy with a BMI of 23 would be in the obese category (95th percentile or greater).

A 10-year-old boy with a BMI of 21 would be in the overweight category (85th to less than 95th percentile).

A 10-year-old boy with a BMI of 18 would be in the healthy weight category (5th percentile to less than 85th percentile).

A 10-year-old boy with a BMI of 13 would be in the underweight category (less than 5th percentile).

95th percentile
85th percentile
5th percentile

The percentage of children who are obese has been increasing and along with it the incidence of health problems associated with obesity.

Results from the National Health and Nutrition Examination Surveys illustrate the increase in the percentage of children who are obese over the past 20 years. The most recent data from 2011–2012 indicates that although overall obesity rates in children have not changed, rates in very young children may be declining.[23]

Legend:
- 1971–1974
- 1988–1994
- 2007–2008
- 2011–2012

y-axis: Obesity (%)
x-axis: Age (years) — 2–5, 6–11, 12–19

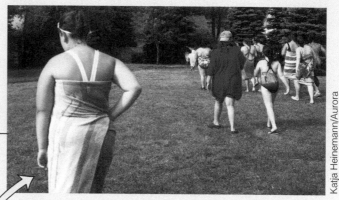

Katja Heinemann/Aurora

Obese children are at risk for depression, unhealthy blood cholesterol levels, high blood pressure, and type 2 diabetes.

Psychosocial problems: Obese children are more likely than others to be socially isolated and to have depression, poor self-image, and low self-esteem. Social isolation, in turn, results in boredom, depression, inactivity, and withdrawal—all of which can increase eating and decrease activity, worsening the problem.

Elevated blood cholesterol: Blood cholesterol screening is recommended between the ages of 9 and 11 and again between 17 and 21 years of age.[25]

Cholesterol levels in children and adolescents 2 to 19 years old[24]		
	Total cholesterol (mg/100 mL)	**LDL cholesterol (mg/100 mL)**
Acceptable	< 170	< 110
Borderline	170–199	110–129
High	≥ 200	≥ 130

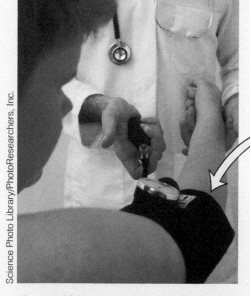

Science Photo Library/PhotoResearchers, Inc.

Elevated blood pressure: The prevalence of hypertension and prehypertension has been increasing in children over the past 20 years. As with adults, blood pressure increases with obesity and can be reduced with weight loss, a DASH-style diet, reductions in sodium intake, and increases in activity level.[25]

Type 2 diabetes: The longer an individual has diabetes, the greater the risk of complications that can lead to blindness, kidney failure, heart disease, or amputations (see Chapter 4).

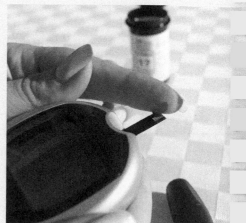

Bambu Productions/Getty Images

help overweight and obese children to stop gaining weight or slowly lose weight. The intensity of the weight-loss programs recommended for children depends on their weight category and their health risks.[26] For overweight children at low risk, weight loss is not recommended; rather, weight gain should be slowed while they continue to grow taller. This allows them to "grow into" their weight. A child who is at the 85th percentile for BMI at age 7 and gains only a few pounds a year can be at the 75th percentile by age 9. For children in the obese BMI range, programs should be designed to promote slow weight loss of no more than 1 pound per month for children 2 to 5 and no more than 2 pounds per week for older children and adolescents. For severely obese youths (BMI > 99th percentile) for whom reduced intake, increased activity, and behavior change have not been successful, weight-loss medications and/or surgery may be recommended.[26]

It can be difficult to modify a child's food consumption patterns. Denying food may promote further overeating by making the child feel that he or she will not obtain enough to satisfy hunger. Thus, restrictions on food intake should be relatively mild, and the focus instead should be on offering nutrient-dense foods.

Public health recommendations, including the 2010 Dietary Guidelines, suggest that children be physically active for at least an hour each day. This may be difficult for overweight children, who are often embarrassed by their bodies and shy away from group activities. Increases in physical activity need to be gradual in order to make exercise a positive experience. A good way to start is to limit time spent watching television and playing video and computer games.

Watching television has a major influence on children's energy balance because it affects both food intake and activity level (**Figure 12.7** and *Thinking It Through*). Sitting in front of the television encourages snacking and reduces activity. Television also affects the quality of the diet because commercials introduce children to foods to which they might otherwise not be exposed. When children are attracted to foods advertised on television, those foods are more likely to be purchased.[27] The American Academy of Pediatrics recommends that children limit television and other screen activities to 2 hours per day or less.[25]

Limiting television and other screen time allows more time for active games, walks after dinner, bike rides, hikes, swimming, volleyball, and other activities that the whole family can enjoy together. The *Let's Move!* initiative, launched by Michelle Obama to combat childhood obesity, provides information to help kids become more physically active within their families, schools, and communities.[28] This information is available at ChooseMyPlate.gov. Learning to enjoy sports and exercise in childhood will set the stage for an active lifestyle in adulthood.

Television affects food intake and activity level • Figure 12.7

Watching television encourages inactivity and unhealthy snacking.

a. Hours spent watching television are hours when physical activity is at a minimum. More time spent watching TV is associated with higher BMI among children and adolescents.[29]

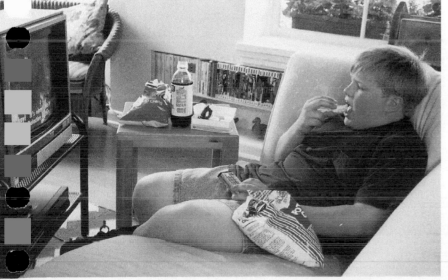

Donna Day/Stone/Getty Images

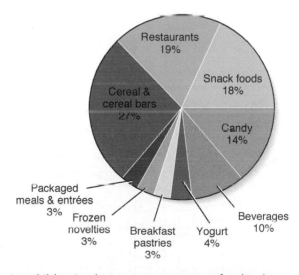

b. During children's television programming, food is the most frequently advertised product category. This chart, which illustrates the types of food advertised on Saturday morning children's television programming, shows that almost half of the commercials advertise candy, snack foods, beverages, and pastries.[30]

A Case Study on Under- and Overnutrition

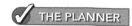 THE PLANNER

Sam is 8 years old and has gained 5 pounds in the past 3 months. His parents are worried because all Sam wants to do is watch TV. Because Sam's parents are both overweight, they are concerned that he will also have a weight problem, so they take him to see his pediatrician.

 1 Based on this growth chart, how has Sam's BMI percentile changed over the past year?

Your answer:

Reviewing Sam's diet and exercise patterns, the doctor learns that Sam has been watching TV or playing video games for about 6 hours a day. A recall of his intake shows that he eats donuts and milk for breakfast, gets lunch from the school lunch program, and then snacks so much on chips and candy when he gets home from school that he doesn't really eat dinner. He likes fruit, refuses to eat vegetables, and drinks 5 to 6 cups of whole milk daily.

 2 What nutrients are likely to be excessive in this dietary pattern? Which are likely to be deficient?

Your answer:

A blood test reveals that Sam has iron deficiency anemia. The pediatrician prescribes an iron supplement and refers Sam and his parents to a dietitian. She recommends that the family switch to 1% milk to reduce Sam's energy and saturated fat intake and to a fortified cereal for breakfast to increase his iron intake. She also recommends that they limit Sam's after-school snacking to fruit so he can eat a better evening meal.

 3 Why might Sam's high intake of milk contribute to his anemia?

Your answer:

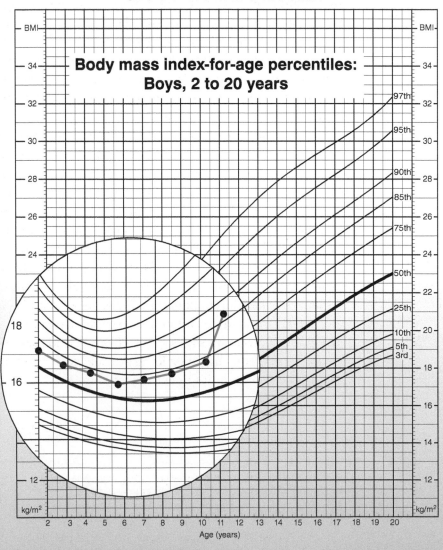

CDC Growth Charts: United States

Body mass index-for-age percentiles: Boys, 2 to 20 years

 4 How might Sam's iron deficiency have contributed to his weight gain?

Your answer:

5 Sam needs to increase his activity to avoid further weight gain. What activity recommendations would you make for Sam?

Your answer:

(Check your answers in online Appendix L)

Dental caries A diet that is high in sugary foods promotes the formation of dental caries (see Chapter 4). Because the primary teeth guide the growth of the permanent teeth, maintaining healthy primary teeth is just as important as preserving the permanent ones. Tooth decay is caused by prolonged contact between sugar and bacteria on the surface of the teeth. When soft drinks and other sweetened beverages, which are a major source of added sugar in children's diets, are sipped slowly between meals they increase the risk of tooth decay.

Attention-deficit/hyperactivity disorder (ADHD) Five to 10% of school-age children have been diagnosed with ADHD; it occurs more frequently in boys than in girls.[31] ADHD involves extreme physical activity, excitability, impulsiveness, distractibility, short attention span, and low tolerance for frustration. Children with ADHD have more difficulty learning but usually are of normal or above-average intelligence.

Although parents of children with ADHD report a worsening of symptoms after excessive ingestion of candy or soda, controlled studies have not found sugar intake to affect children's behavior or cognitive performance.[32] It has been suggested, however, that reactive hypoglycemia (see Chapter 4) following sugar ingestion may contribute to inattention and cognitive impairment in children with ADHD.[32] In some children, the hyperactive behavior observed after sugar consumption may be the result of situational factors. For example, the excitement of a birthday party rather than the sugar in the cake may be what affects behavior.

One cause of hyperactive behavior in children is caffeine. Caffeine is a stimulant that causes sleeplessness, restlessness, and irregular heartbeats. Beverages, foods, and medicines containing caffeine are often part of children's diets. For example, caffeinated beverages such as Coke and Mountain Dew are commonly included in children's fast-food meals.

Other possible causes of hyperactivity include lack of sleep, overstimulation, desire for more attention, or lack of physical activity. Specific foods and food additives have also been implicated as causes of hyperactivity. Numerous studies have failed to provide sufficient evidence for the efficacy of any dietary treatment for ADHD. However, some children are sensitive to specific additives and may benefit from a diet that eliminates them.[32]

Lead toxicity Lead is an environmental contaminant that can be toxic, especially in children under age 6. Children can be exposed to lead in air pollution, old house paint, lead plumbing, and certain ceramics. Children are at particular risk for lead toxicity because they absorb lead much more efficiently than do adults. It is estimated that infants and young children may absorb as much as 50% of ingested lead. Malnourished children are at particular risk because malnutrition increases lead absorption due to the fact that lead is better absorbed from an empty stomach and when other minerals such as calcium, zinc, and iron are deficient. Once it has been absorbed from the gastrointestinal tract, lead circulates in the bloodstream and then accumulates in the bones and, to a lesser extent, the brain, teeth, and kidneys. Lead disrupts the functioning of neurotransmitters and thus interferes with the functioning of the nervous system.

In young children, lead poisoning can affect IQ and cause both learning disabilities and behavior problems. High levels of lead can contribute to iron deficiency anemia, changes in kidney function, nervous system changes, and even seizures, coma, and death. No safe blood lead level has been identified. There are about a half a million U.S. children with blood lead levels above the reference level of 5 μg/100 mL.[33] Medical treatment is recommended for children with blood lead levels greater than or equal to 45 μg/100 mL.

Because of the risks of lead toxicity from environmental contamination, lead is no longer used in house paint, gasoline, or solder. As a result, the number of children ages 1 to 5 with elevated blood lead levels has decreased dramatically. Despite these gains, certain groups remain at elevated risk of high blood lead levels. Low-income children are at particular risk. Low-income families are more likely to live in older buildings that still have lead paint and lead plumbing. Typical blood lead levels are also higher for non-Hispanic black children than those for Mexican American and non-Hispanic white children, in part reflecting differences in socioeconomic status.[33] The effects of lead poisoning are permanent, but if high levels are detected early, the lead can be removed with medical treatment.

CONCEPT CHECK 🛑 STOP

1. **How** do children's energy and protein requirements change as they age?

2. **What** factors affect children's food choices?

3. **What** health risks are associated with obesity in children?

MyPlate recommendations for teens • Figure 12.10

The recommendations shown here are for 11- and 18-year-old boys and girls who engage in more than 60 minutes of activity daily. The 10 oz of grains recommended for an active 18-year-old boy may seem like a huge amount. But when spread over the course of a day (in the form of, say, a large bowl of cereal and toast for breakfast, two tacos for lunch, and a dinner that includes spaghetti and garlic bread), it is an amount that is easily consumed by a teenage boy.

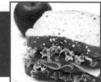

ChooseMyPlate.gov

Food group	Grains Make half your grains whole	Vegetables Vary your veggies	Fruits Focus on fruits	Dairy Get your calcium-rich foods	Protein Go lean with protein
Amount for an 11-yr-old male	7 ounces	3 cups	2 cups	3 cups	6 ounces
Amount for an 11-yr-old female	6 ounces	2½ cups	2 cups	3 cups	5½ ounces
Amount for an 18-yr-old male	10 ounces	4 cups	2½ cups	3 cups	7 ounces
Amount for an 18-yr-old female	8 ounces	3 cups	2 cups	3 cups	6½ ounces

adolescents eat, and skipped meals and meals away from home are common. A food is more likely to be selected because it tastes good, it is easy to grab, or friends are eating it than because it is a healthy choice. No matter when foods are consumed throughout the day, an adolescent's diet should follow the recommendations of MyPlate for the appropriate age, gender, and activity level (**Figure 12.10** and *What Should I Eat?*). The best indicators of adequate intake are satiety and a growth pattern that follows the curve of the growth charts.

Making fast food fit There is nothing wrong with an occasional fast-food meal, but a steady diet of burgers, fries, and pizza will likely contribute to an overall unhealthy diet.

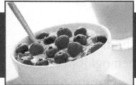 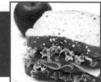 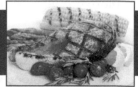

WHAT SHOULD I EAT?

Adolescence

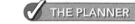 THE PLANNER

Balance unhealthy choices with healthy ones
- Have low-fat milk with your burger and fries.
- Eat an extra vegetable with dinner.
- Put a variety of vegetables on your pizza.
- Try fresh fruit for dessert.

Eat breakfast
- Grab some whole-grain toast with peanut butter.
- Stick a cereal bar or muffin in your backpack.
- Have a yogurt on the go.

Snack well
- Reach for an apple, a pear, or an orange before the cookies and chips.
- Dip your chips in salsa, guacamole, or hummus.

- Nibble on nuts and seeds.
- Crunch some baby carrots.

Count up your calcium
- Drink milk; low-fat milk has fewer calories than soda.
- Put extra milk on your cereal.
- Make a shake by mixing plain nonfat yogurt and fruit in the blender.
- Have cheese with crackers, on pizza, or in tacos.

 Use iProfile to calculate the calcium content of your favorite fast-food meal.

Make healthier fast-food choices Table 12.2	
Instead of . . .	**Choose . . .**
Double-patty hamburger with cheese, mayonnaise, special sauce, and bacon	Regular single-patty hamburger without mayonnaise, special sauce, and bacon
Breaded and fried chicken sandwich	Grilled chicken sandwich
Chicken nuggets or tenders	Grilled chicken strips
Large French fries	Baked potato, side salad, or small order of fries
Fried chicken wings	Baked skinless wings
Crispy-shell chicken taco with extra cheese and sour cream	Grilled-chicken soft taco without sour cream
Nachos with cheese sauce	Tortilla chips with bean dip
12-in. meatball sub	6-in. turkey breast sub with lots of vegetables
Thick-crust pizza with extra cheese and meat toppings	Thin-crust pizza with extra veggies
Donut	Cinnamon and raisin bagel with low-fat cream cheese

Fast food is typically low in fruits and vegetables and high in solid fats and sodium. About 35% of the empty calories consumed by U.S. children are from foods such as sugar-sweetened beverages, dairy desserts, French fries, and pizza served at fast-food restaurants.[39] Most teens in the United States consume more than the recommended amounts of added sugar, solid fat, and sodium and fewer fruits and vegetables than recommended. The lettuce and tomatoes that garnish a burger or taco are not enough to meet the MyPlate recommendations for vegetables. French fries, which are high in fat and salt, are the most frequently consumed vegetable. To fit fast food into a healthy diet, make more nutrient-dense fast-food choices and make sure other meals and snacks eaten throughout the day supply the nutrients that are not obtained from fast food. Many fast-food franchises now offer fruit, salads, yogurt, and low-fat milk. And some of the old standbys are not bad choices. A plain, single-patty hamburger provides a lot less fat and energy than one with two patties and a high-fat sauce. A chicken sandwich can be a healthy choice if it is grilled or barbecued, not breaded and fried (**Table 12.2**).

Keeping vegetarian choices healthy It is not uncommon for a teen to decide to consume a vegetarian diet even if the rest of the family does not. Some give up meat for health reasons or to lose weight, while others give up meat because they are concerned about animals and the environment. A vegetarian diet can be a healthy choice when it is carefully planned to meet nutrient needs, not just to eliminate meat. A poorly planned vegetarian diet will be no healthier than any other poorly planned diet. Adequate protein is generally not a problem, but meatless diets can be low in iron and zinc. Teenagers eating a vegan diet may also be at risk for vitamin B_{12} deficiency and inadequate calcium and vitamin D intake (see Chapter 6). We generally think of vegetarian diets as being low in fat and calories, but one that is based on high-fat dairy products can be high in saturated fat, cholesterol, and calories (**Figure 12.11**).

Healthy vegetarian choices • Figure 12.11

The vegetarian meal on the left is high in saturated fat, cholesterol, and added sugar. In contrast, the whole-grain pita bread stuffed with chickpeas, corn, spinach, and tomatoes served with reduced-fat milk, shown on the right is low in saturated fat, cholesterol, and added sugar, and is high in fiber and a good source of calcium and iron.

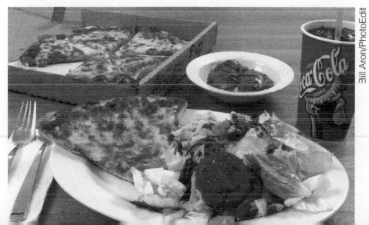
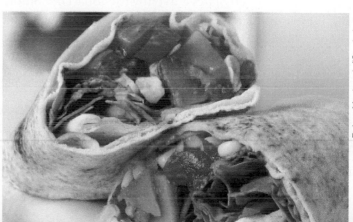

Bill Aron/PhotoEdit

Robyn Mackenzie/iStockphoto

Special Concerns for Teens

Peer pressure to fit in and concern about physical appearance probably have a greater impact on behavior during adolescence than at any other time in life. Many girls want to lose weight even if they are not overweight, and boys want to gain weight in order to achieve a strong, muscular appearance.

Eating disorders As discussed in Chapter 9, the excessive concern about weight, low self-esteem, and poor body image that are common during the teenage years contribute to the development of eating disorders. These disorders can be fatal, but even in less severe cases, the nutritional consequences of an eating disorder can affect growth and development during adolescence and have a lifelong impact on bone health.

The impact of athletics Participation in competitive sports may affect adolescent nutrient needs and eating patterns. Like adult athletes, teen athletes require more water and energy than do their less active peers. Individuals involved in sports, such as football, that require the athlete to be large and heavy, usually do not have trouble eating enough to meet the additional energy needs, but they may be tempted to experiment with anabolic steroids or other ergogenic supplements in an effort to "bulk up," and as a result compromise their health. As discussed in Chapter 10, steroids can stunt growth in adolescence as well as lead to sexual and reproductive disorders, heart disease, liver damage, acne, and aggressive, violent behavior. Teens participating in gymnastics and wrestling may restrict their food intake in order to stay light and lean. Weight restriction at this stage of life may affect nutritional status and maturation and increase the risk of developing an eating disorder. In female athletes, the combination of hard training and weight restriction can lead to the *female athlete triad* (see Chapter 10).

Tobacco use Approximately 23% of high school students in the United States currently use tobacco.[40] Smoking increases the risk of cardiovascular disease and lung cancer. Smoking can limit appetite, and many teens start smoking in order to control their weight and are afraid to quit because they fear that they will gain weight if they do.[41] Smoking may also have an impact on nutrient intake; a study of smokers found that they eat more saturated fat and fewer fruits and vegetables than do nonsmokers.[42] This dietary pattern increases the risk of developing heart disease and cancer.

Alcohol use Alcohol is a drug that has short-term effects that occur soon after ingestion and long-term health consequences that are associated with overuse. These effects are discussed in greater depth in the last section of the chapter.

Although it is illegal to sell alcohol to adolescents, alcoholic beverages are commonly available at teen social gatherings, and peer pressure to consume them is strong. Surveys of American youth suggest that approximately 39% of the nation's high school students drank alcohol during the last month and 22% binge drank.[43] **Binge drinking** involves consumption of five or more drinks in a row for men or four or more in a row for women in about 2 hours. It often leads to dangerous risk-taking behaviors and blood alcohol levels that are high enough to cause loss of consciousness, coma, and even death.

> **binge drinking** A pattern of drinking that brings a person's blood alcohol concentration to 80 mg/100 mL or above.

Consumption of alcohol with caffeinated beverages is common among teens and is particularly dangerous.[44] The stimulant effects of the caffeine counters the depressant effects of the alcohol, but judgment and motor function are still impaired. The person is drunk but does not feel drunk. As a result, he or she may drink to the point of alcohol toxicity or think it is safe to get behind the wheel of a car.

CONCEPT CHECK 🛑 STOP

1. **How** does puberty affect body composition in males and females?

2. **How** do the energy needs of teens compare with those of adults?

3. **What** factors contribute to low calcium intake in teens?

4. **What** could a teen choose at a fast-food restaurant to boost vegetable intake?

12.3 Nutrition for the Adult Years

LEARNING OBJECTIVES

1. **Distinguish** life expectancy from active life expectancy.

2. **Compare** the energy and nutrient requirements of older and younger adults.

3. **Discuss** how the physical, mental, and social changes of aging increase nutritional risks.

4. **Plan** a diet for a sedentary 80-year-old woman, based on MyPlate recommendations.

The benefits of a healthy diet do not stop when you stop growing. Good nutrition throughout your adult years can keep you healthy and active into your 80s and beyond. In the United States, **life expectancy** is 76.3 years for men and 81.1 years for women.[45] However, not all of these years are necessarily active and healthy. The average healthy or **active life expectancy** is 65.1 years for men and 68 years for women.[46] This means that, on average, men spend the last 11 years of life and women the last 13 years physically or socially restricted by disease and disability.

life expectancy The average length of life for a particular population of individuals.

active life expectancy The number of years a person is able to live in an independent state, without being limited by chronic conditions.

The goal of successful aging is to increase not only life expectancy but active life expectancy. Achieving this goal is particularly important because we live in a nation with an aging population (**Figure 12.12a**). Keeping older adults healthy will benefit not only the aging individuals themselves but also the family members who must find the time and resources to care for them and the public health programs that attempt to meet their needs. Although nutrition is not the key to immortality, a healthy diet can prevent malnutrition and delay the onset of chronic diseases that typically begin in middle age and reduce the quality of life in older adults (**Figure 12.12b**).

The number of older adults is rising • Figure 12.12

The number of older adults is increasing, and there is great disparity in their health.

a. About 13% of the U.S. population is 65 years of age or over; by 2040 this percentage is expected to reach 21%.[47] The **oldest old** (≥ 85 years), one of the fastest-growing age groups, have more activity limitations and chronic conditions and require more public health dollars and services than do younger adults.[47]

b. Chronological age is not always the best indicator of a person's health. A person who is 75 may have the vigor and health of someone who is 55, or vice versa. Some older adults are healthy, independent, and active, while others are chronically ill, dependent, and at high risk for malnutrition.

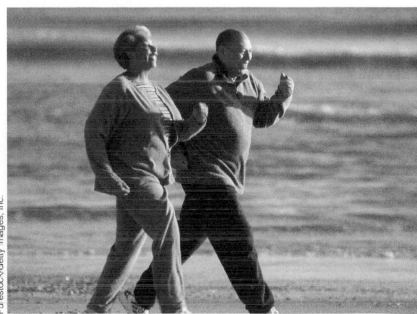

Purestock/Getty Images, Inc.

The Issue: Even before Ponce De Leon searched for the fountain of youth in what is now Florida, humans longed for a way to preserve youth. So far, though, the only dietary intervention that has been shown to slow aging and extend life is cutting calorie intake. Is calorie restriction a good way for people to slow aging and extend their lives?

Most of us eat too much. Eating too many calories and too much salt, saturated fat, and sugar shortens life expectancy by increasing the incidence of obesity, high blood pressure, diabetes, heart disease, and cancer. Eliminating dietary excesses can help us live healthier lives, but many argue that eating even less than what is currently recommended will help us live longer and healthier lives.

It has been known since the 1930s that, for many animals, consuming a calorie-restricted diet (10 to 30% less than recommended intake) that meets the need for all essential nutrients will slow aging and increase longevity.[48] There is good evidence that short-lived species such as insects, worms, mice, and other rodents that are fed a calorie-restricted diet live longer—as much as 150% longer—than animals that eat more calories.[49] The calorie-restricted animals have a lower incidence of age-related chronic diseases, better immune function, lower blood glucose, and better overall organ function than do animals whose diets are not calorie restricted.

There is less evidence for the effectiveness of calorie restriction in humans and other primates. One study in rhesus monkeys, begun in 1989, suggests that calorie restriction does extend lifespan; the animals have lower body fat and less muscle loss, as well as a lower incidence of cancer, heart disease, and type 2 diabetes.[50] A similar study also found beneficial

health effects in rhesus monkeys but no increase in longevity.[50] Short-term studies in humans have shown that calorie restriction causes a reduction in body weight, blood pressure, blood cholesterol, blood glucose, and indices of oxidative stress.[51,52]

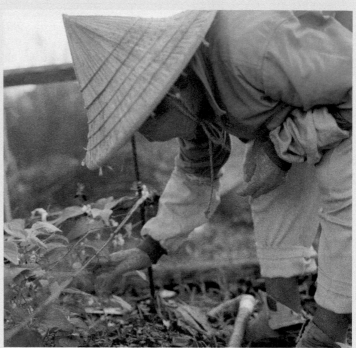

Ana Nance/Redux Pictures

Many Okinawans who followed the traditional dietary and lifestyle pattern lived to be over 100 years old.

What Is Aging?

Aging is universal to all living things, but it is a process that we still don't fully understand (see *Debate: Can Eating Less Help You Live Longer?*). We know that as organisms grow older, the number of cells in their bodies decreases and the functioning of the remaining cells declines. This loss of cells and cell function occurs throughout life, but the effects are not felt for many years because organisms start out life with more cells and cell function than they need. This reserve capacity allows an organism to continue functioning normally despite a decrease in the number and function of cells. In young adults, the reserve capacity of organs is 4 to 10 times that required to sustain life. As a person ages and reserve capacity decreases,

> **aging** The inevitable accumulation of changes associated with and responsible for an ever-increasing susceptibility to disease and death.

the effects of aging become evident in all body systems. With this loss of function comes a reduction in the ability to repair damage and resist infection, so older people may die from diseases from which they could easily have recovered when they were younger.

The human **life span** is about 120 years, but how long individuals live and the rate at which they age are determined by the genes they inherit, their lifestyle, and the extent to which they are able to avoid accidents, disease, and environmental toxins (**Figure 12.13**). A person with a family history of heart disease who eats a healthy diet and exercises regularly may never be limited by heart disease. In contrast, someone with no family history of heart disease who is inactive, smokes, and eats a poor diet may develop heart problems that lead to disability and death.

> **life span** The maximum age to which members of a species can live.

Long-term evidence of the benefits of calorie restriction comes from studying the people of Okinawa.[53] Until recently, Okinawans practiced calorie restriction by eating until they were only 80% full. In addition, they led active lives, worked as farmers, and consumed a nutrient-dense diet, high in green and yellow vegetables, whole grains, soy, fish, and lean meat and low in refined grains, saturated fat, salt, and sugar.[54] Older Okinawans maintain a low BMI and have a lower incidence of chronic diseases than people living in the United States or on mainland Japan (see graph).[53] But this may not be just a life-style consideration; there is also evidence that genetics and climate may contribute to greater life expectancy.[55–57]

So, is calorie restriction something that we should all prac-tice in order to live longer? In a world in which obesity, diabe-tes, and other diet-related conditions are limiting our active life expectancy, the benefits of calorie restriction are intrigu-ing. But calorie restriction is far more difficult than drinking from the mythical fountain of youth. A person whose EER is about 2000 Calories/day could eat only 1200 to 1500 Calo-ries/day when practicing caloric restriction. Meeting nutrient needs would require carefully planned meals and snacks; a poorly planned diet would lead to malnutrition. Side effects would include food cravings, weight loss, a lack of energy, and in some cases psychological consequences. Based on the Okinawan experience, this ascetic lifestyle would add only a few years of life.[52] Would it be worth the sacrifices?

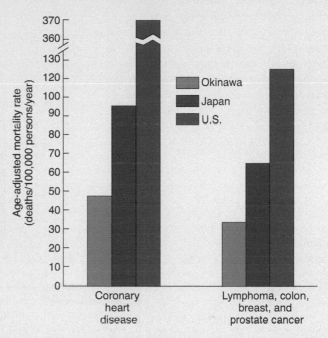

Think Critically Use the graph to compare the incidence of heart disease in Okinawa with that in Japan and the Unit-ed States. Suggest some possible explanations for these differences.

Factors that affect how fast we age • Figure 12.13

Genes determine the efficiency with which cells are maintained and repaired and also determine our susceptibility to age-related diseases, such as cardiovascular disease and cancer, but lifestyle and environment also affect how fast we age.

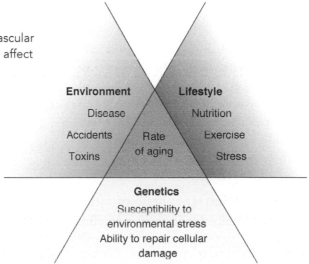

Declining muscle mass • Figure 12.14

With age, the percentage of body weight that is muscle declines and the percentage that is fat increases.[58] Some of the decline in energy needs in older adults is due to this decrease in muscle mass; the less lean muscle a person has, the lower his or her BMR. The EER for an 80-year-old man is almost 600 Calories less than for a 20-year-old man of the same size and activity level. For women, the difference is about 400 Calories/day.

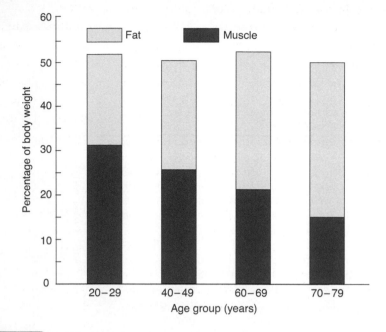

Think Critically How much daily exercise would an 80-year-old woman need in order to expend about the same number of calories per day as a sedentary 20-year-old woman of the same height and weight?

Nutrition and Health Concerns Throughout Adulthood

The physiological and health changes that accompany aging affect energy and nutrient requirements, how some nutrient requirements must be met, and the risk of malnutrition. In order to best recommend nutrient intakes for adults of all ages, the DRIs include four adult age categories: young adulthood (ages 19–30), middle age (ages 31–50), adulthood (ages 51–70), and older adulthood (over age 70). These recommendations are designed to meet the needs of the majority of healthy individuals in each age group. Although the incidence of chronic diseases and disabilities increases with advancing age, these conditions are not considered when making general nutrient intake recommendations for this population.

Energy and energy-yielding nutrient recommendations Adult energy needs typically decline with age, due primarily to decreases in basal metabolic rate (BMR) and activity level (**Figure 12.14**). The need for most nutrients

does not change, however, so in order to meet nutrient needs without exceeding energy needs, older adults must consume a nutrient-dense diet. For example, adult protein requirements do not change with age; therefore, older adults must consume a diet that is higher in protein relative to calories than that of younger adults.

The proportions of carbohydrate and fat recommended in the diet also remain the same in older adults as in younger adults. In order to ensure adequate vitamin, mineral, and fiber intake, most dietary carbohydrate should come from unrefined sources. Adequate fiber, when consumed with adequate fluid, helps prevent constipation, hemorrhoids, and diverticulosis—conditions that are common in older adults. High-fiber diets may also be beneficial in the prevention and management of diabetes, cardiovascular disease, and obesity.

Sources of dietary fat should also be chosen with nutrient density in mind. A diet with 20 to 35% of energy from fat that contains adequate amounts of the essential fatty acids and limits saturated fat, *trans* fat, and cholesterol is recommended.

Meeting the water needs of older adults The recommended water intake for older adults is the same as for younger adults, but meeting these needs may be more challenging for older adults. Advanced age brings a reduction in the sense of thirst, which can decrease fluid intake. In addition, some older adults have mobility limitations that reduce their access to beverages. The risk of dehydration is further increased in older adults by greater water losses. The kidneys are no longer as efficient at conserving water as they once were, and many older adults also take medications that increase water loss.

The risk of vitamin and mineral deficiencies in older adults The physiological changes of aging and the decrease in calorie needs put older adults at risk for deficiency of several vitamins and minerals. Recommended intakes are rarely higher than for younger adults, but for a few nutrients, special recommendations are made about how needs should be met.

Intakes of certain B vitamins are a concern for older adults. The RDA for vitamin B_6 is greater in adults ages 51 and older than for younger adults because higher dietary intakes are needed to maintain the same functional levels in the body. Folate intake is a concern because deficiency of folate alone or in combination with vitamin B_{12} and vitamin B_6 deficiencies may contribute to the development of cancer, cardiovascular disease, and cognitive dysfunction.[59]

The RDA for vitamin B_{12} is not increased in older adults, but it is recommended that people over 50 meet their RDA for vitamin B_{12} by consuming foods that are fortified with this vitamin or by taking a supplement containing vitamin B_{12}. This is because food-bound vitamin B_{12} is not absorbed efficiently in many older adults due to atrophic gastritis, an inflammation of the stomach lining that causes a reduction in stomach acid (see Chapter 7).[60,61] Reduced secretion of stomach acid also allows microbial overgrowth in the stomach and small intestine, and the greater number of microbes compete for available vitamin B_{12}, further reducing the amount of vitamin B_{12} that is absorbed. It is estimated that 10 to 30% of U.S. adults over age 50 and 40% of those in their 80s have atrophic gastritis. The vitamin B_{12} in fortified foods and supplements is not bound to proteins, so it is absorbed even when stomach acid levels are low. Atrophic gastritis may also reduce the absorption of iron, folate, calcium, and vitamin K.

Women over age 50 need less iron than younger women because they no longer lose iron through menstruation. The RDA for women 51 and older is 8 mg, the same as for adult men of all ages. Despite low iron needs, iron deficiency anemia is a concern among women and men in this age group. Common causes are chronic blood loss due to disease and medication and poor iron absorption due to antacid use and low stomach acid.

Calcium status is a problem in elderly people because calcium intake is low and intestinal absorption decreases with age. Without sufficient calcium, bone mass decreases, and the risk of bone fractures due to osteoporosis increases. The reduction in estrogen that occurs with menopause further increases bone loss in women by increasing the rate of bone breakdown and decreasing the absorption of calcium from the intestine. The RDA for adult men age 51 to 70 years is 1000 mg/day. Because of the accelerated bone loss in women during the postmenopausal period, the RDA for women 51 to 70 years is increased to 1200 mg/day. To reduce age-related bone loss, the RDA for men and women over 70 years of age is 1200 mg/day.[6]

Vitamin D, which is necessary for adequate calcium absorption, is also a concern in elderly people. Intake is often low, and synthesis in the skin is reduced due to limited exposure to sunlight and because the capacity to synthesize vitamin D in the skin decreases with age. The RDA for people ages 51 to 70 years is 600 IU (15 µg)/day, the same as for younger adults. For individuals over age 70 years, the RDA is increased to 800 IU (20 µg)/day.[6]

Factors That Increase the Risk of Malnutrition in Older Adults

The aging process usually does not cause malnutrition in healthy, active adults, but nutritional health can be compromised by the physical changes that occur with age, the presence of disease, and economic, psychological, and social circumstances.[62] These factors can increase the risk of malnutrition by altering nutrient needs and decreasing the motivation to eat and the ability to acquire and enjoy food. Malnutrition then exacerbates some of these factors, contributing to a downward health spiral from which it is difficult to recover (**Figure 12.15a**).

Causes and consequences of malnutrition • Figure 12.15

✔ THE PLANNER

Many of the physiological changes and health problems associated with age can affect nutritional status.

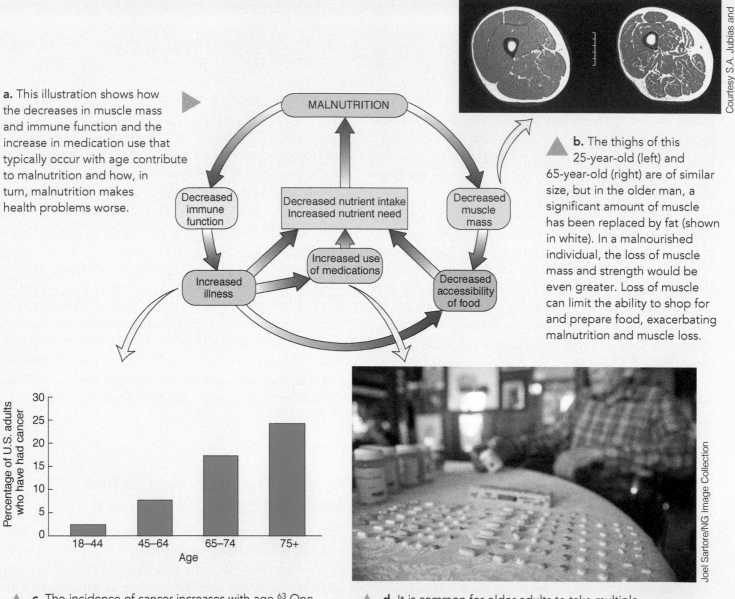

Courtesy S.A. Jubias and K.E. Conley, University of Washington MedicalCenter

a. This illustration shows how the decreases in muscle mass and immune function and the increase in medication use that typically occur with age contribute to malnutrition and how, in turn, malnutrition makes health problems worse.

MALNUTRITION

Decreased immune function

Decreased nutrient intake
Increased nutrient need

Decreased muscle mass

Increased use of medications

Increased illness

Decreased accessibility of food

b. The thighs of this 25-year-old (left) and 65-year-old (right) are of similar size, but in the older man, a significant amount of muscle has been replaced by fat (shown in white). In a malnourished individual, the loss of muscle mass and strength would be even greater. Loss of muscle can limit the ability to shop for and prepare food, exacerbating malnutrition and muscle loss.

Joel Sartore/NG Image Collection

c. The incidence of cancer increases with age.[63] One reason for the higher incidence is that the immune system's ability to destroy cancer cells declines. Reduced immune function also increases the frequency of infectious diseases and reduces the ability to recover from these diseases.

d. It is common for older adults to take multiple medications. Shown here are the pills this 73-year-old man takes each week. Medications can affect nutritional status by interfering with taste, chewing, and swallowing; by causing loss of appetite, gastrointestinal upset, constipation, or nausea; and by increasing nutrient losses or decreasing nutrient absorption.

Physiological changes With age comes a decrease in muscle size and strength (**Figure 12.15b**). This decrease affects both the skeletal muscles needed to move the body and the heart and respiratory muscles needed to deliver oxygen to the tissues. Some of this decline is due to changes in hormone levels and muscle protein synthesis, but lack of exercise is also an important contributor.[64] The decrease in muscle strength contributes not only to **physical frailty**, which is characterized by general weakness, impaired mobility and balance, and poor endurance, but also to the risk of falls and fractures. In the oldest old, those age 85 years and older, loss of muscle strength is the limiting factor that determines whether they can continue to live independently.

The immune system's ability to fight disease declines with age. With this decline, the incidence of infections, cancers, and autoimmune diseases increases, and the effectiveness of immunizations decreases (**Figure 12.15c**). In turn, increases in infections and chronic disease can lead to increased use of medications that affect nutritional status (**Figure 12.15d**). Malnutrition exacerbates the decline in immune function.

Chronic illness About 66% of the older population suffers from multiple chronic conditions.[65] These conditions affect the ability to maintain good nutritional health because they can change nutrient requirements, decrease the appeal of food, and impair the ability to obtain and prepare an adequate diet.

Some illnesses change the type of diet that is recommended. For instance, kidney failure reduces the ability to excrete protein waste products, so the diet must be lower in protein. Blood pressure is affected by sodium intake, so a low-sodium diet is recommended for individuals with high blood pressure. Dietary restrictions such as these limit food choices and can affect the palatability of the diet and thereby contribute to malnutrition in elderly people.

Physical disabilities can limit a person's ability to obtain and prepare food. The nation's most common reason for physical disability among older adults is **arthritis**, a condition that causes pain and stiffness in the joints and limits mobility (**Figure 12.16**). Arthritis affects more than 52 million Americans. Half of all individuals age 70 and older with arthritis need help with the activities of daily living, including shopping for and preparing and eating meals.[66]

> **arthritis** A disease characterized by inflammation of the joints, pain, and sometimes changes in structure.

Osteoarthritis • Figure 12.16

Osteoarthritis, the most common form of arthritis, occurs when the cartilage that cushions the joints degenerates, allowing the bones to rub together and cause pain. Anti-inflammatory medications help reduce the pain. Supplements of glucosamine and chondroitin are marketed to improve symptoms and slow the progression of osteoarthritis, but clinical studies on the effect of these supplements on pain and function have been equivocal.[67]

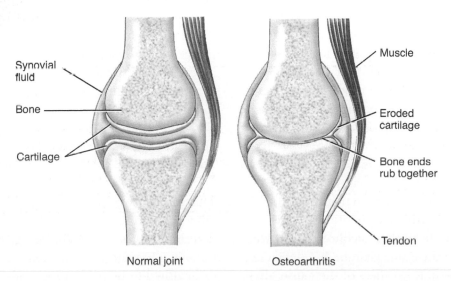

Synovial fluid
Bone
Cartilage
Muscle
Eroded cartilage
Bone ends rub together
Tendon

Normal joint   Osteoarthritis

Cataracts • Figure 12.17

A cataract is a clouding of the lens of the eye that impairs vision. When cataracts obscure vision, the affected lens can be removed and replaced with an artificial plastic lens.

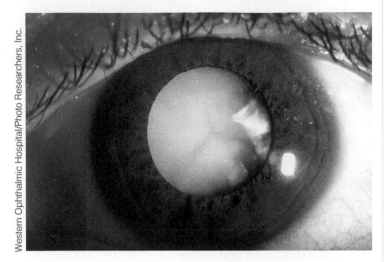

Western Ophthalmic Hospital/Photo Researchers, Inc.

Visual disorders become more common as a person ages. **Macular degeneration** is the most common cause of blindness in older Americans. The **macula** is a small area of the retina of the eye that distinguishes fine detail. If the number of viable cells in the macula is reduced, visual acuity declines, ultimately resulting in blindness. **Cataracts** are another common cause of declining vision (**Figure 12.17**).

> **macular degeneration** Degeneration of a portion of the retina that results in loss of visual detail and eventually blindness.

> **dementia** A deterioration of mental state that results in impaired memory, thinking, and/or judgment.

> **Alzheimer's disease** A disease that results in a relentless and irreversible loss of mental function.

Oxidative damage is believed to cause both macular degeneration and cataracts. Therefore, a diet that is high in foods containing antioxidant nutrients and phytochemicals might slow or prevent these eye disorders.

Changes in mental status can affect nutrition by interfering with the response to hunger and the ability to eat and to obtain and prepare food. The incidence of **dementia** increases with age. Dementia involves impairment in memory, thinking, or judgment that is severe enough to cause personality changes and affect daily activities and relationships with others. Causes of dementia include multiple strokes, alcoholism, dehydration, side effects of medication, vitamin B_{12} deficiency, and **Alzheimer's disease**. Regardless of the cause, these neurological problems can affect the ability to consume a healthy diet.

Another cause of altered mental status in elderly people is depression. Social, psychological, and physical factors all contribute to depression in elderly people. Retirement and the death and relocation of friends and family members can cause social isolation, which contributes to depression. Physical disability causes loss of independence. The inability to engage in normal daily activities, easily visit with friends and family members, and provide for personal needs contributes to depression. Depression can make meals less appetizing and decrease the quantity and quality of foods consumed, thereby increasing the risk of malnutrition.

Use of medications Because elderly people have an increased frequency of acute and chronic illnesses, they are likely to take multiple medications (see Figure 12.15d).[68] Medications can affect nutritional status, and nutritional status can alter the effectiveness of medications. The more medications taken, the greater the chance of side effects that affect nutritional status, such as decreased appetite, changes in taste, and nausea. Diet can also change the effectiveness of medications. For example, vitamin K hinders the action of anticoagulants, which are taken to reduce the risk of blood clots. On the other hand, omega-3 fatty acids, such as those in fish oils, inhibit blood clotting and may intensify the effect of an anticoagulant drug and cause bleeding.

Economic and social issues Almost 3.6 million elderly Americans live below the poverty level, and many live on a fixed income, making it difficult to afford health care, especially medications, and a healthy diet.[69] Food costs and limited food preparation facilities can reduce the types of foods available. In 2013, 8.7% of households in the United States that included elderly people experienced **food insecurity**,[70] which occurs when the availability of nutritionally adequate, safe food or the ability to acquire food in socially acceptable ways is limited. This in turn increases the risk of malnutrition.

Keeping Healthy Throughout the Adult Years

There is no secret dietary factor that will bestow immortality, but good nutrition and an active lifestyle are major determinants of successful aging. A well-planned, nutritionally adequate diet can extend an individual's years of healthy life by preventing malnutrition and delaying the onset of chronic diseases. Regular exercise can help maintain muscle mass, bone strength, and cardiorespiratory function, helping to prolong independent living. The foods consumed by older adults are determined not only by preferences and physiologic changes but also by factors such as living arrangements, finances, transportation, and disability. For those with economic, social, or physical limitations, food assistance programs or assisted living can help prevent food insecurity.

Identifying older adults at risk To address concerns about the nutritional health of elderly individuals, the U.S. Nutrition Screening Initiative promotes screening for nutrition-related problems in older adults. This program is working to increase awareness of nutritional problems among elderly people by involving practitioners and community organizations as well as relatives, friends, and others caring for elderly people in evaluating the nutritional status of the aging population. This program developed the DETERMINE checklist (**Table 12.3**), based on an acronym for the physiological, medical, and socioeconomic situations that increase the risk of malnutrition among elderly people. Older people themselves, as well as family members and caregivers, can use this tool to determine when malnutrition is a potential problem.

Meeting nutrient needs Meeting the nutrient needs of older adults can be challenging (see *What Should I Eat?*).

DETERMINE: A checklist of the warning signs of malnutrition   Table 12.3

Disease	Any disease, illness, or condition that causes changes in eating can predispose a person to malnutrition. Memory loss and depression can also interfere with nutrition if they affect food intake.
Eating poorly	Eating either too little or too much can lead to poor health.
Tooth loss/ mouth pain	Poor health of the mouth, teeth, and gums interferes with the ability to eat.
Economic hardship	Having to, or choosing to, spend less than $25 to $30 per person per week on food interferes with nutrient intake.
Reduced social support	Not having contact with people on a daily basis has a negative effect on morale, well-being, and eating.
Multiple medicines	The more medicines a person takes, the greater the chances of side effects such as weakness, drowsiness, diarrhea, changes in taste and appetite, nausea, and constipation.
Involuntary weight loss or gain	Unintentionally losing or gaining weight is a warning sign that should not be ignored. Being overweight or underweight also increases the risk of malnutrition.
Needs assistance in self-care	Difficulty walking, shopping, and cooking increases the risk of malnutrition.
Elder above age 80	The risks of frailty and health problems increase with increasing age.

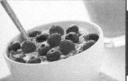   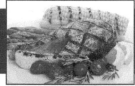

WHAT SHOULD I EAT?

© Sara Winter/iStockphoto   © Jill Chen/iStockphoto   © Steve Mcsweeny/iStockphoto

Advancing Age

Consume plenty of fluids and fiber
- Drink a beverage with every meal.
- Keep a bottle of water handy and sip on it.
- Choose whole grain breads and cereals.
- Add extra veggies to your soup.

Pay attention to vitamin B$_{12}$, calcium, and vitamin D
- Make sure your cereal is fortified with vitamin B$_{12}$.
- Drink milk; it provides both calcium and vitamin D.
- Spend a few minutes in the sun to get some vitamin D with no calories at all.
- Add some canned salmon to a salad for lunch.

Antioxidize
- Have a bowl of strawberries or blueberries – they are full of antioxidant phytochemicals.
- Choose colorful vegetables to boost carotenoids.
- Use a healthy vegetable oil and add nuts and seeds to your salads to get your vitamin E.
- Select seafood to boost selenium intake.

Work on meals for one
- Ask the grocer to break up larger packages of eggs and meats.
- Buy in bulk and share with a friend.
- Make a whole pot but freeze it in meal-size portions.
- Top a baked potato with leftover vegetables or sauces.

Use iProfile to find foods that are fortified with vitamin B$_{12}$.

Because energy needs are reduced while protein and most micronutrient needs remain the same or increase, food choices must be nutrient dense. Diets need to provide adequate fiber and fluid to prevent constipation; fiber intake in older adults is often below recommendations and dehydration is a problem, especially in persons 85 and older.[62] The medical, social, and economic challenges that often accompany aging make it more difficult to meet nutrient needs. Many older adults need supplements of vitamin D, vitamin B_{12}, and calcium to meet their nutrient needs. However, supplements should not take the place of a balanced, nutrient-dense diet that is high in whole grains, fruits, and vegetables (**Figure 12.18**). In addition to essential nutrients, these foods contain fiber, phytochemicals, and other substances that may protect against disease.

Older adults who have physical limitations need to choose foods that they can easily prepare and consume. For those who have difficulty preparing foods, precooked foods, frozen dinners, and canned soup or dry soup mixes can provide a meal with almost no preparation. Medical nutritional products, such as Ensure or Boost, can also be used to supplement intake.

Physical activity for older adults Regular physical activity can extend years of active, independent life, reduce the risk of disability, and improve the quality of life for older adults. Exercise also allows an increase in food intake without weight gain, so micronutrient needs are met more easily. A physical activity program for older adults should improve endurance, strength, flexibility, and balance.[71] Endurance activities such as walking, biking, and swimming provide protection against chronic disease. Recommendations are the same as for younger adults: a minimum of 150 minutes per week of moderate-intensity aerobic activity (**Figure 12.19**). Muscle-strengthening exercise is recommended 2 or more days per week to increase strength and lean body mass. Lifting small weights or stretching elastic bands at an intensity that requires some physical effort can provide strength training. Flexibility makes the tasks of everyday life easier. Flexibility exercises should include those that move the muscles through a full range of motion, such as arm circles, as well as those that stretch muscles their full length. Improvements in strength, endurance, and flexibility all enhance balance, which reduces the risk of falls. Specific balance exercises such as backward walking, heel

MyPlate for older adults • Figure 12.18

The MyPlate recommendations shown here are for 20- and 70-year-old men and women who get less than 30 minutes of activity per day. The older adults need to consume fewer servings from most food groups and are allotted fewer empty calories: only 120 Calories/day for a 70-year-old woman and 260 Calories/day for a 70-year-old man compared to 260 and 360 Calories/day, respectively, for their 20-year-old counterparts.

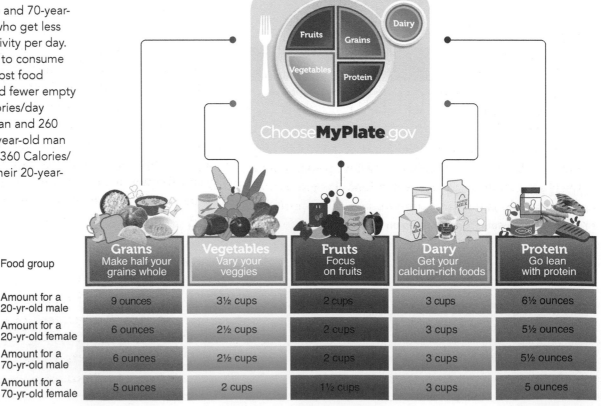

Food group	Grains Make half your grains whole	Vegetables Vary your veggies	Fruits Focus on fruits	Dairy Get your calcium-rich foods	Protein Go lean with protein
Amount for a 20-yr-old male	9 ounces	3½ cups	2 cups	3 cups	6½ ounces
Amount for a 20-yr-old female	6 ounces	2½ cups	2 cups	3 cups	5½ ounces
Amount for a 70-yr-old male	6 ounces	2½ cups	2 cups	3 cups	5½ ounces
Amount for a 70-yr-old female	5 ounces	2 cups	1½ cups	3 cups	5 ounces

Physical activity for older adults • Figure 12.19

Exercise classes and other group-based activities can be a good way for older adults to start an exercise program. Water activities, such as water aerobics and swimming, do not stress the joints and hence can be used to improve endurance in individuals with arthritis or other bone and joint disorders. Some weight-bearing activity, such as walking, is encouraged to promote bone health.

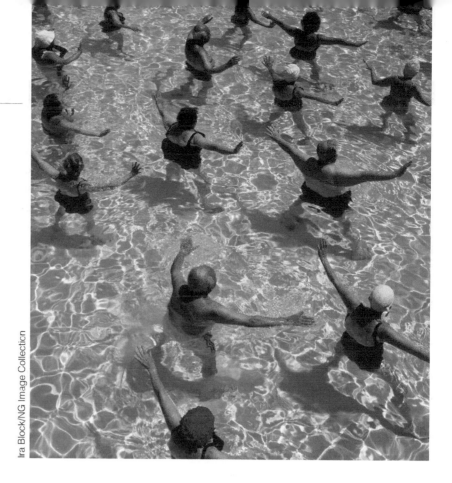

Ira Block/NG Image Collection

walking, and those practiced in tai chi and yoga can further improve balance.

Overcoming economic and social issues

Overcoming socioeconomic limitations may involve providing education about economics and food preparation or providing assistance with shopping and food preparation. Options for people with limited incomes include reduced-cost meals at senior centers, federal food assistance programs (discussed in Chapter 14), food banks, and soup kitchens.

Another problem that contributes to poor nutrient intake in older adults is loneliness. Living, cooking, and eating alone can decrease interest in food. Programs that provide nutritious meals in communal settings promote social interaction and can improve nutrient intake. For those who are unable to attend communal meals, home-delivered meals are available.

Overcoming physical limitations: Assisted living

The physical and psychological declines associated with aging eventually cause many people to require assistance in everyday living. Assisted living facilities allow individuals to live in their own apartments but provide help, as needed, with activities such as eating, bathing, dressing, housekeeping, and taking medications. These facilities provide an interim level of care for those who cannot live safely on their own but do not require the total care provided in a nursing home. Eventually, many older adults will need to live in nursing homes. Even though nursing homes provide access to food and medical care, their residents are at increased risk for malnutrition because they are more likely to have medical conditions that increase nutrient needs or interfere with food intake or nutrient absorption; in addition, they are at risk because they are dependent on others to provide for their care. Even when adequate meals are provided, many nursing home residents require assistance in eating and frequently do not consume all the food served, thus increasing their likelihood of developing deficits of energy, water, and other nutrients.[72]

CONCEPT CHECK   STOP

1. **What** is the goal of successful aging?
2. **How** do the energy needs of older adults compare to those of younger adults?
3. **Why** are older adults at risk for malnutrition?
4. **How** do the MyPlate recommendations change as adults age?

Alcohol Metabolism

In people who occasionally consume moderate amounts of alcohol, most of the alcohol is broken down in the liver by the enzyme alcohol dehydrogenase (ADH) (**Figure 12.22**). This enzyme has also been found in all parts of the gastrointestinal tract.[74] When greater amounts of alcohol are consumed, a second pathway in the liver, called the microsomal ethanol-oxidizing system (MEOS), also metabolizes alcohol. The rate at which ADH breaks down alcohol is fairly constant, but MEOS activity increases when more alcohol is consumed.[74] MEOS also metabolizes other drugs, so as activity increases in response to high alcohol intake, it can alter the metabolism of other drugs.

Adverse Effects of Alcohol

The consumption of alcohol has short-term effects that interfere with organ function for several hours after ingestion. Chronic alcohol consumption has long-term effects that cause disease both because the alcohol interferes with nutritional status and because alcohol metabolism produces toxic compounds.

Short-term effects of alcohol When alcohol intake exceeds the liver's ability to break it down, the excess accumulates in the bloodstream. The circulating alcohol acts as a depressant, impairing mental and physical abilities. First, alcohol affects reasoning; if drinking continues, the brain's vision and speech centers are affected. Next, large-muscle control becomes impaired, causing lack of coordination. Finally, if alcohol consumption continues, it can result in **alcohol poisoning**, a serious condition that can slow breathing, heart rate, and the gag reflex, leading to loss of consciousness, choking, coma, and even death. This most frequently occurs in cases of binge drinking. Even if an individual does not experience a loss of consciousness, excess drinking may still cause memory loss.

PROCESS DIAGRAM

Metabolizing alcohol • Figure 12.22

✓ THE PLANNER

The ADH pathway predominates when small amounts of alcohol are consumed. The MEOS becomes important when larger amounts of alcohol are consumed. The MEOS reaction requires oxygen and the input of energy (ATP) to break down alcohol. It also generates reactive oxygen molecules that can contribute to liver disease.

HOW IT WORKS

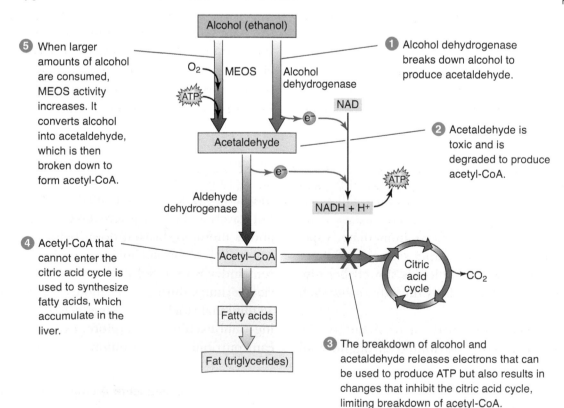

❺ When larger amounts of alcohol are consumed, MEOS activity increases. It converts alcohol into acetaldehyde, which is then broken down to form acetyl-CoA.

❶ Alcohol dehydrogenase breaks down alcohol to produce acetaldehyde.

❷ Acetaldehyde is toxic and is degraded to produce acetyl-CoA.

❹ Acetyl-CoA that cannot enter the citric acid cycle is used to synthesize fatty acids, which accumulate in the liver.

❸ The breakdown of alcohol and acetaldehyde releases electrons that can be used to produce ATP but also results in changes that inhibit the citric acid cycle, limiting breakdown of acetyl-CoA.

Drinking enough alcohol to cause amnesia is called **blackout drinking**. Blackout drinking puts people at risk because they have no memory of events that occurred during the blackout. During alcohol-related memory blackouts, people may engage in risky behaviors such as having unprotected sexual intercourse, vandalizing property, or driving a car—and have no memory of it afterward.

The effects of alcohol on the central nervous system are what make driving while under the influence of alcohol so dangerous. Alcohol affects reaction time, eye-hand coordination, and balance. Not only does alcohol impair one's ability to operate a motor vehicle, but it also impairs one's judgment in making the decision to drive. Abuse of alcohol also contributes to domestic violence and is a factor in more than 100,000 deaths per year, including almost 40% of all traffic fatalities.[75]

Alcoholism One risk associated with regular alcohol consumption is the possibility of alcohol addiction, or **alcoholism**. The risk of alcoholism is increased in individuals who begin drinking at a younger age. Alcoholism, like any other drug addiction, is a physiological condition that needs treatment. It is believed to have a genetic component that makes some people more likely to become addicted, but environmental factors also play a significant role.[76] Thus, someone with a genetic predisposition toward alcoholism whose family and peers do not consume alcohol is much less likely to become addicted than someone with the same genes who drinks regularly with friends.

Alcoholic liver disease The most significant physiological effects of chronic alcohol consumption occur in the liver. The metabolism of alcohol by ADH promotes fat synthesis (see Figure 12.22), which leads to the accumulation of fat in the liver. Metabolism by the MEOS generates reactive oxygen molecules, which cause oxidation of lipids, membrane damage, and altered enzyme activities. Whether alcohol is broken down by ADH or the MEOS, toxic acetaldehyde is formed. Acetaldehyde binds to proteins and inhibits chemical reactions and mitochondrial function, allowing more acetaldehyde to accumulate and causing further liver damage.

Chronic alcohol consumption leads to three types of alcoholic liver disease. **Fatty liver** is the accumulation of fat in liver cells. It occurs in almost all people who drink heavily due to increased synthesis and deposition of fat. If drinking continues, this condition may progress to **alcoholic hepatitis**. Both of these conditions are reversible if alcohol consumption is stopped and good nutritional and health practices are followed. If alcohol consumption continues, **cirrhosis** may develop (**Figure 12.23**).

> **alcoholic hepatitis** Inflammation of the liver caused by alcohol consumption.
>
> **cirrhosis** Chronic and irreversible liver disease characterized by loss of functioning liver cells and accumulation of fibrous connective tissue.

Malnutrition and other health problems Malnutrition is one of the complications of long-term excessive alcohol consumption. Alcohol contributes energy—7 Calories/g—but few nutrients; it may replace more nutrient-dense energy sources in the diet. Alcoholic beverages are also often consumed with high-sugar mixers, which add more empty calories to the diet. In addition to decreasing nutrient intake, alcohol interferes with nutrient absorption. Alcohol causes inflammation of the stomach, pancreas, and intestine, impairing digestion of food and absorption of nutrients into the blood. Deficiency of the B vitamin thiamin is a particular concern related to chronic alcohol consumption. Alcohol also contributes to malnutrition by altering the storage, metabolism, and excretion of other vitamins and some minerals.

Alcoholic cirrhosis • Figure 12.23

The liver on the left is normal. The one on the right has cirrhosis. This is an irreversible condition in which fibrous deposits scar the liver and interfere with its functioning. Because the liver is the primary site of many metabolic reactions, cirrhosis is often fatal.

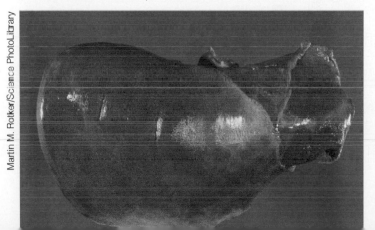
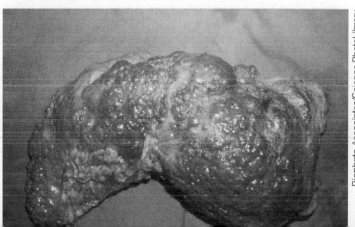

Martin M. Rotker/Science PhotoLibrary

Biophoto Associates/Science PhotoLibrary

In addition to causing liver disease and malnutrition, heavy drinking is associated with cancer of the oral cavity, pharynx, esophagus, larynx, breast, liver, colon, rectum, and stomach.[77] Even moderate alcohol consumption has been found to increase the risk of certain cancers in women.[78] Excess alcohol use also increases the risk of hypertension, heart disease, and stroke.[79] Some of this effect is related to the fact that calories consumed as alcohol are more likely to be deposited as fat in the abdominal region, and excess abdominal fat increases the risk of high blood pressure, heart disease, and diabetes.

Benefits of Alcohol Consumption

For some adults, moderate alcohol consumption may be beneficial. Consuming alcoholic beverages can stimulate appetite, improve mood, and enhance social interactions. Light to moderate drinking can also reduce the risk of heart disease and stroke.[80] The primary mechanisms by which alcohol lowers cardiovascular risk are by raising blood levels of HDL cholesterol and by inhibiting the formation of blood clots. The phytochemicals in red wine are thought to make it more cardioprotective than other alcoholic beverages.[81] Moderate alcohol consumption is associated with reduced risk of death among middle-aged and older adults and may help to keep cognitive function intact with age.[9]

Whether or not the benefits of alcohol consumption outweigh the risks, drinking is a personal decision that must take into account medical and social considerations. If you do not drink, you should not begin drinking to reduce cardiovascular risk or achieve other potential health benefits. Anyone who chooses to drink should do so in moderation. Alcohol should be consumed slowly—at a rate of no more than one drink every 1.5 hours. Sipping, not gulping, allows the liver time to break down what has already been consumed. Alternating nonalcoholic and alcoholic drinks will also slow down the rate of alcohol intake and prevent dehydration. Alcohol absorption is most rapid on an empty stomach. Consuming alcohol with meals slows its absorption and may also enhance its protective effects on the cardiovascular system.

CONCEPT CHECK STOP

1. **How** much beer per day constitutes moderate drinking for a man?
2. **How** can alcohol metabolism lead to a fatty liver?
3. **What** are the symptoms of alcohol poisoning?
4. **How** does moderate alcohol intake reduce the risk of cardiovascular disease?

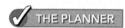 THE PLANNER

Summary

1 Nutrition for Children 402

- A child's diet should meet the needs for growth, development, and activity as well as reduce the risk of chronic disease later in life. Energy and protein needs per kilogram of body weight decrease as children grow, but total needs increase. The acceptable range of fat intake is higher for young children than for adults. Calcium, vitamin D, and iron intakes are often low in children's diets, putting them at risk for low bone density and anemia.

- To help children meet their nutrient needs and develop nutritious habits, caregivers should offer a variety of healthy foods at meals and snacks throughout the day. Children can then choose what and how much they consume. The **National School Lunch Program** provides low-cost school lunches designed to meet nutrient needs and promote healthy diets.

- Obesity rates among children in the United States have been rising, as shown in the graph. Poor diet contributes

to obesity and obesity along with a poor diet increase the incidence of diabetes, high blood cholesterol, and high blood pressure. Watching television contributes to childhood obesity by promoting the intake of foods that are high in calories, fat, and sugar and by reducing the amount of exercise children get. A diet high in sugary foods can increase the risk of dental caries. Children are at particular risk for lead toxicity. Reductions in the use of lead in paint and gasoline have decreased the incidence of high blood lead levels.

Obesity and the health of America's children • Figure 12.6

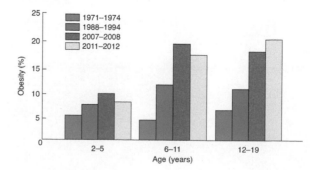

2 Nutrition for Adolescents 412

- During adolescence, the changes associated with **puberty** and the **adolescent growth spurt** have an impact on nutrient requirements. Body composition and the nutritional requirements of boys and girls diverge. Energy and protein requirements are higher during adolescence than during adulthood, and vitamin requirements increase to meet the needs of rapid growth. Calcium intake is often low in the adolescent diet, particularly if more sweetened beverages than milk are consumed, as shown. Iron deficiency anemia is common in adolescent girls due to low intake and iron losses through menstruation.

Beverage choices in children and teens • Figure 12.9

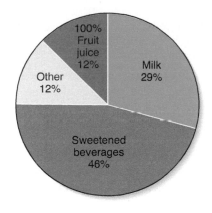

- The food choices of adolescents are usually determined more by social activities, peer pressure, and participation in athletics than by nutrient needs. Teens can improve their diets by making healthier fast-food choices. Poorly planned vegetarian diets can be low in iron, zinc, calcium, vitamin D, and vitamin B_{12} and high in saturated fat and cholesterol.

- Psychological and social changes occurring during the adolescent years make eating disorders more common than at any other time of life. Adolescent nutritional status may also be affected by weight-loss diets, supplements to enhance athletic performance, and the use of cigarettes or alcohol.

3 Nutrition for the Adult Years 417

- As a population, Americans are living longer but not necessarily healthier lives. Increasing **active life expectancy** is an important public health goal. The genes people inherit, as well as their diet, lifestyle, and other environmental factors, determine how long they live.

- Energy needs decrease with age, but the needs for protein, water, fiber, and most micronutrients remain the same. Decreases in nutrient intake and changes in the metabolism or absorption of certain micronutrients, including vitamin B_{12}, vitamin D, and calcium, put older adults at risk for deficiency. Iron requirements decrease in women after menopause, but many older adults are at risk for iron deficiency due to poor absorption or blood loss from disease or medications.

- Older adults are at risk for malnutrition due to the physiological changes that accompany **aging**, such as a decrease in muscle mass, illustrated here, and a decline in immune function. Chronic illnesses, which are more common in elderly people than in younger people, may change nutrient requirements, decrease the appeal of food, and impair a person's ability to obtain and prepare an adequate diet. Medications to treat diseases may also affect nutritional status in older adults. Physical disabilities such as **arthritis** and **macular degeneration**, changes in mental status caused by **dementia** or depression, and social and economic factors increase the risk of **food insecurity**.

Causes and consequences of malnutrition • Figure 12.15b

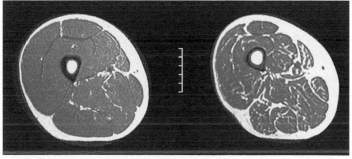

Courtesy S.A. Jubias and K.E. Conley,University of Washington MedicalCenter

- A nutrient-dense diet and regular physical activity can prevent malnutrition, delay the chronic diseases associated with aging, and increase independence in older adults. The DETERMINE checklist helps identify older adults who are at risk for malnutrition. Economic or physical assistance may be required to meet nutritional needs.

4 The Impact of Alcohol Throughout Life 428

- **Alcohol**, which refers to **ethanol**, is absorbed rapidly, causing the blood alcohol level to rise and its effects to be felt almost immediately. Absorption is slowed when there is food in the stomach. Alcohol is metabolized primarily in the liver. Some is excreted in urine and exhaled in expired air.

- Moderate amounts of alcohol are broken down by the enzyme alcohol dehydrogenase (ADH). When greater amounts of alcohol are consumed, a second pathway in the liver, called the microsomal ethanol-oxidizing system (MEOS), also metabolizes alcohol. Alcohol metabolism increases fat synthesis in the liver and generates reactive oxygen molecules that can contribute to liver disease.

- In the short term, excess alcohol consumption causes **alcohol poisoning**, which interferes with brain function. Chronic alcohol consumption can lead to **alcoholism** and can damage the liver, resulting in **fatty liver, alcoholic hepatitis**, and eventually **cirrhosis**, shown in the photo. Excess alcohol consumption also increases the risks of malnutrition and of developing hypertension, heart disease, and stroke, as well as certain types of cancer.

Alcoholic cirrhosis • Figure 12.23

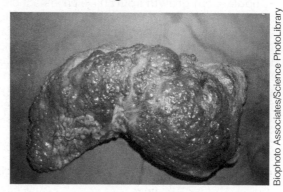

Biophoto Associates/Science PhotoLibrary

- Moderate alcohol consumption can decrease the risk of heart disease by increasing HDL cholesterol and reducing blood clot formation.

Key Terms

- active life expectancy 417
- adolescent growth spurt 412
- aging 418
- alcohol 429
- alcohol poisoning 430
- alcoholic hepatitis 431

- alcoholism 431
- Alzheimer's disease 424
- arthritis 423
- binge drinking 416
- blackout drinking 430
- cataracts 424
- cirrhosis 431

- dementia 424
- ethanol 429
- fatty liver 431
- food insecurity 424
- life expectancy 417
- life span 418
- macula 424

- macular degeneration 424
- National School Lunch Program 406
- oldest old 417
- physical frailty 423
- puberty 412

What is happening in this picture?

Riding your bike makes you thirsty. This boy in Virginia has interrupted his bike ride to purchase a soda.

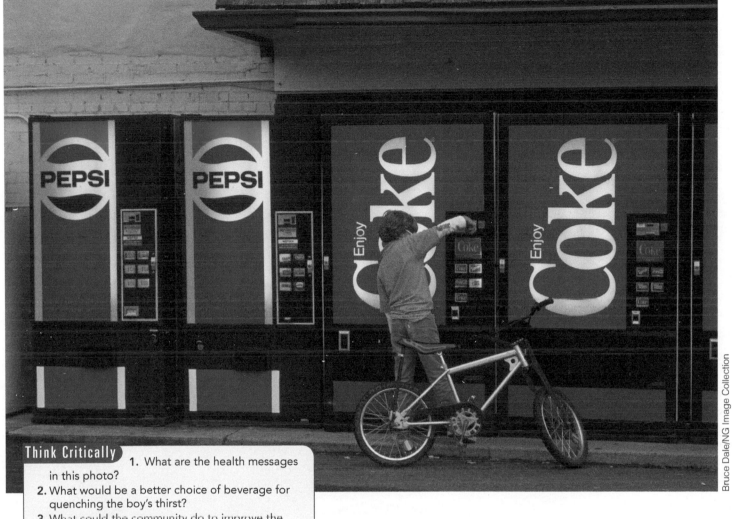

Bruce Dale/NG Image Collection

Think Critically

1. What are the health messages in this photo?
2. What would be a better choice of beverage for quenching the boy's thirst?
3. What could the community do to improve the boy's beverage options?

THE PLANNER ✓

Review your Chapter Planner on the chapter opener and check off you completed work.

How Safe Is Our Food Supply?

Americans believe that much, if not all, of the food they purchase has been inspected for safety, and that the facilities in which their food is prepared and processed are certified to be sanitary and disease- and contaminate-free. Of course it is cost-prohibitive and impractical to inspect every single facility and every product every minute of every day, so sometimes food reaches us that is not safe. And sometimes it reaches us completely uninspected by anyone.

In February of 2014, a California-based beef producer recalled almost nine million pounds of product that had never been inspected: The animals the meat came from were diseased. A month earlier, the same company had been forced to recall 40 tons of uninspected beef. In the

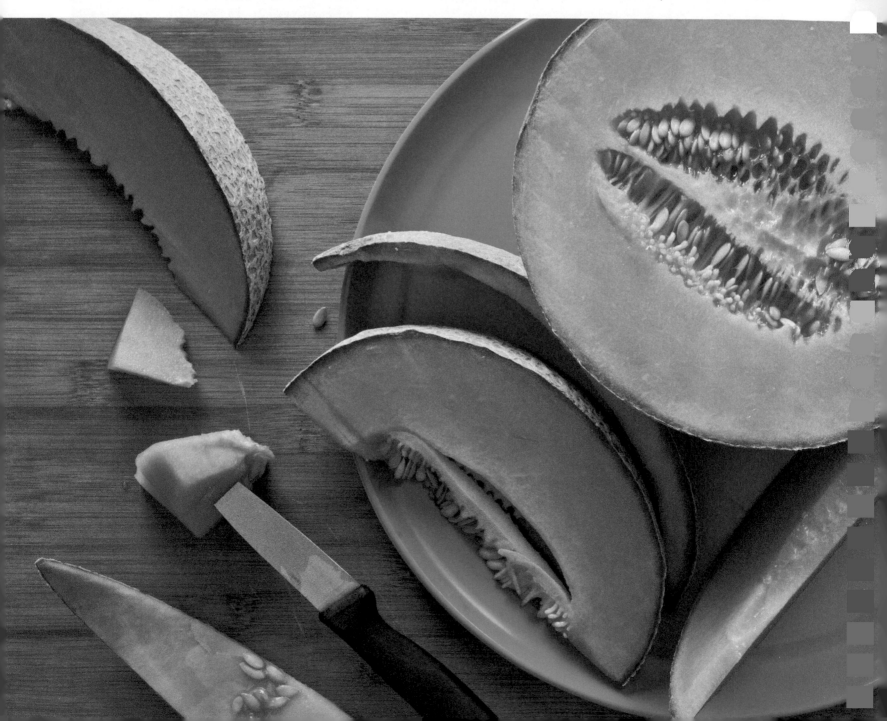

fall of 2013, two Colorado cantaloupe farmers pled guilty to criminal charges in connection with a *Listeria* outbreak that killed 33: They claimed they did not operate a melon-washing system properly. Food-borne illnesses annually sicken 48 million Americans and kill 3000 of us. Even our water is sometimes threatened. A third of a million West Virginians started out 2014 with contaminated tap water because of a chemical spill in the Elk River.

Despite these frightening incidents, most food arrives in our homes safe and fit to eat, and it remains that way if we handle it properly. The modern U.S. food supply is perhaps the safest in human history, but danger still lurks if adequate food-handling practices are not in place from farm or feedlot to table.

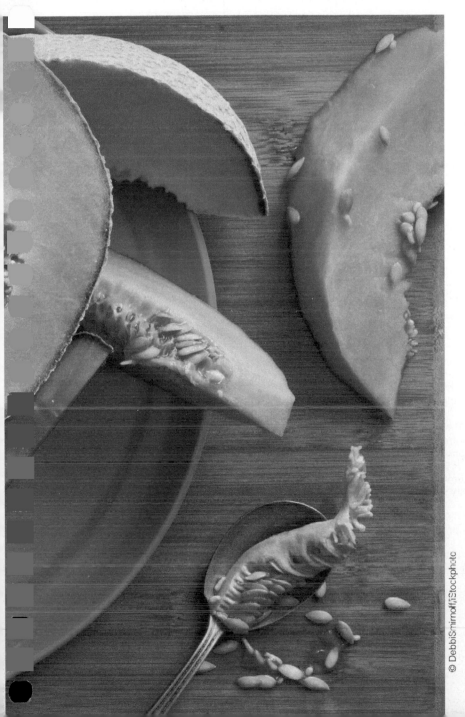
© DebbiSmirnoff/iStockphoto

CHAPTER OUTLINE

CHAPTER PLANNER ✓

- ❏ Stimulate your interest by reading the introduction and looking at the visual.
- ❏ Scan the Learning Objectives in each section: p. 438 ❏   p. 442 ❏   p. 453 ❏   p. 459 ❏   p. 465 ❏
- ❏ Read the text and study all figures and visuals. Answer any questions.

Analyze key features

- ❏ Process Diagram, p. 439 ❏   p. 440 ❏   p. 445 ❏ p. 447 ❏   p. 466 ❏
- ❏ Nutrition InSight, p. 443 ❏   p. 450 ❏   p. 467 ❏
- ❏ Thinking it Through, p. 451 ❏
- ❏ What a Scientist Sees, p. 452 ❏
- ❏ Debate, p. 455 ❏
- ❏ Stop: Answer the Concept Checks before you go on: p. 441 ❏   p. 452 ❏   p. 459 ❏   p. 465 ❏   p. 469 ❏

End of chapter and online review:

- ❏ Review the Summary, Key Terms, and online links to Additional Resources.
- ❏ Answer the Critical and Creative Thinking Questions.
- ❏ Answer What's happening in this picture?
- ❏ Complete the online Self-Test and check your answers.

13.1 Keeping Food Safe

LEARNING OBJECTIVES

1. **Name** the primary cause of food-borne illness.
2. **Explain** why a contaminated food does not cause illness in everyone who eats it.
3. **Discuss** the roles of the federal agencies responsible for the safety of the U.S. food supply.
4. **Explain** how a HACCP system helps prevent food-borne illness.

Have you ever had food poisoning? Whether you know it or not, you probably have. Oftentimes what we call the 24-hour flu is actually food poisoning, also called **food-borne illness**. Most food-borne illness is caused by consuming food that has been contaminated by disease-causing **microbes**; occasionally, it is caused by toxic chemicals or other contaminants that find their way into food.

Whether or not you get sick from eating a contaminated food depends on how potent the contaminant is, how much of it you consume, and how often you consume it, as well as on your age, size, and health. Some food contaminants cause harm even when minute amounts are consumed, and almost any substance can be toxic if a large enough amount of it is consumed. How well a substance is absorbed and how it is metabolized by the body affect toxicity. Dietary factors and nutritional status can affect absorption. For example, mercury, which is extremely toxic, is not absorbed well if the diet is high in selenium, and lead absorption is decreased by the presence of iron and calcium in the diet. Contaminants that are stored in the body after being absorbed are more likely to be toxic because they accumulate over time, eventually causing symptoms of toxicity. Contaminants that are easily excreted from the body are less likely to cause toxicity.

> **food-borne illness** An illness caused by consumption of contaminated food.
>
> **microbes** Microscopic organisms, or microorganisms, including bacteria, viruses, and fungi.

Agencies that monitor the food supply   Table 13.1

International Organizations

Food and Agriculture Organization of the United Nations (FAO)	Promotes and shares knowledge in all aspects of food quality and safety and in all stages of food production: harvest, postharvest handling, storage, transport, processing, and distribution.
World Health Organization (WHO)	Develops international food safety policies, food inspection programs, and standards for hygienic food preparation; promotes technologies that improve food safety and consumer education about safe food practices. Works closely with the FAO.

Federal Organizations

U.S. Food and Drug Administration (FDA)	Ensures the safety and quality of all foods sold across state lines with the exception of red meat, poultry, and egg products; inspects food processing plants; inspects imported foods with the exception of red meat, poultry, and egg products; sets standards for food composition; oversees use of drugs and feed in food-producing animals; enforces regulations for food labeling, food and color additives, and food sanitation.
U.S. Department of Agriculture (USDA) Food Safety and Inspection Service (FSIS)	Enforces standards for the wholesomeness and quality of red meat, poultry, and egg products produced in the United States and imported from other countries. If an imported food is suspect, it can be tested for contamination and denied entry into the country.
U.S. Environmental Protection Agency (EPA)	Regulates pesticide levels and must approve all pesticides before they can be sold in the United States; establishes water quality standards.
National Marine Fisheries Service	Oversees the management of fisheries and fish harvesting; operates a voluntary program of inspection and grading of fish products.
National Oceanic and Atmospheric Administration (NOAA)	Oversees fish and seafood products. Its Seafood Inspection Program inspects and certifies fishing vessels, seafood processing plants, and retail facilities for compliance with federal sanitation standards.
Centers for Disease Control and Prevention (CDC)	Monitors and investigates the incidence and causes of food-borne illnesses.

State and Local Governments

Oversee all food within their jurisdiction; also inspect restaurants, grocery stores, and other retail food establishments, as well as dairy farms and milk processing plants, grain mills, and food manufacturing plants within local jurisdictions.

An individual's size, overall health and nutritional status, and immune function affect his or her risk of food-borne illness. Infants and children are at greater risk than adults because their immune systems are immature and their small size means that a given amount of contaminant represents a greater amount per unit of body weight than it would in an adult. Elderly people, people with AIDS, and those receiving chemotherapy or other immunosuppressant drugs are at increased risk because their immune systems may be compromised. Pregnancy weakens the immune system, putting pregnant women and their unborn babies at risk. Poor nutritional status and chronic conditions such as diabetes and kidney disease may decrease the body's ability to detoxify harmful substances.

The Role of Government

Agencies at international, federal, state, and local levels monitor the safety of the food supply (**Table 13.1**). Federal agencies set standards and establish regulations for the safe handling of food and water and for the information included on food labels. They regulate the use of additives, packaging materials, and agricultural chemicals; inspect food processing and storage facilities; monitor domestic and imported foods for contamination; and investigate outbreaks of food-borne illness.

Each year, 1 in 6 Americans, or about 48 million people, get sick, 128,000 are hospitalized, and 3000 die from food-borne illnesses.[1] Media coverage of outbreaks of food-borne illness on cruise ships, of deaths from *E. coli* infection, and of cows infected with mad cow disease have heightened public concern and led to the development of the National Food Safety Initiative. The goal of this initiative is to reduce the incidence of food-borne illness by improving food safety practices and policies throughout the United States. Because food can be contaminated anywhere in the supply chain—from where it is grown to when it is served in your home—the program targets food safety from farm to table (**Figure 13.1**). In 2011, in

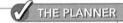

PROCESS DIAGRAM

Keeping food safe from farm to table • Figure 13.1

✔ THE PLANNER

Keeping food safe involves identifying possible points of contamination along a food's journey from the farm to the dinner table and implementing controls to prevent or contain contamination.

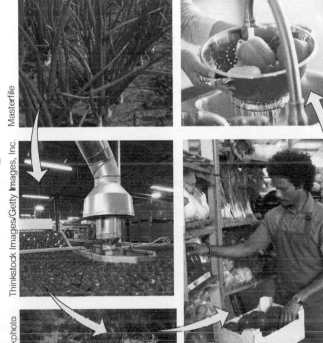

1 Farm Crops can be contaminated with bacteria before they are even harvested. Good agricultural practices help minimize contamination during growing, harvesting, sorting, packing, and storage.

2 Processing Contamination of processing equipment can transfer microbes to food. To prevent contamination, processors must follow guidelines concerning cleanliness and training of workers; develop a protocol that anticipates how biological, chemical, or physical hazards are most likely to occur; and establish appropriate measures to prevent them from occurring.

3 Transportation During transport, poor sanitation and inadequate refrigeration can contaminate food and allow microbes to grow. Clean containers and vehicles, plus refrigeration, can prevent the growth of food-borne bacteria.

5 Table Even a safe food can be contaminated in the home. Consumers can prevent food-borne illness at their table by carefully washing hands and food preparation equipment, as well as by handling, storing, and preparing food properly.

4 Retail Food can become contaminated during handling or storage in grocery stores or during preparation in restaurants. The FDA's Food Code provides recommendations for the handling and service of food in an effort to help owners and employees at retail establishments prevent food-borne illness. Local health inspections ensure cleanliness and proper procedures.

Ask Yourself

Why does contamination that occurs during processing have the potential to make more people sick than contamination that occurs at home?

439

response to the continued threat from our food supply, the FDA Food Safety Modernization Act was passed. This legislation focuses on preventing food-borne illness, not just reacting to problems as they occur. It gives the FDA an inspection mandate and new legal powers to ensure that companies are doing their part and to stop potentially unsafe food from entering the marketplace.[2]

The Role of Food Manufacturers and Retailers

The responsibility for providing safe food to the marketplace falls on the shoulders of food manufacturers, processors, and distributors. To meet this responsibility, they must establish and implement a **Hazard Analysis Critical Control Point (HACCP)** system. A HACCP system analyzes food production, processing, and transport, with the goal of identifying potential sources of

> **Hazard Analysis Critical Control Point (HACCP)** A food safety system that focuses on identifying and preventing hazards that could cause food-borne illness.

contamination and points where measures can be taken to control contamination. Then, by monitoring these **critical control points**, contamination can be prevented or eliminated (**Figure 13.2**). Unlike traditional methods of protecting the food supply, which use visual spot checks and random testing to catch contamination after it occurs, HACCP systems are designed to *prevent* contamination.

The Role of the Consumer

Although government agencies, manufacturers, and retailers are involved in creating a safe food supply, consumers also need to assume responsibility for their food. Even a food that has been manufactured, packaged, and transported with great care can cause food-borne illness if it is not handled carefully at home. Consumers can prevent most food-borne illness through careful food handling, storage, and preparation (discussed in depth later in the chapter). They can also protect themselves and others by reporting incidents involving unsanitary, unsafe, deceptive, or mislabeled food to the appropriate agencies (**Table 13.2**).

HACCP in liquid egg production • Figure 13.2

The scrambled eggs served in your cafeteria at school or work most likely came out of a carton rather than a shell. To produce this product, eggs are shelled, mixed together in large vats, heated to kill microbial contaminants, packaged, and either refrigerated or frozen. A contaminated batch could sicken hundreds of people. This example shows how a HACCP system might be used to prevent contaminated eggs from reaching the consumer.

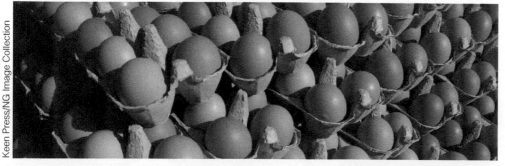

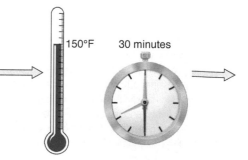

150°F   30 minutes

① **Conduct a hazard analysis** The manufacturer analyzes its processing steps for potential hazards and determines what preventive measures can be taken. In the case of eggs, there is a large potential for contamination with the bacterium *Salmonella*. Adequate heating is a preventive measure that can eliminate this hazard.

② **Identify the critical control points** Critical control points are the steps in a food's processing at which the hazard can be eliminated. In the case of egg processing, the critical control point is heating the shelled egg mixture in a large chamber.

③ **Set critical limits** Critical limits are the parameters that will prevent the hazard. In the case of these eggs, the critical limits are sufficient heating time and temperature to ensure that *Salmonella* bacteria are killed.

How to report food-related issues   Table 13.2

Before reporting a food-related issue, get all the facts. Determine whether you have used the product as intended and according to the manufacturer's instruction. Check to see if the item is past its expiration date. After these steps have been taken, report the incident to the appropriate agency:

• **Problems related to any food except meat and poultry, including adverse reactions:** Report emergencies to the FDA's main emergency number, which is staffed 24 hours a day: 301-443-1240. Nonemergencies can be reported to the FDA consumer complaint coordinator in your area, which you can find at www.fda.gov/Safety/ReportaProblem/default.htm.

• **Issues related to meat and poultry:** Report first to your state department of agriculture and then to the USDA Meat and Poultry Hotline (888-MPHotline or mphotline.fsis@usda.gov).

• **Restaurant food and sanitation problems:** Report directly to your local or state health department.

• **Issues related to alcoholic beverages:** Report to the U.S. Department of the Treasury's Bureau of Alcohol, Tobacco, Firearms, and Explosives.

• **Pesticide, air, and water pollution:** Report first to your state environmental protection department and then to the U.S. EPA.

• **Products purchased at the grocery store:** Return to the store. Grocery stores are concerned with the safety of the foods they sell, and they will take responsibility for tracking down and correcting the problem. They will either refund your money or replace the product.

CONCEPT CHECK   STOP

1. **What** causes food-borne illness?
2. **Why** might the same food make one person sick and not another person?
3. **Who** is responsible for the safety of the food you eat?
4. **How** does HACCP differ from traditional visual food inspection?

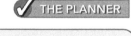
THE PLANNER

Ask Yourself

What is the critical control point for the elimination of *Salmonella* in liquid egg production?

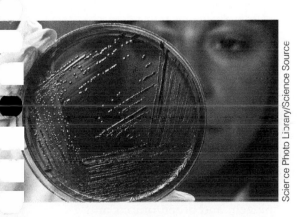

Science Photo Library/Science Source

Egg Pasteurization Record

Date	Batch number	Time	Temp.

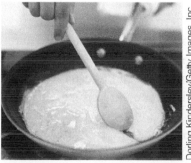

Dorling Kindersley/Getty Images, Inc.

④ **Monitor the critical control points** Procedures need to be in place to continually monitor the critical control points. With egg processing, each batch is tested for *Salmonella*. If the temperature is not hot enough or the heating is not continued long enough, *Salmonella* can survive, as shown here by the growing bacterial colonies.

⑤ **Establish corrective action** If a critical limit is not met, corrective action is necessary. Batches of eggs that are contaminated with *Salmonella* are discarded, and the temperature of the heat chamber is adjusted to ensure that *Salmonella* in the next batch will be killed.

⑥ **Maintain record-keeping procedures** Extensive records are kept, documenting the monitoring of critical control points and corrective actions taken. This enables the source of a problem to be traced in the event of an outbreak of food-borne illness.

⑦ **Institute verification procedures** Plans and records are continuously reviewed to ensure that the HACCP plan is working and only safe eggs are reaching consumers.

13.2 Pathogens in Food

Most cases of food-borne illness in the United States are caused by food that has been contaminated with **pathogens**. The pathogens that most commonly affect the food supply include bacteria, viruses, molds, and parasites. A typical case of food-borne illness causes a short bout of flulike symptoms, including abdominal pain, nausea, diarrhea, and vomiting. However, more severe symptoms, such as kidney failure, arthritis, paralysis, miscarriage, and even death, sometimes occur.

pathogen A biological agent that causes disease.

Any food-borne illness caused by pathogens that multiply in the human body is called a **food-borne infection**. Contracting a food-borne infection usually involves consumption of a large number of pathogens that infect the body or produce toxins within the body. Any food-borne illness caused by consuming a food that contains toxins produced by pathogens is referred to as **food-borne intoxication**. Even food that contains only a few pathogens can cause food-borne intoxication if the pathogens have produced enough toxin. Avoiding food-borne illness—both infection and intoxication—requires knowing how to handle and store food in ways that will prevent contamination and prevent or minimize the growth of pathogens that may already be present in the food. Even a food that is contaminated with pathogens can be safe if it is prepared in a manner that destroys any pathogens or toxins that are present.

Bacteria in Food

Bacteria are present in the soil, on our skin, on most surfaces in our homes, and in the food we eat. Most are harmless, some are beneficial, and a few are pathogenic, causing food-borne infection or intoxication.[3]

Bacterial food-borne infection *Salmonella* is the most common cause of bacterial food-borne illness in the United States.[4] Although poultry and eggs are the foods most often contaminated with *Salmonella*, it has also been found in a variety of foods ranging from peanut butter, ground meat, fruits, and vegetables to processed foods such as frozen pot pies (**Figure 13.3a** and **b**).[5] Because *Salmonella* is killed by heat, foods that are likely to be contaminated should be cooked thoroughly.

Campylobacter jejuni is a leading cause of acute bacterial diarrhea in the United States, affecting about 845,000 people annually.[4] Common sources are undercooked chicken, unpasteurized milk, cheeses made from unpasteurized milk, and untreated water (**Figure 13.3b** and **c**). A sampling of raw chicken from supermarkets from 2005 to 2011 found that about 40% of samples were contaminated with *Campylobacter*.[6] This organism grows slowly in cold temperatures and is killed by heat, so careful storage and thorough cooking are key to preventing infection.

Escherichia coli, commonly called *E. coli*, is a bacterium that inhabits the gastrointestinal tracts of humans and other animals. It comes into contact with food through fecal contamination of water or unsanitary handling of food. Some strains of *E. coli* are harmless, but others can cause serious food-borne infection. One strain of *E. coli*, found in water contaminated by human or animal feces, is the cause of "travelers' diarrhea." Another strain, *E. coli* O157:H7, produces a toxin in the body that causes abdominal pain, bloody diarrhea, and in severe cases a form of kidney failure called **hemolytic-uremic syndrome**, which can be fatal.

E. coli O157:H7 entered the public spotlight in 1993, when it led to the deaths of several children who had consumed undercooked, contaminated hamburgers from a fast-food restaurant (**Figure 13.3d**).[7] Thorough cooking of the hamburgers would have killed the bacteria that caused these deaths. *E. coli* can also contaminate produce such as lettuce, spinach, and green onions and cause illness if the produce is eaten raw (**Figure 13.3e**). In 2013, *E. coli* contamination of ready-to-eat salads sickened people in four states.[8] In 2011, infected bologna, another food that we don't typically cook, sickened people in five different states.[9] In addition to concerns about *E. coli* O157:H7 in our meat and produce, a new,

Nutrition InSight How bacteria contaminate our food • Figure 13.3

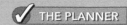

Pathogenic bacteria can enter the food supply in a number of ways.

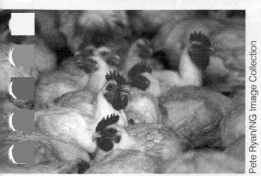

a. Because poultry farms house large numbers of chickens in close proximity, one infected chicken can infect thousands of others. *Salmonella* can infect the ovaries of hens and contaminate the eggs before the shells are formed, so that the bacteria are present inside the shell when the eggs are laid. Therefore, eggs should never be eaten raw.

Pete Ryan/NG Image Collection

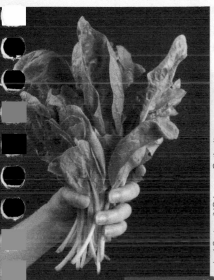

David Arnold/NG Image Collection

c. *Campylobacter* can be carried by healthy cattle and by flies on farms. As a result, the bacteria are commonly present in unpasteurized (raw) milk. Unpasteurized milk is also a common source of *Listeria*. During pasteurization, milk is heated to a temperature that is high enough to kill both *Campylobacter* and *Listeria*. Avoiding products made with unpasteurized milk will reduce the risk of *Campylobacter* and *Listeria* infection.

e. *E. coli* and other bacteria can also contaminate fruits and vegetables if they are fertilized with raw or improperly composted manure or irrigated with water containing untreated sewage or manure. Produce may also be contaminated by wash water or through direct or indirect contact with cattle, deer, or sheep. Thoroughly washing fruits and vegetables can reduce the number of pathogens but does not make contaminated produce risk free.

Joel Sartore/NG Image Collection

Think Critically Why should hamburger be cooked more thoroughly than steak to prevent *E coli* infection?

b. In processing plants, *Salmonella* and *Campylobacter* from infected birds can be transferred to the meat of healthy birds. Consumers should always handle raw chicken as if it contains pathogens. ▼

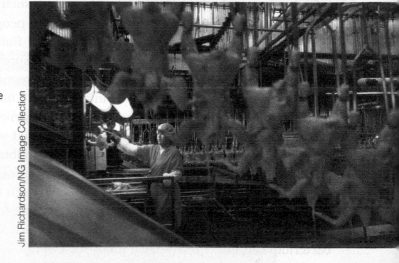

Jim Richardson/NG Image Collection

d. *E. coli* O157:H7 can live in the intestines of healthy cattle and contaminate the meat after slaughter. *E. coli*-contaminated meat that comes into contact with a grinder may contaminate hundreds of pounds of ground beef. Contaminated ground beef is a particular concern because the pathogens are mixed throughout during grinding rather than remaining on the surface, as they do on steaks and chops. The *E. coli* on the outside of the meat are quickly killed during cooking, but those in the interior survive if the meat is not cooked thoroughly. ▼

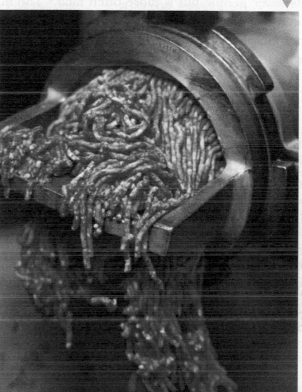

John A. Rizzo /Photodisc/GettyImages, Inc.

Shellfish can be contaminated with norovirus if the water in which they live is polluted with human or animal feces. Cooking destroys noroviruses, so water and uncooked foods such as leafy vegetables, fruits, and nuts are the most common causes of norovirus food-borne illness. Most outbreaks are caused by food contaminated during preparation and service; one study found that infected food handlers may have contributed to 82% of the outbreaks examined.[15] Norovirus infection can be spread from one infected person to another, so it spreads swiftly where many people congregate in a small area. You may have heard of it as a cause of food-borne illness aboard cruise ships. These outbreaks make headlines, but norovirus outbreaks are just as likely in nursing homes, restaurants, hotels, and dormitories as they are aboard cruise ships.

Hepatitis A is another viral infection that can be contracted from food or water that is contaminated with fecal matter. Hepatitis A infection causes liver inflammation, jaundice, fever, nausea, fatigue, and abdominal pain. The infection can require a recovery period of several months, but it does not require treatment and does not cause permanent liver damage. Hepatitis in drinking water is destroyed by chlorination. Cooking destroys the virus in food, and good sanitation can prevent its spread. A vaccine that protects against hepatitis A infection is available.

Moldy Foods

Many types of **mold** grow on foods such as bread, cheese, and fruit. Under certain conditions, these molds produce toxins (**Figure 13.6**). More than 250 different mold toxins have been identified. Cooking and freezing stop mold growth but do not destroy toxins that have already been produced. If a food is moldy, it should be discarded, the area where it was stored should be cleaned, and neighboring foods should be checked to see if they have also become contaminated.

> **mold** Multicellular fungi that form filamentous branching growths.

Parasites in Food

Some **parasites** are microscopic single-celled animals, and others are worms large enough to be seen with the naked eye. Parasites that can be transmitted through consumption of contaminated food and water cause food-borne illness. *Giardia lamblia* is a single-celled parasite that causes diarrhea and other GI symptoms. It is often contracted by hikers who drink untreated water from streams contaminated with animal feces. *Giardia* infection is also becoming a problem in day-care centers where diapers are changed and hands and surfaces are not thoroughly washed.[3] *Cryptosporidium parvum* is

> **parasite** An organism that lives at the expense of another.

Mold toxin and liver cancer • Figure 13.6

The mold *Aspergillus flavus* produces *aflatoxin*, which is among the most potent carcinogens and mutagens known. The level of aflatoxin that may be present in foods in the United States is regulated, so there has never been an outbreak of illness caused by aflatoxin in the United States, but it is a problem in developing countries.

> **Interpret the Data**
>
> Which continents have the highest incidence of liver cancer? Are these areas also at risk for aflatoxin exposure?

a. The filamentous growths seen in this electron micrograph belong to the mold *Aspergillus flavus*, which produces aflatoxin. This mold commonly grows on corn, rice, wheat, peanuts, almonds, walnuts, sunflower seeds, and spices such as black pepper and coriander.

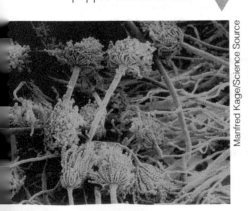

Manfred Kage/Science Source

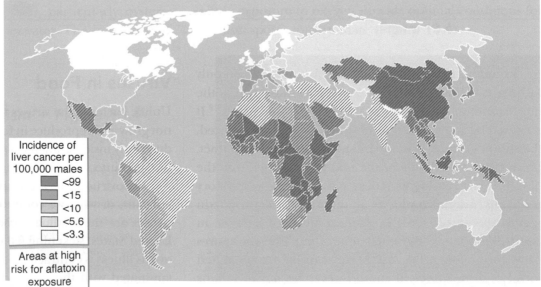

Incidence of liver cancer per 100,000 males
- <99
- <15
- <10
- <5.6
- <3.3

Areas at high risk for aflatoxin exposure

b. Exposure to aflatoxin can lead to liver cancer. Many regions with high rates of liver cancer also have high exposure to aflatoxin.[16]

Herring worm • Figure 13.7

The body cavity of this herring contains the larval form of the small roundworm *Anisakis simplex*, also called herring worm. When consumed in raw fish, these parasites burrow into the wall of the esophagus, stomach, or intestinal tract, causing *Anisakiasis*, which is characterized by severe abdominal pain.[3] The fresher the fish when it is eviscerated, the less likely it is to cause this disease because the larvae move from the fish's stomach to its flesh only after the fish dies.

another single-celled parasite that causes diarrhea. It is commonly contracted from and spread by contaminated water, and the life stage of the parasite that causes infection is resistant to chlorine.[3]

Trichinella spiralis is a parasite that is found in raw and undercooked pork and game meats. Once ingested, these small, wormlike organisms find their way to the muscles, where they grow, causing flulike symptoms. Fish are another common source of parasitic infections because they carry the larvae of parasites such as roundworms, flatworms, flukes, and tapeworms (**Figure 13.7**). As the popularity of eating raw fish has increased, so has the incidence of parasitic infections from fish. Parasites, including those in fish, are killed by thorough cooking. When consuming raw fish, parasitic infections can be avoided by eating fish that has been frozen.

Prions in Food

The strangest and scariest, yet rarest, food-borne illness is caused not by a microbe but by a protein, called a **prion**, that has folded improperly. Abnormal prions are believed to be the cause of mad cow disease, or **bovine spongiform encephalopathy (BSE)**, a deadly degenerative neurological disease that affects cattle. The human form of this disease is **variant Creutzfeldt-Jakob Disease (vCJD)**. People are believed to contract it by eating tissue from a cow infected with BSE (**Figure 13.8**).[17] Symptoms of vCJD begin as mood swings and numbness and within about 14 months progress to dementia and death.

> **prion** A pathogenic protein that is the cause of degenerative brain diseases called spongiform encephalopathies. *Prion* is short for *proteinaceous infectious particle*.

How prions multiply • Figure 13.8

The abnormal prions that cause BSE differ from normal proteins in the way they are folded—that is, in their three-dimensional structure. When the improperly folded form of a prion is introduced into the brain after a person has eaten contaminated tissue, it can reproduce by corrupting neighboring proteins, essentially changing their shape so that they, too, become abnormal prions. Because the abnormal prions are not degraded normally, they accumulate and form clumps called plaques. These plaques cause deadly nervous tissue damage.

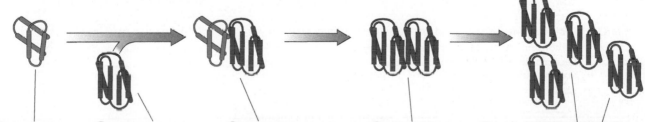

1. Normal prion proteins are present in the brain.
2. Abnormal prion proteins arise spontaneously or enter from the diet.
3. Normal and abnormal prion proteins come into contact with each other.
4. Normal prions are converted into abnormal prions.
5. Abnormal prion proteins accumulate in the brain, leading to the formation of plaques that damage brain tissue.

PROCESS DIAGRAM

Pathogens in Food **447**

Summary of bacterial, viral, and parasitic food-borne illnesses   Table 13.3

Microbe	Sources	Symptoms	Onset (time after consumption)	Duration
Bacteria				
Campylobacter jejuni	Unpasteurized milk, untreated water, undercooked meat and poultry	Fever, headache, diarrhea, abdominal pain	2–5 days	2–10 days
Clostridium botulinum	Improperly canned foods, deep-dish casseroles, honey	Lassitude, weakness, vertigo, respiratory failure, paralysis	18–36 hours	10 days or longer (must administer antitoxin)
Clostridium perfringens	Fecal contamination, deep-dish casseroles	Nausea, diarrhea, abdominal pain	about 16 hours	12–24 hours
Escherichia coli O157:H7	Fecal contamination, undercooked ground beef	Abdominal pain, bloody diarrhea, kidney failure	1–9 days	2–9 days in uncomplicated cases
Listeria monocytogenes	Raw milk products; soft ripened cheeses; deli meats and cold cuts, raw and undercooked poultry; meats; raw and smoked fish; raw vegetables	Fever, headache, stiff neck, chills, nausea, vomiting. May cause spontaneous abortion or stillbirth in pregnant women and meningitis and blood infections in the fetus.	Hours to weeks	Days to weeks
Salmonella	Fecal contamination; raw or undercooked eggs and meat, especially poultry; contaminated produce	Nausea, abdominal pain, diarrhea, headache, fever	6–72 hours	4–7 days
Shigella	Fecal contamination of water or foods, especially salads such as chicken, tuna, shrimp, and potato salads	Diarrhea, abdominal pain, fever, vomiting	8–50 hours	5–7 days
Staphylococcus aureus	Human contamination from coughs and sneezes; eggs, meat, potato and macaroni salads	Severe nausea, vomiting, diarrhea	1–7 hours	Hours–1 day
Vibrio parahaemolyticus	Raw seafood from contaminated water	Cramps, diarrhea, fever, nausea, vomiting	4–90 hours	2–6 days
Yersinia enterocolitica	Pork, unpasteurized milk, and oysters	Diarrhea, vomiting, fever, abdominal pain; often mistaken for appendicitis	1–11 days	A few days – 3 weeks
Viruses				
Hepatitis A	Human fecal contamination of food or water, raw shellfish	Jaundice, liver inflammation, fatigue, fever, nausea, anorexia, abdominal discomfort	15–50 days	1–2 weeks to several months
Norovirus	Fecal contamination of water or foods, especially shellfish and salad ingredients	Diarrhea, nausea, vomiting	24–48 hours	12–60 hours
Parasites				
Anisakis simplex	Raw fish	Severe abdominal pain	24 hours–2 weeks	3 weeks
Cryptosporidium parvum	Fecal contamination of food or water	Severe watery diarrhea	7–10 days	2–14 days, but may become chronic
Giardia lamblia	Fecal contamination of water and uncooked foods	Diarrhea, abdominal pain, gas, anorexia, nausea, vomiting	1–2 weeks	2–6 weeks, but may be chronic
Toxoplasma gondii	Meat, primarily pork	Toxoplasmosis (can cause central nervous system disorders, flulike symptoms, and birth defects in the offspring of women exposed during pregnancy; see Chapter 11)	5–23 days	Several weeks, but may become chronic
Trichinella spiralis	Undercooked pork, game meat	Muscle weakness, flulike symptoms	1–4 weeks	Several weeks

vCJD is believed to be transmitted by consumption of the brain and nervous tissue, intestines, eyes, or tonsils of contaminated animals, but thus far meat (if free of central nervous system tissue) and milk have not been found to transmit either BSE or vCJD.[3] Even though cooking does not destroy prions, the risk of acquiring vCJD is extremely small. Safeguards are in place to prevent cattle in the United States from contracting BSE. These include restrictions on the import of animals and animal products from countries where BSE has occurred, restrictions on what can be included in cattle feed, and testing for BSE before meat is released into the food supply.[18] Several cows with BSE have been identified in the United States, but meat from these animals did not enter the food supply. Thus far there has been no known instance of U.S. beef causing a case of vCJD.

What Bug Has You Down?

There are certainly a wide variety of food-borne pathogens that can make you sick (**Table 13.3**). Recent improvements in governmental outbreak surveillance, attentiveness by health-care professionals, and testing frequency and accuracy have made it possible to identify even more cases of food-borne illness than was possible a few years ago. Despite the added attention, data that measures trends in food-borne disease indicate that there has not been much progress in reducing food-borne infections; the incidence of infection with nine key pathogens was not significantly different in 2013 than in 2006–2008.[19] Public awareness of the problem and education on how to handle food safely can help reduce the incidence of food-borne illness in the future.

Preventing Microbial Food-Borne Illness

Microbes in food multiply when they are presented with the right conditions for growth. Choosing food carefully can help reduce the risk of microbial food-borne illness by minimizing the number of food-borne pathogens brought into the home (**Table 13.4**). Once at home, preparing food in a clean kitchen reduces **cross-contamination**. Storing food at refrigerator or freezer temperatures either limits or stops microbial growth. Heating foods to the recommended temperature kills microbes and destroys toxins

> **cross-contamination**
> The transfer of contaminants from one food or object to another.

Safe grocery choices **Table 13.4**

- Purchase food from reputable vendors.

- Select jars that are securely closed: Seals should not be broken and safety "buttons" on jar lids should not be popped.

- Avoid cans that are rusted, dented, or bulging.

- Do not purchase food unless packaging is secure.

- Select frozen foods from below the frost line in the freezer.

- Choose frozen foods that are solidly frozen and avoid those that contain frost or ice crystals.

- Check voluntary freshness dates and avoid foods with expired dates:

  - **Sell-by or pull-by date:** Used by manufacturers to tell grocers when to remove their product from the shelves. You should buy the product before this date, but if the food has been handled and stored properly, it is usually still safe for consumption after it. For example, milk is usually still good at least a week beyond its sell-by date if it has been properly refrigerated.

  - **Best if used by, use-by, quality assurance, or freshness date:** Used to specify the last date on which the product will retain maximum freshness, flavor, and texture. Beyond this date, the product's quality may diminish, but the food may still be safe if it has been handled and stored properly.

  - **Expiration date:** Used to specify the last day on which a product should be eaten. State governments regulate these dates for perishable items, such as milk and eggs. The FDA regulates only the expiration dates of infant formula.

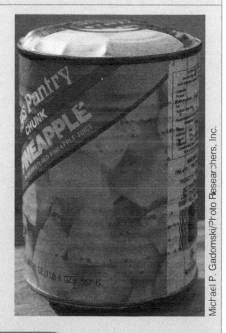

Michael P. Gadomski/Proto Researchers, Inc.

> **Ask Yourself**
> Is the canned pineapple in this photo a safe choice? Why or why not?

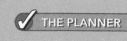
The Fight Bac! educational campaign recommends that consumers follow four steps—clean, separate, cook, and chill—to prevent food-borne illness (see www.fightbac.org).[20]

The Fight Bac! icon illustrates food-handling practices that will keep food safe from bacteria and prevent food-borne illness. ▼

Hands, countertops, cutting boards, and utensils should be washed with warm, soapy water before each step in food preparation.

Foods that are going to be cooked should not be prepared on the same surfaces as foods that are eaten raw.

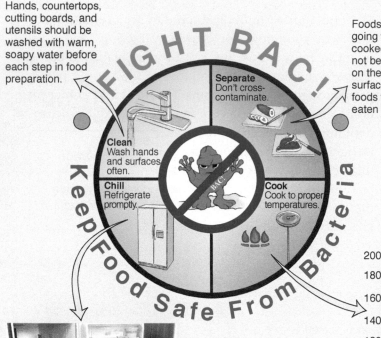

FIGHT BAC!
Keep Food Safe From Bacteria

Separate
Don't cross-contaminate.

Clean
Wash hands and surfaces often.

Chill
Refrigerate promptly.

Cook
Cook to proper temperatures.

Minimum internal temperature for safety

165 — Poultry, stuffing, casseroles, reheated leftovers
160 — Ground meat, dishes containing egg

145 — Beef, pork, lamb, veal roasts, steaks and chops*
Fish**

*Allow meat to rest 3 minutes before carving or consuming
**Cook until flesh is opaque and separates easily with a fork

200°
180°
160°
140° — Cooked foods should be held at 140° or above.
Eggs should be cooked until the white and yolk are firm, not runny.

120°
100° — **DANGER ZONE** — Temperatures in this zone allow rapid bacterial growth and production of bacterial toxins. Foods should only be allowed to remain in this temperature range for minimal amounts of time, generally less than 2 hrs. When cooling hot foods, temperature should be reduced to 40° within 2 hours
80°
60°
40° — Refrigerator temperature: Stops the growth of all but a few cold-tolerant organisms
20°
0° — Freezer temperature: Prevents bacterial growth, but some bacteria are able to survive

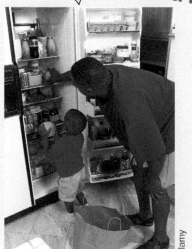

Fresh and frozen foods brought from the store should be refrigerated or frozen immediately. Fresh meat, poultry, and fish should be frozen if it will not be used within a day or two. Processed meats such as hot dogs and bologna should be refrigerated but can be kept longer than fresh meat. Freezers should be set to 0°F and refrigerators to less than 40°F.

▲ Temperature is one of the best weapons consumers have for preventing food-borne illness. Minimizing the time food temperatures remain in the danger zone—between 40 and 140°F—reduces bacterial growth and therefore the risk of food-borne illness. Use a food thermometer to make sure that the food is cooked to a safe internal temperature; color is not a good indicator of safety.

Alamy

(**Figure 13.9**). Foods that are served cold should be kept cold until they are served. Frozen foods should be kept frozen and then thawed in the refrigerator or microwave before cooking, not thawed at room temperature, which favors microbial growth. Cooked food should be handled with care and kept hot until it is served and chilled quickly before storage. When in doubt about the safety of a food, throw it out

Cross-contamination can occur when uncooked foods containing live microbes come into contact with foods that have already been cooked. Therefore, cooked meat should never be returned to the same dish that held the raw meat, and sauces used to marinate uncooked foods should never be used as sauces on cooked food. Leftover cooked food should be refrigerated as soon as possible after it has been served. As a general rule, food should not be left unrefrigerated for more than 2 hours, or for more than an hour if the ambient temperature is above 90°F.[21] The temperature range that is most favorable for microbial growth is the range at which food usually sits between service and storage. Large portions of food should be divided before refrigeration so they will cool quickly. Most leftovers should be kept for only a few days.

Although much of the food-borne illness in the United States is caused by food prepared in homes, an outbreak in a commercial or institutional establishment usually involves more people and is more likely to be reported (see *Thinking It Through*). Food in retail establishments has many opportunities to be contaminated because of the large volume of food handled and the large number

A Case Study on Tracking Food-Borne Illness

On Friday, more than half of the 200 children enrolled at the local elementary school were either absent or went home sick sometime during the school day. They had symptoms that included nausea and vomiting, diarrhea, abdominal pain, and fever. Food-borne illness was suspected, and the local health department was notified. Inspectors were able to trace the source of the outbreak to the Spring Celebration held at the school on Thursday. For this event, the first-graders made cupcakes; the second-graders, cookies; the third-graders, fruit salad; and the fourth-graders, frozen custard. All the children were interviewed about which of these foods they had eaten that day, and the information was used to compile the following graph:

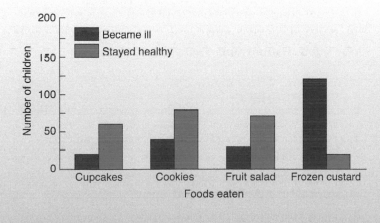

 1 Based on the graph, which food is the most likely cause of the illness? Why?

Your answer:

The children's physicians found that their stool samples contained the bacterium *Salmonella enteritidis*. The health inspectors determined that the frozen custard recipe that the children used included raw eggs.

 2 How can eggs become contaminated with *Salmonella*?

Your answer:

 3 The cookie and cupcake recipes also called for eggs. Why are these unlikely to be the cause of the food-borne illness?

Your answer:

 4 Suggest a reason why 20 of the children who consumed the frozen custard did not get ill.

Your answer:

 5 Suggest a food for next year's celebration that would be a safer choice.

Your answer:

(Check your answers in online Appendix L.)

THINKING IT THROUGH

WHAT A SCIENTIST SEES

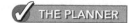

A Picnic for Bacteria

James Shaffer/Photo Edit

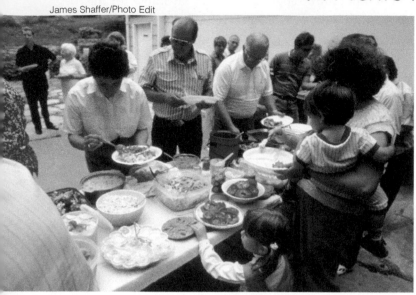

Looks great—lots of food and people together on a warm, sunny day. Most people see lunch, but those concerned with food-borne illness see trouble. If a food is contaminated with pathogenic bacteria, it won't take long before enough bacteria are present to cause food-borne illness. The number of bacterial cells doubles each time the cells divide, resulting in an exponential growth curve like the one shown here. If 10 bacterial cells contaminate the egg salad during preparation and then it sits in the warm sun for 4 hours, during which time the cells divide every 20 minutes, there will be 40,960 bacterial cells in the salad when you scoop a portion of it onto your plate.

Limiting bacterial growth is a consideration any time food must be carried out of the home. Any food that is transported should be kept cold. Lunches should be transported to and from work or school in a cooler or an insulated bag and refrigerated upon arrival. Perishable foods that are brought home from work or school uneaten should be thrown out and not saved for another day.

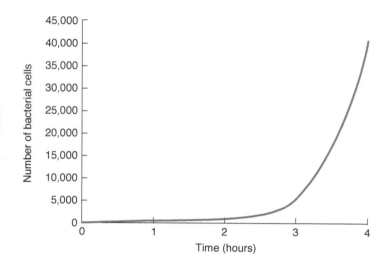

Think Critically What foods would be the safest to include in lunch boxes and serve at picnics? Why?

---

of people involved in its preparation. Consumers should choose restaurants with safety in mind. Restaurants should be clean, and cooked foods should be served hot. Cafeteria steam tables should be kept hot enough that the water is steaming and food is kept above 140°F. Cold foods, such as salad bar items, should be kept either refrigerated or on ice to keep the food at 40°F or colder.

Picnics, potluck suppers, and other large events where food is served provide a prime opportunity for bacteria to flourish because food is often left at room temperature or in the sun for long periods before it is consumed. Whether you are at a picnic, a potluck, or at home, food should not be left out of refrigeration for more than 2 hours, or for more than 1 hour if the air temperature is over 90°F. When diners serve themselves, cross-contamination from dirty hands or used plates and utensils is possible. Unlike the

food in salad bars at restaurants, the food at a family picnic is not placed under a sneeze guard to prevent contamination from coughs and sneezes. All food that is served outdoors at a picnic or county fair should be approached with food safety in mind (see *What a Scientist Sees*).

CONCEPT CHECK

1. **How** does *Clostridium botulinum* cause food-borne illness?

2. **What** pathogenic bacteria commonly contaminate chicken and eggs?

3. **How** do viruses make us sick?

4. **How** does refrigeration help prevent food-borne illness?

13.3 Agricultural and Industrial Chemicals in Food

LEARNING OBJECTIVES

1. **Illustrate** how contaminants move through the food chain and into our foods.

2. **Compare** the risks and benefits of using pesticides with those of growing food organically.

3. **Describe** how to minimize the risks of exposure to chemical contaminants.

Chemicals used in agricultural production and industrial wastes contaminate the environment and can find their way into the food supply. How harmful these chemicals are depends on whether they persist in the environment and whether they accumulate in the organisms that consume them or can be broken down and excreted by those organisms. Some contaminants are eliminated from the environment quickly because they are broken down by microorganisms or chemical reactions. Others remain in the environment for very long periods, and when taken up by plants and small animals, they are not metabolized or excreted. When these plants or small animals are consumed by larger animals that are in turn eaten by still larger animals, the contaminants accumulate, reaching higher concentrations at each level of the food chain (**Figure 13.10**). This process is called **bioaccumulation**. Because the toxins are not eliminated from the body, the greater the

> **bioaccumulation**
> The process by which compounds accumulate or build up in an organism faster than they can be broken down or excreted.

Contamination throughout the food chain • Figure 13.10

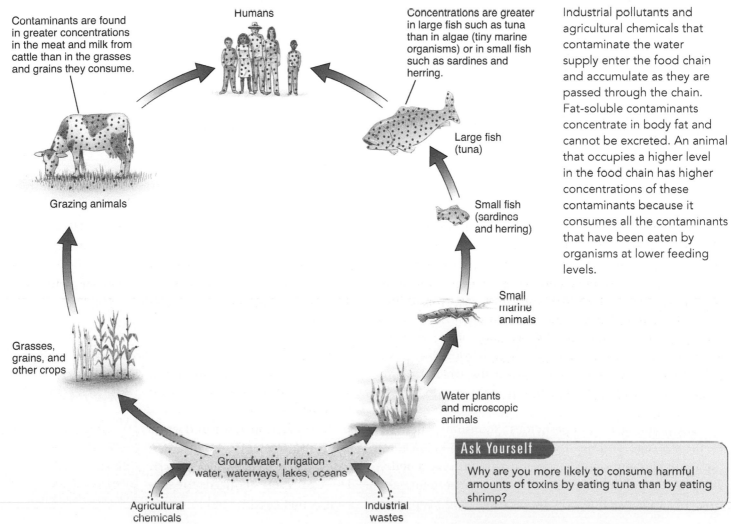

Contaminants are found in greater concentrations in the meat and milk from cattle than in the grasses and grains they consume.

Humans

Concentrations are greater in large fish such as tuna than in algae (tiny marine organisms) or in small fish such as sardines and herring.

Grazing animals

Large fish (tuna)

Small fish (sardines and herring)

Small marine animals

Grasses, grains, and other crops

Water plants and microscopic animals

Groundwater, irrigation water, waterways, lakes, oceans

Agricultural chemicals

Industrial wastes

Industrial pollutants and agricultural chemicals that contaminate the water supply enter the food chain and accumulate as they are passed through the chain. Fat-soluble contaminants concentrate in body fat and cannot be excreted. An animal that occupies a higher level in the food chain has higher concentrations of these contaminants because it consumes all the contaminants that have been eaten by organisms at lower feeding levels.

Ask Yourself

Why are you more likely to consume harmful amounts of toxins by eating tuna than by eating shrimp?

Pesticide tolerances • Figure 13.11

As shown in these pie charts from an analysis of samples of domestically produced food and imported food from 100 countries, only a small percentage of foods exceed tolerances.[22] To further reduce pesticide risks and exposure in the United States, more effective, less toxic chemical pesticides are being developed; the use of older, more toxic products is decreasing; and production methods that result in low-pesticide and pesticide-free produce are being implemented.

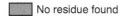 No residue found

Residue found but levels are below tolerances

Residue found that exceeds tolerance or for which no tolerance has been established in the sampled food.

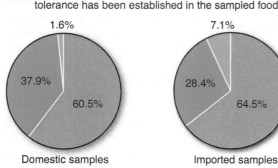

1.6%   7.1%

37.9%   28.4%

60.5%   64.5%

Domestic samples   Imported samples

Interpret the Data

What percentage of imported food samples was free of pesticide residues?

amount consumed, the greater the amount present in the body.

Pesticides: Risks and Benefits

Pesticides are used to prevent plant diseases and insect infestations. They are applied both to crops in the fields and to harvested produce in order to prevent spoilage and extend shelf life. Crops that are grown using pesticides generally produce higher yields and look more appealing because they have less insect damage. Once they have been applied, however, pesticides can travel into water supplies, soil, and other parts of the environment. Because pesticides enter the environment, pesticide residues are found not only on the treated plants but also in meat, poultry, fish, and dairy products (see Figure 13.10).

The potential risks of pesticides to consumers depend on the size, age, and health of the person who consumes the pesticides and on the type and amount consumed.[23] To protect public health and the environment, the types of pesticides that may be used on food crops, the

frequency of their use, and the amount of residue that may remain when foods reach consumers are regulated. The EPA approves and registers pesticides that are used in food production and establishes **tolerances**. Pesticide tolerances are the maximum amounts of pesticide residues that may remain in or on a food.[24] To establish tolerances that are safe for both children and adults, the EPA considers tests done in experimental animals and on cells growing in the laboratory, as well as the amount of the pesticide to which consumers are likely to be exposed. Tolerances are then usually set at least 100 times lower than the highest dose that has no harmful effects in test animals.

The FDA and the USDA monitor pesticide residues in foods. In general, pesticide residue levels in both domestic and imported foods have been found to be well below federally permitted limits (**Figure 13.11**).[22] Although repeated consumption of large doses of any one pesticide could be harmful, such a situation is unlikely because most people consume a variety of foods that have been produced in many different locations.

Integrated pest management One way to limit pesticide use is through **integrated pest management (IPM)**. IPM is an agricultural pest control method that combines chemical and nonchemical methods and emphasizes the use of natural toxins and more effective pesticide application. For example, increasing the use of naturally pest-resistant crop varieties that thrive without the use of pesticides can reduce costs and do less environmental damage. IPM programs use information about the life cycles of pests and their interaction with the environment to manage pest damage economically and with the least possible hazard to people, property, and the environment.

> **integrated pest management (IPM)** A method of agricultural pest control that integrates nonchemical and chemical techniques.

Organic food production Organic food is produced using methods that minimize the use of synthetic pesticides and promote recycling of resources and conservation of soil and water to protect the environment (see *Debate: Should You Go Organic?*). The USDA sets standards for substances that can be used in or are

> **organic food** Food that is produced, processed, and handled in accordance with the standards of the USDA National Organic Program.

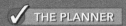
The Issue: As people become more and more concerned about food safety, nutritional health, and the environment, they are turning to organic food. Should you be choosing organic over conventionally produced food?

The sale of organic foods is on the rise. Most of this increase has been from organic fruits and vegetables, which now represent just over 10% of all U.S. fruit and vegetable sales.[25] Organic foods are chosen because they are often perceived as safer, more nutritious, and better for the environment. If safer means fewer synthetic pesticides, then organic produce is a good choice. It contains fewer pesticides and is significantly lower in nitrates than traditionally grown foods.[26] But it can be argued that there is little evidence that the current levels of pesticide exposure from conventional produce present risks to human health (see Figure 13.11). Moreover, other contamination risks are associated with organic foods. For example, manure is often used for fertilizer, and if the manure is not treated properly, it can contain pathogenic bacteria.[27]

Many consumers believe that organically produced food is not only safer but also more nutritious. *Nutritious* can mean that it is more effective at preventing nutrition-related diseases.[28] When consumption of organic food is compared with consumption of conventionally produced foods, the majority of studies do not show organic foods to be beneficial in terms of preventing nutrition-related diseases. Research data on the nutrient content of organically produced food are ambivalent. Some studies report that organically produced foods contain more nutrients than conventionally produced food, and others have found no consistent differences in nutrient content.[29] This confusion is not surprising because many factors—including growing conditions, season, the fertilizer regime,

and the methods used for crop protection (for example, use of pesticides and herbicides)—affect the nutritional composition of fruits and vegetables. Nutrient content is also affected by how the food is stored, transported, and processed prior to consumption.

What about the environment? It is hard to argue that organic farming is not better for the environment. Instead of synthetic pesticides and fertilizer, it relies on natural methods of pest control, crop rotation, compost, and cover crops to maintain the soil. The result is preservation of the soil, so crops can be grown far into the future, and reduction in the amounts of chemicals released into the environment. But organic growing still impacts the environment. As occurs with conventionally grown produce, runoff from manure can pollute waterways, and organic food, like conventional food, is often shipped long distances, using energy and generating pollution.

Is a diet based on organic foods safer, more nutritious, and better for the environment? We can assume that both conventional and organic foods sold in the United States are generally safe. Whether organic is more nutritious depends not only on individual foods but on the diet as a whole. If your choices of organic foods are limited by availability or cost, then choosing only organic may limit nutrient intake. Are organic foods better for the environment? They reduce pesticide and fertilizer use, but if organic foods are not available locally the environmental cost of transporting them is no different than it is for conventional foods.

Think Critically Are these organic onions that were shipped across the country a better environmental choice than conventionally grown onions from the farm across town?

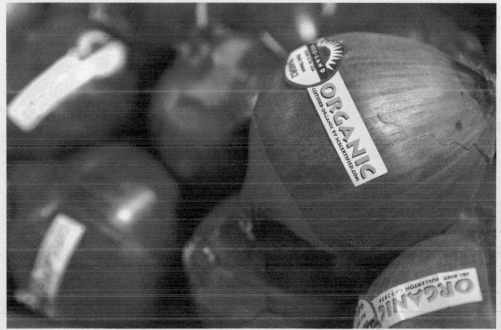

Drew Rush/NG Image Collection

prohibited from use in organic food production. Most conventional pesticides, fertilizers made with synthetic ingredients, sewage sludge, genetically modified ingredients, irradiation, antibiotics, and growth hormones are prohibited from use in organic food production. Before a food can be labeled "organic," the USDA must certify the farming and processing operations that produce and handle the food (**Figure 13.12**).

Organic farming techniques reduce farm workers' exposure to pesticides and decrease the quantity of pesticides introduced into the food supply and the environment. Organic foods, however, are not completely free of synthetic pesticides and other agricultural chemicals not approved for organic use because irrigation water, rain, and a variety of other sources can introduce trace amounts into organically grown foods. The threshold for pesticide residues in organic foods is set at 5% of the EPA's pesticide-residue tolerance.[30] Choosing organic food will reduce pesticide exposure, but it will not make your food risk free.

Industrial Contaminants

Industrial chemicals that contaminate the environment find their way into the food supply. Fish accumulate substances from the water in which they live and feed. Shellfish accumulate contaminants because they feed by passing large volumes of water through their bodies.

Pollutants in the water can also contaminate crops and move through the food chain into meat and milk (see Figure 13.10).

One group of carcinogenic compounds that pollutes the environment is **polychlorinated biphenyls (PCBs)**. Prior to the 1970s, these chemicals were used in the manufacture of electrical capacitors and transformers, plasticizers, waxes, and paper. PCBs in runoff from manufacturing plants contaminated water, particularly near the Great Lakes. PCBs are no longer produced, but because they do not degrade, they are still in the environment and accumulate in fish caught in contaminated waters. PCBs are a particular problem for pregnant and lactating women because prenatal exposure to PCBs and consumption of contaminated breast milk can damage the fetal and infant nervous system and cause learning deficits. Pregnant and breastfeeding women should check with their local health department for recommendations regarding fish consumption.

Other contaminants from manufacturing, such as chlordane (used to control termites); radioactive substances such as strontium-90; and toxic metals such as cadmium, lead, arsenic, and mercury, have found their way into fish and shellfish. Cadmium and lead can interfere with the absorption of other minerals. Cadmium can cause kidney damage, and lead can impair brain development. Arsenic is believed to increase the risk of cancer. Mercury, which has been found in large fish, particularly

Labeling organic foods • Figure 13.12 _____

Products that meet the definition of "100% organic" or "organic" may display the USDA "organic" seal shown here.

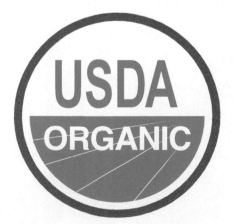

Labeling term	Meaning
100% organic	Contains 100% organically produced raw or processed ingredients.
Organic	Contains at least 95% organically produced raw or processed ingredients.
Made with organic ingredients	Contains at least 70% organically produced ingredients.

Mercury poisoning • Figure 13.13

This Japanese boy has Minamata disease, a neurological syndrome caused by mercury poisoning. The disease first appeared in Minamata, Japan, in 1956 and was caused by the release of mercury into the water by a local chemical factory. The mercury accumulated in the fat of fish and shellfish that were eaten by the local population.

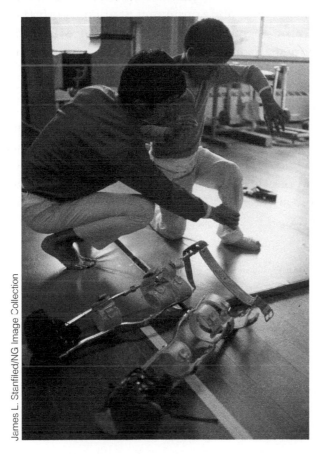

James L. Stanfiled/NG Image Collection

swordfish, king mackerel, tilefish, and shark, damages nerve cells (**Figure 13.13**).[31] Because mercury is especially damaging during prenatal development, pregnant women are advised to avoid certain types of fish and limit their consumption of others (see Chapter 11).

Antibiotics and Hormones

Antibiotics and hormones are administered to animals to improve health, increase growth, or otherwise enhance food production. To prevent these chemicals from being passed on to consumers, both the types of drugs used and when they can be administered are regulated, and animal tissues are monitored for drug residues.[32]

Animals are treated with antibiotics when they are sick, but for decades animals have also been given antibiotics to prevent disease and promote growth. This treatment increases the amount of meat produced and reduces costs, but if it is used improperly, antibiotic residues can remain in the meat. In addition, the overuse of antibiotics in animals can contribute to the development of antibiotic-resistant strains of bacteria. When exposed to an antibiotic, bacteria that are resistant to it survive and produce offspring that are also resistant. If these antibiotic-resistant bacteria infect humans, the resulting illness cannot be treated with that antibiotic. In order to limit antibiotic use, in 2013, the FDA took steps that will make the use of antibiotics for growth enhancement of healthy livestock illegal; antibiotics will still be available to treat sick animals, but only with a veterinary prescription.[33]

Hormones are used to increase weight gain in sheep and cattle and milk production in dairy cows. Some hormones, such as estrogen and testosterone, occur naturally. Generally, these are administered in slow-release form, and their levels are no higher in treated animals than in untreated animals. Before a synthetic hormone can be used, it must be demonstrated that hormone residues in meat from treated animals are within safe limits.

A synthetic hormone that has created public concern is genetically engineered **bovine somatotropin (bST)**. Cows naturally produce bST, which stimulates milk production. Genetically engineered bST is produced by bacteria and injected into cows to further increase milk production (**Figure 13.14**). Milk from cows that have been treated with genetically engineered bST is indistinguishable from other milk.[34]

Bovine somatotropin • Figure 13.14

Consumer groups are concerned that the injection of cows with bST may cause health problems for humans who consume the milk. The FDA has concluded that bST causes no serious long-term health effects, and it does not require milk from bST-treated cows to be specially labeled. Some dairies voluntarily label their products as bST free.

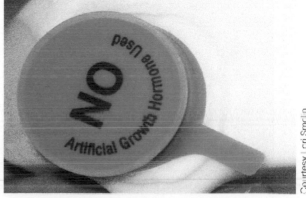

Courtesy Lori Smolin

Choosing Wisely to Minimize Agricultural and Industrial Contaminants

Even though individual consumers cannot detect chemical contaminants in food, care in selection and preparation can reduce the amounts consumed. One of the easiest ways to reduce risk is to choose a wide variety of foods, thus avoiding excessive consumption of contaminants that may be present in any one food. Because chemicals accumulate through the food chain, eating lower on the food chain can minimize consumption of contaminants (see Figure 13.10).

To reduce exposure to pesticide residues in fruits and vegetables, consumers can choose organic foods or locally grown produce. Locally grown produce contains fewer pesticides because the pesticides used to prevent spoilage and extend the shelf life of shipped produce are not needed. Exposure to pesticide residues on conventionally grown produce can be minimized by washing and in some cases peeling (**Figure 13.15a**). Pesticides and other toxins that are ingested by animals concentrate in fat, so intake can be reduced by trimming all fat from meat and removing the skin from poultry.

Intake of pesticides and other chemical pollutants from fish and seafood products can also be minimized by choosing wisely and consuming a variety of fish (**Figure 13.15b**). To minimize consumption of contaminants, remove the skin, fatty material, and dark meat from fish. Use cooking methods such as broiling, poaching, boiling, and baking, which allow contaminants from the fatty portions of fish to drain out. Do not eat the "tomale" in lobster. The tomale, a green paste inside the abdominal cavity of a cooked lobster, serves as the liver and pancreas and is the organ in which toxins accumulate. The analogous organ in blue crabs, called the "mustard" because of its yellow color, should also be avoided (see *What Should I Eat?*).

Reducing exposure to pesticides and pollutants • Figure 13.15

Proper food selection and preparation can reduce exposure to pesticides and other pollutants.

a. Pesticide residues on fruits and vegetables can be removed or reduced by peeling or washing with tap water and scrubbing with a brush, if appropriate. In the case of leafy vegetables such as lettuce and cabbage, the outer leaves can be removed and discarded. Washing apples, cucumbers, eggplant, squash, and tomatoes may not remove all the pesticides because these fruits and vegetables are coated with wax in order to maintain freshness by sealing in moisture, but wax also seals in pesticides. The wax and pesticides can be removed by peeling, but removing the peel also eliminates fiber and some micronutrients.

b. Exposure to chemical contaminants can be minimized by choosing saltwater fish caught well offshore, away from polluted coastal waters. Fish that live near the shore or spend part of their life cycle in fresh water are more likely to contain contaminants. Smaller species of fish are safer because they are earlier in the food chain, and smaller fish within a species are safer because they are younger and hence have had less time to accumulate contaminants (see Figure 13.10).

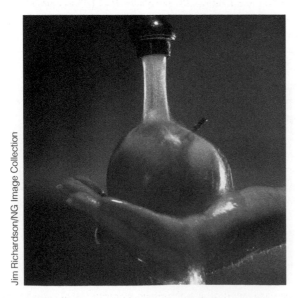

Jim Richardson/NG Image Collection

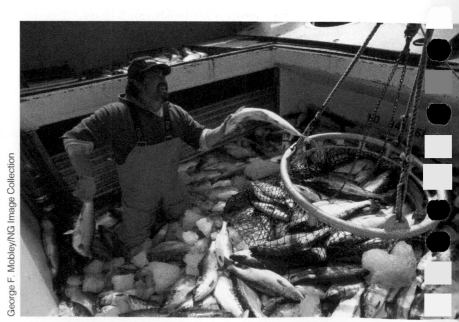

George F. Mobley/NG Image Collection

WHAT SHOULD I EAT?

Food Safety

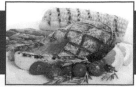

© Sara Winter/iStockphoto   © Jill Chen/iStockphoto   © Steve Mcsweeny/iStockphoto

Avoid ingesting pathogenic microbes
- Make sure your burger is well done.
- Skip the runny eggs and have them scrambled.
- Pass on the dough! Treat yourself to chocolate chip cookies only after they come out of the oven.
- Slice up some melon, but make sure the knife, the cutting board, and the skin of the melon are clean before you slice it.

Reduce pesticides and pollutants in your food
- Buy locally grown produce.
- Look for the organic symbol.

- Try the small fish in the pond.
- Make a salad after you have washed the lettuce and peeled off the outer leaves.
- Trim the fat and don't eat the skin of poultry and fish.

Use iProfile to compare the calories and grams of fat in a chicken breast with and without skin.

CONCEPT CHECK   **STOP**

1. **How** can a pesticide used on broccoli plants end up in milk?

2. **How** can organic food cause food-borne illness?

3. **What** can you do to minimize PCBs in your diet?

13.4 Technology for Keeping Food Safe

LEARNING OBJECTIVES

1. **Describe** how temperature is used to prevent food spoilage.

2. **Discuss** how irradiation preserves food.

3. **Explain** how packaging protects food.

4. **Discuss** the risks and benefits of food additives.

ood spoils when its taste, texture, or nutritional value is changed either by enzymes that are naturally present in the food or by microbes that grow on the food. For thousands of years, humans have treated food in order to prevent spoilage. Techniques that preserve food work by destroying enzymes present in the food, by killing microbes, or by slowing microbial growth (**Table 13.5**).

FAT TOM	Table 13.5
The acronym FAT TOM reminds us of the conditions required for microbial growth. Most food preservation techniques modify one or more of these factors to stop or slow microbial growth.	
Food	Food contains nutrients that promote bacterial growth.
Acidity	Most bacteria grow best at a pH near neutral. Some food additives, such as citric acid and ascorbic acid (vitamin C), are acids, which prevent microbial growth by lowering the pH of food.
Time	The longer a food sits at an optimum growth temperature, the more bacteria it will contain. Food should not be left in the temperature danger zone for more than 2 hours.
Temperature	The high temperatures of canning, cooking, and pasteurization kill microbes, and the low temperatures of freezing and refrigeration slow or stop microbial growth.
Oxygen	In order to grow, most bacteria need oxygen, so packaging that eliminates oxygen prevents their growth.
Moisture	Bacteria need water to grow, so preservation methods such as drying or use of high concentrations of salt or sugar, which draw water away by osmosis, prevent bacteria from growing.

Because irradiation can be used in place of chemical treatments, it reduces consumers' exposure to chemical pesticides and preservatives. It is one of the technologies promoted by the National Food Safety Initiative because of its potential for improving the safety of food and reducing the incidence of food-borne illness.

Food Packaging

Packaging plays an important role in food preservation; it keeps molds and bacteria out, keeps moisture in, and protects food from physical damage. An open package of refrigerated cheddar cheese will be moldy in a few days, but an unopened package will stay fresh for weeks.

Food packaging is continually being improved. In the past two decades, for instance, consumer demand for fresh and easy-to-prepare foods has led manufacturers to offer partially cooked pasta, vegetables, seafood, fresh and cured meats, and dry products such as whole-bean and ground coffee in packaging that, if unopened, will keep perishable food fresh much longer than will conventional packaging. Vacuum packaging and **modified atmosphere packaging (MAP)** use plastics or other packaging materials that are impermeable to oxygen. In vacuum packaging, the air inside the package is removed prior to sealing in order

> **modified atmosphere packaging (MAP)** A preservation technique used to prolong the shelf life of processed or fresh food by changing the gases surrounding the food in the package.

to eliminate the oxygen. In modified atmosphere packaging, the air is flushed out and replaced with another gas, such as carbon dioxide or nitrogen. In both types of packaging, the low oxygen level prevents the growth of aerobic bacteria, slows the ripening of fruits and vegetables, and slows down oxidation reactions, which cause discoloration in fruits and vegetables and rancidity in fats.

Packaging can protect food from spoilage, but even the best packaging can introduce risk if it becomes part of the food. A variety of substances found in paper and plastic containers and packaging, and even dishes, can leach into food (**Figure 13.18**). Substances that are known to contaminate food are regulated by the EPA and the FDA. However, these regulations apply only to the intended use of the product. When a product is used improperly, substances from its packaging can migrate into food. For instance, some plastics migrate into food when heated in a microwave oven. Thus, only containers designed for microwave cooking should be used for microwaving food.

Food Additives

What keeps bread from molding, gives margarine its yellow color, and keeps Parmesan cheese from clumping in the shaker? The answer to all these questions is food additives. Substances that are intentionally added to foods are called **direct food additives**. Other substances

> **direct food additive** A substance that is intentionally added to food. Direct food additives are regulated by the FDA.

Bisphenol A from plastics • Figure 13.18

Bisphenol A (BPA) is a chemical in the plastic used in hard, transparent water bottles, baby bottles, and food containers as well as the coating inside cans. Some but not all plastic containers marked with recycle codes 3 or 7 are made with BPA. There is some concern that BPA could adversely affect development in fetuses, infants, and children.[39] The FDA supports efforts to eliminate the use of BPA in baby bottles and infant feeding cups and to replace BPA or minimize BPA levels in food can linings.

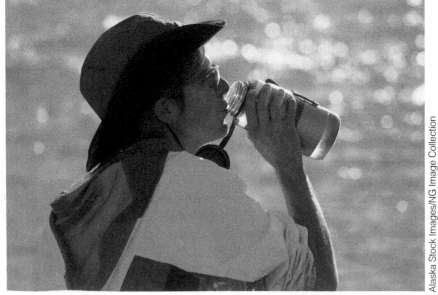

Alaska Stock Images/NG Image Collection

Reducing nitrosamine risk • Figure 13.19

To minimize the risk posed by nitrosamines without increasing the risk of bacterial food-borne illness, the FDA limits the amount of nitrate and nitrite that can be added to food and requires the addition of antioxidants such as vitamin C, which reduce nitrosamine formation, to foods that contain these additives. Consumers can reduce nitrosamine exposure by limiting their consumption of cured meat to 3 to 4 ounces per week and maintaining adequate intakes of the antioxidant vitamins C and E.

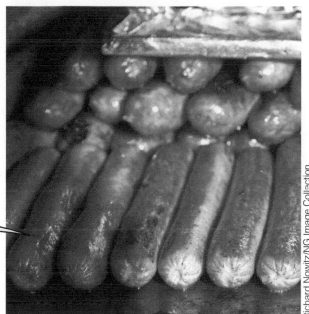

INGREDIENTS: MECHANICALLY SEPARATED CHICKEN, WATER, PORK, MODIFIED CORN STARCH, DEXTROSE, SALT, BEEF, CONTAINS 2% OR LESS OF THE FOLLOWING: CORN SYRUP, FLAVORINGS, SODIUM PHOSPHATES, POTASSIUM LACTATE, SODIUM DIACETATE, SODIUM ASCORBATE (VITAMIN C), OLEO RESIN OF PAPRIKA, SODIUM NITRITE

Richard Nowitz/NG Image Collection

that get into food unintentionally—such as the oil used to lubricate food processing machinery—are referred to as **indirect food additives**. The FDA regulates the amounts and types of direct and indirect food additives in food.

indirect food additive A substance that is expected to unintentionally enter food during manufacturing or from packaging. Indirect food additives are regulated by the FDA.

Regulating food additives

Food additives improve food quality and help protect us from disease, but if the wrong additive is used or the wrong amount is added, it could do more harm than good. A manufacturer that wants to use a new food additive must submit to the FDA a petition that describes the chemical composition of the additive, how it is manufactured, and how it is detected in food. The manufacturer must prove that the additive will be effective for its intended purpose at the proposed levels, that it is safe for its intended use, and that its use is necessary. Additives may not be used to disguise inferior products or deceive consumers. They cannot be used if they significantly destroy nutrients or if the same effect can be achieved through sound manufacturing processes.

More than 600 chemicals defined as food additives were already in common use when legislation regulating food additives was passed. To accommodate substances that the FDA or the USDA had already determined to be safe, they were designated as **prior-sanctioned** substances and are exempt from regulation. The nitrates and nitrites used to retard the growth of *Clostridium botulinum* in cured meats are prior-sanctioned substances, for instance. However, their use has been controversial because they form carcinogenic **nitrosamines** in the digestive tract. They are still allowed in foods, however, because they prevent botulism, and there is little evidence that they pose a serious risk in the amounts consumed in the human diet (**Figure 13.19**).[40]

A second category that is not subject to food additive regulation consists of substances **generally recognized as safe (GRAS)**, based either on their history of use in food before 1958 or on published scientific evidence. However, just because a substance is on the GRAS or prior-sanctioned list doesn't mean that it is safe or that it will stay on these

generally recognized as safe (GRAS) A group of chemical additives that are considered safe, based on their long-standing presence in the food supply without harmful effects.

lists. If new evidence suggests that a substance in either category is unsafe, the FDA may take action to require that the substance be removed from food products.

Substances that are toxic at some level of consumption may be harmless at a lower level. To ensure that additives are safe, most of those that are allowed in foods can be added only at levels 100 times below the highest level that has been shown to have no harmful effects. This is a greater margin of safety than exists for many vitamins and other naturally occurring substances.

Type of additive	What's on the label	What they do	Where they are used
Preservatives	Ascorbic acid, citric acid, sodium benzoate, calcium propionate, sodium erythorbate, sodium nitrite, calcium sorbate potassium sorbate, BHA, BHT, EDTA, tocopherols	Maintain freshness; prevent spoilage caused by bacteria, molds, fungi, or yeast; slow or prevent changes in color, flavor, or texture; and delay rancidity	Jellies, beverages, baked goods, cured meats, oils and margarines, cereals, dressings, snack foods, fruits and vegetables
Sweeteners	Sucrose, glucose, fructose, sorbitol, mannitol, corn syrup, high-fructose corn syrup, saccharin, aspartame, sucralose, acesulfame potassium (acesulfame-K), neotame	Add sweetness with or without extra calories	Beverages, baked goods, table-top sweeteners, many processed foods
Color additives	FD&C blue nos. 1 and 2, FD&C green no. 3, FD&C red nos. 3 and 40, FD&C yellow nos. 5 and 6, orange B, citrus red no. 2, annatto extract, beta-carotene, grape skin extract, cochineal extract or carmine, paprika oleoresin, caramel color, fruit and vegetable juices, saffron, colorings or color added	Prevent color loss due to exposure to light, air, temperature extremes and moisture; enhance colors; give color to colorless and "fun" foods	Processed foods, candies, snack foods, margarine, cheese, soft drinks, jellies, puddings, and pie fillings
Flavors, spices, and flavor enhancers	Natural flavoring, artificial flavor, spices, monosodium glutamate (MSG), hydrolyzed soy protein, autolyzed yeast extract, disodium guanylate or inosinate	Add specific flavors or enhance flavors already present in foods	Many processed foods, puddings and pie fillings, gelatin mixes, cake mixes, salad dressings, candies, soft drinks, ice cream, BBQ sauce
Nutrients	Thiamine hydrochloride, riboflavin (vitamin B_2), niacin, niacinamide, folate or folic acid, beta-carotene, potassium iodide, iron or ferrous sulfate, alpha-tocopherols, ascorbic acid, vitamin D, amino acids (L-tryptophan, L-lysine, L-leucine, L-methionine)	Replace vitamins and minerals lost in processing; add nutrients that may be lacking in the diet	Flour, breads, cereals, rice, pasta, margarine, salt, milk, fruit beverages, energy bars, instant breakfast drinks
Emulsifiers	Soy lecithin, mono- and diglycerides, egg yolks, polysorbates, sorbitan monostearate	Allow smooth mixing and prevent separation; reduce stickiness; control crystallization; keep ingredients dispersed	Salad dressings, peanut butter, chocolate, margarine, frozen desserts
Stabilizers and thickeners, binders, and texturizers	Gelatin, pectin, guar gum, carrageenan, xanthan gum, whey	Produce uniform texture, improve "mouth-feel"	Frozen desserts, dairy products, cakes, pudding and gelatin mixes, dressings, jams and jellies, sauces
pH control agents and acidulants	Lactic acid, citric acid, ammonium hydroxide, sodium carbonate	Control acidity and alkalinity, prevent spoilage	Beverages, frozen desserts, chocolate, low-acid canned foods, baking powder
Leavening agents	Baking soda, monocalcium phosphate, calcium carbonate	Promote rising of baked goods	Breads and other baked goods
Anti-caking agents	Calcium silicate, iron ammonium citrate, silicon dioxide	Keep powdered foods free-flowing, prevent moisture absorption	Salt, baking powder, confectioners' sugar
Humectants	Glycerin, sorbitol	Retain moisture	Shredded coconut, marshmallows, soft candies, confections

The regulations for substances that cause cancer are far more rigid because of the **Delaney Clause**, part of the 1958 Food Additives Amendment. It states that a substance that induces cancer in either an animal species or humans, at any dosage, may not be added to food. Debate continues regarding whether the Delaney Clause should be liberalized to allow the use of substances that are added at a level so low that they would not represent a significant health risk.

Identifying food additives Food additives are used to make food safer; maintain palatability and wholesomeness; improve color, flavor, or texture; aid in processing; and enhance nutritional value (**Table 13.6**). Their use ensures the availability of wholesome, appetizing, and affordable foods that meet consumer demands throughout the year. The FDA's database *Everything Added to Food in the United States* lists more than 3000 additives.[42] Many of these, such as sugar and spices, are used in homes every day. Other additives may sound like a chemical soup: calcium propionate in bread, disodium EDTA in kidney beans, and BHA in potato chips. Understanding what these chemicals are used for can help make the ingredient list a source of information rather than a cause for concern.

Sensitivities to additives Some individuals are allergic or sensitive to certain food additives. For example, the flavor enhancer monosodium glutamate (MSG), commonly used in Chinese food, can cause adverse reactions known as *MSG symptom complex* or *Chinese restaurant syndrome* in sensitive individuals (see Chapter 6). Sulfites can cause symptoms ranging from stomachache and hives to severe asthma. Sulfites are used as preservatives in baked goods, canned foods, condiments, and dried fruits. Sensitive individuals can identify foods that contain sulfites by checking food labels. The forms of sulfites allowed in packaged foods include sulfur dioxide, sodium sulfite, sodium and potassium bisulfite, and sodium and potassium metabisulfite. Foods served in restaurants may also contain sulfites. For example, a potato dish served in a restaurant may be prepared using potatoes that were peeled and soaked in a sulfite solution before cooking.

Color additives can also cause adverse reactions. FD&C yellow no. 5, for instance, listed as tartrazine on medicine labels, may cause itching and hives in sensitive people. It is found in beverages, desserts, and processed vegetables. Color additives are listed in the ingredient list along with other food additives. Colors in foods are classified as certified or exempt. Certified colors are human-made, meet strict specifications for purity, and must be listed by name in the ingredient list. Colors that are exempt from certification include pigments from natural sources such as dehydrated beets and carotenoids; these may be listed collectively in the ingredient list as "artificial color."

CONCEPT CHECK STOP

1. **What** is pasteurization?
2. **How** does irradiation help extend the shelf life of food?
3. **How** does modified atmosphere packaging prevent food spoilage?
4. **Why** are food additives regulated?

13.5 Biotechnology

LEARNING OBJECTIVES

1. **Explain** how genetic engineering introduces new traits into plants.
2. **List** ways in which genetic engineering is being used to enhance the food supply.
3. **Discuss** some potential risks associated with genetic engineering.
4. **Describe** how genetically modified foods and crops are regulated to ensure safety.

Biotechnology alters the characteristics of organisms by making selective changes in their DNA. The concept is not new. For centuries, farmers have selected seeds from plants with the most desirable characteristics to plant for the next year's crop, bred the animals that grew fastest or produced the most milk to improve the productivity of the next generation of animals, and

biotechnology The process of manipulating life forms via genetic engineering in order to provide desirable products for human use.

Engineering a genetically modified plant • Figure 13.20

✓ THE PLANNER

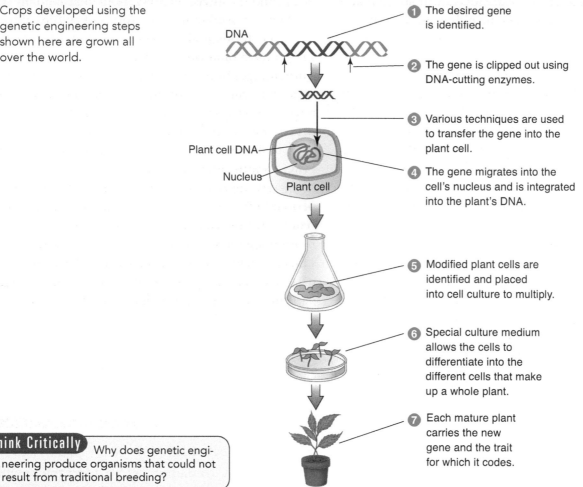

Crops developed using the genetic engineering steps shown here are grown all over the world.

DNA

Plant cell DNA

Nucleus

Plant cell

1 The desired gene is identified.

2 The gene is clipped out using DNA-cutting enzymes.

3 Various techniques are used to transfer the gene into the plant cell.

4 The gene migrates into the cell's nucleus and is integrated into the plant's DNA.

5 Modified plant cells are identified and placed into cell culture to multiply.

6 Special culture medium allows the cells to differentiate into the different cells that make up a whole plant.

7 Each mature plant carries the new gene and the trait for which it codes.

Think Critically Why does genetic engineering produce organisms that could not result from traditional breeding?

---

crossbred plant varieties to combine the desired traits of each. However, these traditional methods may require many generations to produce the desired results. Biotechnology uses **genetic engineering** or **genetic modification (GM)** to select genes for specific traits. Genetic engineering has significantly sped up the process of modifying the traits of organisms. Like all other new technologies, however, it may introduce new risks.

> **genetic engineering or genetic modification (GM)** A set of techniques used to manipulate DNA for the purpose of changing the characteristics of an organism or creating a new product.

How Biotechnology Works

Genetically modified organisms (GMOs) are created through genetic engineering. To modify a plant such as corn, a piece of DNA containing the gene for a desired characteristic is taken from plant, animal, or bacterial cells and transferred to corn plant cells (**Figure 13.20**). The DNA is then referred to as **recombinant DNA** because the new DNA is a combination of the DNA from two organisms. The modified corn cells are then allowed to divide into more and more cells and eventually differentiate into the various types of cells that make up a whole corn plant. The new plant is a **transgenic** organism. Each cell in the new plant contains the transferred gene for the desired trait. This technique is used to introduce characteristics such as disease and drought resistance into plants. Genetic engineering is more difficult in animals because animal cells do not take up genes as easily as plant cells do,

> **recombinant DNA** DNA that has been formed by joining DNA from different sources.
>
> **transgenic** An organism with a gene or group of genes intentionally transferred from another species or breed.

and making copies of these cells (clones) is also more difficult. However, these techniques have been used to produce cows that yield more milk, cattle and pigs that have more meat on them, and sheep that grow more wool.[43]

Applications of Biotechnology

The techniques of biotechnology can be used in a variety of ways in food production to alter quantity, quality, cost, safety, and shelf life. By making plants resistant to herbicides, insects, and various plant diseases, this technology has increased crop yields and reduced damage from insects and plant diseases (**Figure 13.21a** and **b**). By altering enzyme activity and other traits, biotechnology is being used to increase the shelf life of fresh fruits and vegetables and create products that have greater consumer appeal, such as seedless grapes and watermelons.

Biotechnology is also used in food processing. For example, many foods are produced with the help of enzymes. Rennet, an enzyme used in cheese production; enzymes used in the production of high-fructose corn syrup; and the enzyme lactase, used to reduce the lactose content of milk, are now all produced by GM microbes.

Biotechnology also has great potential for addressing the problem of world hunger and malnutrition. Although world hunger is rooted in political, economic, and cultural issues that cannot be resolved by agricultural technology alone, GM crops that target some of the major nutritional deficiencies worldwide are being developed. To address protein deficiency, varieties of corn, soybeans, and sweet potatoes with enhanced levels of essential amino acids are being developed. To address vitamin A deficiency, genes that code for the production of enzymes needed for the synthesis of the vitamin A precursor ß-carotene have been inserted into rice (**Figure 13.21c**).[44] To address multiple nutrient deficiencies, the BioCassava Plus program has used biotechnology to develop cassava with increased zinc, iron, protein, and vitamin A levels.[45]

Nutrition InSight — The potential of biotechnology • Figure 13.21

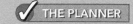 THE PLANNER

Biotechnology has led to the creation of insect-resistant corn, virus-resistant papayas, and rice that is a source of ß-carotene.

a. Insect-resistant corn is created by inserting a gene from the bacterium *Bacillus thuringiensis* (or Bt). The gene produces a protein called Bt toxin that is toxic to certain insects, such as this European corn borer, but safe for humans and other animals. The presence of the new gene improves the crop yield and also reduces the amounts of chemical pesticides that need to be applied.

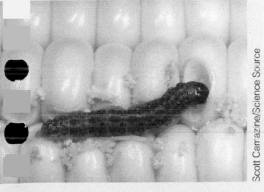

Scott Camazine/Science Source

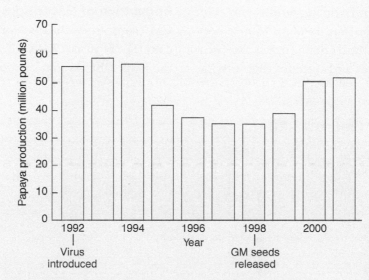

b. In the 1990s, the papaya crop in Hawaii was severely diminished by the papaya ring-spot virus (PRSV). In response, researchers developed papaya that is genetically modified to resist PRSV. The seeds were released for commercialization in 1998, allowing Hawaiian papaya production to rebound.[46] This was the first genetically enhanced fruit crop on the market. Genes for resistance to various viruses have also been used to create virus-resistant strains of potatoes, squash, cucumbers, and watermelons. [47]

c. Half the world's population depends on rice as a dietary staple, but rice is a poor source of vitamin A. Genetically modified rice, called Golden Rice (seen here compared with white rice) for the color imparted by the ß-carotene pigment, has the potential to significantly increase vitamin A intake (discussed further in Chapter 14 *Debate*). One variety contains enough provitamin A in 1 cup of cooked rice to meet the needs of a child.[48]

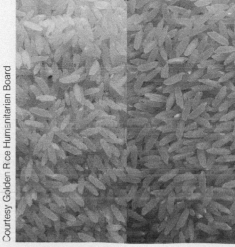

Courtesy Golden Rice Humanitarian Board

Risks and Regulation of Biotechnology

The rapid advancement of biotechnology during the past decade has created the potential for health problems and environmental damage. Regulations are in place to control the use of genetic engineering and GMOs. Despite these precautions, many consumers and scientists believe that the impact of this booming technology has not yet become apparent. They urge that this technology be used with caution to avoid health or environmental impacts that outweigh the benefits.

Consumer concerns Consumer safety concerns related to GM foods include the possibility that the nutrient content of a food may have been negatively affected or that an allergen or a toxin may have inadvertently been introduced into a food that was previously safe. For example, if DNA from fish or nuts—foods that commonly cause allergic reactions—were introduced into soybeans or corn, these foods would then be dangerous to individuals allergic to fish or nuts. To prevent this kind of situation from occurring unintentionally, biotechnology companies have established systems for monitoring the allergenic potential of proteins used for plant genetic engineering. In 1996, allergy testing successfully prevented soybeans containing a gene from a Brazil nut from entering the market.[49]

Environmental concerns An environmental concern about GM crops is that they will be used to the exclusion of other varieties, thereby reducing biodiversity. The ability of populations of organisms to adapt to new conditions, diseases, or other hazards depends on the presence of many different species and varieties that provide a diversity of genes. If farmers plant only GM insect-resistant, high-yielding crops, other species and varieties may eventually become extinct, and the genes for the traits they possess may be lost forever.

Another environmental issue is the possibility that GM crops will create "superweeds." This might occur, for example, if a trait such as increased rate of growth introduced into a domesticated plant species were passed on to a related wild species. This could produce a fast-growing weed, or superweed, that would compete with the domesticated species. As a safeguard, plant developers are avoiding introducing genes for traits that could increase a plant's competitiveness or other undesirable properties in weedy relatives.

There is also concern that crops that have been engineered to produce pesticides will promote the evolution of pesticide-resistant insects. An illustration is the case of insects that feed on plants modified to produce the Bt toxin (see Figure 13.21a). As more and more of the insects' food supply consists of plants that produce this pesticide, only insects that carry genes that make them resistant to Bt toxin survive and reproduce. This increases the number of Bt-resistant insects and therefore reduces the effectiveness of Bt toxin as a method of pest control. Although an important concern when growing GM crops, pesticide-resistant insects may also evolve when pesticides are sprayed on crops.

Regulation of GM food products The most common GM crops are soybeans, corn, cotton, and rapeseed (or canola) (**Figure 13.22**). Therefore, foods produced in the United States that contain corn or high-fructose corn

---

Growth of GM crops • Figure 13.22

Despite concerns about the impact of GM crops, the number of acres planted with them worldwide has risen steadily.[50]

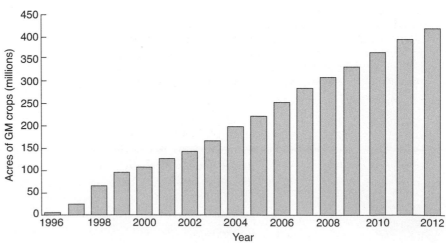

syrup, such as many breakfast cereals, snack foods, and soft drinks; foods made with soybeans; and foods made with cottonseed and canola oils are likely to contain GM ingredients. You don't recognize these foods as genetically modified because they appear no different from other foods, and food manufacturers are not required to provide special labeling unless the food is known to pose a potential risk.

To ensure that GMOs cause no harm to consumers or to the environment, the FDA, the USDA, and the EPA are all involved in overseeing plant biotechnology. Safety and environmental issues are monitored at all stages of the process. The FDA regulates the safety and labeling of foods containing GM ingredients. Labeling of foods containing GM ingredients is required only if the nutritional composition of the food has been altered; if it contains potentially harmful allergens, toxins, pesticides, or herbicides; if it contains ingredients that are new to the food supply; or if it has been changed significantly enough that its traditional name no longer applies. Premarket approval is required when the new food contains a substance that is not commonly found in foods or when it contains a substance that does not have a history of safe use in foods. To prevent material from a new plant variety intended for food use from inadvertently entering the food supply before its safety has been established, the FDA has asked developers to provide information about the safety of the new plants at a relatively early stage of development.[51]

The USDA regulates agricultural products and research concerning the development of new plant varieties, including those developed through genetic engineering. The EPA regulates any pesticides that may be present in foods and sets tolerances for these pesticides. This includes GM plants containing proteins that protect them from insects or disease.

CONCEPT CHECK STOP

1. **Where** does the DNA introduced into GMOs come from?

2. **How** does biotechnology increase crop yields?

3. **Why** might a GM food cause an allergic reaction when the unmodified food does not?

4. **What** types of GM foods carry special labels?

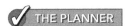 THE PLANNER

Summary

1 Keeping Food Safe 438

- Most **food-borne illness** is caused by food contaminated with disease-causing **microbes**; occasionally, it can be caused by chemical contaminants in food. The harm caused by contaminants in the food supply depends on the type of toxin, dose, length of time over which the contaminant is consumed, how it is metabolized and excreted, and the size, age, and health of the consumer.

- The food supply is monitored for safety by food manufacturers and regulatory agencies at the international, federal, state, and local levels. Federal programs promote the use of **Hazard Analysis Critical Control Point (HACCP)** systems, which monitor critical limits such as the time and temperature shown here, to prevent and eliminate food contamination rather than catch it after it occurs. Consumers can prevent most cases of food-borne illness by following safe food-handling and preparation guidelines.

HACCP in liquid egg production • Figure 13.2

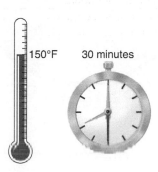

150°F   30 minutes

2 Pathogens in Food 442

- The **pathogens** that affect the food supply include bacteria, viruses, molds, parasites, and prions. Some bacteria cause **food-borne infection** because they are able to grow in the gastrointestinal tract when ingested. Others produce toxins in food, and consumption of the toxin causes **food-borne intoxication.**

- Viruses do not grow on food, but when consumed in food, they can reproduce in human cells and cause food-borne illness.

- **Molds** that grow on foods produce toxins that can harm consumers.

- **Parasites** include microscopic single-celled animals, as well as worms that can be seen with the naked eye. They are consumed in contaminated water or food.

- Improperly folded **prion** proteins cause **bovine spongiform encephalopathy (BSE)** in cattle. The risk of acquiring the human form of this deadly degenerative neurological disease is extremely low.

- The risk of food-borne illness can be decreased through proper food selection, preparation, and storage to kill pathogens or minimize their growth. These steps are emphasized by the Fight Bac! Campaign, illustrated here.

**Safe food handling, storage, and preparation •
Figure 13.9**

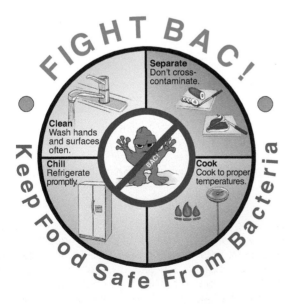

3 Agricultural and Industrial Chemicals in Food 453

- Contaminants in the environment can find their way into the food supply. Those that deposit in the fatty tissue of animals are not eliminated, leading to **bioaccumulation** as they pass through the food chain, as illustrated here.

**Contamination throughout the food chain •
Figure 13.10**

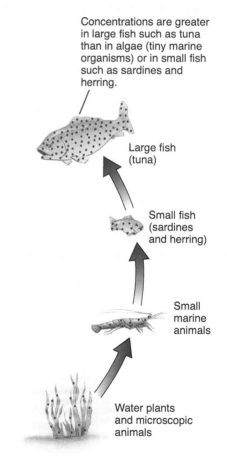

Concentrations are greater in large fish such as tuna than in algae (tiny marine organisms) or in small fish such as sardines and herring.

Large fish (tuna)

Small fish (sardines and herring)

Small marine animals

Water plants and microscopic animals

- Pesticides help increase crop yields and the quality of produce. To decrease the risk of pesticide toxicity, **tolerances** are established, and foods are monitored for pesticide residues. Safer pesticides are being developed, and U.S. farmers are reducing the amounts applied by using **integrated pest management (IPM)** and **organic food** production methods.

- Industrial pollutants such as **PCBs** have contaminated some waterways and the fish and shellfish that live in them. Larger, longer-lived fish and those that live in contaminated waters have the highest concentrations.

- Antibiotics and hormones are used in animal food production. The amounts entering the food supply pose little risk, but the overuse of antibiotics contributes to the development of antibiotic-resistant strains of bacteria. Changes are underway to reduce the treatment of animals with antibiotics for growth enhancement.

- Consumers can reduce the amounts of pesticides and other environmental contaminants in food by carefully selecting and handling produce, selecting saltwater varieties of fish caught far offshore in unpolluted waters, and trimming fat from meat, poultry, and fish before cooking.

4 Technology for Keeping Food Safe 459

- Heating foods to high temperatures, cooling them to low temperatures, and altering levels of acidity, moisture, and oxygen prevent food spoilage and lengthen shelf life by killing microbes or slowing their growth.

- **Irradiation** preserves food by exposing it to radiation. This process kills microbes, destroys insects, and slows the germination and ripening of fruits and vegetables. Irradiated foods can be identified by the symbol shown here.

Irradiated foods •Figure 13.17a

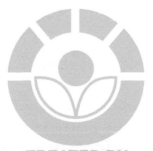

TREATED BY IRRADIATION

- Packaging keeps molds and bacteria out of foods, keeps moisture in, and protects food from physical damage. Vacuum packaging and **modified atmosphere packaging (MAP)** reduce the oxygen available for microbial growth. The safety of packaging materials must be considered because components of packaging can leach into food.

- **Direct food additives** are used to preserve or enhance the appeal of food. **Indirect food additives** are substances known to find their way into food during cooking, processing, and packaging. Both are FDA regulated. **Accidental contaminants**, which enter food when it is handled or prepared incorrectly, are not regulated by the FDA.

5 Biotechnology 465

- **Biotechnology** produces **genetically modified organisms (GMOs)** by transferring a gene for a desired characteristic from one organism to another, as shown here. The result is a **transgenic** organism.

Engineering a genetically modified plant • Figure 13.20

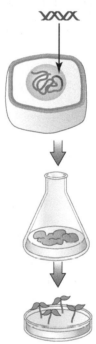

- Biotechnology has the potential to improve the volume, safety, and quality of the food supply, but it also has the potential to introduce allergens or toxins into foods or to negatively affect nutrient content. Environmental concerns about the use of GMOs include reduction of biologic diversity, creation of "superweeds," and evolution of pesticide-resistant insects. Regulations are in place to control the use of genetic engineering and GMOs.

Key Terms

- accidental contaminant 460
- acrylamide 461
- aseptic processing 460
- bioaccumulation 453
- biotechnology 465
- botulism 444
- bovine somatotropin (bST) 457
- bovine spongiform encephalopathy (BSE) 447
- critical control point 440
- cross-contamination 449
- Delaney Clause 465
- direct food additive 462
- food additive 460
- food-borne illness 438
- food-borne infection 442
- food-borne intoxication 442

- generally recognized as safe (GRAS) 463
- genetic engineering or genetic modification (GM) 466
- Hazard Analysis Critical Control Point (HACCP) 440
- hemolytic-uremic syndrome 442
- heterocyclic amines (HCAs) 460
- indirect food additive 463
- infant botulism 445
- integrated pest management (IPM) 454
- irradiation 461
- microbes 438
- modified atmosphere packaging (MAP) 462
- mold 446
- nitrosamine 463

- organic food 454
- parasite 446
- pasteurization 460
- pathogen 442
- polychlorinated biphenyls (PCBs) 456
- polycyclic aromatic hydrocarbons (PAHs) 460
- prion 447
- prior-sanctioned substance 463
- recombinant DNA 466
- spore 444
- tolerance 454
- transgenic 466
- variant Creutzfeldt-Jakob Disease (vCJD) 447

What is happening in this picture?

The non-GMO label on this bag of popcorn indicates that it does not contain any genetically modified ingredients. Whether GMO-labeling is voluntary or mandatory, designing an appropriate label is a complex issue. Simple labels such as this one may imply that the product is better than other products. However, a more detailed label that describes how a particular product was modified would be too lengthy and would not be understood by many consumers.

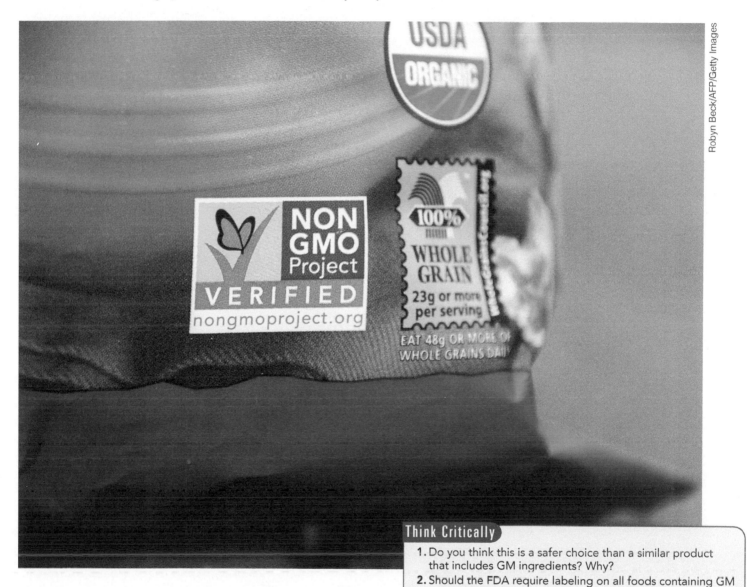

Robyn Beck/AFP/Getty Images

Think Critically

1. Do you think this is a safer choice than a similar product that includes GM ingredients? Why?
2. Should the FDA require labeling on all foods containing GM ingredients?
3. Why might food companies oppose this type of labeling?

THE PLANNER ✓

Review your Chapter Planner on the chapter opener and check off your completed work.

Feeding the World

Fantasists often consider how growing populations will face a world of limited food supplies. In the 1966 novel *Make Room! Make Room!*, New York City's 35 million people subsist on seaweed, oatmeal, rationed water, and soy; meat is a rarity, illegally procured from "meatleggers." In the 1999 film *The Matrix*, a character betrays his comrades for a *virtual* steak dinner.

The 1990s are history, along with the rest of the 20th century, and one may argue that we are not in the dire straits anticipated by these fantasies. Even though disaster has been averted thus far, the production, distribution, safety, consumption, and sustainability of the world's food and water resources remain matters of great concern to all. A large part of the world's population faces

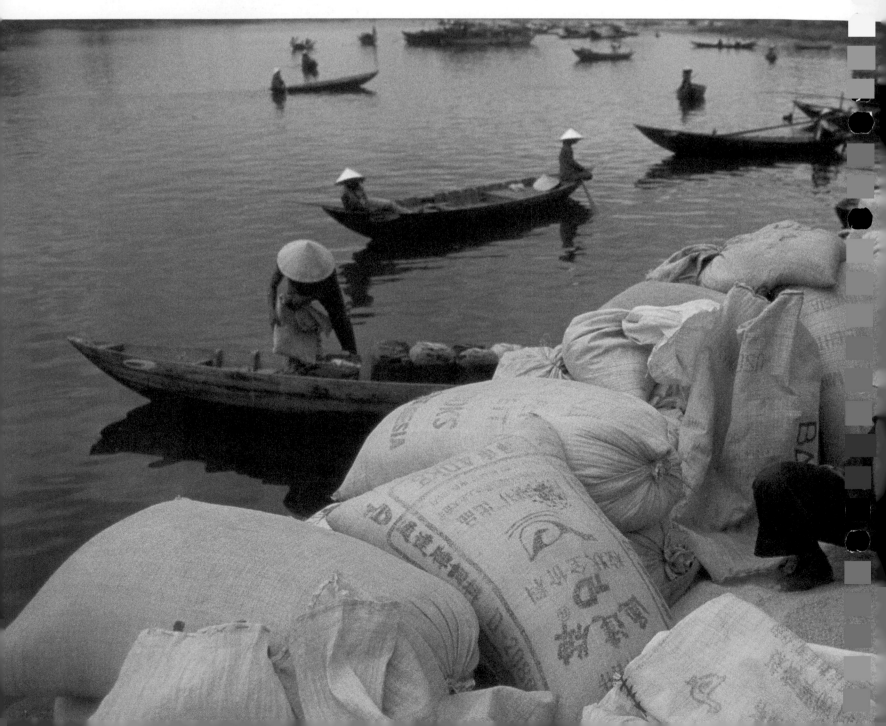

undernutrition and starvation on a daily basis, leading to a plethora of public health issues. Another portion faces problems caused by too rich a diet, leading to overnutrition, obesity, and a different—but equally dangerous and costly—set of public health issues.

Governments have historically concerned themselves with adequate food production and distribution for burgeoning populations, but individual self-interest has often defeated more altruistic—and sensible—nutrition objectives. Global and national economic and political interests may alleviate or exacerbate world nutrition conditions.

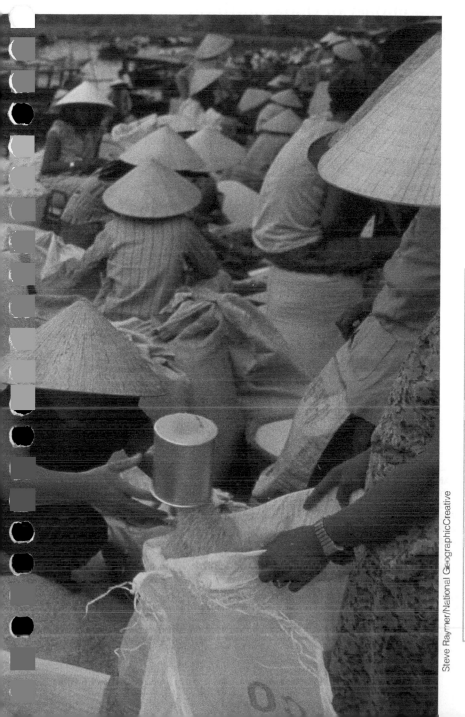

Steve Raymer/National GeographicCreative

As countries develop economically, they face many of the problems that are common in industrialized countries, including nutrition-related noncommunicable diseases (NCDs) such as obesity, diabetes, heart disease, and cancer.[10, 12]

a. This schematic represents the dietary changes that occur with nutrition transition and the health consequences associated with these changes.[13] The traditional rural diet is often inadequate in energy, protein, or micronutrients. The affluent Western diet meets nutrient needs but is high in fat and sugar and low in fiber. A diet that falls somewhere between these extremes is optimal for health.

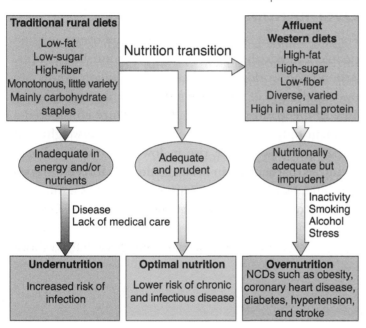

b. This graph shows the percentage of the total years of productive life that were lost due to NCDs in low-, middle-, and high-income countries in 2008 and the percentage projected by 2030.[12]

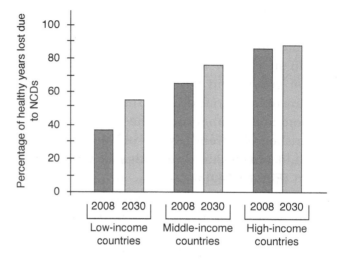

Interpret the Data

Comparing 2008 and 2030 projections, in which income group is the increase in lost healthy years due to NCDs greatest?

obesity increases the risk of cardiovascular disease, hypertension, stroke, type 2 diabetes, certain cancers, and arthritis, among other conditions, it is a major contributor to the global burden of chronic disease and disability

The prevalence of overweight and obesity is also growing among children worldwide. According to recent estimates, more than 40 million children under age 5 are overweight; more than 30 million of these children live in developing countries.[9] In some countries, a high prevalence of overweight children now exists alongside a high prevalence of undernourished children. Overweight and obese children are likely to stay obese into adulthood and are more likely to develop diseases such as diabetes and cardiovascular diseases at a younger age.

Why Do Undernutrition and Overnutrition Exist Side by Side?

We see the problems of undernutrition and overnutrition existing side by side because diets and lifestyles change as economic conditions improve. Traditional diets in developing countries are based on a limited number of foods—primarily starchy grains and root vegetables. As incomes increase and food availability improves, the diet becomes more varied, and energy intake increases with the addition of meat, milk, and other more calorie-dense foods. Along with these dietary changes, there is a decrease in activity due to occupations that are less physically demanding, greater access to transportation, more labor-saving technology, and more passive leisure time (**Figure 14.2a**).

Some of the effects of this **nutrition transition** are positive: Life expectancy increases, and the frequencies of low birth weight, stunting, infectious diseases, and nutrient deficiencies decrease. However, at the same time, rates of heart disease, cancer, diabetes, obesity, and childhood obesity increase (**Figure 14.2b**).[10] Transition to a diet high in animal protein and refined foods also increases the use of natural resources and in the long term may deplete nonrenewable resources.

nutrition transition A series of changes in diet, physical activity, health, and nutrition that occur as poor countries become more prosperous.

1. **How** prevalent are undernutrition and overnutrition around the world?

2. **What** is the impact of stunting on the health and productivity of a population?

3. **How** does nutrition transition affect a population's health?

14.2 Causes of Hunger Around the World

LEARNING OBJECTIVES

1. **Explain** the concept of food insecurity.

2. **Discuss** the factors that cause food shortages for populations and individuals.

3. **Describe** the consequences of three nutrient deficiencies that are common worldwide.

The specific reasons for hunger and **food insecurity** vary with time and location, but the underlying cause is that the available food is not distributed equitably. This inequitable distribution results in either a shortage of food or the wrong combination of foods to meet nutrient needs. This situation, in turn, results in protein–energy malnutrition and individual nutrient deficiencies.

food insecurity A situation in which people lack adequate physical, social, or economic access to sufficient, safe, nutritious food that meets their dietary needs and food preferences for an active and healthy life.

famine A widespread lack of access to food due to a disaster that causes a collapse in food production and marketing systems.

natural causes of famines. Human causes include wars and civil conflicts (**Figure 14.3**).

Food shortages due to famine are very visible because they cause many deaths in an area during a short period, but chronic food shortages take a greater toll. Chronic shortages occur when economic inequities result in lack of money, health care, and education for individuals or populations; when the population outgrows the food supply; when cultural and religious practices limit food choices; or when environmental damage limits the amount of food that can be produced.

Food Shortages

The most obvious example of a food shortage is **famine**. Drought, floods, earthquakes, and crop destruction due to diseases or pests are

Poverty   Twenty-one percent of people around the world live below the international

Famine • Figure 14.3

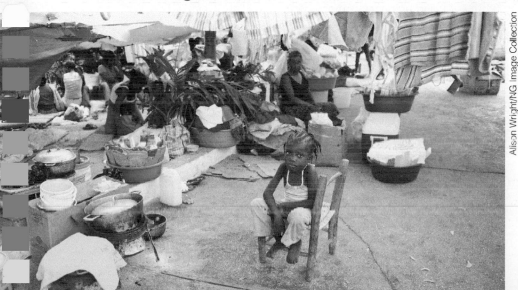

Alison Wright/NG Image Collection

Many survivors of the earthquakes in Haiti live in makeshift camps such as this one. This natural disaster destroyed the infrastructure that once distributed food throughout the country. Regions that have barely enough food to survive under normal conditions are vulnerable to famine. This situation is analogous to a man standing in water up to his nostrils: If all is calm, he can breathe, but if there is a ripple, he will drown. A ripple such as a natural or civil disaster reduces the margin of survival and creates famine.

The impact of poverty •

Figure 14.4

Poverty increases undernutrition not only by limiting the availability of food but also by reducing access to health care and education.

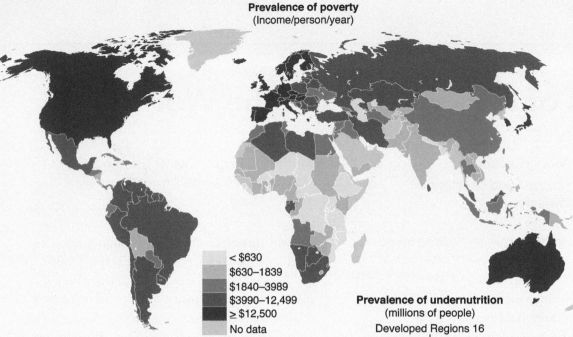

Prevalence of poverty
(Income/person/year)

< $630
$630–1839
$1840–3989
$3990–12,499
≥ $12,500
No data

The regions of the world where poverty is the most prevalent (see map) correspond to the regions where there are the greatest number of undernourished people (see chart). Developing countries, where one in four people subsists on less than $1.25 a day, account for 98% of the world's undernourished people.[1,14] In wealthy countries, hungry people can usually obtain help to get food or money to buy food, but in poor countries, a family that cannot grow enough food or earn enough money to buy food may have nowhere to turn for help.

Clinics, such as this one in Ghana, are not accessible to many people in the developing world. Lack of immunizations and treatment for infections and other illnesses results in an increase in infectious disease and a decrease in survival rates from chronic diseases such as cancer. Lack of health care also increases infant mortality and the incidence of low-birth-weight births.

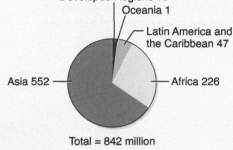

Prevalence of undernutrition
(millions of people)
Developed Regions 16
Oceania 1
Latin America and the Caribbean 47
Asia 552
Africa 226

Total = 842 million

Interpret the Data

What percentage of the world's undernourished people live in Africa?
a. 26.8%   c. 62.5%
b. 50%   d. 4%

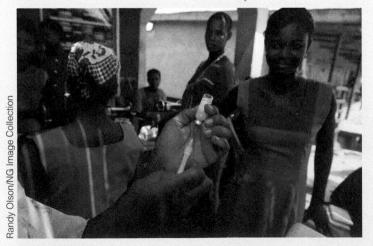

Randy Olson/NG Image Collection

Ask Yourself

How can lack of health care increase the incidence of undernutrition?

These young Indonesian girls are working in a textile factory rather than going to school. Lack of education prevents people from escaping poverty and contributes to undernutrition and disease because it leads to inadequate care for infants, children, and pregnant women. ▼

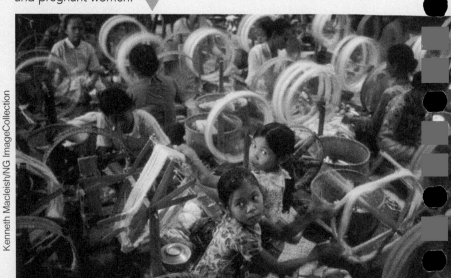

Kenneth Macleish/NG ImageCollection

poverty line, earning less than $1.25 per day.[14] Poverty is central to the problem of hunger and undernutrition (**Figure 14.4**). In addition to creating food insecurity, poverty reduces access to health care, increasing the prevalence of disease and disability. When diseases go untreated, nutrient needs are increased, a situation that further limits the ability to obtain an adequate diet and contributes to malnutrition. Those who are poor also have less access to education, and this lack of access contributes to undernutrition and disease and reduces opportunities to escape poverty. Lack of education about food preparation and storage can affect food safety and the health of the household: Unsanitary food preparation increases the incidence of gastrointestinal diseases, which contribute to malnutrition.

Overpopulation Overpopulation exists when a region has more people than its natural resources can support. A fertile river valley can support more people per acre than can a desert environment. But even in fertile regions of the world, if the number of people increases excessively, resources are overwhelmed, and food shortages occur. At present, enough food is produced throughout the world to prevent hunger if that food is distributed equitably, but demand is rising. The human population is currently growing at a rate of more than 86 million persons per year (**Figure 14.5**).[15] This rate of growth could eventually outstrip the planet's ability to produce enough food to nourish the world's population.

In addition to overpopulation, food production methods and the search for new energy sources are affecting our ability to feed the world's population. For example, more grain-intensive livestock production and the recent acceleration in the use of grain to produce ethanol to fuel cars, have increased the demand for grain.[16] The increased demand has contributed to dramatic increases in food prices, which have made it even more challenging for low- and middle-income families worldwide to obtain enough food. The rising price of grain and fuel oil has also reduced the amount of food aid, widening the gap between the amount of food available and the amount needed to meet nutritional needs.[17]

Cultural practices In some cultures, access to food may be limited for certain individuals in households. For example, because they are viewed as less important, women and girls may receive less food than men and boys. How much food is available to an individual within a

World population growth • Figure 14.5

About 90% of the world's population growth is occurring in less developed countries. Developing countries cannot escape poverty because their economies cannot keep pace with such rapid population growth. Efforts to produce enough food can damage the soil and deplete environmental resources, further reducing the capacity to produce food in the future.

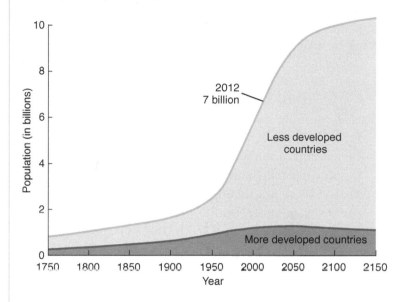

household depends on gender, control of income, education, age, birth order, and genetic endowments.

The cultural acceptability or unacceptability of foods also contributes to food shortages and undernutrition. If available foods are culturally unacceptable, a food shortage exists unless the population can be educated to accept the new food. For example, insects are eaten in some cultures and are an excellent source of protein, but in other cultures they are unacceptable as food.

Limited environmental resources The land and other resources available to produce food are limited. Some resources, such as minerals and fossil fuels, are present in finite amounts and are nonrenewable—that is, once they have been used, they cannot be replaced within a reasonable amount of time. Others, such as soil and water, are **renewable resources** because they will be available indefinitely if they are used at a rate at which the Earth can restore them. For example, when agricultural land is used wisely—that is, when crops are rotated, erosion is prevented, and contamination is limited—it

> **renewable resource** A resource that is restored and replaced by natural processes and can therefore be used forever.

Environmental impact on the oceans • Figure 14.6

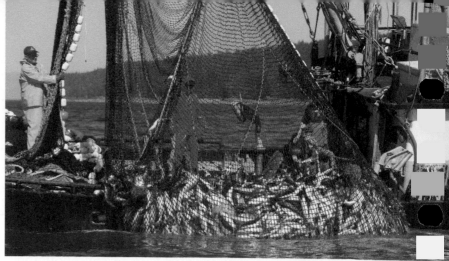

Overfishing has severely reduced the numbers of many marine species. Pollution also threatens the world's fishing grounds. Oil spills and deliberate dumping occur offshore, and sewage, pesticides, organic pollutants, and sediments from erosion wash into coastal waters, where most fish spend at least part of their lives. Even aquaculture, designed to increase fish production, produces wastes that can pollute ocean water and harm other marine organisms.

can be reused almost endlessly. However, if land is not used carefully, damage caused by soil erosion, nutrient depletion, and accumulation of pollutants may reduce the amount of usable land over the long term.

Modern mechanized agricultural methods have increased food production but use more energy and resources than more traditional labor-intensive farming. Large-scale farming can erode the soil and deplete its nutrients. Fertilizers and pesticides can contaminate groundwater and eventually pollute waterways. And if a product is shipped over long distances, requires refrigeration or freezing, or needs other types of processing, the environmental costs are increased even more.

As more countries undergo nutrition transition, the demand for meat-based diets will increase, as will the use of natural resources and energy. In general, the environmental cost of producing plant-based foods is lower than that of producing animal products.[18] Raising cattle creates both air and water pollution. The animals themselves produce methane, a greenhouse gas, in their gastrointestinal tracts. Large-scale "factory farming" makes the problem worse because more methane is produced when animal sewage is stored in ponds and heaps. In fact, livestock is responsible for a larger percentage of greenhouse gas emissions than all the cars in the world combined. Livestock production also accounts for over 8% of global human water use and releases nutrients, pathogens, and other pollutants into waterways.[19] It is not only the resources of the land that are at risk. Population growth has increased the demand for fish to the point that the earth's oceans are being depleted (**Figure 14.6**).

Poor-Quality Diets

Even when there is enough food, malnutrition can occur if the quality of the diet is poor. The typical diet in developing countries is based on high-fiber grain products or root vegetables and has little variety. Adults who are able to consume a relatively large amount of this diet may be able to meet their nutrient needs. But individuals with high nutrient needs because they are ill or pregnant and those with limited capacity to consume this bulky grain diet, such as children and elderly individuals, are at risk for nutrient deficiencies. Deficiencies of protein, iron, iodine, and vitamin A are common with poor-quality diets.[20] The images in **Figure 14.7** will help you recall these common deficiencies that were discussed in greater detail in earlier chapters.

Several other vitamin and mineral deficiencies have recently emerged or reemerged as problems throughout the world. Beriberi, pellagra, and scurvy—diseases caused by deficiencies of thiamin, niacin, and vitamin C, respectively—are rare in the developed world but still occur among extremely poor and underprivileged people and in large refugee populations.[20] In many parts of the world, folate deficiency causes macrocytic anemia during pregnancy and often compounds existing iron deficiency anemia. Deficiencies of vitamin B_6 and vitamin B_{12} are also associated with anemia. About a third of the world's population lives in countries with a high prevalence of zinc deficiency. Subclinical zinc deficiency is now recognized as a significant factor that may limit growth among children in both the developing and developed world.[21]

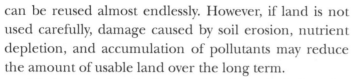

CONCEPT CHECK   STOP

1. **What** causes food insecurity?
2. **How** can environmental damage lead to food shortages?
3. **Why** do children develop protein and micronutrient deficiencies more often than adults?

Protein and micronutrient deficiencies • Figure 14.7

Deficiencies of protein and energy as well as vitamin A, iodine, and iron are common throughout the developing world.

Protein–energy malnutrition is most common in children. When there is a general lack of food, the wasting associated with *marasmus* results, and when the diet is limited to starchy grains and vegetables, *kwashiorkor*, characterized by a bloated belly, can predominate (see Chapter 6). Other factors, such as metabolic changes caused by infection, may also play a role in the development of kwashiorkor.

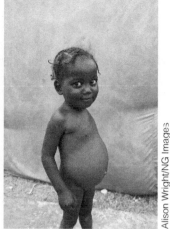

Think Critically Why are children who consume a starchy, low-protein diet less likely to meet their protein needs than adults consuming the same diet?

Marasmus

Kwashiorkor

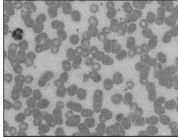

Normal red blood cells

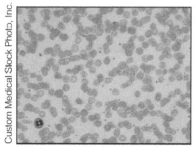

Iron deficiency anemia

More than 2 billion people worldwide suffer from iron deficiency anemia, which is characterized by small, pale red blood cells (see Chapter 8).[23] The lack of iron reduces the amount of hemoglobin produced, and the lack of hemoglobin lowers the blood's ability to deliver oxygen. In developing countries, intestinal parasites, which cause gastrointestinal blood loss, and acute and chronic infections, such as malaria, increase the risk and severity of dietary iron deficiency. Iron deficiency can have a major impact on the health and productivity of a population.

Although goiter, seen here, is a more visible manifestation of iodine deficiency, the subtle effects of deficiency on mental performance and work capacity may have a greater impact on the population as a whole. Iodine-deficient children have lower IQs and impaired school performance.[22] Iodine deficiency in children and adults is associated with apathy and decreased initiative and decision-making capabilities (see Chapter 8).

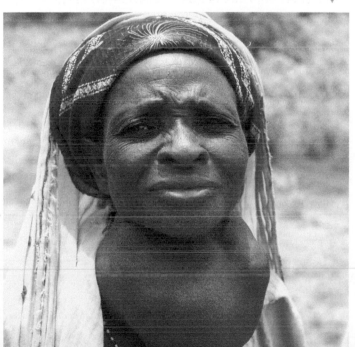

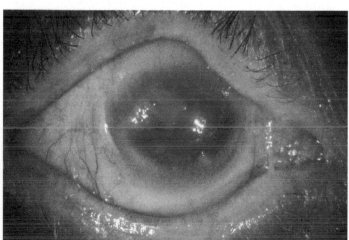

It is estimated that more than 250 million preschool children worldwide suffer from vitamin A deficiency.[24] Vitamin A deficiency leads to *xerophthalmia*, shown here. Vitamin A deficiency is the leading cause of preventable blindness among children. It also depresses immune function, thus increasing the risk of illness and death from infections, particularly measles and diarrheal disease (see Chapter 7).

Causes of Hunger in the United States

LEARNING OBJECTIVES

1. **Discuss** the causes of food insecurity in the United States.

2. **Describe** how lack of access to health care, education, and transportation prevent people from escaping poverty.

3. **List** the population groups that are at greatest risk for undernutrition in the United States.

Most of the nutritional problems in the United States are related to overnutrition. However, 14.5% of households in the United States experience food insecurity (**Figure 14.8**).[25] This situation is caused not by a general food shortage but by an inequitable distribution of food and money. The incidence of hunger and food insecurity is highest among women, infants, children, elderly individuals, and those who are poor, homeless, ill, or disabled. However, a sudden decrease in income or increase in living expenses can put anyone at risk for food insecurity.

Poverty and Food Insecurity

In the United States, as elsewhere in the world, poverty is the main cause of food insecurity. Poverty reduces access to food, education, and health care. Fifteen percent of Americans (46.5 million people) live at or below the poverty level.[26] These individuals have little money to spend on food and often have limited access to affordable food.

The high price of real estate in cities has driven supermarkets into the suburbs, and because many low-income city families do not own cars, they must shop at small, expensive corner stores or pay cab fares if they wish to take advantage of lower prices at more distant, larger stores. This has created areas referred to as **food deserts**. Food deserts also exist in rural and low-income communities where grocery stores may be great distances away. Lack of easy access to transportation and/or financial resources limits the ability to acquire affordable, healthy foods, and increases the risk of nutrient deficiencies and nutrition-related chronic diseases.[27]

food desert An area that lacks access to affordable fruits, vegetables, whole grains, low-fat milk, and other foods that make up a healthy diet.

Poverty also limits access to health care, leading to poorer health status. Iron deficiency is more than twice as frequent in low-income children as in children in

higher-income families, and the incidence of heart disease, cancer, hypertension, and obesity increases with decreasing income.[28] As in developing nations, poverty is reflected in infant mortality rates. The average infant mortality in the U.S. population is about 6.14 per 1000 live births.[29] However, there are groups within the population that have infant mortality rates as high as those in impoverished nations. Among African Americans, the infant mortality rate is 11.46 per 1000 live births—almost twice that of the general population. This difference may reflect differences in infant mortality risk factors, such as poverty and lack of access to medical care.

Lack of education, which is both a cause and a consequence of poverty, also contributes to food insecurity. For people at or below the poverty level, educational opportunities are fewer and lower in quality than those for people with higher incomes. In the short term, lack of knowledge about food selection, food safety, and home

Food insecurity in the United States • Figure 14.8

Current data show that 14.5% of U.S. households experienced food insecurity at some point during the year.[25]

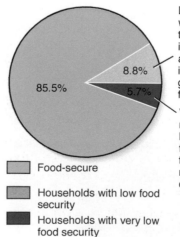

Low food security means that families were able to avoid substantially disrupting their eating patterns or reducing food intake by using coping strategies, such as eating a less varied diet, participating in federal food assistance programs, or getting emergency food from community food pantries.

Very low food security means that the normal eating patterns of one or more household members were disrupted and food intake was reduced at times during the year because families had insufficient money or other resources to use for obtaining food.

85.5%   8.8%   5.7%

☐ Food-secure

☐ Households with low food security

☐ Households with very low food security

Education and poverty • Figure 14.9

A lack of education limits the types of jobs available and hence the income level a person can attain.

a. Income level in the United States is directly correlated with level of education.[30]

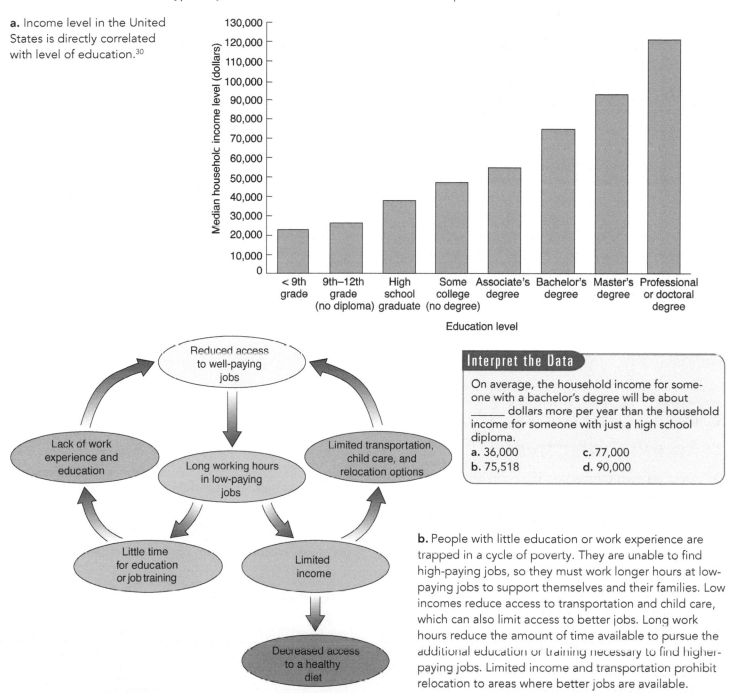

Interpret the Data

On average, the household income for someone with a bachelor's degree will be about _____ dollars more per year than the household income for someone with just a high school diploma.

a. 36,000   **c.** 77,000
b. 75,518   **d.** 90,000

b. People with little education or work experience are trapped in a cycle of poverty. They are unable to find high-paying jobs, so they must work longer hours at low-paying jobs to support themselves and their families. Low incomes reduce access to transportation and child care, which can also limit access to better jobs. Long work hours reduce the amount of time available to pursue the additional education or training necessary to find higher-paying jobs. Limited income and transportation prohibit relocation to areas where better jobs are available.

economics can contribute to malnutrition. Too little food may cause the diet to be deficient in energy or particular nutrients, but poor food choices also allow food insecurity to coexist with obesity. Lack of education about food safety can also increase the incidence of food-borne illness. In the long term, lack of education prevents people from getting the higher-paying jobs that could allow them to escape poverty (**Figure 14.9**).

Poor families must use most of their income to pay for shelter, a situation that seriously reduces the chances that they will be adequately fed. The high cost of housing not only limits food budgets but also contributes to the growing problem of homelessness in the United States. Over 600,000 Americans are homeless; two-thirds of these people live in shelters, and the remainder live in unsheltered locations such as in abandoned buildings, under bridges, or in their cars.[31] Homeless people are at high risk of food insecurity because they lack not only money but also cooking and food storage facilities.

Vulnerable Stages of Life

The high nutrient needs of pregnant and lactating women and small children put them at particular risk for undernutrition. Almost one-third of households with children headed by single women live below the poverty line.[32] Poverty and food insecurity place these women and children at risk for undernutrition, and their special nutritional needs magnify this risk. Because of their increased need for some nutrients, undernutrition may occur in pregnant women, infants, and children even when the rest of the household is adequately fed. For example, the amount of iron in the family's diet may be enough to prevent anemia in all the family's members except a pregnant teenager.

Elderly individuals are vulnerable to food insecurity and undernutrition due to the higher frequency of diseases and disabilities in this population group. Disease and disability may limit their ability to purchase, prepare, and consume food. Greater nutritional risk among older adults is associated with more hospital admissions and hence higher health-care costs. The number of individuals over age 85 is expected to triple by 2050; as the number of elderly people increases, so will the number of people at risk for food insecurity.[33]

CONCEPT CHECK — STOP

1. **Why** are some Americans hungry in a land of plenty?
2. **How** are education and poverty related?
3. **Who** is at risk for undernutrition in the United States?

14.4 Eliminating Hunger

LEARNING OBJECTIVES

1. **Discuss** two strategies that can help reduce population growth.
2. **Discuss** the role of sustainable agriculture in maintaining the food supply.
3. **Explain** how international trade can help eliminate hunger.
4. **Describe** five federal programs designed to alleviate hunger in the United States.

Solving the problem of world hunger is a daunting task. In 1996, the World Food Summit set a goal of cutting world hunger in half by 2015. Current estimates put the number of undernourished people in the world at 842 million. While this indicates that some progress has been made, it is far from the World Summit's goal of less than 500 million.[1]

Solutions to world hunger need to address population growth, ensure that the nutrient needs of a large and diverse population are met with culturally acceptable foods, and increase food production without damaging the global ecosystem (**Figure 14.10**). Meeting these goals will require input from politicians, nutrition scientists, economists, and the food industry. Economic policies,

Millennium Development Goals • Figure 14.10

The Millennium Development Goals, illustrated here, have been the most successful global antipoverty effort in history. Since they were established by the United Nations (UN) Millennium Summit in 2000, the number of people living in extreme poverty and the proportion of people without access to safe drinking water have been cut in half. Visible improvements have been made in primary education and all health areas, including significant progress in the fight against malaria and tuberculosis.[34]

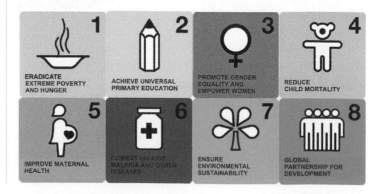

Emergency food relief • Figure 14.11

Many organizations are working to combat world hunger. The American Red Cross and High Commissioner for Refugees of the UN concentrate on famine relief. The Food and Agriculture Organization (FAO) works to improve the production, intake, and distribution of food worldwide. The World Health Organization (WHO) focuses on international health and emphasizes the prevention of nutrition problems, and the UN Children's Fund (UNICEF) targets education and vaccination and responds to crisis situations to improve the lives of children.

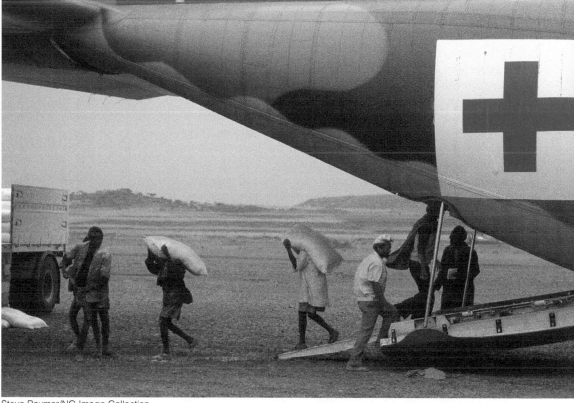

Steve Raymer/NG Image Collection

technical advances, and legislative measures must put in place programs and policies to provide food in the short term, and in the long term provide education and establish sustainable programs to allow the continued production and distribution of acceptable foods.

Providing Short-Term Food Aid

When people are starving, short-term food and medical aid must be provided right away. The standard approach has been to bring food into stricken areas (**Figure 14.11**). This food generally consists of agricultural surpluses from other countries and often is not well planned in terms of its nutrient content. Although this type of relief is necessary for a population to survive an immediate crisis such as famine, it does little to prevent future hunger.

Controlling Population Growth

In the long term, solving the problem of world hunger requires balancing the number of people and the amount of food that can be produced. The world's population has increased dramatically since the middle of the 20th century, but population growth has recently begun to slow. The birth rate worldwide has declined—from 5 children per woman in 1950 to 2.5 in 2012.[35] This downward trend in population growth must continue to ensure that food production and natural resources can support the population. Changes in cultural and economic factors as well as family planning and government policies can be used to influence the birth rate.

Economic and cultural factors that affect birth rate In many cultures, a large family is expected. A major reason for this expectation is high infant and child mortality rates. When infant mortality rates are high, people choose to have many children in order to ensure that some will survive. Higher birth rates in some developing countries are also due to the economic and societal roles of children. Children are needed to work farms, support the elders, and otherwise contribute to the economic survival of families. Programs that foster economic development and ensure access to food, shelter, and medical care

WHAT A SCIENTIST SEES

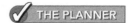

Education and Birth Rate

The large number of children in this impoverished Indonesian family is indicative of the uneven burden of population growth in the developing world. A scientist sees that one of the reasons for the many children in this family is lack of education for women. Education increases the likelihood that women will have control over their fertility and gives them knowledge that can be used to improve the family's health and economic situation. Education builds job skills that allow women to join the workforce, marry later in life, and have fewer children. The graph shows that higher literacy among women is associated with lower birth rates. Women who are better educated have options other than having numerous children.

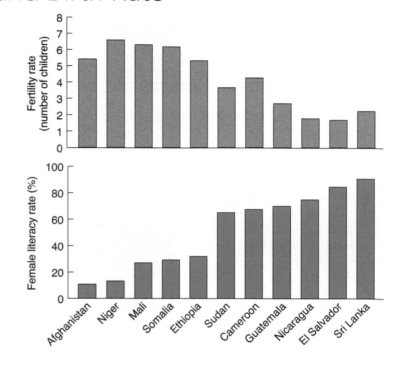

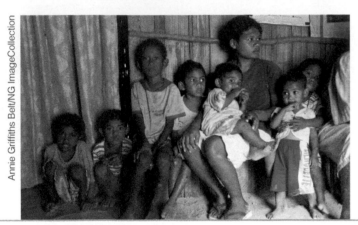

Annie Griffiths Belt/NG ImageCollection

Think Critically Based on the trends illustrated in the graph, how do you think the birth rate for high school dropouts in the United States compares to the birth rate for college graduates?

---

have been shown to cause a decline in birth rates because people feel secure having fewer children. Economic development also reduces the need for children as workers.

Another cultural factor that influences birth rate is gender inequality. Girls are often kept at home to work rather than being sent to school. In most developing countries, the literacy rate is lower for women than for men, and fewer women attend primary and secondary school. This lack of education leaves women few options other than remaining home and having children. Providing education for girls has been shown to reduce birth rates (see *What a Scientist Sees*).[36]

Family planning and government policies Changes in cultural and economic factors may reduce the desire for large families, but reducing the birth rate also requires the availability of health and family-planning services. To be successful, family-planning efforts must be acceptable to the population and compatible with

cultural and religious beliefs. Governments around the world have used a number of approaches, such as provision of contraceptives, education, and economic incentives, to decrease population growth (**Figure 14.12**).

Increasing Food Production While Protecting the Environment

Advances in agricultural technology have allowed food production to keep pace with population growth. However, the use of energy-intensive modern agricultural techniques has contributed to serious environmental problems. Commercial inorganic fertilizers and pesticides and modern farm machinery increase food production but at the same time pollute the air and water. Overuse of land causes deterioration of soil quality, which will limit food production in the future. For food production to continue to meet the needs of future generations, we must figure out how to continue to increase food yields and availability while conserving the

Access to birth control • Figure 14.12

Access to birth control has reduced the fertility rate over the last several decades.

a. A birth control vendor explains condoms to women at a market in the Ivory Coast. The birth rate in this West African country declined from nearly 7 children per woman in 1988 to an estimated 3.63 in 2014,[37] due in part to increased use of modern methods of birth control. Increased knowledge and availability of contraceptives is linked to a decrease in birth rate.

b. As seen in the graph, the percentage of women in the developing countries who are using contraception has been increasing but still lags behind use in the developed world. The availability of contraceptives gives women more control over the number of children they have and hence have to support.[38]

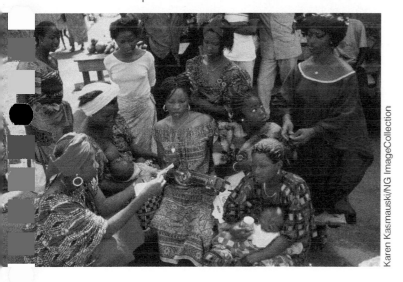

Karen Kasmauski/NG ImageCollection

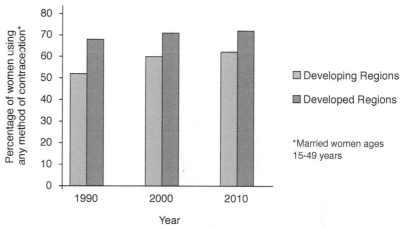

- Developing Regions
- Developed Regions

*Married women ages 15-49 years

world's natural resources (see *Thinking It Through* on the next page).

Sustainable agriculture uses food production methods that prevent damage to the environment and allow the land to restore itself so that food can be produced indefinitely. For example, contour plowing and terracing help prevent erosion, keeping the soil available for future crops. Rotating the crops grown in a field prevents the depletion of nutrients in the soil, reducing the need for fertilizers. Sustainable agriculture uses environmentally friendly chemicals that degrade quickly and do not persist as residues in the environment. It also relies on diversification. This approach to farming maximizes natural methods of pest control and fertilization and protects farmers from changes in the marketplace (**Figure 14.13**).

> **sustainable agriculture**
> Agricultural methods that maintain soil productivity and a healthy ecological balance while having minimal long-term impacts.

A sustainable farm • Figure 14.13

A sustainable farm consists of a total agricultural ecosystem rather than a single crop. It may include field crops, fruit- and nut-bearing trees, herds of livestock, and forests.

Increasing biological diversity in crops and animals protects the farmer, maximizes natural pest control, and minimizes pesticide input.

Wetlands

Sustainable agriculture

Orchard

Certified sustainable timber

Crops

Pasture

Growing a different crop in a field each year helps keep the soil healthy and minimizes soil erosion. It reduces problems caused by crop diseases, insect pests, and weeds.

Having both crops and livestock allows the farmer to recycle crop nutrients by spreading livestock manure on a field. Animals can feed on weeds and crop waste that cannot be used as human food.

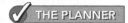
THE PLANNER

A Case Study on What One Person Can Do

Keesha is concerned about the problems of hunger and malnutrition and the impact her choices have on the environment. Although she is a college student who cannot afford to make monetary contributions to relief organizations, she would like her everyday choices to have a minimal impact on the environment.

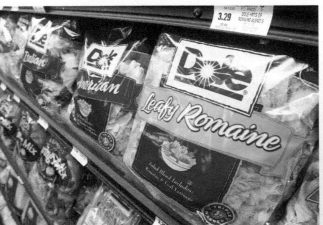

Waltraud Ingerl/iStockphoto

Liba Taylor/Robert Harding Justin Sullivan/Getty Images, Inc.

 1 What are the advantages and disadvantages of the salad options shown in the photos in terms of convenience, food safety, and environmental impact?

Your answer:

Keesha likes fish but has heard that some fish are endangered.

 2 Go to the National Geographic Web site http://ocean.nationalgeographic.com/ocean/take-action/seafood-substitutions/ to find some ocean-friendly substitutes for her seafood choices.

Fish	Substitute variety
Atlantic cod	
Chilean sea bass	
Orange roughy	

The following are some inexpensive changes Keesha can make to reduce her impact on the environment.

 3 What are the advantages and disadvantages of each?

Action	Advantages	Disadvantages
Bike instead of drive on short trips around town.		
Buy a canvas bag for carrying groceries.		
Carry a reusable water bottle rather than buy bottled water.		
Compost vegetable scraps.		
Buy locally grown produce.		
Buy organically grown produce.		

(Check your answers in online Appendix L)

Sustainable agriculture is not a single program but involves choosing options that mesh well with local soil, climate, and farming techniques. In some cases, organic farming, which does not use synthetic pesticides, herbicides, and fertilizers (see Chapter 13), may be a more sustainable option. Organic techniques have a smaller environmental impact because they reduce the use of agricultural chemicals and the release of pollutants into the environment. Organic farming is also advantageous in terms of soil quality and biodiversity, but it has a disadvantage in terms of land use because crop yields are often lower. A combination of organic and conventional techniques, as is used with integrated pest management (see Chapter 13), might improve land use and protect the environment.

Other sustainable programs include agroforestry, in which techniques from forestry and agriculture are used together to restore degraded areas; natural systems agriculture, which attempts to develop agricultural systems that include many types of plants and therefore function like natural ecosystems; and the technique of reducing fertilizer use by matching nutrient resources with the demands of the particular crop being grown. One modern technology that may be integrated with sustainable systems is genetic engineering. As discussed in Chapter 13, genetic engineering can increase crop yields by inserting genes that improve the efficiency with which plants convert sunlight into food or genes that make plants resistant to herbicides, insects, and plant diseases.

Increasing Food Availability Through Economic Development and Trade

Hunger will exist as long as there is poverty. Even when food is plentiful, the poor do not have access to enough of the right foods to maintain their nutritional health. Economic development that leads to safe and sanitary housing, access to health care and education, and the resources to acquire enough food are essential if hunger is to be eliminated. Government policies can help reduce poverty and improve food security by increasing the population's income, lowering food prices, or funding food programs for those who are poor.

Economic development in the form of industrialization can also help provide food for a country's population by increasing access to international trade. The newly industrialized countries of Asia, such as South Korea, rely on imported food to provide a varied food supply

for their populations. In general, countries around the world are becoming more dependent on food imports and on exports of food and other goods to pay for the food they import. This trade can increase the availability of food for the world's population as a whole.

Whether a country's agricultural emphasis is on producing **subsistence crops** or **cash crops** influences the availability of food for its people. Shifting to cash crops improves the country's cash flow but uses local resources to produce crops for export and limits the ability of its people to produce enough food to feed their families. For example, if a large portion of the arable land in a country is used to grow cash crops such as coffee and tea, little agricultural land remains for growing grains and vegetables that nourish the local population. If, however, the cash from the crop is used to purchase nutritious foods from other countries, this decision may help alleviate undernutrition.

> **subsistence crop** A crop that is grown as food for a farmer's family, with little or nothing left-over to sell.
>
> **cash crop** A crop that is grown to be sold for monetary return rather than as food for the local population.

Ensuring a Nutritious Food Supply

To ensure the nutritional health of a population, the foods that are grown or imported must supply both sufficient energy and adequate amounts of all essential nutrients. If the diet does not provide enough of all the essential nutrients, either the dietary pattern must be changed, commonly consumed foods must be fortified, or supplements containing deficient nutrients must be provided. For these changes to be beneficial, consumers must know how to choose foods that provide the needed nutrients and how to handle them safely.

Nutrition education Education can help improve nutrient intake by teaching consumers what foods to grow, which foods to choose, and how to prepare foods safely.

Education is particularly important when introducing a new crop. No matter how nutritious it may be, a new plant variety is not beneficial unless local farmers know how to grow it and the population accepts it as a food source and knows how to prepare it for consumption. For instance, white yams are common in some regions but are a poor source of β-carotene, which the body can use to make vitamin A. If sweet potatoes, which are rich in

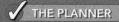
The Issue: Golden Rice is a genetically modified (GM) variety of rice developed to increase the vitamin A in the food supply of populations in which this deficiency is prevalent. Its development has stimulated debate about whether it is an effective way to prevent vitamin A deficiency and whether any genetically modified product is an appropriate and safe way to help alleviate malnutrition.

Each year vitamin A deficiency takes the sight and lives of hundreds of thousands of children worldwide. The deficiency is most common in impoverished populations where the dietary staple is deficient in vitamin A. Currently, this deficiency is addressed using vitamin A supplementation, fortification of the food supply, and interventions that increase the variety of the diet to include foods that are rich in vitamin A. A more controversial solution is growing rice that has been genetically engineered to synthesize β-carotene, a yellow-orange pigment that is a precursor to vitamin A. If it replaced white rice as a staple, Golden Rice could alleviate vitamin A deficiency. However, the controversy that ensued after it was developed has kept the preventive potential of Golden Rice from being fully assessed.

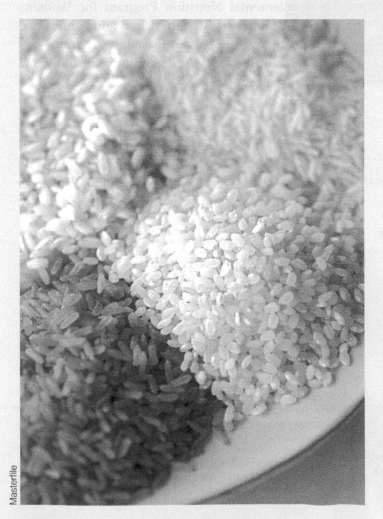

Masterfile

Initial concerns about Golden Rice focused on whether it would provide enough vitamin A to alleviate deficiency. The original variety provided so little β-carotene that a 2-year-old child would need to eat 3 kilograms of it each day to get enough vitamin A.[43] However, a newer variety contains enough β-carotene in ½ cup of dry rice to provide about 430 μg of retinol, more than enough to meet the RDA for an 8-year-old child.[44] Critics of Golden Rice have expressed concern that the β-carotene in the rice might not provide usable vitamin A to the body. However, a recent study that compared the vitamin A value of the β-carotene in Golden Rice to that of a β-carotene supplement found that both resulted in similar blood levels of retinol.[44] Even though Golden Rice can provide enough vitamin A, many still argue that it may not necessarily be a solution to vitamin A malnutrition. Deficient populations typically suffer from other nutrient deficiencies in addition to vitamin A and when protein, fat, or zinc is deficient, the body can't efficiently use vitamin A.[45,46]

There is also concern that introducing Golden Rice, which is a GM organism, into the environment will cause harm. The worry is that its use will decrease the diversity of rice varieties grown. Reducing diversity increases the risk of crop destruction due to insects and disease.[45] Proponents of GM crops argue that this concern occurs whenever a new crop that is preferred by farmers is introduced and that the potential health benefits outweigh the environmental concerns. Opponents of Golden Rice also argue that it could exacerbate malnutrition by encouraging a diet based solely on rice.[47] Although the use of Golden Rice rather than white rice is unlikely to affect dietary diversity, switching to Golden Rice does little to address the underlying causes of malnutrition, which are poverty and lack of access to a varied diet.

While debate over the usefulness of Golden Rice continues, vitamin A deficiency remains a major public health issue. Opponents to this approach argue that work on Golden Rice has diverted resources from proven programs that address multiple nutrient deficiencies. Proponents contend that the problem is not the rice but rather the regulatory climate that has prevented it from being introduced.[48] In efforts to move production forward, former Greenpeace leaders have now endorsed the Golden Rice NOW campaign in Europe to promote its use.[49,50] Even the Pope has gotten involved, and although the Vatican has not endorsed the use of Golden Rice, the Pope has given it his personal blessing.[51]

Science, politics, and now even religion are weighing in on Golden Rice. Everyone would likely agree that the goal is to prevent malnutrition and in the long term eliminate poverty, which reduces access to a healthy diet. GM crops such as Golden Rice alone may not be the solution to malnutrition. Supplementation may be necessary for those in immediate need, and fortification and supplementation may work better in urban settings. However, the question remains, should Golden Rice be part of the arsenal available to eliminate vitamin A deficiency?

Think Critically Do the risks of GM crops outweigh the risks of vitamin A deficiency? Defend your position.

Programs to prevent undernutrition in the United States   **Table 14.1**

Program	Target population	Goals and methods
Supplemental Nutrition Assistance Program (SNAP)	Low-income individuals	Increases access to food by providing coupons or debit cards that can be used to purchase food at a grocery store
Commodity Supplemental Food Program (CSFP)	Low-income pregnant women, breast-feeding and non–breast-feeding postpartum women, infants and children under age 6, and elderly people	Provides food by distributing U.S. Department of Agriculture commodity foods
Special Supplemental Nutrition Program for Women, Infants, and Children (WIC)	Low-income pregnant women, breast-feeding and non–breast-feeding postpartum women, and infants and children under age 5	Provides vouchers for the purchase of foods (including infant formula and infant cereal) high in nutrients that are typically lacking in the program's target population; provides nutrition education and referrals for health care
WIC Farmers' Market Nutrition Program	WIC participants	Increases access to fresh produce by providing vouchers that can be used to purchase produce at authorized local farmers' markets
School Breakfast Program	Low-income children	Provides free or low-cost breakfasts at school to improve the nutritional status of children
National School Lunch Program	Low-income children	Provides free or low-cost lunches at school to improve the nutritional status of children
Special Milk Program	Low-income children	Provides milk for children in schools, camps, and child-care institutions with no federally supported meal program
Summer Food Service Program	Low-income children	Provides free meals and snacks for children when school is not in session
Child and Adult Care Food Program	Children up to age 12 and elderly and disabled adults	Provides nutritious meals to children and adults in day-care settings
Team Nutrition	School-age children	Provides nutrition education, training and technical assistance, and resources to participating schools, with the goal of improving children's lifelong eating and physical activity habits
Head Start	Low-income preschool children and their families	Provides meals and education, including nutrition education
Nutrition Program for the Elderly	Individuals age 60 and over and their spouses	Provides free congregate meals in churches, schools, senior centers, or other facilities and delivers food to homebound people
Senior Farmers' Market Program	Low-income seniors	Provides coupons that can be exchanged for eligible foods at farmers' markets, roadside stands, and community-supported agricultural programs
Homeless Children Nutrition Program	Preschoolers living in shelters	Reimburses providers for meals served
Emergency Food Assistance Program	Low-income people	Provides commodities to soup kitchens, food banks, and individuals for home use
Healthy People 2020	U.S. population	Sets national health promotion objectives to improve the health of the U.S. population through the health-care system and industry involvement, as well as individual actions
Expanded Food and Nutrition Education Program (EFNEP)	Low-income families	Provides education in all aspects of food preparation and nutrition
Temporary Assistance for Needy Families (TANF)	Low-income households	Provides assistance and work opportunities to needy families by granting states federal funds to implement welfare programs
Food Distribution Program on Indian Reservations	Low-income households living on reservations and Native Americans living near reservations	Provides food by distributing USDA commodity foods

Field gleaning • Figure 14.16

These oranges were harvested in California as part of a local gleaning program. Field gleaning is a type of food recovery that involves collecting crops that are not harvested because it is not economically profitable to harvest them or that remain in fields after mechanical harvesting. The word *gleaning* means "gathering after the harvest" and dates back at least as far as biblical times.

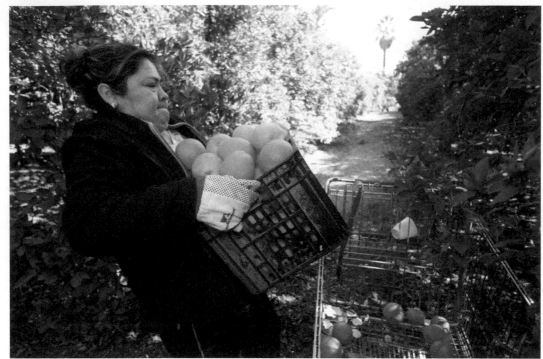

© Damian Dovarganes/AP Photos

In addition to federal nutrition assistance programs, church, community, and charitable emergency food shelters provide for the basic nutritional needs of many Americans. In the United States, about 150,000 nonprofit food distribution programs help direct food to those in need.[54] The leading hunger-relief charity in the United States is Feeding America, which provides food assistance to more than 37 million low-income people per year. It includes a network of food banks across the country and supports thousands of local charitable organizations, such as food pantries and soup kitchens, which distribute food directly to hungry Americans.

Virtually all these food distribution programs use food obtained through **food recovery**, which involves collecting food that is wasted in fields, commercial kitchens, restaurants, and grocery stores and distributing it to those in need (**Figure 14.16**). It is estimated that 40% of America's food goes uneaten. Reducing losses by 15% would provide enough food to feed 25 million people.[55]

Nutrition education People who have more nutrition information and greater awareness of the relationship between diet and health consume healthier diets. Healthy diets not only improve current health by optimizing growth, productivity, and well-being but are essential for preventing chronic diseases. Increasing knowledge about nutrition can reduce medical costs and improve the quality of life.

Education can help individuals with lower incomes stretch their limited food dollars by making wise choices at the store and reducing food waste at home. It can promote community gardens to increase the availability of seasonal vegetables. It can teach people how to prepare foods received from commodity distribution programs and food banks. It can explain safe food handling and preparation methods. Knowing which foods to choose and how to handle them safely is as important in preventing malnutrition as having the money to buy enough food. In addition to the programs described in Table 14.1, the *Dietary Guidelines for Americans*, MyPlate, and food labels educate the general public about making wise food choices (see *What Should I Eat?*).

WHAT SHOULD I EAT?

Make Your Meals Green

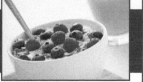
© Sara Winter/iStockphoto

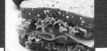
© Jill Chen/iStockphoto

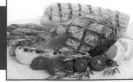
© Steve Mcsweeny/iStockphoto

✓ THE PLANNER

Eat more plants
- Reduce the amount of meat in your meal.
- Eat vegetarian at least some of the time.
- Eat lower on the food chain—more plant foods and small fish.
- Grow and eat some of your own vegetables.

Cut down on your contribution to pollution
- Buy in bulk in order to cut down on packaging.
- Use reusable bags to take your groceries home.
- Choose locally grown and organically produced foods.
- Cook from scratch—use fewer processed foods.

Use iProfile to compare the nutrients in a vegetarian versus a meat-based meal.

CONCEPT CHECK   STOP

1. **How** does educating women help control population growth?

2. **What** impact does sustainable agriculture have on the world's food supply?

3. **How** can growing cash crops improve a nation's food supply?

4. **What** is the nutrition safety net?

✓ THE PLANNER

Summary

1 The Two Faces of Malnutrition 476

- In poorly nourished populations, a **cycle of undernutrition** exists in which poorly nourished women give birth to low-birth-weight infants at risk for disease and early death. If these children survive, they grow into adults who are physically unable to fully contribute to society. In populations where undernutrition is prevalent, low birth weight, a high **infant mortality rate**, **stunting**, and infections are more common.

- Overnutrition coexists with **hunger** and **starvation** in both developed and developing nations around the world. As economic conditions improve, **nutrition transition** to more Western diet and lifestyle patterns contribute to the growing problem of nutrition-related noncommunicable diseases (NCDs), as shown in the graph.

Nutrition transition • Figure 14.2b

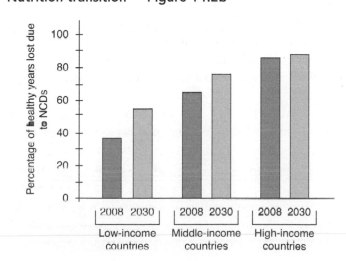

2 Causes of Hunger Around the World 479

- The underlying cause of hunger and **food insecurity** is that the food available in the world is not distributed equitably. **Famine** results from natural and human-caused disasters that temporarily disrupt food production and distribution. Chronic food shortage is most common in the developing world, as shown in the chart. It occurs when economic inequities result in lack of money, health care, and education; when overpopulation and limited natural resources create a situation in which there are more people than food; when cultural practices limit food choices; and when **renewable resources** are misused, limiting the ability to continue to produce food.

The impact of poverty • Figure 14.4

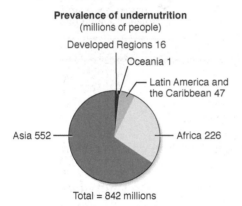

Prevalence of undernutrition
(millions of people)

Developed Regions 16
Oceania 1
Latin America and the Caribbean 47
Asia 552
Africa 226

Total = 842 millions

- Deficiencies of protein, iron, iodine, and vitamin A are common worldwide when the quality of the diet is poor. Pregnant women, children, elderly individuals, and those who are ill may not be able to meet their nutrient needs with the available diet.

3 Causes of Hunger in the United States 484

- Both undernutrition and overnutrition are problems in the United States. As in developing nations, in the United States undernutrition and food insecurity are associated with poverty, which limits education and access to health care and adequate housing, as depicted here.

Education and poverty • Figure 14.9b

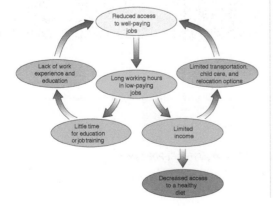

Reduced access to well-paying jobs

Lack of work experience and education

Long working hours in low-paying jobs

Limited transportation, child care, and relocation options

Little time for education or job training

Limited income

Decreased access to a healthy diet

- High nutrient needs increase the risk of undernutrition in women and children, and disease and disability increase risk in elderly individuals.

4 Eliminating Hunger 486

- Short-term solutions to eliminating hunger provide food through relief at local, national, and international levels, as shown here.

Emergency food relief • Figure 14.11

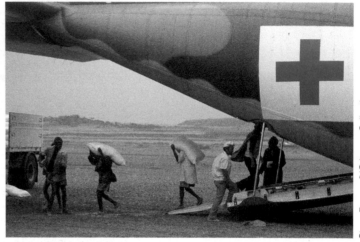

Steve Raymer/NG Image Collection

- Eliminating world hunger in the long term requires controlling population growth. This can be addressed by improving economic conditions, providing education, particularly for women, and ensuring access to family planning services.

- **Sustainable agriculture** helps eliminate hunger by allowing food to be produced without damaging the environment.

- Economic development helps prevent hunger by eliminating poverty and ensuring access to health care and education. It also increases access to international trade, which can be used to import food or to export **cash crops** to bring more money into the country.

- Food fortification and dietary supplementation can be used to increase protein quality, eliminate micronutrient deficiencies, and improve the overall quality of the diet.

- Nutrition programs in the United States focus on maintaining a nutrition safety net that provides access to affordable food and education to promote healthy eating.

Key Terms

- cash crop 491
- cycle of undernutrition 476
- famine 479
- food desert 484

- food insecurity 479
- food recovery 496
- hunger 476
- infant mortality rate 477

- nutrition transition 478
- renewable resource 481
- starvation 476
- stunting 477

- subsistence crop 491
- sustainable agriculture 489

What is happening in this picture?

This 250-fold magnification shows the mouth of a hookworm, which it uses to attach to the lining of the small intestine and feed on blood. Hookworm larvae penetrate the skin, infecting people when they walk barefoot in contaminated soil. Hookworm infection affects about 576 to 740 million people worldwide.[56]

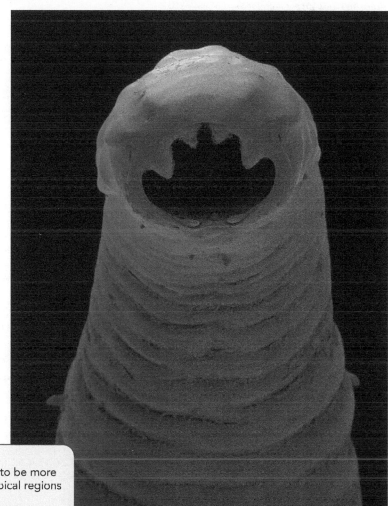

David Scharf/Science Source

Think Critically

1. Why might you expect this infection to be more common in poor tropical and subtropical regions than elsewhere?
2. How would hookworm infection affect iron status? Why?
3. How would hookworm infection affect a population's productivity? Why?

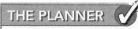

THE PLANNER ✓

Review your Chapter Planner on the chapter opener and check off your completed work.

DRI recommended intake tables for Vitamins and for Minerals are on the front and back covers of this text.

Acceptable Macronutrient Distribution Ranges (AMDR) for Healthy Diets as a Percent of Energy

Age	Carbohydrate	Added Sugars	Total Fat	Linoleic Acid	α- Linolenic Acid	Protein
1–3 y	45–65	≤25	30–40	5–10	0.6–1.2	5–20
4–18 y	45–65	≤25	25–35	5–10	0.6–1.2	10–30
≥19 y	45–65	≤25	20–35	5–10	0.6–1.2	10–35

Source: Institute of Medicine, Food and Nutrition Board. "Dietary Reference Intakes for Energy, Carbohydrate, Fiber, Fat, Fatty Acids, Cholesterol, Protein, and Amino Acids." Washington, D.C.: National Academies Press, 2002, 2005.

Dietary Reference Intakes: Recommended Intakes for Individuals: Carbohydrates, Fiber, Fat, Fatty Acids, Protein, and Water

Life Stage Group	Carbohydrate (g/day)	Fiber (g/day)	Fat (g/day)	Linoleic Acid (g/day)	α-Linolenic Acid (g/day)	Protein (g/kg/day)[a]	Protein (g/day)	Water[b] (L/day)
Infants								
0–6 mo	60*	ND	31*	4.4*†	0.5*‡	1.52*	9.1*	0.7*
6–12 mo	95*	ND	30*	4.6*†	0.5*‡	1.50	11.0	0.8*
Children								
1–3 y	130	19*	ND	7*	0.7*	1.10	13	1.3*
4–8 y	130	25*	ND	10*	0.9*	0.95	19	1.7*
Males								
9–13 y	130	31*	ND	12*	1.2*	0.95	34	2.4*
14–18 y	130	38*	ND	16*	1.6*	0.85	52	3.3*
19–30 y	130	38*	ND	17*	1.6*	0.80	56	3.7*
31–50 y	130	38*	ND	17*	1.6*	0.80	56	3.7*
51–70 y	130	30*	ND	14*	1.6*	0.80	56	3.7*
>70 y	130	30*	ND	14*	1.6*	0.80	56	3.7*
Females								
9–13 y	130	26*	ND	10*	1.0*	0.95	34	
14–18 y	130	26*	ND	11*	1.1*	0.85	46	2.1*
19–30 y	130	25*	ND	12*	1.1*	0.80	46	2.3*
31–50 y	130	25*	ND	12*	1.1*	0.80	46	2.7*
51–70 y	130	21*	ND	11*	1.1*	0.80	46	2.7*
>70 y	130	21*	ND	11*	1.1*	0.80	46	2.7*
Pregnancy	175	28*	ND	13*	1.4*	1.10	71	3.0*
Lactation	210	29*	ND	13*	1.3*	1.10	71	3.8*

ND = not determined. *Values are AI (Adequate Intakes), † Refers to all ω-6 polyunsaturated fatty acids, ‡Refers to all ω-3 polyunsaturated fatty acids.

Source: Institute of Medicine, Food and Nutrition Board. "Dietary Reference Intakes for Energy, Carbohydrate, Fiber, Fat, Fatty Acids, Cholesterol, Protein, and Amino Acids" (2002/2005); "Dietary Reference Intakes for Water, Potassium, Sodium, Chloride, and Sulfate" (2005) Washington, D.C.: National Academies Press.

[a] Based on g protein per kg of body weight for the reference body weight, e.g., for adults 0.8 g/kg body weight for the reference body weight.

[b] Total water includes all water contained in food, beverages, and drinking water.

Dietary Reference Intake Values for Energy: Estimated Energy Requirement (EER) Equations and Values for Active Individuals by Life Stage Group

Life Stage Group	EER Prediction Equation	EER for Active Physical Activity Level (kCal\day)[a]	
		Male	Female
0–3 mo	$EER = (89 \times \text{weight of infant in kg} - 100) + 175$	538	493 (2 mo)[c]
4–6 mo	$EER = (89 \times \text{weight of infant in kg} - 100) + 56$	606	543 (5 mo)[c]
7–12 mo	$EER = (89 \times \text{weight of infant in kg} - 100) + 22$	743	676 (9 mo)[c]
1–2 y	$EER = (89 \times \text{weight of infant in kg} - 100) + 20$	1046	992 (2 y)[c]
3–8 y			
Male	$EER = 88.5 - (61.9 \times \text{Age in yrs}) + PA^b[(26.7 \times \text{Weight in kg}) + (903 \times \text{Height in m})] + 20$	1742 (6 y)[c]	
Female	$EER = 135.3 - (30.8 \times \text{Age in yrs}) + PA^b[(10.0 \times \text{Weight in kg}) + (934 \times \text{Height in m})] + 20$		1642 (6 y)[c]
9–13 y			
Male	$EER = 88.5 - (61.9 \times \text{Age in yrs}) + PA^b[(26.7 \times \text{Weight in kg}) + (903 \times \text{Height in m})] + 25$	2279 (11 y)[c]	
Female	$EER = 135.3 - (30.8 \times \text{Age in yrs}) + PA^b[(10.0 \times \text{Weight in kg}) + (934 \times \text{Height in m})] + 25$		2071(11 y)[c]
14–18 y			
Male	$EER = 88.5 - (61.9 - \text{Age in yrs}) + PA^b[(26.7 \times \text{Weight in kg}) + (903 \times \text{Height in m})] + 25$	3152 (16 y)[c]	
Female	$EER = 135.3 - (30.8 \times \text{Age in yrs}) + PA^b[(10.0 \times \text{Weight in kg}) + (934 \times \text{Height in m})] + 25$		2368 (16 y)[c]
19 and older			
Males	$EER = 662 - (9.53 \times \text{Age in yrs}) + PA^b[(15.91 \times \text{Weight in kg}) + (539.6 \times \text{Height in m})]$	3067 (19 y)[c]	
Females	$EER = 354 - (6.91 \times \text{Age in yrs}) + PA^b[(9.36 \times \text{Weight in kg}) + (726 \times \text{Height in m})]$		2403 (19 y)[c]
Pregnancy			
14–18 y			
1st trimester	Adolescent EER + 0		2368 (16 y)[c]
2nd trimester	Adolescent EER + 340		2708 (16 y)[c]
3rd trimester	Adolescent EER + 452		2820 (16 y)[c]
19–50 y			
1st trimester	Adult EER + 0		2403 (19 y)[c]
2nd trimester	Adult EER + 340		2743 (19 y)[c]
3rd trimester	Adult EER + 452		2855 (19 y)[c]
Lactation			
14–18 y			
1st 6 mo	Adolescent EER + 330		2698 (16 y)[c]
2nd 6 mo	Adolescent EER + 400		2768 (16 y)[c]
19–50 y			
1st 6 mo	Adult EER + 330		2733 (19 y)[c]
2nd 6 mo	Adult EER + 400		2803 (19 y)[c]

[a] The intake that meets the average energy expenditure of active individuals at a reference height, weight, and age.

[b] See table entitle "Physical Activity Coefficients (PA Values) for Use in EER Equations" to determine the PA value for various ages, genders, and activity levels.

[c] Value is calculated for an individual at the age in parentheses.

Physical Activity Coefficients (PA Values) for Use in EER Equations

Age and Gender	Sedentary	Low Active	Active	Very Active
3 to 18 y				
Boys	1.00	1.13	1.26	1.42
Girls	1.00	1.16	1.31	1.56
≥19 y				
Men	1.00	1.11	1.25	1.48
Women	1.00	1.12	1.27	1.45

Source: Institute of Medicine, Food and Nutrition Board. "Dietary Reference Intakes for Energy, Carbohydrate, Fiber, Fat, Fatty Acids, Cholesterol, Protein, and Amino Acids." Washington, D.C.: National Academies Press, 2002, 2005.

Dietary Reference Intakes: Tolerable Upper Intake Levels (UL[a]): Vitamins

Life Stage Group	Vitamin A (μg/day)[b]	Vitamin C (mg/day)	Vitamin D (μg/day)	Vitamin E (mg/day)[c,d]	Vitamin K	Thiamin	Riboflavin	Niacin (mg/day)[d]	Vitamin B$_6$ (mg/day)	Folate (μg/day)[d]	Vitamin B$_{12}$	Pantothenic Acid	Biotin	Choline (g/day)	Carotenoids[e]
Infants															
0–6 mo	600	ND[f]	25	ND	ND	ND	ND	ND	ND	ND	ND	ND	ND	ND	ND
6–12 mo	600	ND	38	ND	ND	ND	ND	ND	ND	ND	ND	ND	ND	ND	ND
Children															
1–3 y	600	400	63	200	ND	ND	ND	10	30	300	ND	ND	ND	1.0	ND
4–8 y	900	650	75	300	ND	ND	ND	15	40	400	ND	ND	ND	1.0	ND
Males, Females															
9–13 y	1,700	1,200	100	600	ND	ND	ND	20	60	600	ND	ND	ND	2.0	ND
14–18 y	2,800	1,800	100	800	ND	ND	ND	30	80	800	ND	ND	ND	3.0	ND
19–70 y	3,000	2,000	100	1,000	ND	ND	ND	35	100	1,000	ND	ND	ND	3.5	ND
>70 y	3,000	2,000	100	1,000	ND	ND	ND	35	100	1,000	ND	ND	ND	3.5	ND
Pregnancy															
14–18 y	2,800	1,800	100	800	ND	ND	ND	30	80	800	ND	ND	ND	3.0	ND
19–50 y	3,000	2,000	100	1,000	ND	ND	ND	35	100	1,000	ND	ND	ND	3.5	ND
Lactation															
14–18 y	2,800	1,800	100	800	ND	ND	ND	30	80	800	ND	ND	ND	3.0	ND
19–50 y	3,000	2,000	100	1,000	ND	ND	ND	35	100	1,000	ND	ND	ND	3.5	ND

[a] UL = The maximum level of daily nutrient intake that is likely to pose no risk of adverse effects. Unless otherwise specified, the UL represents total intake from food, water, and supplements. Due to lack of suitable data, ULs could not be established for vitamin K, thiamin, riboflavin, vitamin B$_{12}$, pantothenic acid, biotin, or carotenoids. In the absence of ULs, extra caution may be warranted in consuming levels above recommended intakes.

[b] As preformed vitamin A only.

[c] As α-tocopherol; applies to any form of supplemental α-tocopherol.

[d] The ULs for vitamin E, niacin, and folate apply to synthetic forms obtained from supplements, fortified foods, or a combination of the two.

[e] β-Carotene supplements are advised only to serve as a provitamin A source for individuals at risk of vitamin A deficiency.

[f] ND = Not determinable due to lack of data of adverse effects in this age group and concern with regard to lack of ability to handle excess amounts. Source of intakes should be from food only to prevent high levels of intake.

Source: Dietary Reference Intake Tables: The Complete Set. Institute of Medicine, National Academy of Sciences. Available online at www.nap.edu. Reprinted with permission from *Dietary Reference Intakes: The Essential Guide to Nutrient Requirements*, 2006, by the National Academy of Sciences, Washington, D.C. Institute of Medicine, Food and Nutrition Board, Dietary Reference Intakes for Calcium and Vitamin D (2011), National Academies Press, Washington. DC, 2011.

Dietary Reference Intakes: Tolerable Upper Intake Levels (UL[a]): Minerals

Life Stage Group	Arsenic[b]	Boron (mg/day)	Calcium (g/day)	Chromium	Copper (μg/day)	Fluoride (mg/day)	Iodine (μg/day)	Iron (mg/day)	Magnesium (mg/day)[c]	Manganese (mg/day)	Molybdenum (μg/day)	Nickel (mg/day)	Phosphorus (g/day)	Selenium (μg/day)	Silicon[d]	Vanadium (mg/day)[e]	Zinc (mg/day)	Sodium (g/day)	Chloride (g/day)	Potassium
Infants																				
0–6 mo	ND[f]	ND	1.0	ND	ND	0.7	ND	40	ND	ND	ND	ND	ND	45	ND	ND	4	ND	ND	ND
6–12 mo	ND	ND	1.5	ND	ND	0.9	ND	40	ND	ND	ND	ND	ND	60	ND	ND	5	ND	ND	ND
Children																				
1–3 y	ND	3	2.5	ND	1,000	1.3	200	40	65	2	300	0.2	3	90	ND	ND	7	1.5	2.3	ND
4–8 y	ND	6	2.5	ND	3,000	2.2	300	40	110	3	600	0.3	3	150	ND	ND	12	1.9	2.9	ND
Males, Females																				
9–13 y	ND	11	3.0	ND	5,000	10	600	40	350	6	1,100	0.6	4	280	ND	ND	23	2.2	3.4	ND
14–18 y	ND	17	3.0	ND	8,000	10	900	45	350	9	1,700	1.0	4	400	ND	ND	34	2.3	3.6	ND
19–30 y	ND	20	2.5	ND	10,000	10	1,100	45	350	11	2,000	1.0	4	400	ND	1.8	40	2.3	3.6	ND
31–50 y	ND	20	2.5	ND	10,000	10	1,100	45	350	11	2,000	1.0	4	400	ND	1.8	40	2.3	3.6	ND
51–70 y	ND	20	2.0	ND	10,000	10	1,100	45	350	11	2,000	1.0	4	400	ND	1.8	40	2.3	3.6	ND
>70 y	ND	20	2.0	ND	10,000	10	1,100	45	350	11	2,000	1.0	3	400	ND	1.8	40	2.3	3.6	ND
Pregnancy																				
14–18 y	ND	17	3.0	ND	8,000	10	900	45	350	9	1,700	1.0	3.5	400	ND	ND	34	2.3	3.6	ND
19–50 y	ND	20	2.5	ND	10,000	10	1,100	45	350	11	2,000	1.0	3.5	400	ND	ND	40	2.3	3.6	ND
Lactation																				
14–18 y	ND	17	3.0	ND	8,000	10	900	45	350	9	1,700	1.0	4	400	ND	ND	34	2.3	3.6	ND
19–50 y	ND	20	2.5	ND	10,000	10	1,100	45	350	11	2,000	1.0	4	400	ND	ND	40	2.3	3.6	ND

[a] UL = the maximum level of daily nutrient intake that is likely to pose no risk of adverse effects. Unless otherwise specified, the UL represents total intake from food, water, and supplements. Due to lack of suitable data, ULs could not be established for arsenic, chromium, silicon, and potassium. In the absence of ULs, extra caution may be warranted in consuming levels above recommended intakes.

[b] Although the UL was not determined for arsenic, there is no justification for adding arsenic to food or supplements.

[c] The ULs for magnesium represent intake from a pharmacological agent only and do not include intake from food and water.

[d] Although silicon has not been shown to cause adverse effects in humans, there is no justification for adding silicon to supplements.

[e] Although vanadium in food has not been shown to cause adverse effects in humans, there is no justification for adding vanadium to food and vanadium supplements should be used with caution. The UL is based on adverse effects in laboratory animals and this data could be used to set a UL for adults but not children and adolescents.

[f] ND = Not determinable due to lack of data of adverse effects in this age group and concern with regard to lack of ability to handle excess amounts. Source of intake should be from food only to prevent high levels of intake.

Source: Dietary Reference Intake Tables: The Complete Set. Institute of Medicine, National Academy of Sciences. Available online at www.nap.edu. Reprinted with permission from *Dietary Reference Intakes: The Essential Guide to Nutrient Requirements,* 2006, by the National Academy of Sciences, Washington, D.C. Institute of Medicine, Food and Nutrition Board. Dietary Reference Intakes for Calcium and Vitamin D (2011), National Academies Press, Washington, DC, 2011.

Dietary Reference Intake Values for Energy: Total Energy Expenditure (TEE) Equations for Overweight and Obese Individuals

Life Stage Group	TEE Prediction Equation (Cal/day)	PA Values
Overweight boys aged 3–18 years	TEE = 114 − (50.9 × age in yrs) + PA[(19.5 × weight in kg) + (1161.4 × height in m)]	Sedentary = 1.00 Low active = 1.12 Active = 1.24 Very active = 1.45
Overweight girls aged 3–18 years	TEE = 389 − (41.2 × age in yrs) + PA[(15.0 × weight in kg) + (701.6 × height in m)]	Sedentary = 1.00 Low active = 1.18 Active = 1.35 Very active = 1.60
Overweight and obese men aged 19 years and older	TEE = 1086 − (10.1 × age in yrs) + PA[(13.7 × weight in kg) + (416 × height in m)]	Sedentary = 1.00 Low active = 1.12 Active = 1.29 Very active = 1.59
Overweight and obese women aged 19 years and older	TEE = 448 − (7.95 × age in yrs) + PA[(11.4 × weight in kg) + (619 × height in m)]	Sedentary = 1.00 Low active = 1.16 Active = 1.27 Very active = 1.44

Source: Institute of Medicine, Food and Nutrition Board "Dietary Reference Intakes for Energy, Carbohydrate, Fiber, Fat, Fatty Acids, Cholesterol, Protein, and Amino Acids," Washington, DC: National Academy Press, 2002, 2005.

USDA Food Patterns

For each food group or subgroup,[a] recommended average daily intake amounts[b] at all calorie levels. Recommended intakes from vegetable and protein foods subgroups are per week. For more information and tools for application go to MyPlate.gov

Calorie level of pattern	1,000	1,200	1,400	1,600	1,800	2,000	2,200	2,400	2,600	2,800	3,000	3,200
Fruits	1 c	1 c	1½c	1½ c	1½ c	2 c	2 c	2 c	2 c	2 ½ c	2 ½ c	2 ½ c
Vegetables	1 c	1½ c	1½ c	2 c	2½ c	2 ½ c	3 c	3 c	3 ½ c	3 ½ c	4 c	4 c
Dark-green vegetables	½ c/wk	1 c/wk	1 c/wk	1½ c/wk	1½ c/wk	1½ c/wk	2 c/wk	2 c/wk	2½ c/wk	2½ c/wk	2½ c/wk	2½ c/wk
Red and orange vegetables	2½ c/wk	3 c/wk	3 c/wk	4 c/wk	5½ c/wk	5½ c/wk	6 c/wk	6 c/wk	7 c/wk	7 c/wk	7½ c/wk	7½ c/wk
Beans and peas (legumes)	½ c/wk	½ c/wk	½ c/wk	1 c/wk	1½ c/wk	1½ c/wk	2 c/wk	2 c/wk	2 ½ c/wk	2 ½ c/wk	3 c/wk	3 c/wk
Starchy vegetables	2 c/wk	3 ½ c/wk	3 ½ c/wk	4 c/wk	5 c/wk	5 c/wk	6 c/wk	6 c/wk	7 c/wk	7 c/wk	8 c/wk	8 c/wk
Other vegetables	1½ c/wk	2½ c/wk	2½ c/wk	3½ c/wk	4 c/wk	4 c/wk	5 c/wk	5 c/wk	5½c/wk	5½ c/wk	7 c/wk	7 c/wk
Grains	3 oz-eq	4 oz-eq	5 oz-eq	5 oz-eq	6 oz-eq	6 oz-eq	7 oz-eq	8 oz-eq	9 oz-eq	10 oz-eq	10 oz-eq	10 oz-eq
Whole grains	1 ½ oz-eq	2 oz-eq	2 ½ oz-eq	3 oz-eq	3 oz-eq	3 oz-eq	3 ½ oz-eq	4 oz-eq	4 ½ oz-eq	5 oz-eq	5 oz-eq	5 oz-eq
Enriched grains	1 ½ oz-eq	2 oz-eq	2 ½ oz-eq	2 oz-eq	3 oz-eq	3 oz-eq	3 ½ oz-eq	4 oz-eq	4 ½ oz-eq	5 oz-eq	5 oz-eq	5 oz-eq
Protein foods	2 oz-eq	3 oz-eq	4 oz-eq	5 oz-eq	5 oz-eq	5 ½ oz-eq	6 oz-eq	6 ½ oz-eq	6 ½ oz-eq	7 oz-eq	7 oz-eq	7 oz-eq
Seafood	3 oz/wk	5 oz/wk	6 oz/wk	8 oz/wk	8 oz/wk	8 oz/wk	9 oz/wk	10 oz/wk	10 oz/wk	11 oz/wk	11 oz/wk	11 oz/wk
Meat, poultry, eggs	10 oz/wk	14 oz/wk	19 oz/wk	24 oz/wk	24 oz/wk	26 oz/wk	29 oz/wk	31 oz/wk	31 oz/wk	34 oz/wk	34 oz/wk	34 oz/wk
Nuts, seeds, soy products	1 oz/wk	2 oz/wk	3 oz/wk	4 oz/wk	4 oz/wk	4 oz/wk	4 oz/wk	5 oz/wk	5 oz/wk	5 oz/wk	5 oz/wk	5 oz/wk
Dairy	2 c	2 ½ c	2 ½ c	3 c	3 c	3 c	3 c	3 c	3 c	3 c	3 c	3 c
Oils	15 g	17 g	17 g	22 g	24 g	27 g	29 g	31 g	34 g	36 g	44 g	51 g
Maximum SoFAS[c] limit, calories (% of calories)	137 (14%)	121 (10%)	121 (9%)	121 (8%)	161 (9%)	258 (13%)	266 (12%)	330 (14%)	362 (14%)	395 (14%)	459 (15%)	596 (19%)

[a] All foods are assumed to be in nutrient-dense forms, lean or low-fat and prepared without added fats, sugars, or salt. Solid fats and added sugars may be included up to the daily maximum limit identified in the table.

[b] Food group amounts are shown in cup (c) or ounce-equivalents (oz-eq). Oils are shown in grams (g). Quantity equivalents for each food group are:
- Grains, 1 ounce-equivalent is 1 one-ounce slice bread; 1 ounce uncooked pasta or rice: 1/2 cup cooked rice, pasta, or cereal; 1 tortilla (6" diameter); 1 pancake (5" diameter); 1 ounce ready-to-eat cereal (about 1 cup cereal flakes).
- Vegetables and fruits, 1 cup equivalent is: 1 cup raw or cooked vegetable or fruit; 1/2 cup dried vegetable or fruit; 1 cup vegetable or fruit juice; 2 cups leafy salad greens.
- Protein foods, 1 ounce-equivalent is: 1 ounce lean meat, poultry, seafood; 1 egg; 1 Tbsp peanut butter; 1/2 ounce nuts or seeds. Also, 1/4 cup cooked beans or peas may also be counted as 1 ounce equivalent.
- Dairy, 1 cup equivalent is: 1 cup milk, fortified soy beverage, or yogurt; 1 1/2 ounce natural cheese (e.g., cheddar); 2 ounces of processed cheese

[c] SoFAS are calories from solid fats and added sugars. The limit for SoFAS is the remaining amount of calories in each food pattern after selecting the specified amount in each food group in nutrient-dense forms (forms that are fat-free or low-fat and with no added sugars). The number of SoFAS is lower in the 1,200, 1,400, and 1,600 calorie patterns than in the 1,000 calorie pattern. The nutrient goals for the 1,200 to 1,600 calorie patterns are higher and require that more calories be used for nutrient-dense foods from the food groups.

Recommended Dietary Intakes (RDIs)* Used to Establish Daily Values

Vitamins and Minerals	Units of Measurement	Adults and Children 4 or more Years of Age	Infants	Children Under 4 Years of Age	Pregnant or Lactating Women
Vitamin A	International Units†	5000 (1000 μg)	1500	2500	8000
Vitamin D	International Units†	400 (10 μg)	400	400	400
Vitamin E	International Units†	30 (10 μg)	5	10	30
Vitamin C	Milligrams	60	35	40	60
Folic acid	Micrograms	400	0.1	0.2	0.8
Thiamin	Milligrams	1.5	0.5	0.7	1.7
Riboflavin	Milligrams	1.7	0.6	0.8	2.0
Niacin	Milligrams	20	8	9	20
Vitamin B_6	Milligrams	2.0	0.4	0.7	2.5
Vitamin B_{12}	Micrograms	6.0	2	3	8
Biotin	Micrograms	300	0.05	0.15	0.30
Pantothenic acid	Milligrams	10	3	5	10
Calcium	Milligrams	1000	0.6	0.8	1.3
Phosphorous	Milligrams	1000	0.5	0.8	1.3
Iodine	Micrograms	150	45	70	150
Iron	Milligrams	18	15	10	18
Magnesium	Milligrams	400	70	200	450
Copper	Milligrams	2.0	0.6	1.0	2.0
Zinc	Milligrams	15	5	8	15
Vitamin K	Micrograms	80	—‡	—‡	—‡
Chromium	Micrograms	120	—	—	—
Selenium	Micrograms	70	—	—	—
Molybdenum	Micrograms	75	—	—	—
Manganese	Milligrams	2	—	—	—
Chloride	Milligrams	3400	—	—	—

*Based on National Academy of Sciences' 1968 Recommended Dietary Allowances.

†The RDIs for fat-soluble vitamins are expressed in International Units (IU). Values that are approximately equivalent in micrograms are given in parentheses.

‡No values yet established for vitamin K, chromium, selenium, molybdenum, manganese, or chloride for this population.

Source: USDA Food Labeling Guide. Available online at http://www.cfsan.fda.gov/~dms/2lg-xf.htm

Energy Expenditure for Various Activities

Type of Activity	Calories per Hour (by body weight)				
	100 lb	120 lb	150 lb	180 lb	200 lb
Aerobics (heavy)	363	435	544	653	726
Aerobics (medium)	227	272	340	408	454
Aerobics (light)	136	163	204	245	272
Archery	159	190	238	286	317
Backpacking	408	490	612	735	816
Badminton (doubles)	181	218	272	327	363
Badminton (singles)	231	278	347	416	463
Basketball (nonvigorous)	431	517	646	776	862
Basketball (vigorous)	499	599	748	898	998
Bicycling (6 mph)	159	190	238	286	317
Bicycling (10 mph)	249	299	374	449	499
Bicycling (11 mph)	295	354	442	531	590
Bicycling (12 mph)	340	408	510	612	680
Bicycling (13 mph)	385	463	578	694	771
Billiards	91	109	136	163	181
Bowling	177	212	265	318	354
Boxing—competition	603	724	905	1086	1206
Boxing—sparring	376	452	565	678	753
Calisthenics (heavy)	363	435	544	653	726
Calisthenics (light)	181	218	272	327	363
Canoeing (2.5 mph)	150	180	224	269	299
Canoeing (5 mph)	340	408	510	612	680
Carpentry	227	272	340	408	454
Climbing (mountain)	454	544	680	816	907
Disco dancing	272	327	408	490	544
Ditch digging (hand)	263	316	395	473	526
Fencing	340	408	510	612	680
Fishing (bank/boat)	159	190	238	286	317
Fishing (in waders)	249	299	374	449	499
Football (touch)	340	408	510	612	680
Gardening	145	174	218	261	290
Golf (carry clubs)	227	272	340	408	454
Golf (pull cart)	163	196	245	294	327
Golf (ride in cart)	113	136	170	204	227
Handball (vigorous)	454	544	680	816	907
Hiking (X-country)	249	299	374	449	499
Hiking (mountain)	340	408	510	612	680
Horseback trotting	231	278	317	416	463

(continued)

atrophy Wasting or decrease in the size of a muscle or other tissue caused by lack of use.

attention-deficit/hyperactivity disorder (ADHD) A condition characterized by a short attention span and a high level of activity, excitability, and distractibility.

autoimmune disease A disease that results from immune reactions that destroy normal body cells.

basal metabolic rate (BMR) The rate of energy expenditure under resting conditions. It is measured after 12 hours without food or exercise.

basal metabolism The energy expended to maintain an awake, resting body that is not digesting food.

behavior modification A process that is used to gradually and permanently change habitual behaviors.

beriberi A thiamin deficiency disease that manifests in one of two forms: dry beriberi, which causes weakness and nerve degeneration, or wet beriberi, which causes heart changes.

beta-carotene (β-carotene) A carotenoid found in many yellow and red-orange fruits and vegetables that is a precursor of vitamin A. It is also an antioxidant.

beta-cryptoxanthin (β-cryptoxanthin) A carotenoid found in corn, green peppers, and lemons that can provide some vitamin A activity.

bicarbonate A chemical released by the pancreas into the small intestine that neutralizes stomach acid.

bile A digestive fluid made in the liver and stored in the gallbladder that is released into the small intestine, where it aids in fat digestion and absorption.

binge drinking A pattern of drinking that brings a person's blood alcohol concentration to 80 mg/100mL or above.

binge-eating disorder An eating disorder characterized by recurrent episodes of binge eating accompanied by a loss of control over eating in the absence of purging behavior.

bioaccumulation The process by which compounds accumulate or build up in an organism faster than they can be broken down or excreted.

bioavailability The extent to which the body can absorb and use a nutrient.

biotechnology The process of manipulating life forms via genetic engineering in order to provide desirable products for human use.

biotin One of the B vitamins, needed in energy metabolism.

blackout drinking Amnesia following a period of excessive alcohol consumption.

blood pressure The amount of force exerted by the blood against the walls of arteries.

body composition The term used to describe the different components (lean versus fat tissues) that when taken together make up an individual's body weight.

body image The way a person perceives and imagines his or her body.

body mass index (BMI) A measure of body weight relative to height that is used to compare body size with a standard.

bone remodeling The process whereby bone is continuously broken down and reformed to allow for growth and maintenance.

bone resorption The process by which bone is broken down by osteoclasts releasing calcium from bone to the blood.

botulism A severe food-borne intoxication that results from consuming the toxin produced by *Clostridium botulinum*.

bovine somatotropin (bST) A hormone naturally produced by cows that stimulates the production of milk. A synthetic version of this hormone is now being produced by genetic engineering.

bovine spongiform encephalopathy (BSE) A fatal neurological disease that affects cattle (mad cow disease) and may be transmitted to humans by consuming contaminated beef by-products.

bran The protective outer layers of whole grains. It is a concentrated source of dietary fiber.

brush border The microvilli surface of the intestinal mucosa, which contains some digestive enzymes.

bulimia nervosa An eating disorder characterized by the consumption of a large amount of food at one time (binge eating) followed by purging behaviors such as self-induced vomiting to prevent weight gain.

calcitonin A hormone produced by the thyroid gland that stimulates bone mineralization and inhibits bone breakdown, thus lowering blood calcium levels.

calorie A unit of measure used to express the amount of energy provided by food.

capillary A small, thin-walled blood vessel through which blood and the body's cells exchange gases and nutrients.

carbohydrate loading See glycogen supercompensation

carbohydrates A class of nutrients that includes sugars, starches, and fibers. Chemically, they all contain carbon, along with hydrogen and oxygen, in the same proportions as in water (H_2O).

cardiorespiratory endurance The efficiency with which the body delivers to cells the oxygen and nutrients needed for muscular activity and transports waste products from cells.

cardiovascular disease Any disease affecting the heart and blood vessels.

cardiovascular system The organ system that includes the heart and blood vessels and circulates blood throughout the body.

carotenoids Yellow, orange, and red pigments synthesized by plants and many microorganisms. Some can be converted to vitamin A.

cash crop A crop that is grown to be sold for monetary return rather than as food for the local population.

cataracts A disease of the eye that results in cloudy spots on the lens (and sometimes the cornea), which obscure vision.

celiac disease A disorder that causes damage to the intestines when the protein gluten is eaten.

cell The basic structural and functional unit of living things.

cell differentiation Structural and functional changes that cause cells to mature into specialized cells.

cellular respiration The reactions that break down carbohydrates, fats, and proteins to produce carbon dioxide, water, and energy in the form of ATP.

cellulose An insoluble fiber that is the most prevalent structural material of plant cell walls.

cesarean section The surgical removal of the fetus from the uterus.

Chinese restaurant syndrome See MSG symptom complex

Choice Lists A new term for Exchange Lists; a system of grouping foods based on their carbohydrate, protein, fat, and energy content.

cholesterol A sterol, produced by the liver and consumed in the diet, that is needed to build cell membranes and make hormones and other essential molecules. High blood levels increase the risk of heart disease.

choline A compound needed for the synthesis of the phospholipid phosphatidylcholine, the neurotransmitter acetylcholine, and a number of other biochemical reactions. It is not a vitamin, but is considered an essential nutrient.

chylomicron A lipoprotein that transports lipids from the mucosal cells of the small intestine and delivers triglycerides to other body cells.

chyme A mixture of partially digested food and stomach secretions.

cirrhosis A chronic and irreversible liver disease characterized by loss of functioning liver cells and accumulation of fibrous connective tissue.

cobalamin The chemical term for vitamin B_{12}.

coenzyme An organic nonprotein substance that binds to an enzyme to promote its activity.

cofactor An inorganic ion or coenzyme that is required for enzyme activity.

collagen The major protein in connective tissue.

colostrum The first milk, produced by the breast late in pregnancy and for up to a week after delivery. Compared to mature milk, it contains more water, protein, immune factors, minerals, and vitamins and less fat.

complete dietary protein See high-quality protein

complex carbohydrates Carbohydrates composed of sugar molecules linked together in straight or branching chains. They include oligosaccharides, starches, and fibers.

conditionally essential amino acids Amino acids that are essential in the diet only under certain conditions or at certain times of life; also called semiessential amino acids.

constipation Infrequent or difficult defecation.

control group In a scientific experiment, the group of participants used as a basis of comparison. They are similar to the participants in the experimental group but do not receive the treatment being tested.

creatine phosphate A compound stored in muscle that can be broken down quickly to make ATP.

creatine A compound that can be converted into creatine phosphate, which replenishes muscle ATP during short bursts of activity. Creatine is a dietary supplement used by athletes to increase muscle mass and delay fatigue during short intense exercise.

cretinism A condition resulting from poor maternal iodine intake during pregnancy that impairs mental development and growth in the offspring.

crib death See sudden infant death syndrome

critical control point A possible point in food production, manufacturing, and transportation where contamination could occur or be prevented or eliminated.

critical period Time in growth and development when an organism is more susceptible to harm from poor nutrition or other environmental factors.

cross-contamination The transfer of contaminants from one food or object to another.

cycle of undernutrition A cycle in which undernutrition is perpetuated by an inability to meet nutrient needs at all life stages.

Daily Value A reference value for the intake of nutrients used on food labels to help consumers see how a given food fits into their overall diet.

DASH (Dietary Approaches to Stop Hypertension) eating plan A dietary pattern recommended to lower blood pressure. It is abundant in fruits and vegetables; includes low-fat dairy products, whole grains, legumes, and nuts; and incorporates moderate amounts of lean meat.

deamination The removal of the amino group from an amino acid.

dehydration A state that occurs when not enough water is present to meet the body's needs.

Delaney Clause A clause added to the 1958 Food Additives Amendment of the Pure Food and Drug Act that prohibits the intentional addition to foods of any compound that has been shown to induce cancer in animals or humans at any dose.

dementia A deterioration of mental state that results in impaired memory, thinking, and/or judgment.

denaturation Alteration of a protein's three-dimensional structure.

dental caries Cavities, or decay of the tooth enamel caused by acid produced when bacteria growing on the teeth metabolize carbohydrate.

designer food or **nutraceutical** A food or supplement thought to have health benefits in addition to its nutritive value.

diabetes mellitus A disease characterized by elevated blood glucose due to either insufficient production of insulin or decreased sensitivity of cells to insulin.

diarrhea An intestinal disorder characterized by frequent or watery stools.

dietary folate equivalent (DFE) The amount of folate equivalent to 1 μg of folate naturally occurring in food, 0.6 μg of synthetic folic acid from fortified food or supplements consumed with food, or 0.5 μg synthetic folic acid consumed on an empty stomach.

Dietary Guidelines for Americans A set of nutrition recommendations designed to promote population-wide dietary changes to reduce the incidence of nutrition-related chronic disease.

Dietary Reference Intakes (DRIs) A set of reference values for the intake of energy, nutrients, and food components that can be used for planning and assessing the diets of healthy people in the United States and Canada.

dietary supplement A product designed to supplement the diet; may include nutrients (vitamins, minerals, amino acids, fatty acids), enzymes, herbs, or other substances.

diet-induced thermogenesis See thermic effect of food

diffusion The movement of molecules from an area of higher concentration to an area of lower concentration without the expenditure of energy.

digestion The process by which food is broken down into components small enough to be absorbed into the body.

dipeptide Two amino acids linked by a peptide bond.

direct food additive A substance intentionally added to food. Direct food additives are regulated by the FDA.

disaccharide A carbohydrate made up of two sugar units.

dispensable amino acid See nonessential amino acid

diuretic A substance that increases the amount of urine passed from the body.

diverticula Sacs or pouches that protrude from the wall of the large intestine.

diverticulitis A condition in which diverticula in the large intestine become inflamed.

diverticulosis A condition in which outpouches (or sacs) form in the wall of the large intestine.

docosahexaenoic acid (DHA) A 22-carbon omega-3 polyunsaturated fatty acid found in fish that may be needed in the diet of newborns. It can be synthesized from α-linolenic acid.

Down syndrome A disorder caused by extra genetic material that results in distinctive facial characteristics, mental impairment, and other abnormalities.

eating disorder A psychological illness characterized by specific abnormal eating behaviors, often intended to control weight.

eclampsia Convulsions or seizures during or immediately after pregnancy. Untreated, it can lead to coma or death.

edema Swelling due to the buildup of extracellular fluid in the tissues.

eicosanoids Regulatory molecules that can be synthesized from omega-3 and omega-6 fatty acids.

eicosapentaenoic acid (EPA) A 20-carbon-omega-3 polyunsaturated fatty acid found in fish that can be synthesized from α-linolenic acid but may be essential in humans under some conditions.

electrolyte A positively or negatively charged ion that conducts an electrical current in solution. Commonly refers to sodium, potassium, and chloride.

element A substance that cannot be broken down into products with different properties.

embryo The developing human from two through eight weeks after fertilization.

empty calories Calories from solid fats and/or added sugars, which add calories to the food but few nutrients.

emulsifier A substance with both water-soluble and fat-soluble portions that can break fat into tiny droplets and suspend it in a watery fluid.

endorphins Compounds that cause a natural euphoria and reduce the perception of pain under certain stressful conditions.

endosperm The largest portion of a kernel of grain. It is primarily starch and serves as a food supply for the sprouting seed.

energy balance The amount of energy consumed in the diet compared with the amount expended by the body over a given period.

energy-yielding nutrients Nutrients that can be metabolized to provide energy in the body. They include carbohydrates, fats, and proteins.

enrichment The addition of specific amounts of nutrients to replace those lost during processing.

enzyme A protein molecule that accelerates the rate of a chemical reaction without itself being changed.

epidemiology The branch of science that studies health and disease trends and patterns in populations.

epiglottis A piece of elastic connective tissue that covers the opening to the lungs during swallowing.

ergogenic aid A substance, appliance, or procedure that improves athletic performance.

essential amino acid or **indispensable amino acid** An amino acid that cannot be synthesized by the body in sufficient amounts to meet its needs and therefore must be included in the diet.

essential fatty acid A fatty acid that must be consumed in the diet because it cannot be made by the body or cannot be made in sufficient quantities to meet the body's needs.

essential fatty acid deficiency A condition characterized by dry, scaly skin and poor growth that results when the diet does not supply sufficient amounts of linoleic acid and α-linolenic acid.

essential nutrient A nutrient that must be consumed in the diet because it cannot be made by the body or cannot be made in sufficient quantities to maintain body functions.

Estimated Average Requirements (EARs) Nutrient intakes estimated to meet the needs of 50% of the healthy individuals in a given gender and life-stage group.

Estimated Energy Requirements (EERs) Energy intakes that are predicted to maintain body weight in healthy individuals.

ethanol The alcohol in alcoholic beverages; it is produced by yeast fermentation of sugar.

evidence-based practice Using the compiled evidence from all available well-controlled, peer-reviewed studies to develop recommendations and policies regarding nutrition and health care.

Exchange Lists A system of grouping foods based on their carbohydrate, protein, fat, and energy content. These have been revised as "Choice Lists".

experimental group In a scientific experiment, the group of participants who undergo the treatment being tested.

extreme obesity or **morbid obesity** A body mass index greater than 40 km/m².

facilitated diffusion Assisted diffusion of a substance across a cell membrane.

failure to thrive Inability of a child's growth to keep up with normal growth curves.

famine A widespread lack of access to food due to a disaster that causes a collapse in the food production and marketing systems.

fasting Abstinence from food for a period of at least 8 to 12 hours.

fasting hypoglycemia Low blood sugar that is not related to food intake; often caused by an insulin-secreting tumor.

fat The common term for lipid, or more specifically triglyceride, the most abundant lipid in our food and our bodies.

fatigue Inability to continue an activity at an optimal level.

fat-soluble vitamin A vitamin that does not dissolve in water; includes vitamins A, D, E, and K.

fatty acid A molecule made up of a chain of carbons linked to hydrogens, with an acid group at one end of the chain.

fatty liver The accumulation of fat in the liver. An early symptom of excess alcohol consumption.

feasting Consumption of a large amount of food.

feces Body waste, including unabsorbed food residue, bacteria, mucus, and dead cells, which is eliminated from the gastrointestinal tract by way of the anus.

female athlete triad The combination of energy restriction, changes in hormone levels that affect the menstrual cycle, and low bone mineral density that occurs in some female athletes, particularly those involved in sports in which low body weight and appearance are important.

fertilization The union of a sperm and an egg.

fetal alcohol spectrum disorders (FASDs) A range of physical and behavioral disorders or conditions and functional or mental impairments linked to prenatal alcohol exposure. One of the most severe FASDs is fetal alcohol syndrome.

fetal alcohol syndrome (FAS) A characteristic group of physical and mental abnormalities in an infant resulting from maternal alcohol consumption during pregnancy.

fetus A developing human from the ninth week after fertilization to birth.

fiber A type of carbohydrate that cannot be broken down by human digestive enzymes.

fibrin The protein produced during normal blood clotting that forms an interlacing fibrous network that is essential for formation of the clot.

fitness A set of attributes related to the ability to perform routine physical activities without undue fatigue.

fluorosis A condition affecting the teeth that is caused by chronic overconsumption of fluoride. It is characterized by black and brown stains and cracking and pitting of the teeth.

foam cell A cholesterol-filled white blood cell.

folate A general term that refers to the many forms of this B vitamin, which is needed for the synthesis of DNA and the metabolism of some amino acids.

folic acid An easily absorbed form of the vitamin folate that is present in dietary supplements and fortified foods.

food additive A substance that is intentionally added to or can reasonably be expected to become a component of a food during processing.

food allergy An adverse immune response to a specific food protein.

food desert An area that lacks access to affordable fruits, vegetables, whole grains, low-fat milk, and other foods that make up a healthy diet.

food guide A food group system that suggests amounts of different types of foods needed to meet nutrient intake recommendations.

food insecurity A situation in which people lack adequate physical, social, or economic access to sufficient, safe, nutritious food that meets their dietary needs and food preferences for an active and healthy life.

food intolerance or **food sensitivity** An adverse reaction to a food that does not involve the production of antibodies by the immune system.

food recovery The collection of wholesome food for distribution to the poor and hungry, including collection of crops from farmers' fields that have already been mechanically harvested or on fields where it is not economically profitable to harvest.

food sensitivity See food intolerance

food-borne illness An illness caused by consumption of contaminated food.

food-borne infection Illness caused by the ingestion of food containing microorganisms that can multiply inside the body and produce effects that are injurious.

food-borne intoxication Illness caused by consuming a food containing a toxin.

fortification The addition of nutrients to foods.

fortified food A food to which one or more nutrients has been added.

free radical A type of highly reactive atom or molecule that causes oxidative damage.

fructose A monosaccharide found in fruits and honey that is composed of six carbon atoms arranged in a ring structure; commonly called fruit sugar.

functional food A food that has health-promoting properties beyond basic nutritional functions.

galactose A monosaccharide composed of six carbon atoms arranged in a ring structure; when combined with glucose, it forms the disaccharide lactose.

gallstone A stone formed in the gallbladder or bile duct when substances in the bile harden.

gastric banding See adjustable gastric banding

gastric bypass A surgical procedure that reduces the size of the stomach and bypasses a portion of the small intestine.

gastric juice A substance produced by the gastric glands of the stomach that contains an inactive form of pepsin and hydrochloric acid.

gastric sleeve surgery A bariatric surgical procedure that removes part of the stomach leaving a thin vertical sleeve about the size of a banana. The smaller stomach restricts the amount of food that can be consumed at one session and therefore reduces caloric intake.

gastrin A hormone secreted by the mucosa of the stomach that stimulates the secretion of enzymes and acid in the stomach.

gastroesophageal reflux disease (GERD) A chronic condition in which acidic stomach contents leak into the esophagus, causing pain and damaging the esophagus.

gastrointestinal tract A hollow tube consisting of the mouth, pharynx, esophagus, stomach, small intestine, and large intestine in which digestion of food and absorption of nutrients occur; also called the alimentary canal, GI tract or digestive tract.

gene A length of DNA that contains the information needed to synthesize a polypeptide chain; responsible for inherited traits.

gene expression The events of protein synthesis in which the information coded in a gene is used to synthesize a protein or a molecule of RNA.

generally recognized as safe (GRAS) A group of chemical additives that are considered safe, based on their long-standing presence in the food supply without harmful effects.

genetic engineering or **genetic modification (GM)** A set of techniques used to manipulate DNA for the purpose of changing the characteristics of an organism or creating a new product.

genetically modified organism (GMO) An organism whose genetic material has been altered using genetic engineering techniques.

germ The embryo or sprouting portion of a kernel of grain. It contains vegetable oil, vitamins, and minerals.

gestational diabetes A condition characterized by high blood glucose levels that develops during pregnancy.

gestational hypertension High blood pressure that develops after the 20th week of pregnancy and returns to normal after delivery. It may be an early sign of preeclampsia.

ghrelin A hormone produced by the stomach that affects food intake.

glucagon A hormone made in the pancreas that raises blood glucose levels by stimulating the breakdown of liver glycogen and the synthesis of glucose.

glucose A 6-carbon monosaccharide that is the primary form of carbohydrate used provide energy in the body. Also known as blood sugar.

glutathione peroxidase A selenium-containing enzyme that protects cells from oxidative damage by neutralizing peroxides.

glycemic index A ranking of the effect that the consumption of a single carbohydrate-containing food has on blood glucose in relation to consumption of a reference carbohydrate such as white bread or glucose.

glycemic load An index of the glycemic response that occurs after eating specific foods. It is calculated by multiplying a food's glycemic index by the amount of available carbohydrate in a serving of the food.

glycemic response The rate, magnitude, and duration of the rise in blood glucose that occurs after food is consumed.

glycogen The storage form of carbohydrate in animals, made up of many glucose molecules linked together in a highly branched structure.

glycogen supercompensation or **carbohydrate loading** A regimen designed to increase muscle glycogen stores beyond their usual level.

glycolysis An anaerobic metabolic pathway that splits glucose into two three-carbon pyruvate molecules; the energy released from one glucose molecule is used to make two molecules of ATP.

goiter An enlargement of the thyroid gland caused by a deficiency of iodine.

goitrogen A substance that interferes with the utilization of iodine or the function of the thyroid gland.

Hazard Analysis Critical Control Point (HACCP) A food safety system that focuses on identifying and preventing hazards that could cause food-borne illness.

health claim A food label claim that describes the relationship between a nutrient or food and a disease or health condition. Only approved health claims may appear on food labels.

Healthy People A set of national health promotion and disease prevention objectives for the U.S. population.

heartburn A burning sensation in the chest or throat caused when acidic stomach contents leak back into the esophagus.

heat cramps Muscle cramps caused by an imbalance of sodium and potassium; may result from excessive exercise without adequate fluid and electrolyte replacement.

heat exhaustion Low blood pressure, rapid pulse, fainting, and sweating caused when dehydration decreases blood volume so much that blood can no longer both cool the body and provide oxygen to the muscles.

heat stroke Elevated body temperature as a result of fluid loss and the failure of the temperature regulatory center of the brain.

heat-related illnesses Conditions, including heat cramps, heat exhaustion, and heat stroke, that can occur due to an unfavorable combination of exercise, hydration status, and climatic conditions.

heme iron A readily absorbable form of iron found in meat, fish, and poultry that is chemically associated with certain proteins.

hemochromatosis An inherited disorder that results in increased iron absorption.

hemoglobin An iron-containing protein in red blood cells that binds and transports oxygen through the bloodstream to cells.

hemolytic anemia A condition in which there is an insufficient number of red blood cells because many have burst.

hemolytic-uremic syndrome A disorder, usually in children, that occurs when an infection in the digestive system produces toxic substances that destroy red blood cells causing them to block capillaries, eventually resulting in kidney failure.

hemorrhoid A swollen vein in the anal or rectal area.

hepatic portal vein The vein that transports blood from the gastrointestinal tract to the liver.

heterocyclic amines (HCAs) A class of mutagenic substances produced when there is incomplete combustion of amino acids during the cooking of meats—for example, when meat is charred.

high-density lipoprotein (HDL) A lipoprotein that picks up cholesterol from cells and transports it to the liver so that it can be eliminated from the body.

high quality protein or **complete dietary protein** An easily digestible protein that contains all of the amino acids needed for protein synthesis in amounts similar to those found in body proteins.

hormone A chemical messenger that is produced in one location in the body, released into the blood, and travels to other locations, where it elicits responses.

hunger A desire to consume food that is triggered by internal physiological signals or the recurrent involuntary lack of food that over time may lead to malnutrition.

hydrogenation A process used to make partially hydrogenated oils in which hydrogen atoms are added to the carbon–carbon double bonds of unsaturated fatty acids, making them more saturated. *Trans* fatty acids are formed during the process.

hydrolyzed protein or **protein hydrolysate** A mixture of amino acids or amino acids and polypeptides that results when a protein is completely or partially broken down by treatment with acid or enzymes.

hypercarotenemia A condition caused by the accumulation of carotenoids in the adipose tissue, causing the skin to appear yellow-orange.

hypertension Blood pressure that is consistently elevated to 140/90 millimeters (mm) mercury or greater.

hypertensive disorders of pregnancy A spectrum of conditions involving a rise in blood pressure during pregnancy.

hypertrophy An increase in the size of a muscle or organ.

hypoglycemia Abnormally low blood glucose levels.

hyponatremia Abnormally low concentration of sodium in the blood.

hypothesis A proposed explanation for an observation or a scientific problem that can be tested through experimentation.

implantation The process through which a developing embryo embeds itself in the uterine lining.

incomplete dietary protein A protein that is deficient in one or more of the amino acids required for protein synthesis in humans.

indirect food additive A substance that is expected to unintentionally enter food during manufacturing or from packaging. Indirect food additives are regulated by the FDA.

indispensable amino acid See essential amino acid

infancy The period of early childhood, generally from birth to 1 year of age.

infant botulism A potentially life-threatening disease in which the bacteria *Clostridium botulinum* grows within the baby's gastrointestinal tract.

infant mortality rate The number of deaths during the first year of life per 1000 live births.

inflammation A protective response to injury or destruction of tissues; signs of acute inflammation include pain, heat, redness, swelling, and loss of function.

insoluble fiber Fiber that does not dissolve in water and is less readily be broken down by bacteria in the large intestine. It includes cellulose, some hemicelluloses, and lignin.

insulin A hormone made in the pancreas that allows glucose to enter cells and stimulates the synthesis of protein, fat, and liver and muscle glycogen.

insulin resistance A condition in which the normal amount of insulin produces a subnormal effect in the body.

integrated pest management (IPM) A method of agricultural pest control that integrates nonchemical and chemical techniques.

intestinal microflora Microorganisms that inhabit the large intestine.

intrinsic factor A protein produced in the stomach that aids in the absorption of adequate amounts of vitamin B_{12}.

iodized salt Table salt to which a small amount of sodium iodide or potassium iodide has been added in order to supplement the iodine content of the diet.

ion An atom or a group of atoms that carries an electrical charge.

iron deficiency anemia An iron deficiency disease that occurs when the oxygen-carrying capacity of the blood is decreased because there is insufficient iron to make hemoglobin.

iron overload A condition in which iron accumulates in the tissues; characterized by bronzed skin, enlarged liver, diabetes mellitus, and abnormalities of the pancreas and the joints.

irradiation A process that exposes foods to radiation in order to kill contaminating organisms and retard the ripening and spoilage of fruits and vegetables.

Keshan disease A heart disease that occurs in an area of China where the soil is very low in selenium.

ketoacidosis A life-threatening condition in which ketone levels in the blood are high enough to increase blood acidity.

ketone or **ketone body** An acidic molecule formed when there is not sufficient carbohydrate to break down acetyl-CoA.

ketone body See ketone

ketosis High levels of ketones in the blood.

kilocalorie (kcal) A unit of heat that is used to express the amount of energy provided by foods. It is the amount of heat required to raise the temperature of 1 kilogram of water 1 degree Celsius (1 kcalorie = 1000 calories. When Calorie is spelled with a capital C it denotes kilocalorie).

kwashiorkor A form of protein-energy malnutrition in which only protein is deficient.

lactation Production and secretion of milk.

lacteal A lymph vessel in the villi of the small intestine that picks up particles containing the products of fat digestion.

lactic acid An end product of anaerobic metabolism and an additive used in food to maintain acidity or form curds.

lactose intolerance The inability to completely digest lactose due to a reduction in the levels of the enzyme lactase.

lactose A disaccharide made of glucose linked to galactose that is found in milk.

large for gestational age Weighing more than 4 kg (8.8 lbs) at birth.

LDL receptor See Low-density lipoprotein receptor.

lean body mass Body mass attributed to nonfat body components such as bone, muscle, and internal organs; also called *fat-free mass*.

lecithin A phosphoglyceride composed of a glycerol backbone, two fatty acids, a phosphate group, and a molecule of choline; often used as an emulsifier in foods.

legume The starchy seed of a plant that produces bean pods; includes peas, peanuts, beans, soybeans, and lentils.

leptin A protein hormone produced by adipocytes that signals information about the amount of body fat.

let-down The release of milk from the milk-producing glands and its movement through the ducts and storage sinuses.

life expectancy The average length of life for a particular population of individuals.

life span The maximum age to which members of a species can live.

limiting amino acid The essential amino acid that is available in the lowest concentration relative to the body's needs.

linoleic acid An omega-6 essential fatty acid with 18 carbons and 2 carbon–carbon double bonds.

lipases Fat-digesting enzymes.

lipid bilayer Two layers of phosphoglyceride molecules oriented so that the fat-soluble fatty acid tails are sandwiched between the water-soluble phosphate-containing heads.

lipids A class of nutrients, commonly called fats, that includes fatty acids, triglycerides, phospholipids, and sterols; most do not dissolve in water.

lipoprotein A particle that transports lipids in the blood.

lipoprotein lipase An enzyme that breaks down triglycerides into free fatty acids and glycerol; attached to the outside of the cells that line the blood vessels.

liposuction A procedure that suctions out adipose tissue from under the skin; used to decrease the size of local fat deposits such as on the abdomen or hips.

low birth weight A birth weight less than 2.5 kg (5.5 lbs).

low-density lipoprotein (LDL) A lipoprotein that transports cholesterol to cells.

low-density lipoprotein receptor A protein on the surface of cells that binds to LDL particles and allows their contents to be taken up for use by the cell.

lumen The inside cavity of a tube, such as the gastrointestinal tract.

lymphatic system The system of lymph vessels and other lymph organs and tissues that drains excess fluid from the spaces between cells and provides immune function.

lymphocyte A small white blood cell (leukocyte) that plays a large role in defending the body against disease.

macrocytic anemia A reduction in the blood's hemoglobin content and hence capacity to carry oxygen that is characterized by abnormally large immature and mature red blood cells.

macronutrients Nutrients needed by the body in large amounts. These include water and the energy-yielding nutrients carbohydrates, lipids, and proteins.

macrophage A type of white blood that ingests foreign material as part of the immune response to foreign invaders such as infectious microorganisms.

macula an oval, yellow-pigmented area on the central retina, that is the central point of sharpest vision.

macular degeneration Degeneration of a portion of the retina that results in loss of visual detail and eventually in blindness.

major mineral A mineral required in the diet in an amount greater than 100 mg/day or present in the body in an amount greater than 0.01% of body weight.

malnutrition A condition resulting from an energy or nutrient intake either above or below that which is optimal.

maltose A disaccharide made of two glucose molecules linked together.

marasmus A form of protein-energy malnutrition in which a deficiency of energy in the diet causes severe body wasting.

maximal oxygen consumption See aerobic capacity

maximum heart rate The maximum number of beats per minute that the heart can attain.

menopause The time in a woman's life when the menstrual cycle ends.

metabolic pathway A series of chemical reactions inside of a living organism that results in the transformation of one molecule into another.

metabolism The sum of all the chemical reactions that take place in a living organism.

micelle A particle that is formed in the small intestine when the products of fat digestion are surrounded by bile. It facilitates the absorption of lipids.

microbes Microscopic organisms, or microorganisms, including bacteria, viruses, and fungi.

micronutrients Nutrients needed by the body in small amounts. These include vitamins and minerals.

microvillus (plural, **microvilli**) A minute projection on the mucosal cell membrane that increases the absorptive surface area in the small intestine.

mineral In nutrition, an element needed by the body to maintain structure and regulate chemical reactions and body processes.

mitochondrion (plural, **mitochondria**) A cellular organelle that is responsible for providing energy in the form of ATP via aerobic metabolism; the citric acid cycle and electron transport chain are located here.

modified atmosphere packaging (MAP) A preservation technique used to prolong the shelf life of processed or fresh food by changing the gases surrounding the food in the package.

mold Multicellular fungi that form filamentous branching growths.

molecule A group of two or more atoms of the same or different elements bonded together.

monoglyceride A glycerol molecule with one fatty acid attached.

monosaccharide A carbohydrate made up of a single sugar unit.

monosodium glutamate (MSG) A food additive used as a flavor enhancer, commonly used in Chinese food; made up of the amino acid glutamate bound to sodium.

monounsaturated fatty acid A fatty acid containing one carbon–carbon double bond.

morbid obesity See extreme obesity

morning sickness Nausea and vomiting that affects many women during the first few months of pregnancy and that in some women can continue throughout the pregnancy.

MSG symptom complex or **Chinese restaurant syndrome** A group of symptoms including headache, flushing, tingling, burning sensations, and chest pain reported by some individuals after consuming monosodium glutamate (MSG).

mucosa The layer of tissue lining the gastrointestinal tract and other body cavities.

mucosal cell A type of epithelial cell that makes up the lining of the gastrointestinal tract and other body cavities.

mucus A viscous fluid secreted by glands in the digestive tract and other parts of the body. It lubricates, moistens, and protects cells from harsh environments.

muscle endurance The ability of a muscle group to continue muscle movement over time.

muscle strength The amount of force that can be produced by a single contraction of a muscle.

muscle-strengthening exercise Activities that are specifically designed to increase muscle strength, endurance, and size; also called strength-training exercise or resistance-training exercise.

myelin A soft, white fatty substance that covers nerve fibers and aids in nerve transmission.

myoglobin An iron-containing protein in muscle cells that binds oxygen.

MyPlate A plate-shaped food guide released in 2011 that suggests amounts and types of food from five food groups to meet the recommendations of the Dietary Guidelines.

National School Lunch Program A federally funded program designed to provide free or reduced cost lunches to school-age children.

neural tube defect An abnormality in the brain or spinal cord that results from errors that occur during prenatal development.

neurotransmitter A chemical substance produced by a nerve cell that can stimulate or inhibit another cell.

niacin A B vitamin needed in energy metabolism.

niacin equivalent (NE) A unit used to express the amount of niacin present in food, including that which can be made from its precursor, tryptophan. One NE is equal to 1 mg of niacin or 60 mg of tryptophan.

night blindness Inability to see clearly in dim light.

nitrogen balance The amount of nitrogen consumed in the diet compared with the amount excreted over a given period.

nitrosamine A carcinogenic compound produced by reactions between nitrites and amino acids.

nonessential or **dispensable amino acid** Amino acid that can be synthesized by the human body in sufficient amounts to meet needs.

nonexercise activity thermogenesis (NEAT) The energy expended for everything we do other than sleeping, eating, or sports-like exercise.

nonnutritive sweetener or **artificial sweetener** A substance used to sweeten food that provides few or no calories.

nursing bottle syndrome Extreme tooth decay in the upper teeth resulting from putting a child to bed with a bottle containing milk or other sweet liquids.

nutraceutical See designer food

nutrient A substance in food that provides energy and structure to the body and regulates body processes.

nutrient content claim A claim on food labels used to describe the level of a nutrient in a food. The Nutrition Labeling and Education Act of 1990 defines these terms and regulates the circumstances under which they can be used.

nutrient density A measure of the nutrients provided by a food relative to its calorie content.

nutrients Substances in food that provide energy and structure to the body and regulate body processes.

nutrigenetics The study of how the genes people inherit affect the impact their diet has on health.

nutrigenomics The study of how the nutrients and other food components people consume affect gene activity.

Nutrition Facts The portion of a food label that provides information about the nutritional composition of a food and how that food fits into the overall diet.

nutrition transition A series of changes in diet, physical activity, health, and nutrition that occurs as poor countries become more prosperous.

nutritional genomics The study of how our genes affect the impact of nutrients or other food components on health (nutrigenetics) and how nutrients affect the activity of our genes (nutrigenomics).

nutritional programming The concept that the nutritional conditions that exist while a baby is developing in the womb, and in infancy, affect future development and health.

nutritional status An individual's health, as it is influenced by the intake and utilization of nutrients.

obese Having excess body fat. Obesity is defined as having a body mass index (ratio of weight to height squared) of 30 kg/m² or greater.

obesity genes Genes that code for proteins involved in the regulation of body fat. When they are abnormal, the result is abnormal amounts of body fat.

oldest old Individuals 85 years of age and older.

oligosaccharide A carbohydrate made up of 3 to 10 sugar units.

omega-3 fatty acid A fatty acid containing a carbon–carbon double bond between the third and fourth carbons from the omega end; includes α-linolenic acid found in vegetable oils and eicosapentaenoic acid (EPA) and docosahexaenoic acid (DHA) found in fish oils.

omega-6 fatty acid A fatty acid containing a carbon–carbon double bond between the sixth and seventh carbons from the omega end; includes linoleic and arachidonic acid.

organ A discrete structure composed of more than one tissue that performs a specialized function.

organ system A group of cooperative organs.

organic compound A substance that contains carbon bonded to hydrogen.

organic food Food that is produced, processed, and handled in accordance with the standards of the USDA National Organic Program.

osmosis The unassisted diffusion of water across the cell membrane.

osteomalacia A vitamin D deficiency disease in adults, characterized by loss of minerals from bone, bone pain, muscle aches, and an increase in bone fractures.

osteopenia A reduction in bone density to below normal levels.

osteoporosis A bone disorder characterized by reduced bone mass, increased bone fragility, and increased risk of fractures.

overload principle The concept that the body adapts to the stresses placed on it.

overnutrition Poor nutritional status resulting from a dietary intake in excess of that which is optimal for health.

overtraining syndrome A collection of emotional, behavioral, and physical symptoms that occurs when the amount and intensity of exercise exceeds an athlete's capacity to recover.

overweight Being too heavy for one's height, usually due to an excess of body fat. Overweight is defined as having a body mass index (ratio of weight to height squared) of 25 to 29.9 kilograms/meter^2 (kg/m^2).

oxidative damage Damage caused by highly reactive oxygen molecules that steal electrons from other compounds, causing changes in structure and function.

oxidized LDL cholesterol A substance formed when the cholesterol in LDL particles is oxidized by reactive oxygen molecules. It is key in the development of atherosclerosis because it is taken up by macrophages, transforming them into foam cells.

oxytocin A hormone released by the posterior pituitary that stimulates the ejection or let-down of milk during lactation.

pancreatic amylase A starch-digesting enzyme found in pancreatic juice.

pancreatic juice Fluid secreted by the pancreas that contains bicarbonate to neutralize acid and enzymes for the digestion of carbohydrates, fats, and proteins.

pantothenic acid One of the B vitamins, needed in energy metabolism.

parasite An organism that lives at the expense of others.

parathyroid hormone (PTH) A hormone released by the parathyroid gland that acts to increase blood calcium levels.

partially hydrogenated oils Liquid oils that have undergone a process that adds hydrogen atoms to the carbon–carbon double bonds of unsaturated fatty acids to make the oil more solid and/or increase the shelf life of the product.

pasteurization The process of heating food products in order to kill disease-causing organisms.

pathogen A biological agent that causes disease.

peak bone mass The maximum bone density attained at any time in life, usually occurring in young adulthood.

peer-review process The review of the design and validity of a research experiment by experts in the field of study who did not participate in the research.

pellagra A disease resulting from niacin deficiency, which causes dermatitis, diarrhea, dementia, and, if not treated, death.

pepsin A protein-digesting enzyme produced by the stomach. It is secreted in the gastric juice in an inactive form (pepsinogen) and activated by acid in the stomach.

peptic ulcer An open sore in the lining of the stomach, esophagus, or upper small intestine.

peptide Two or more amino acids joined by peptide bonds.

peptide bond The chemical linkage between the amino group of one amino acid and the acid group of another.

peristalsis Coordinated muscular contractions that move material through the GI tract.

pernicious anemia A macrocytic anemia resulting from vitamin B_{12} deficiency that occurs when dietary vitamin B_{12} cannot be absorbed due to a lack of intrinsic factor.

phagocyte A type of white blood cell that engulfs and consumes foreign particles such as bacteria.

pharynx A funnel-shaped opening that connects the nasal passages and mouth to the respiratory passages and esophagus. It is a common passageway for food and air and is responsible for swallowing.

phenylketonuria (PKU) A genetic disease in which the amino acid phenylalanine cannot be metabolized normally, causing it to build up in the blood. If untreated, the condition results in brain damage.

phosphate group A chemical group consisting of one phosphorus atom and four oxygen atoms.

phospholipid A type of lipid whose structure includes a phosphorus atom.

photosynthesis The metabolic process by which plants trap energy from the sun and use it to make sugars from carbon dioxide and water.

physical frailty Impairment in function and reduction in physiologic reserves severe enough to cause limitations in the basic activities of daily living.

phytochemical A substance found in plant foods that is not an essential nutrient but may have health-promoting properties.

pica An abnormal craving for and ingestion of nonfood substances that have little or no nutritional value.

placebo A fake medicine or supplement that is indistinguishable in appearance from the real thing. It is used to disguise the control and experimental groups in an experiment.

placenta An organ produced from maternal and embryonic tissues. It secretes hormones, transfers nutrients and oxygen from the mother's blood to the fetus, and removes metabolic wastes.

plant sterol A compound found in plant cell membranes that resembles cholesterol in structure. It can lower blood cholesterol by competing with cholesterol for absorption in the gastrointestinal tract.

polychlorinated biphenyls (PCBs) Carcinogenic industrial compounds that have found their way into the environment and, subsequently, the food supply. Repeated exposure causes them to accumulate in biological tissues over time.

polycyclic aromatic hydrocarbons (PAHs) A class of mutagenic substances produced during cooking when there is incomplete combustion of organic materials—for example, when fat drips on a grill.

polypeptide A chain of amino acids linked by peptide bonds that is part of the structure of a protein.

polysaccharide A carbohydrate made up of many sugar units linked together.

polyunsaturated fatty acid A fatty acid that contains two or more carbon–carbon double bonds.

postmenopausal bone loss Accelerated bone loss that occurs in women for about 5 to 10 years surrounding menopause.

prebiotic A substance that passes undigested into the colon and stimulates the growth and/or activity of certain types of bacteria.

prediabetes A consistent elevation of blood glucose levels to between 100 and 125 mg/dl of blood, a level above normal but not high enough to be diagnostic of diabetes but thought to increase the risk of developing diabetes.

preeclampsia A condition characterized by elevated blood pressure, a rapid increase in body weight, protein in the urine, and edema. Also called *toxemia*.

prehypertension Blood pressures of 120 to 139 millimeters of mercury systolic (top number) or 80 to 89 diastolic (bottom number). It increases the risk of developing hypertension as well as the risk of artery damage and heart disease.

premature See preterm

preterm or **premature** An infant born before 37 weeks of gestation.

prion A pathogenic protein that is the cause of degenerative brain diseases called spongiform encephalopathies. *Prion* is short for proteinaceous infectious particle.

prior-sanctioned substance A substance that the FDA or the USDA had determined was safe for use in a specific food prior to the 1958 Food Additives Amendment.

probiotic A product that contains live bacteria, which when consumed temporarily lives in the colon and confers health benefits on the host.

prolactin A hormone released from the anterior pituitary that stimulates the mammary glands to produce milk.

protease A protein-digesting enzyme.

protein A class of nutrients that includes molecules made up of one or more intertwining chains of amino acids. They contain carbon, hydrogen, oxygen, and nitrogen.

protein complementation The process of combining proteins from different sources so that they collectively provide the proportions of amino acids required to meet the body's needs.

protein hydrolysate See hydrolyzed protein

protein quality A measure of how efficiently a protein in the diet can be used to make body proteins.

protein-energy malnutrition (PEM) A condition characterized by loss of muscle and fat mass and an increased susceptibility to infection that results from the long-term consumption of insufficient amounts of energy and/or protein to meet the body's needs.

prothrombin A blood protein required for blood clotting.

provitamin or **vitamin precursor** A compound that can be converted into the active form of a vitamin in the body.

puberty A period of rapid growth and physical changes that ends in the attainment of sexual maturity.

pyridoxal phosphate The major coenzyme form of vitamin B_6 that functions in more than 100 enzymatic reactions, many of which involve amino acid metabolism.

qualified health claim A health claim on a food label that has been approved based on emerging but not well-established evidence of a relationship between a food, food component, or dietary supplement and reduced risk of a disease or health-related condition.

reactive hypoglycemia Low blood sugar that occurs an hour or so after the consumption of high-carbohydrate foods; results from an overproduction of insulin.

recombinant DNA DNA that has been formed by joining DNA from different sources.

Recommended Dietary Allowances (RDAs) Nutrient intakes that are sufficient to meet the needs of almost all healthy people in a specific gender and life-stage group.

refined Refers to foods that have undergone processing that changes or removes various components of the original food.

renewable resource A resource that is restored and replaced by natural processes and can therefore be used forever.

resistance-training exercise See muscle-strengthening exercise

resistant starch Starch that escapes digestion in the small intestine of healthy people.

resting heart rate The number of times that the heart beats per minute while a person is at rest.

resting metabolic rate (RMR) The rate of energy expenditure at rest. It is measured after 5 to 6 hours without food or exercise.

retinoids The chemical forms of preformed vitamin A: retinol, retinal, and retinoic acid.

retinol activity equivalent (RAE) The amount of retinol, α-carotene, β-carotene, or β-crytoxanthin that must be consumed to equal the vitamin A activity of 1 μg of retinol.

retinol-binding protein A protein that is necessary to transport vitamin A from the liver to tissues in need.

rhodopsin A light-sensitive compound found in the retina of the eye that is composed of the protein opsin loosely bound to retinal.

riboflavin A B vitamin needed in energy metabolism.

rickets A vitamin D deficiency disease in children, characterized by poor bone development because of inadequate calcium absorption.

saliva A watery fluid that is produced and secreted into the mouth by the salivary glands. It contains lubricants, enzymes, and other substances.

salivary amylase An enzyme secreted by the salivary glands that breaks down starch into smaller units.

satiety The feeling of fullness and satisfaction caused by food consumption that eliminates the desire to eat.

saturated fat A type of lipid that is most abundant in solid animal fats and is associated with an increased risk of heart disease.

saturated fatty acid A fatty acid in which the carbon atoms are bonded to as many hydrogen atoms as possible; it therefore contains no carbon–carbon double bonds.

scientific method The general approach of science that is used to explain observations about the world around us.

scurvy A vitamin C deficiency disease characterized by bleeding gums, tooth loss, joint pain, bleeding into the skin and mucous membranes, and fatigue.

segmentation Rhythmic local constrictions of the intestine that mix food with digestive juices and speed absorption by repeatedly moving the food mass over the intestinal wall.

set point A level at which body fat or body weight seems to resist change despite changes in energy intake or output.

simple carbohydrates Carbohydrates known as sugars that include monosaccharides and disaccharides.

simple diffusion The unassisted diffusion of a substance across the cell membrane.

small for gestational age An infant born at term weighing less than 2.5 kg (5.5 lb).

sodium chloride The chemical formula of table salt.

soluble fiber Fiber that dissolves in water or absorbs water and is readily broken down by intestinal microflora. It includes pectins, gums, and some hemicelluloses.

solute A dissolved substance.

solvent A fluid in which one or more substances dissolve.

Special Supplemental Nutrition Program for Women, Infants, and Children (WIC) A program funded by the federal government that provides nutrition education and food vouchers to pregnant and lactating women and their young children.

sphincter A muscular valve that helps control the flow of materials in the gastrointestinal tract.

spina bifida A neural tube defect in which part of the spinal cord is exposed through a gap in the backbone, causing varying degrees of disability.

spore The dormant state of some bacteria that is resistant to heat but can germinate and produce a new organism when environmental conditions are favorable.

sports anemia A temporary decrease in hemoglobin concentration that occurs during exercise training. It occurs as an adaptation to training and does not impair delivery of oxygen to tissues.

starch A carbohydrate found in plants, made up of many glucose molecules linked in straight or branching chains.

starvation A severe reduction in nutrient and energy intake that impairs health and eventually causes death. It is the most extreme form of malnutrition.

steroid precursor An androgenic hormone produced primarily by the adrenal glands and gonads that acts as precursor in the production of testosterone and estrogen.

sterol A type of lipid with a structure composed of multiple chemical rings.

strength-training exercise See muscle-strengthening exercise

structure/function claim A claim on a food label that describes the role of a nutrient or dietary ingredient in maintaining normal structure or function in humans.

stunting A low height for age; less than 5th percentile of height on a reference growth curve.

subcutaneous fat Adipose tissue located under the skin, which is not associated with a great increase in the risk of chronic diseases.

subsistence crop A crop that is grown as food for a farmer's family, with little or nothing left to sell.

sucrose A disaccharide commonly known as table sugar that is made of glucose linked to fructose.

sudden infant death syndrome (SIDS, or crib death) The unexplained death of an infant, usually during sleep.

sugar unit A sugar molecule that cannot be broken down to yield other sugars.

Supplement Facts The portion of a dietary supplement label that includes information about, serving size, ingredients, amount per serving size (by weight), and percent of Daily Value, if established.

sustainable agriculture Agricultural methods that maintain soil productivity and a healthy ecological balance while having minimal long-term impacts.

teratogen A chemical, biological, or physical agent that causes birth defects.

theory A formal explanation of an observed phenomenon made after a hypothesis has been tested and supported through extensive experimentation.

thermic effect of food (TEF) or diet-induced thermogenesis The energy required for the digestion of food and absorption, metabolism, and storage of nutrients.

thiamin A B vitamin needed in energy metabolism.

thirst A sensation of dryness in the mouth and throat associated with a desire for liquids.

thyroid gland A gland located in the neck that produces thyroid hormones and calcitonin.

thyroid hormones Hormones produced by the thyroid gland that regulate metabolic rate.

thyroid-stimulating hormone A hormone that stimulates the synthesis and secretion of thyroid hormones from the thyroid gland.

tissue A collection of similar cells that together carry out a specific function.

tocopherol The chemical name for vitamin E.

Tolerable Upper Intake Levels (ULs) Maximum daily nutrient intake levels that are unlikely to pose risks of adverse health effects to almost all individuals in a given gender and life-stage group.

tolerances The maximum amount of pesticide residues that may legally remain in food, set by the EPA.

total energy expenditure The sum of basal energy expenditure, the thermic effect of food, and the energy used in physical activity, regulation of body temperature, deposition of new tissue, and production of milk.

trace mineral A mineral required in the diet in an amount of 100 mg or less per day or present in the body in amounts of 0.01% of body weight or less.

trans **fatty acid** An unsaturated fatty acid in which the hydrogens are on opposite sides of the carbon–carbon double bond.

transamination The process by which an amino group from one amino acid is transferred to a carbon compound to form a new amino acid.

transcription The process of copying the information in DNA to a molecule of mRNA.

transgenic An organism with a gene or group of genes intentionally transferred from another species or breed.

transit time The time between the ingestion of food and the elimination of the solid waste from that food.

translation The process of translating the mRNA code into the amino acid sequence of a polypeptide chain.

triglyceride The major type of lipid in food and the body, consisting of three fatty acids attached to a glycerol molecule.

trimester A term used to describe each third or three-month period of a pregnancy.

tripeptide Three amino acids linked together by peptide bonds.

tropical oils A term used in the popular press to refer to the saturated plant oils—coconut, palm, and palm kernel oil—that are derived from plants grown in tropical regions.

type 1 diabetes The form of diabetes caused by autoimmune destruction of insulin-producing cells in the pancreas, usually leading to absolute insulin deficiency.

type 2 diabetes The form of diabetes characterized by insulin resistance and relative (rather than absolute) insulin deficiency.

undernutrition Poor nutritional status resulting from a dietary intake below that which meets nutritional needs.

underweight A body mass index of less than 18.5 kg/m^2, or a body weight 10% or more below the desirable body weight standard.

unrefined food A food eaten either just as it is found in nature or with only minimal processing.

unsaturated fat A type of lipid that is most abundant in plant oils and is associated with a reduced risk of heart disease.

unsaturated fatty acid A fatty acid that contains one or more carbon–carbon double bonds; may be either monounsaturated or polyunsaturated.

urea A nitrogen-containing waste product from the breakdown of proteins that is excreted in the urine.

variable A factor or condition that is changed in an experimental setting.

variant Creutzfeldt-Jakob Disease (vCJD) A rare, degenerative, fatal brain disorder in humans. It is believed that the persons who have developed vCJD became infected through their consumption of cattle products contaminated with BSE.

vegan diet A plant-based diet that eliminates all animal products.

vegetarian diet A diet that includes plant-based foods and eliminates some or all foods of animal origin.

vein A vessel that carries blood toward the heart.

venule A small vein that drains blood from capillaries and passes it to larger veins for return to the heart.

very low birth weight A birth weight less than 1.5 kg (3.3 lbs).

very-low-density lipoprotein (VLDL) A lipoprotein assembled by the liver that carries lipids from the liver and delivers triglycerides to body cells.

villus (plural, **villi**) A fingerlike protrusion of the lining of the small intestine that participates in the digestion and absorption of foodstuffs.

visceral fat Adipose tissue deposited in the abdominal cavity around the internal organs. High levels are associated with an increased risk of heart disease, high blood pressure, stroke, diabetes, and breast cancer.

vitamin An organic compound needed in the diet in small amounts to promote and regulate the chemical reactions and processes needed for growth, reproduction, and the maintenance of health.

vitamin A A fat-soluble vitamin needed in cell differentiation, reproduction, and vision.

vitamin B$_{12}$ One of the B vitamins, only found in animal foods.

vitamin B$_6$ One of the B vitamins, needed in protein metabolism.

vitamin C A water-soluble vitamin needed for the maintenance of collagen.

vitamin D A fat-soluble vitamin needed for calcium absorption that can be made in the body when there is exposure to sunlight.

vitamin E A fat-soluble vitamin that functions as an antioxidant.

vitamin K A fat-soluble vitamin needed for blood clotting.

vitamin precursor See provitamin

VO$_2$ max See aerobic capacity

water intoxication A condition that occurs when a person drinks enough water to significantly lower the concentration of sodium in the blood.

water-soluble vitamin A vitamin that dissolves in water; includes the B vitamins and vitamin C.

Wernicke-Korsakoff syndrome A form of thiamin deficiency associated with alcohol abuse that is characterized by mental confusion, disorientation, loss of memory, and a staggering gait.

whole-grain product A product made from the entire kernel of a grain including the bran, endosperm, and germ.

WIC See Special Supplemental Nutrition Program for Women, Infants, and Children

xerophthalmia A spectrum of eye conditions resulting from vitamin A deficiency that may lead to blindness.

zoochemical A substance found in animal food (zoo means animal) that is not an essential nutrient but may have health-promoting properties.

References

Chapter 1

[1] American Dietetic Association. Position of the American Dietetic Association: Nutrient supplementation. *J Am Diet Assoc 109*:2073–2085, 2009.

[2] Schroder, B.G., Griffin, I., Specker, B.L., and Abrams, S.A. Absorption of calcium from the carbonated dairy soft drink is greater than that from fat-free milk and calcium fortified orange juice in women. *Nutritional Research 25*:737–742, 2005.

[3] He, K. Fish, long-chain omega-3 polyunsaturated fatty acids and prevention of cardiovascular disease—Eat fish or take fish oil supplement? *Prog Cardiovasc Dis 52*:95–114, 2009.

[4] Zhou, X.F., Ding, Z.S., and Liu, N.B. Allium vegetables and risk of prostate cancer: evidence from 132,192 subjects. *Asian Pac J Cancer Prev14*:4131–4134, 2013.

[5] Antony, M.L., and Singh, S.V. Molecular mechanisms and targets of cancer chemoprevention by garlic-derived bioactive compound diallyl trisulfide. *Indian J Exp Biol 49*:805–816, 2011.

[6] Andres, S., Abraham, K., Appel, K.E., and Lampen, A. Risks and benefits of dietary isoflavones for cancer. *Crit Rev Toxicol 41*:463–506, 2011.

[7] Gencel, V.B., Benjamin, M.M., Bahou, S.N., and Khalil, R.A. Vascular effects of phytoestrogens and alternative menopausal hormone therapy in cardiovascular disease. *Mini Rev Med Chem 12*:149–174, 2012.

[8] Böhm, F., Edge, R., and Truscott, T.G. Interactions of dietary carotenoids with singlet oxygen (1O2) and free radicals: Potential effects for human health. *Acta Biochim Pol 59*:27–30, 2012.

[9] Nile, S.H., and Park, S.W. Edible berries: Review on bioactive components and their effect on human health. *Nutrition 30*:134–144, 2014.

[10] Toh, J.Y., Tan, V.M., Lim, P.C., et al. Flavonoids from fruit and vegetables: A focus on cardiovascular risk factors. *Curr Atheroscler Rep 15*:368, 2013.

[11] Rodriguez-Matcos, A., Heiss, C., Borges, G., and Crozier, A. Berry (Poly)phenols and Cardiovascular Health. *J Agric Food Chem* 2013 Oct 7. [Epub ahead of print]

[12] Rodriguez-Leyva, D., Dupasquier, C.M., McCullough, R., and Pierce, G.N. The cardiovascular effects of flaxseed and its omega-3 fatty acid, alpha-linolenic acid. *Can J Cardiol 26*:489–496, 2010.

[13] Nogueira Lde, P., Knibel, M.P., Torres, M.R., et al. Consumption of high-polyphenol dark chocolate improves endothelial function in individuals with stage 1 hypertension and excess body weight. *Int J Hypertens 2012*:147321, 2012.

[14] Khatua, T.N., Adela, R., and Banerjee, S.K. Garlic and cardioprotection: insights into the molecular mechanisms. *Can J Physiol Pharmacol 91*:448–458, 2013.

[15] Ma, L., Dou, H.L., Wu, Y.Q., et al. Lutein and zeaxanthin intake and the risk of age-related macular degeneration: a systematic review and meta-analysis. *Br J Nutr 107*:350–359, 2012.

[16] Eussen, S.R., de Jong, N., Rompelberg, C.J., et al. Dose-dependent cholesterol-lowering effects of phytosterol/phytostanol-enriched margarine in statin users and statin non-users under free-living conditions. *Public Health Nutr 14*:1823–1832, 2011.

[17] Alexiadou, K., and Katsilambros, N. Nuts: anti-atherogenic food? *Eur J Intern Med 22*:141–146, 2011.

[18] Zhang, J., Li, L., Song, P., et al. Randomized controlled trial of oatmeal consumption versus noodle consumption on blood lipids of urban Chinese adults with hypercholesterolemia. *Nutr J 11*:54–61, 2012.

[19] Calder, P.C. The role of marine omega-3 (n-3) fatty acids in inflammatory processes, atherosclerosis and plaque stability. *Mol Nutr Food Res 56*:1073–1080, 2012.

[20] Yuan, J.M., Sun, C., and Butler, L.M. Tea and cancer prevention: epidemiological studies. *Pharmacol Res 64*:123–135, 2011.

[21] Borneo, R., and León, A.E. Whole grain cereals: functional components and health benefits. *Food Funct 3*:110–119, 2012.

[22] Crowe, K.M., and Francis, C. Position of the Academy of Nutrition and Dietetics: Functional Foods. *J Acad Nutr Diet 113*:1096–1103, 2013.

[23] Ogden, C.L., Carroll, M.D., Kit, B.K., and Flagel, K.M. Prevalence of childhood and adult obesity in the United States, 2011–2012. *JAMA 311*:806–814, 2014.

[24] U.S. Department of Agriculture and U.S. Department of Health and Human Services. *Dietary Guidelines for Americans, 2010*, 7th Edition. Washington, DC: U.S. Government Printing Office, December, 2010.

[25] U.S. Burden of Disease Collaborators. The state of US health, 1990–2010: burden of diseases, injuries, and risk factors. *JAMA 310*:591–608, 2013.

[26] Murphy, S.L., Xu, J., and Kochanek, K.D. Deaths: Final data for 2010. *National Vital Statistics Reports 61(4)*, May 2013. Available online at http://www.cdc.gov/nchs/data/nvsr/nvsr61/nvsr61_04.pdf. Accessed May 3, 2014.

[27] Kaput, J. Nutrigenomics—2006 update. *Clin Chem Lab Med 45*:279–287, 2007.

[28] Division of Nutrition and Physical Activity. *Research to practice series No. 2: Portion size*. Atlanta: Centers for Disease Control and Prevention, 2006. Available online at http://www.cdc.gov/nccdphp/dnpa/nutrition/pdf/portion_size_research.pdf. Accessed May 3, 2014.

Chapter 2

[1] Davis, C., and Saltos, E. Dietary recommendations and how they have changed over time. In *America's Eating Habits: Changes and Consequences*. Frazao, E., ed. Agriculture Information Bulletin No. (AIB-750), May 1999, page 33–50. Available online at http://www.ers.usda.gov/publications/aib-agricultural-information-bulletin/aib750.aspx#.U2zqcyhfG2N. Accessed May 7, 2014.

[2] U.S. Department of Agriculture and U.S. Department of Health and Human Services. *Dietary Guidelines for Americans, 2010*. 7th ed. Washington, DC: U.S. Government Printing Office, December 2010.

[3] U.S. Department of Agriculture, Economic Research Service. Major trends in the U.S. food supply, 1909–1999. *Food Review 23*:12, 2000.

[4] Wells, H.F., and Buzby, J.C. Dietary assessment of major trends in U.S. food consumption, 1970–2005. *Economic Information Bulletin No. 33*. Economic Research Service, U.S. Department of Agriculture, March 2008.

[5] HealthyPeople.gov. *About Healthy People*. Available online at http://www.healthypeople.gov/2020/about/default.aspx. Accessed May 7, 2014.

[6] Institute of Medicine, Food and Nutrition Board. *Dietary Reference Intakes for Energy, Carbohydrate, Fiber, Fat, Fatty Acids, Cholesterol, Protein, and Amino Acids*. Washington, DC: National Academies Press, 2002.

[7] Finkelstein, E.A., Trogdon, J.G., Cohen, J.W., and Dietz, W. Annual medical spending attributable to obesity: Payer- and service-specific estimates. *Health Affairs* 28:w822–w831, 2009.

[8] Cawley, J., and Maclean, J.C. Report: Unfit for service: the implications of rising obesity for U.S. military recruitment, *NBER Working Paper No. 16408*, September 2010. Available online at http://www.nber.org/papers/w16408. Accessed November 30, 2013.

[9] Vaitheeswaran, V. Food policy debate, *The Economist*, December 8, 2009. Available online at http://www.economist.com/debate/days/view/427. Accessed February 3, 2011.

[10] Ogden, C.L., Carroll, M.D., Kit, B.K., and Flegal, K.M. Prevalence of childhood and adult obesity in the United States, 2011–2012. *JAMA 311*:806–814, 2014.

[11] Freeland-Graves, J.H., and Nitzke, S. Position of the Academy of Nutrition and Dietetics: Total diet approach to healthy eating. *J Acad Nutr Diet 113*:307–317, 2013.

[12] Centers for Disease Control and Prevention. *CDC Estimates of Foodborne Illness in the United States*. Available online at http://www.cdc.gov/foodborneburden/. Accessed May 9, 2014.

[13] U.S. Food and Drug Administration. *A Key to Choosing Healthful Foods: Using the Nutrition Facts on The Food Label*. Available online at http://www.fda.gov/downloads/Food/ResourcesForYou/Consumers/UCM079504.pdf. Accessed April 22, 2014.

[14] U.S. Food and Drug Administration. *Menu and Vending Machines Labeling Requirements*. Available online at http://www.fda.gov/Food/IngredientsPackagingLabeling/LabelingNutrition/ucm217762.htm. Accessed May 9, 2014.

[15] U.S. Food and Drug Administration, *Proposed Changes to the Nutrition Facts Label*. Available online at http://www.fda.gov/Food/GuidanceRegulation/GuidanceDocumentsRegulatoryInformation/LabelingNutrition/ucm385663.htm#Summary. Accessed April 15, 2014.

[16] U.S. Food and Drug Administration. *Food Labeling Guide, Guidance for Industry: A Food Labeling Guide,* January, 2013. Available online at http://www.fda.gov/Food/GuidanceRegulation/GuidanceDocumentsRegulatoryInformation/LabelingNutrition/ucm2006828.htm. Accessed May 9, 2014.

[17] U.S. Food and Drug Administration. *Guidance for Industry: A Labeling Guide For Restaurants and Other Retail Establishments Selling Away-From-Home Foods*, April 2008. Available online at http://www.fda.gov/food/guidanceregulation/ucm053455.htm. Accessed May 9, 2014.

[18] U.S. Food and Drug Administration, *Dietary Supplement Labeling Guide, Guidance for Industry: A Dietary Supplement Labeling Guide*. April 2005. Available online at http://www.fda.gov/food/guidanceregulation/guidancedocumentsregulatoryinformation/dietarysupplements/ucm2006823.htm. Accessed May 9, 2014.

Chapter 3

[1] Frank, D.N., St. Amand, A.L., Feldman, R.A., et al. Molecular-phylogenetic characterization of microbial community imbalances in human inflammatory diseases. *Proc Natl Acad Sci USA 104*:13780–13785, 2007.

[2] Sellers, R.S., and Morton, D. The colon: From banal to brilliant. *Toxicol Pathol 42*:67–81, 2014.

[3] Hempel, S., Newberry, S.J., Maher, A.R., et al. Probiotics for the prevention and treatment of antibiotic-associated diarrhea: A systematic review and meta-analysis *JAMA 307*:1959–1969, 2012.

[4] Isolauri, E., and Salminen, S.; Nutrition, Allergy, Mucosal Immunology, and Intestinal Microbiota (NAMI) Research Group Report. Probiotics: Use in allergic disorders: A Nutrition, Allergy, Mucosal Immunology, and Intestinal Microbiota (NAMI) Research Group Report. *J Clin Gastroenterol 42*(Suppl. 2):S91–S96, 2008.

[5] Dai, C., Zheng, C.Q., Jiang, M., et al. Probiotics and irritable bowel syndrome. *World J Gastroenterol 19*:5973–5980, 2013.

[6] Chong, E.S. A potential role of probiotics in colorectal cancer prevention: Review of possible mechanisms of action. *World J Microbiol Biotechnol 30*:351–374, 2014.

[7] Tremaroli, V., and Backhed, F. Functional interactions between the gut microbiota and host metabolism. *Nature 489*:242–249, 2012.

[8] Bosscher, D., Breynaert, A., Pieters, L., and Hermans, N. Food-based strategies to modulate the composition of the intestinal microbiota and their associated health effects. *J Physiol Pharmacol 60*(Suppl. 6):5–11, 2009.

[9] Centers for Disease Control and Prevention. *Food allergies*. Available online at www.cdc.gov/HealthyYouth/foodallergies. Accessed October 31, 2013.

[10] Gupta, R., Springston, E., Warrier, M.R., et al. The prevalence, severity, and distribution of childhood food allergy in the United States. *Pediatrics 128*:e9–e17, 2011.

[11] National Institute of Diabetes, Digestive and Kidney Diseases. *Celiac disease*. Available online at http://digestive.niddk.nih.gov/ddiseases/pubs/celiac. Accessed October 31, 2013.

[12] van der Windt, D.A., Jellema, P., Mulder, C.J., et al. Diagnostic testing for celiac disease among patients with abdominal symptoms: A systematic review. *JAMA 303*:1738–1746, 2010.

[13] Wu, J., Xu, S., and Zhu, Y. Helicobacter pylori CagA: A critical destroyer of the gastric epithelial barrier. *Dig Dis Sci 58*:1830–1837, 2013.

[14] National Institutes of Health, National Institute of Diabetes and Digestive and Kidney Diseases, National Digestive Disease Information Clearinghouse. *H. pylori and peptic ulcers*. NIH Publication No. 10–4225, April 2010. Available online at http://digestive.niddk.nih.gov/ddiseases/pubs/hpylori. Accessed February 10, 2013.

[15] Marieb, E.N., and Hoehn, K. *Human Anatomy and Physiology*, 9th ed. Menlo Park, CA: Pearson, 2013.

Chapter 4

[1] Welsh, J.A., Sharma, A.J., Grellinger, L., and Vos, M.B. Consumption of added sugars is decreasing in the United States. *Am J Clin Nutr 94*:726–734, 2011.

[2] The National Digestive Diseases Information Clearinghouse (NDDIC), National Institute of Diabetes and Digestive and Kidney Diseases (NIDDK), and National Institutes of Health of the U.S. Department of Health and Human Services. *Lactose intolerance*. Available online at http://digestive.niddk.nih.gov/ddiseases/pubs/lactoseintolerance/. Accessed May 13, 2014.

[3] Kumar, V., Sinha, A.K., Makkar, H.P., et al. Dietary roles of non-starch polysaccharides in human nutrition: A review. *Crit Rev Food Sci Nutr 52*:899–935, 2012.

4 Burkitt, D.P., Walker, A.R.P., and Painter, N.S. Dietary fiber and disease. *JAMA* 229:1068–1074, 1974.

5 Kim, B.S, Jeon, Y.S., and Chun, J. Current status and future promise of the human microbiome. *Pediatr Gastroenterol Hepatol Nutr* 16:71–79, 2013 .

6 Willett, W.C., and Stampfer, M.J. Current evidence on healthy eating. *Annu Rev Public Health* 34:77–95, 2013.

7 Centers for Disease Control and Prevention. *National Diabetes Statistics Report: Estimates of Diabetes and Its Burden in the United States, 2014.* Atlanta, GA: US Department of Health and Human Services; 2014.

8 American Diabetes Association. Standards of medical care in diabetes—2014. *Diabetes Care* 37:S14–S80, 2014.

9 Greenwood, D.C., Threapleton, D.E., Evans, C.E., et al. Glycemic index, glycemic load, carbohydrates, and type 2 diabetes: Systematic review and dose-response meta-analysis of prospective studies. *Diabetes Care* 36: 4166–4171, 2013.

10 Oba, S., Nanri, A., Kurotani, K., et al.; Japan Public Health Center-based Prospective Study Group. Dietary glycemic index, glycemic load and incidence of type 2 diabetes in Japanese men and women: The Japan Public Health Center-based Prospective Study. *Nutr J* 12:165–169, 2013.

11 Salas-Salvadó, J., Martinez-González, M.Á., Bulló, M., and Ros, E. The role of diet in the prevention of type 2 diabetes. *Nutr Metab Cardiovasc Dis* 21(Suppl 2):B32-B48, 2011.

12 Silva, F.M., Kramer, C.K., de Almeida J.C., et al. Fiber intake and glycemic control in patients with type 2 diabetes mellitus: A systematic review with meta-analysis of randomized controlled trials. *Nutr Rev* 71:790–801, 2013.

13 InterAct consortium. Consumption of sweet beverages and type 2 diabetes incidence in European adults: Results from EPIC-InterAct. *Diabetologia* 56:1520–1530, 2013

14 Bradshaw, D.J., and Lynch, R.J. Diet and the microbial aetiology of dental caries: New paradigms. *Int Dent J* 63(Suppl 2):64–72, 2013

15 van Dam, R.M., and Seidell, J.C. Carbohydrate intake and obesity. *Eur J Clin Nutr* 61(Suppl 1):S75–S99, 2007.

16 Giacco, R., Della Pepa, G., Luongo, D., and Riccardi, G. Whole grain intake in relation to body weight: From epidemiological evidence to clinical trials. *Nutr Metab Cardiovasc Dis* 21:901–908, 2011.

17 Aller, E.E., Abete, I., Astrup, A., et al. Starches, sugars and obesity. *Nutrients* 3:341–369, 2011.

18 Te Morenga, L., Mallard, S., and Mann, J. Dietary sugars and body weight: systematic review and meta-analyses of randomised controlled trials and cohort studies. *BMJ* 346:e7492, 2012.

19 Gaby, A. R. Adverse effects of dietary fructose. *Altern Med Rev* 10:294–306, 2005.

20 Tappy, L., and Lê, K. A. Metabolic effects of fructose and the worldwide increase in obesity. *Physiol Rev* 90:23–46, 2010.

21 Stanhope, K.L., Schwarz, J.M., Keim, N.L., et al. Consuming fructose-sweetened, not glucose-sweetened, beverages increases visceral adiposity and lipids and decreases insulin sensitivity in overweight/obese humans. *J Clin Invest* 119:1322–1334, 2009.

22 Rippe, J.M., and Angelopoulos, T.J. Sucrose, high-fructose corn syrup, and fructose, their metabolism and potential health effects: What do we really know? *Adv Nutr* 4:236–245, 2013.

23 Bocarsly, M.E., Powell, E.S., Avena, N.M., and Hoebel, B.G. High-fructose corn syrup causes characteristics of obesity in rats: Increased body weight, body fat and triglyceride levels. *Pharmacol Biochem Behav* 97:101–106, 2010.

24 Lowndes, J., Kawiecki, D., Pardo, S., et al. The effects of four hypocaloric diets containing different levels of sucrose or high fructose corn syrup on weight loss and related parameters. *Nutr J* 11:55, 2012.

25 Bray, G.A. Energy and fructose from beverages sweetened with sugar or high-fructose corn syrup pose a health risk for some people. *Adv Nutr* 4:220–225, 2013.

26 American Dietetic Association. Position of the American Dietetic Association: Use of nutritive and non-nutritive sweeteners. *J Am Diet Assoc* 112:739–758, 2012.

27 Pereira, M. Diet beverages and the risk of obesity, diabetes, and cardiovascular disease: A review of the evidence. *Nutr Rev* 71:433–440, 2013.

28 Anderson, G.H., Foreyt, J., Sigman-Grant, M., and Allison, D.B. The use of low-calorie sweeteners by adults: Impact on weight management. *J Nutr* 142:1163S–1169S, 2013.

29 Renwick, A.G., and Molinary, S.V. Sweet-taste receptors, low-energy sweeteners, glucose absorption and insulin release. *Br J Nutr* 104:1415–1420, 2010.

30 de Koning, L., Malik, V.S., Kellogg, M.D., et al. Sweetened beverage consumption, incident coronary heart disease, and biomarkers of risk in men. *Circulation* 125:1735–1741, 2012.

31 Cho, S.S., Qi, L., Fahey, G.C. Jr, and Klurfeld, D.M. Consumption of cereal fiber, mixtures of whole grains and bran, and whole grains and risk reduction in type 2 diabetes, obesity, and cardiovascular disease. *Am J Clin Nutr* 98:594–619, 2013.

32 Threapleton, D.E., Greenwood, D.C., Evans, C.E.L., et al. Dietary fibre intake and risk of cardiovascular disease: Systematic review and meta-analysis. *BMJ* 347:f6879, 2013.

33 Gunness, P., and Gidley, M.J. Mechanisms underlying the cholesterol-lowering properties of soluble dietary fibre polysaccharides. *Food Funct* 1:149–155, 2010.

34 Cohn, J.S., Kamili, A., Wat, E., et al. Reduction in intestinal cholesterol absorption by various food components: mechanisms and implications. *Atheroscler Suppl* 11:45–48, 2010.

35 Aune, D., Chan, D.S., Lau, R., et al. Dietary fibre, whole grains, and risk of colorectal cancer: Systematic review and dose-response meta-analysis of prospective studies. *BMJ* 343:d6617, 2011.

36 Klement, R.J. and Kämmerer, U. Is there a role for carbohydrate restriction in the treatment and prevention of cancer? *Nutr Metab (Lond)* 8: 75, 2011.

37 Institute of Medicine, *Food and Nutrition Board. Dietary Reference Intakes for Energy, Carbohydrates, Fiber, Fat, Protein and Amino Acids.* Washington, DC: National Academies Press, 2002.

38 U.S. Department of Agriculture and U.S. Department of Health and Human Services. *Dietary guidelines for Americans, 2010,* 7th ed., Washington, DC: U.S. Government Printing Office, December 2010.

39 Johnson, R.K., Appel, L.J., Brands, M., et al. Dietary sugars intake and cardiovascular health: A scientific statement from the American Heart Association on behalf of the American Heart Association Nutrition Committee of the Council on

American Dietetic Association: Vegetarian diets. *J Am Diet Assoc 109*:1266–1282, 2009.

Chapter 7

[1] Miller, D.F. Enrichment programs: Helping mother nature along. *Food Product Development 12*:30–38, 1978.

[2] Butte, N.F., Fox, M.K., Briefel, R.R., et al. Nutrient intakes of US infants, toddlers, and preschoolers meet or exceed dietary reference intakes. *J Am Diet Assoc 110* (12 Suppl.):S27–S37, 2010.

[3] Institute of Medicine, Food and Nutrition Board. *Dietary Reference Intakes for Vitamin C, Vitamin E, Selenium, and Carotenoids.* Washington, DC: National Academies Press, 2000.

[4] Food and Drug Administration. Code of Federal Regulations, Title 21, volume 2. Section 101.45 Guidelines for voluntary nutrition labeling of raw fruits, vegetables, and fish, Revised April 1, 2013. Available online at http://www.accessdata.fda.gov/scripts/cdrh/cfdocs/cfcfr/CFRSearch.cfm?fr=101.45. Accessed January 28, 2014.

[5] Institute of Medicine, Food and Nutrition Board. *Dietary Reference Intakes for Thiamin, Riboflavin, Niacin, Vitamin B-6, Folate, Vitamin B-12, Pantothenic Acid, Biotin, and Choline.* Washington, DC: National Academies Press, 1998.

[6] Becker, D.A., Ingala, E.E., Martinez-Lage, M., et al. Dry Beriberi and Wernicke's encephalopathy following gastric lap band surgery. *J Clin Neurosci 19*:1050–1052, 2012.

[7] Saffert, A., Pieper, G., and Jetten, J. Effect of package light transmittance on vitamin content of milk. *Packing Technology and Science 21*:47–55, 2008.

[8] Kavitha, B., Balasubramanian, R., and Kumar, T. Electrocardiographic enigma of a classical disease: pellagra. *Trop Doct 42*:211–213, 2012.

[9] Debreceni, B., and Debreceni, L. Why do homocysteine-lowering B vitamin and antioxidant E vitamin supplementations appear to be ineffective in the prevention of cardiovascular diseases? *Cardiovasc Ther 30*:227–233, 2012.

[10] LeBlanc, K.E., and Cestia, W. Carpal tunnel syndrome. *Am Fam Physician 83*:952–958, 2011.

[11] Biggs, W.S., and Demuth, R.H. Premenstrual syndrome and premenstrual dysphoric disorder. *Am Fam Physician 84*:918–924, 2011.

[12] Berry, R.J., Bailey, L., Mulinare, J., Bower, C., and Folic Acid Working Group. Fortification of flour with folic acid. *Food Nutr Bull 31*(1 Suppl.):S22–S35, 2010.

[13] Blencowe, H., Cousens, S., Modell, B., and Lawn, J. Folic acid to reduce neonatal mortality from neural tube disorders. *Int J Epidemiol. 39*(Suppl. 1):i110–i121, 2010.

[14] Craig, W.J., Mangels, A.R., and American Dietetic Association. Position of the American Dietetic Association: Vegetarian diets. *J Am Diet Assoc 109*:1266–1282, 2009.

[15] Hemilä, H., and Chalker, E. Vitamin C for preventing and treating the common cold. *Cochrane Database Syst Rev 1*:CD000980, 2013.

[16] Thomas, L.D., Elinder, C.G., Tiselius, H.G., et al. Ascorbic acid supplements and kidney stone incidence among men: a prospective study. *JAMA Intern Med. 173*:386–388, 2013.

[17] Zeisel, S.H., and da Costa, K.A. Choline: An essential nutrient for public health. *Nutr Rev 67*:615–623, 2009.

[18] Patterson, K.Y., Bhagwat, S.A., Williams, J.R., et al. *USDA Database for the Choline Content of Common Foods, Release Two, January 2008.* Available online at www.ars.usda.gov/SP2UserFiles/Place/12354500/Data/Choline/Choln02.pdf. Accessed January 28, 2014.

[19] Institute of Medicine, Food and Nutrition Board. *Dietary Reference Intakes: Vitamin A, Vitamin K, Arsenic, Boron, Chromium, Copper, Iodine, Iron, Manganese, Molybdenum, Nickel, Silicon, Vanadium, and Zinc.* Washington, DC: National Academies Press, 2001.

[20] World Health Organization. *Micronutrient Deficiencies: Vitamin A Deficiency: The Challenge.* Available online at www.who.int/nutrition/topics/vad/en/index.html. Accessed January 28, 2014.

[21] Penniston, K.L., and Tanumihardjo, S.A. The acute and chronic toxic effects of vitamin A. *Am J Clin Nutr 83*:191–201, 2006.

[22] Castaño, G., Etchart, C., and Sookoian, S. Vitamin A toxicity in a physical culturist patient: A case report and review of the literature. *Ann Hepatol 5*:293–395, 2006.

[23] Druesne-Pecollo, N., Latino-Martel, P., Norat, T., et al. Beta-carotene supplementation and cancer risk: A systematic review and metaanalysis of randomized controlled trials. *Int J Cancer 127*:172–184, 2010.

[24] Holick, M.F. Vitamin D: Extraskeletal health. *Rheum Dis Clin North Am 38*:141–160, 2012.

[25] Institute of Medicine, Food and Nutrition Board. *Dietary Reference Intakes for Calcium and Vitamin D.* Washington, DC: National Academies Press, 2011.

[26] Autier, P., Boniol, M., Pizot, C., and Mullie, P. Vitamin D status and ill health: a systematic review. *Lancet Diabetes Endocrinol 2*:76–89, 2014.

[27] Holick, M.F. Vitamin D deficiency: What a pain it is. *Mayo Clin Proc 78*:1457–1459, 2003.

[28] Holick, M.F., and Chen, T.C. Vitamin D deficiency: A worldwide problem with health consequences. *Am J Clin Nutr 87*(Suppl.):1080S–1086S, 2008.

[29] Sabat, R., Guthmann, F., and Rüstow, B. Formation of reactive oxygen species in lung alveolar cells: Effect of vitamin E deficiency. *Lung 186*:115–122, 2008.

[30] Cordero, Z., Drogan, D., Weikert, C., and Boeing, H. Vitamin E and risk of cardiovascular diseases: A review of epidemiologic and clinical trial studies. *Crit Rev Food Sci Nutr 50*:420–440, 2010.

[31] Fortmann, S.P., Burda, B.U., Senger, C.A., et al. Vitamin and mineral supplements in the primary prevention of cardiovascular disease and cancer: An updated systematic evidence review for the U.S. Preventive Services Task Force. *Ann Intern Med 159*:824–834, 2013.

[32] Riccioni, G., D'Orazio, N., Salvatore, C., et al. Carotenoids and vitamins C and E in the prevention of cardiovascular disease. *Int J Vitam Nutr Res 82*:15–26, 2012 .

[33] U.S. Department of Agriculture, Agricultural Research Service, *What We Eat in America*, NHANES 2009-2010. Table 1. Nutrient intakes form food. Available online at http://www.ars.usda.gov/SP2UserFiles/Place/12355000/pdf/0910/tables_1-40_2009-2010.pdf Accessed January 27, 2014.

[34] Vermeer, C. Vitamin K: The effect on health beyond coagulation—an overview. *Food Nutr Res 56*, doi: 10.3402/fnr.v56i0.5329. Epub 2012.

[35] Theuwissen, E., Magdeleyns, E.J., Braam, L.A., et al. Vitamin K status in healthy volunteers. *Food Funct*, December 2, 2013.

[36] Council for Responsible Nutrition. *Supplement Usage, Consumer Confidence*

Remains Steady. Available online at www.crnusa.org/CRNPR10ConsumerSurvey_Usage+Confidence.html. Accessed December 23, 2013.

[37] Guallar, E., Stranges, S., Mulrow, C., et al. Enough is enough: Stop wasting money on vitamin and mineral supplements. *Ann Intern Med 159*:850–851, 2013.

[38] American Dietetic Association. Position of the American Dietetic Association: Nutrient supplementation. *J Am Diet Assoc 109*:2073–2085, 2009.

[39] Bruno, R.S., and Traber, M.G. Cigarette smoke alters human vitamin E requirements. *J Nutr 135*:671–674, 2005.

[40] Gershwin, M.E., Borchers, A.T., Keen, C.L., et al. Public safety and dietary supplementation. *Ann N Y Acad Sci 1190*:104–117, 2010.

[41] Laws, K.R., Sweetnam, H., and Kondel, T.K. Is *Ginkgo biloba* a cognitive enhancer in healthy individuals? A meta-analysis. *Hum Psychopharmacol 27*:527–533, 2012.

[42] Ihl, R. *Cingko biloba* extract ECb 761®: Clinical data in dementia. *Int Psychogeriatr 24* (Suppl. 1):S35–S40, 2012.

[43] Birks, J., and Grimley Evans, J. *Ginkgo biloba* for cognitive impairment and dementia. *Cochrane Database Syst Rev* CD003120, 2009.

[44] National Center for Complementary and Alternative Medicine. *Herbs at a Glance: Ginko*. Available online at http://nccam.nih.gov/health/ginkgo/ataglance.htm. Accessed December 25, 2013.

[45] Diamond, B.J., and Bailey, M.R. Ginkgo biloba: Indications, mechanisms, and safety. *Psychiatr Clin North Am 36*:73–83, 2013.

[46] Nahas, R., and Sheikh, O. Complementary and alternative medicine for the treatment of major depressive disorder. *Can Fam Physician 57*:659–663, 2011.

[47] National Center for Complimentary and Alternative Medicine. *Herbs at a Glance: St. John's wort* Available online at http://nccam.nih.gov/health/stjohnswort/ataglance.htm. Accessed December 25, 2013.

[48] Shergis, J.L., Zhang, A.L., Zhou, W., and Xue, C.C. Panax ginseng in randomised controlled trials: A systematic review *Phytother Res 27*:949–965, 2013.

[49] Zeng, T., Guo, F.F., Zhang, C.L., et al. A meta-analysis of randomized, double-blind, placebo-controlled trials for the effects of garlic on serum lipid profiles. *J Sci Food Agric 92*:1892–1902, 2012.

[50] National Center for Complementary and Alternative Medicine. *Herbs at a Glance: Garlic* Available online at http://nccam.nih.gov/health/garlic/ataglance.htm. Accessed December 25, 2013.

[51] National Center for Complementary and Alternative Medicine. *Herbs at a Glance: Echinachea* Available online at http://nccam.nih.gov/health/echinacea/ataglance.htm. Accessed December 25, 2013.

[52] Gershwin, M.E., Borchers, A.T., Keen, C.L., et al. Public safety and dietary supplementation. *Ann N Y Acad Sci 1190*:104–117, 2010.

[53] Ribnicky, D.M., Poulev, A., Schmidt, B., et al. Evaluation of botanicals for improving human health. *Am J Clin Nutr 87*:472S–475S, 2008.

[54] Newmaster, S.G., Grguric, M., Shanmughanandhan, D., et al. DNA barcoding detects contamination and substitution in North American herbal products. *BMC Medicine 11*:222, 2013

[55] Food and Drug Administration. *Dietary Supplement Warnings and Safety Information*. Available online at www.fda.gov/Food/DietarySupplements/Alerts/default.htm. Accessed January 21, 2011.

[56] Zhang, J., Wider, B., Shang, H., et al. Quality of herbal medicines: challenges and solutions. *Complement Ther Med 20*:100–106, 2012.

[57] Kennedy, D.A., and Seely, D. Clinically based evidence of drug-herb interactions: A systematic review. *Expert Opin Drug Saf 9*:79–124, 2010.

[58] Food and Drug Administration. Current good manufacturing practice in manufacturing, packaging, labeling, or holding operations for dietary supplements; final rule. *Fed Regist 72*:34751–34958, June 25, 2007.

Chapter 8

[1] World Health Organization and United Nations Children's Fund Joint Monitoring Programme for Water Supply and Sanitation (JMP). *Progress on Drinking Water and Sanitation: Special Focus on Sanitation*. Available online at www.who.int/water_sanitation_health/monitoring/jmp_report_7_10_lores.pdf. Accessed June 10, 2014.

[2] Shen, H.-P. Body fluids and water balance. In M.H. Stipanuk and M.A. Caudill (eds.), *Biochemical, Physiological, and Molecular Aspects of Human Nutrition*, 3rd ed. St. Louis: Saunders Elsevier, 2013, pp. 781–800.

[3] Rodwan, J.G. Bottled water 2011: The recovery continues. *BWR* April/May 2012. Available online at http://www.bottledwater.org/files/2011BWstats.pdf. Accessed January 15, 2014.

[4] U.S. Government Accountability Office. *Bottled Water: FDA Safety and Consumer Protections Are Often Less Stringent Than Comparable EPA Protections for Tap Water*, June 2009. Available online at www.gao.gov/new.items/d09610.pdf. Accessed January 14, 2014.

[5] Environmental Working Group. *Bottled Water Quality Investigation: 10 Major Brands, 38 Pollutants*, October 2008. Available online at http://www.ewg.org/research/bottled-water-quality-investigation. Accessed January 14, 2014.

[6] Environmental Working Group. *National Drinking Water Database*. Available online at http://www.ewg.org/tap-water/. Accessed January 15, 2014.

[7] Sierra Club. *Bottled Water Campaign*. Available online at www.sierraclub.org/committees/cac/water/bottled_water/. Accessed January 24, 2014.

[8] Institute of Medicine, Food and Nutrition Board. *Dietary Reference Intakes for Water, Potassium, Sodium, Chloride, and Sulfate*. Washington, DC: National Academies Press, 2004.

[9] Drewnowski, A., Rehm, C.D., and Constant, F. Water and beverage consumption among adults in the United States: Cross-sectional study using data from NHANES 2005-2010. *BMC Public Health 13*:1068, 2013.

[10] Go, A.S., Mozaffarian, D., Roger, V.L., et al.; American Heart Association Statistics Committee and Stroke Statistics Subcommittee. Heart disease and stroke statistics—2014 update: A report from the American Heart Association. *Circulation 129*:e28–e292, 2014.

[11] Carvalho, J.J., Baruzzi, R.G., Howard, P.F., et al. Blood pressure in four remote populations in the Intersalt study. *Hypertension 14*:238–246, 1989.

[12] Appel, L.J., Moore, T.J., Obarzanek, E., et al. A clinical trial of the effects of dietary patterns on blood pressure. *N Engl J Med 336*:1117–1124, 1997.

[13] American Heart Association. *Understanding Your Risk of Developing HBP*. Available online at http://www.heart.org/HEARTORG/Conditions/HighBloodPressure/

20 Norman, R.A., Thompson, D.B., Foroud, T., et al. Genomewide search for genes influencing percent body fat in Pima Indians: Suggestive linkage at chromosome 11q21–q22. *Am J Human Genet 60*:166–173, 1997.

21 Esparza, J., Fox, C., Harper, I.T., et al. Daily energy expenditure in Mexican and USA Pima Indians: Low physical activity as a possible cause of obesity. *Int J Obes Relat Metab Disord 24*:55–59, 2000.

22 Suzuki, K., Jayasena, C.N., and Bloom, S.R. Obesity and appetite control. *Exp Diabetes Res 2012*:824305, 2012.

23 Myers, M.G., Jr., Leibel, R.L., Seeley, R.J., and Schwartz, M.W. Obesity and leptin resistance: Distinguishing cause from effect. *Trends Endocrinol Metab 21*:643–651, 2010.

24 Hill, J.O., Wyatt, H.R., and Peters, J.C. Energy balance and obesity. *Circulation 126*:126–132, 2012.

25 Levine, J.A., Lanningham-Foster, L.M., McCrady, S.K., et al. Interindividual variation in posture allocation: Possible role in human obesity. *Science 307*:584–586, 2005.

26 Stevens, V.L., Jacobs, E.J., Sun, J., et al. Weight cycling and mortality in a large prospective US study. *Am J Epidemiol 175*:785–792, 2012.

27 U.S. Department of Health and Human Services, Office of the Surgeon General. *The Surgeon General's Call to Action to Prevent and Decrease Overweight and Obesity.* Available online at http://www.ncbi.nlm.nih.gov/books/NBK44206/. Accessed June 12, 2014.

28 Martens, E.A., and Westerterp-Plantenga, M.S. Protein diets, body weight loss and weight maintenance. *Curr Opin Clin Nutr Metab Care 17*:75–79, 2014.

29 Acheson, K.J. Carbohydrate for weight and metabolic control: Where do we stand? *Nutrition 26*:141–145, 2010.

30 U.S. Food and Drug Administration. *Beware of Fraudulent Weight-Loss "Dietary Supplements."* Available online at www.fda.gov/ForConsumers/ConsumerUpdates/ucm246742.htm. Accessed February 2, 2014.

31 Manore, M.M. Dietary supplements for improving body composition and reducing body weight: Where is the evidence? *Int J Sport Nutr Exerc Metab 22*:139–154, 2012.

32 Chan, T.Y. Potential risks associated with the use of herbal anti-obesity products. *Drug Saf 32*:453–456, 2009.

33 Lautz, D., Goebel-Fabbri, A., Halperin, F., and Goldfien, A.B. The great debate: Medicine or surgery. What is best for the patient with type 2 diabetes? *Diabetes Care 34*:763–770, 2011.

34 Buchwald, H., Estok, R., Fahrbach, K., et al. Weight and type 2 diabetes after bariatric surgery: Systematic review and meta-analysis. *Am J Med 122*:248–256, 2009.

35 Pontiroli, A.E., and Morabito, A. Long-term prevention of mortality in morbid obesity through bariatric surgery: A systematic review and meta-analysis of trials performed with gastric banding and gastric bypass. *Ann Surg 253*:484–487, 2011.

36 McEwen, L.N., Coelho, R.B., Baumann, L.M., et al. The cost, quality of life impact, and cost-utility of bariatric surgery in a managed care population. *Obes Surg. 20*:919–928, 2010.

37 Mann, D. *Weight Loss Surgery Insurance Coverage.* Consumer Guide to Bariatric Surgery. Available online at www.yourbariatricsurgeryguide.com/insurance/. Accessed June 12, 2014.

38 Smith, B.R., Schauer, P., Nguyen, N.T. Surgical approaches to the treatment of obesity: Bariatric Surgery. *Med Clin N Am 95*:1009–1030, 2011.

39 Online Surgery. *Advantages and Disadvantages of Bariatric Surgery.* Available online at www.onlinesurgery.com/article/advantages-and-disadvantages-of-bariatric-surgery.html. Accessed June 6, 2014.

40 American Psychiatric Association. *Diagnostic and Statistical Manual of Mental Disorders*, 5th ed., Arlington, VA: American Psychiatric Publishing, 2013.

41 Body image worries hit Zulu women. *BBC News*, April 16, 2004. Available online at http://news.bbc.co.uk/2/hi/health/3631359.stm. Accessed June 6, 2014.

42 HealthyPlace. *Eating Disorders: Body Image and Advertising*, December 11, 2008. Available online at www.healthyplace.com/eating-disorders/main/eating-disorders-body-image-and-advertising/menu-id-58/. Accessed June 6, 2014.

43 Keel, P.K., and Forney, K.J. Psychosocial risk factors for eating disorders. *Int J Eat Disord 46*:433–439, 2013.

44 Spann, N., and Pritchard, M. Disordered eating in men: A look at perceived stress and excessive exercise. *Eat Weight Disord 13*:e25–e27, 2008.

45 Anorexia Nervosa and Associated Disorders. *Eating Disorders Statistics.* Available online at http://www.anad.org/get-information/about-eating-disorders/eating-disorders-statistics/ Accessed February 2, 2014.

46 American Dietetic Association, Position of the American Dietetic Association: Nutrition intervention and treatment of eating disorders. *J Am Diet Assoc 111*:1236–1241, 2011.

47 Tozzi, F., Thornton, L.M., Klump, K.L., et al. Symptom fluctuation in eating disorders: Correlates of diagnostic crossover. *Am J Psychiatry 162*:732–740, 2005.

48 Vandereycken, W. History of anorexia nervosa and bulimia nervosa. In Fairburn, C.G., and Brownell, K.D. (eds.), *Eating Disorders and Obesity: A Comprehensive Handbook*, 2nd ed. New York: Guilford Press, 2002, pp. 151–154.

49 Ebeling, H., Tapanainen, P., and Joutsenoja, A. A practice guideline for treatment of eating disorders in children and adolescents. *Ann Med 35*:488–501, 2003.

50 Anorexia Nervosa and Associated Disorders. *Binge Eating Disorder.* Available online at http://www.anad.org/get-information/about-eating-disorders/binge-eating-disorder/ Accessed February 2, 2014.

51 Bratland-Sanda, S., and Sundgot-Borgen, J. Eating disorders in athletes: overview of prevalence, risk factors and recommendations for prevention and treatment. *Eur J Sport Sci 13*:499–508, 2013.

Chapter 10

1 The President's Council on Physical Fitness and Sports. *Physical Activity Protects Against the Health Risks of Obesity.* Available online at https://www.presidentschallenge.org/informed/digest/docs/200012digest.pdf. Accessed September 1, 2014.

2 Dinas, P.C., Koutedakis, Y., and Flouris, A.D. Effects of exercise and physical activity on depression. *Ir J Med Sci 180*:319–325, 2011.

3 Institute of Medicine, Food and Nutrition Board. *Dietary Reference Intakes for Energy, Carbohydrates, Fiber, Fat, Protein and Amino Acids.* Washington, DC: National Academies Press, 2002.

[4] Strasser, B. Physical activity in obesity and metabolic syndrome. *Ann N Y Acad Sci 1281*:141–159, 2013.

[5] Behm, D.G., and Chaouachi, A. A review of the acute effects of static and dynamic stretching on performance. *Eur J Appl Physiol 111*:2633–2651, 2011.

[6] Garber, C.E., Blissmer, B., Deschenes, M. R., et al.; American College of Sports Medicine. American College of Sports Medicine position stand: Quantity and quality of exercise for developing and maintaining cardiorespiratory, musculoskeletal, and neuromotor fitness in apparently healthy adults: Guidance for prescribing exercise. *Med Sci Sports Exerc 43*:1334–1359, 2011.

[7] Gallagher, D., Heymsfield, S., Heo, M., et al. Healthy percentage body fat ranges: An approach for developing guidelines based on body mass index. *Am J Clin Nutr 72*:694–701, 2000.

[8] U.S. Department of Agriculture and U.S. Department of Health and Human Services. *Dietary Guidelines for Americans, 2010*, 7th ed, Washington, DC: U.S. Government Printing Office, December 2010.

[9] U.S. Department of Health and Human Services. *2008 Physical Activity Guidelines for Americans*. Available online at http://www.health.gov/paguidelines/guidelines/. Accessed August 31, 2014.

[10] National Center for Health Statistics. Health, United States, 2012: With Special Feature on Emergency Care. Hyattsville, MD, 2013.

[11] Haskell, W.L., Lee, I-M., Pate, R.R., et al. Physical activity and public health: Updated recommendations for adults from the American College of Sports Medicine and the American Heart Association. *Circulation 116*:1081–1093, 2007.

[12] Matthews, C.E., George, S.M., Moore, S.C., et al. Amount of time spent in sedentary behaviors and cause-specific mortality in US adults. *Am J Clin Nutr 95*:437–445, 2012.

[13] Gulati, M., Shaw, L.J., Thisted, R.A., et al. Heart rate response to exercise stress testing in asymptomatic women: The St. James Women Take Heart Project. *Circulation 122*:130–137, 2010.

[14] Meeusen, R., Duclos, M., Foster, C., et al; European College of Sport Science; American College of Sports Medicine. Prevention, diagnosis, and treatment of the overtraining syndrome: Joint consensus statement of the European College of Sport Science and the American College of Sports Medicine. *Med Sci Sports Exerc 45*:186–205, 2013.

[15] Ament, W., and Verkerke, G.J. Exercise and fatigue. *Sports Med 39*:389–422, 2009.

[16] Finsterer, J. Biomarkers of peripheral muscle fatigue during exercise. *BMC Musculoskelet Disord 13*:218, 2012.

[17] Rivera-Brown, A.M., and Frontera, W.R. Principles of exercise physiology: Response to acute exercise and long-term adaptations to training. *PMR 4*:797–804, 2012.

[18] Bratland-Sanda, S., and Sundgot-Borgen, J. Eating disorders in athletes: overview of prevalence, risk factors and recommendations for prevention and treatment. *Eur J Sport Sci 13*:499–508, 2013.

[19] El Ghoch, M., Soave, F., Calugi, S., and Dalle Grave, R. Eating disorders, physical fitness and sport performance: A systematic review. *Nutrients 5*:5140–5160, 2013.

[20] De Souza, M.J., Nattiv, A., Joy, E., et al.; Expert Panel. 2014 Female Athlete Triad Coalition Consensus Statement on Treatment and Return to Play of the Female Athlete Triad: 1st International Conference held in San Francisco, May 2012 and Second International Conference held in Indianapolis, Indiana, May 2013. *Br J Sports Med 48*:289, 2014.

[21] Remick, D., Chancellor, K., Pederson, J., et al. Hyperthermia and dehydration-related deaths associated with intentional rapid weight loss in three collegiate wrestlers—North Carolina, Wisconsin, and Michigan, November–December, 1997. *MMWR Morb Mortal Wkly Rep 47*:105–108, 1998. Available online at www.cdc.gov/mmwr/preview/mmwrhtml/00051388.htm. Accessed June 15, 2014.

[22] American Dietetic Association. Position of the American Dietetic Association, Dietitians of Canada, and American College of Sports Medicine: Nutrition and athletic performance. *J Am Diet Assoc 109*:509–527, 2009.

[23] Tipton, K.D. Efficacy and consequences of very-high-protein diets for athletes and exercisers. *Proc Nutr Soc 7*:1–10, 2011.

[24] Powers, S.K., Nelson, W.B., and Hudson, M.B. Exercise-induced oxidative stress in humans: cause and consequences. *Free Radic Biol Med 51*:942–950, 2011.

[25] Pendergast, D.R., Meksawan, K., Limprasertkul, A., and Fisher, N.M. Influence of exercise on nutritional requirements. *Eur J Appl Physiol 111*:379–390, 2011.

[26] Latunde-Dada, G.O. Iron metabolism in athletes—achieving a gold standard. *Eur J Haematol 90*:10–15, 2013.

[27] Food and Nutrition Board, Institute of Medicine. *Dietary Reference Intakes: Vitamin A, Vitamin K, Arsenic, Boron, Chromium, Copper, Iodine, Iron, Manganese, Molybdenum, Nickel, Silicon, Vanadium, and Zinc*. Washington, DC: National Academies Press, 2001.

[28] NOAA's National Weather Service. *Heat Index*. Available online at www.weather.gov/os/heat/index.shtml. Accessed February 11, 2014.

[29] Knechtle, B., Gnädinger, M., Knechtle, P., et al. Prevalence of exercise-associated hyponatremia in male ultraendurance athletes. *Clin J Sport Med 23*:226–232, 2011.

[30] Sedlock, D.A. The latest on carbohydrate loading: A practical approach. *Curr Sports Med Rep 7*:209–213, 2008.

[31] Bergstrom, J., Hermansen, L., Hultman, E., and Saltin, B. Diet, muscle glycogen and physical performance. *Acta Physiologica Scandinavica 71*:140–150, 1967.

[32] Spaccarotella, K.J., and Andzel, W.D. Building a beverage for recovery from endurance activity: A review. *J Strength Cond Res 25*:3198–3204, 2011.

[33] Pritchett, K., and Pritchett, R. Chocolate milk: A post-exercise recovery beverage for endurance sports. *Med Sport Sci 59*:127–134, 2012.

[34] Howarth, K.R., Moreau, N.A., Phillips, S.M., and Gibala, M.J. Coingestion of protein with carbohydrate during recovery from endurance exercise stimulates skeletal muscle protein synthesis in humans. *J Appl Physiol 106*:1394–1402, 2009.

[35] Di Luigi, L. Supplements and the endocrine system in athletes. *Clin Sports Med 27*:131–151, 2008.

[36] Nissen, S.L., and Sharp, R.L. Effect of dietary supplements on lean mass and strength gains with resistance exercise: A meta-analysis. *J Appl Physiol 94*:651–659, 2003.

[37] van Amsterdam, J., Opperhuizen, A., and Hartgens, F. Adverse health effects of anabolic androgenic steroids. *Regul Toxicol Pharmacol 57*:117–123, 2010.

38 Liddle, D.G., and Connor, D.J. Nutritional supplements and ergogenic aids. *Prim Care 40*:487–505, 2013.

39 Tokish, J.M., Kocher, M.S., and Hawkins, R.J. Ergogenic aids: A review of basic science, performance, side effects, and status in sports. *Am J Sports Med 32*:1543–1553, 2004.

40 Brown, G.A., Vukovich, M., and King, D.S. Testosterone prohormone supplements. *Med Sci Sports Exerc 38*:1451–1461, 2006.

41 Birzniece, V., Nelson, A.E., and Ho, K.K. Growth hormone and physical performance. *Trends Endocrinol Metab 22*:171–178, 2011.

42 Kanaley, J.A. Growth hormone, arginine and exercise. *Curr Opin Clin Nutr Metab Care 11*:50–54, 2008.

43 Chromiak, J.A., and Antonio, J. Use of amino acids as growth hormone-releasing agents by athletes. *Nutrition 18*:657–661, 2002.

44 Rowlands, D.S., and Thomson, J.S. Effects of beta-hydroxy-beta-methylbutyrate supplementation during resistance training on strength, body composition, and muscle damage in trained and untrained young men: A meta-analysis. *J Strength Cond Res 23*:836–846, 2009.

45 Burke, L.M. Practical considerations for bicarbonate loading and sports performance. *Nestle Nutr Inst Workshop Ser 75*:15–26, 2013.

46 Tarnopolsky, M.A. Caffeine and creatine use in sport. *Ann Nutr Metab 57*(Suppl. 2):1–8, 2010.

47 Gualano, B., Roschel, H., Lancha-Jr, A.H., et al. In sickness and in health: The widespread application of creatine supplementation. *Amino Acids 43*:519–529, 2012.

48 Ganio, M.S., Klau, J.F., Casa, D.J., et al. Effect of caffeine on sport-specific endurance performance: A systematic review. *J Strength Cond Res 23*:315–324, 2009.

49 Berger, A.J., and Alford, K. Cardiac arrest in a young man following excess consumption of caffeinated "energy drinks" *Med J Aust 190*:41–43, 2009.

50 Clauson, K.A., Sheilds, K.M, McQueen, C.E., and Persad, N. Safety issues associated with commercially available energy drinks. *J Am Pharm Assoc 48*:e55–e63, 2008.

51 Ballard, S.L., Wellborn-Kim, J.J., and Clauson, K.A. Effects of commercial energy drink consumption on athletic performance and body composition. *Phys Sportsmen 38*:107–117, 2010.

52 Higgins, J.P., Tuttle, T.D., and Higgins, C.L. Energy beverages: Content and safety. *Mayo Clin Proc 85*:1033–1041, 2010.

53 Duchan, E., Patel, N.D., and Feucht, C. Energy drinks: A review of use and safety. *Phys Sportsmed 38*:171–179, 2010.

54 Kim, H.J., Kim, C.K., Carpentier, A., and Poortmans, J.R. Studies on the safety of creatine supplementation. *Amino Acids 40*:1409–1418, 2011.

55 Jeukendrup, A.E., and Randell, R. Fat burners: Nutrition supplements that increase fat metabolism. *Obes Rev 12*:841–851, 2011.

56 Clegg, M.E. Medium-chain triglycerides are advantageous in promoting weight loss although not beneficial to exercise performance. *Int J Food Sci Nutr 61*:653–679, 2010.

57 Heuberger, J.A., Cohen Tervaert, J.M., Schepers, F.M., et al. Erythropoietin doping in cycling: lack of evidence for efficacy and a negative risk-benefit. *Br J Clin Pharmacol 75*:1406–1421, 2013.

Chapter 11

1 Committee to Reexamine IOM Pregnancy Weight Guidelines, Institute of Medicine, National Research Council. *Weight Gain During Pregnancy: Reexamining the Guidelines.* Washington, DC: National Academies Press, 2009.

2 Iacovidou, N., Varsami, M., and Syggellou, A. Neonatal outcome of preterm delivery. *Ann N Y Acad Sci 1205*:130–134, 2010.

3 Kaiser, L., and Allen, L.A. Position of the American Dietetic Association: Nutrition and lifestyle for a healthy pregnancy outcome. *J Am Diet Assoc 108*:553–561, 2008.

4 Al-Hinai, M., Al-Muqbali, M., Al-Moqbali, A., et al. Effects of pre-pregnancy body mass index and gestational weight gain on low birth weight in Omani infants: A case-control study. *Sultan Qaboos Univ Med J 13*:386–391, 2013.

5 Denison, F.C., Norwood, P., Bhattacharya, S., et al. Association between maternal body mass index during pregnancy, short-term morbidity, and increased health service costs: A population-based study. *BJOG 121*:72–81, 2014.

6 Li, N., Liu, E., Guo, J., et al. Maternal prepregnancy body mass index and gestational weight gain on pregnancy outcomes. *PLoS One 8*:e82310, 2013.

7 Poston, L. Gestational weight gain: Influences on the long-term health of the child. *Curr Opin Clin Nutr Metab Care 15*:252–257, 2012.

8 U.S. Department of Health and Human Services. *2008 Physical Activity Guidelines for Americans.* Available online at http://www.health.gov/paguidelines/guidelines/. Accessed August 31, 2014.

9 Einarson, T.R., Piwko, C., and Koren, G. Prevalence of nausea and vomiting of pregnancy in the USA: A meta analysis. *J Popul Ther Clin Pharmacol 20*:e163–e170, 2013.

10 Maltepe, C., and Koren, G. The management of nausea and vomiting of pregnancy and hyperemesis gravidarum—a 2013 update. *J Popul Ther Clin Pharmacol 20*:e184–e192, 2013.

11 National Center for Health Statistics, Centers for Disease Control and Prevention. *Infant Health.* Available online at www.cdc.gov/nchs/fastats/infant_health.htm. Accessed February 24, 2014.

12 Central Intelligence Agency, The World Fact Book. *Maternal mortality rate.* Available online at https://www.cia.gov/library/publications/the-world-factbook/rankorder/2223rank.html. Accessed February 24, 2014.

13 Lo, J.O., Mission, J.F., and Caughey, A.B. Hypertensive disease of pregnancy and maternal mortality. *Curr Opin Obstet Gynecol 25*:124–132, 2013.

14 Berg, C.J., Callaghan, W.M., Syverson, C., and Henderson, Z. Pregnancy-related mortality in the United States, 1998 to 2005. *Obstet Gynecol 116*:1302–1309, 2010.

15 Mustafa, R., Ahmed, S., Gupta, A., and Venuto, R.C. A comprehensive review of hypertension in pregnancy. *J Pregnancy 2012*:105918, 2012.

16 American College of Obstetricians and Gynecologists, Task Force on Hypertension in Pregnancy. Hypertension in Pregnancy, 2013. Available online at http://www.acog.org/~/media/Task%20Force%20and%20Work%20Group%20Reports/Hypertensionin-Pregnancy.pdf. Accessed March 28, 2014.

17 Food and Nutrition Board, Institute of Medicine. *Dietary Reference Intakes: Water, Potassium, Sodium, Chloride, and Sulfate.*

Washington, DC: National Academies Press, 2004.

[18] Thangaratinam, S., Langenveld, J., Mol, B.W., and Khan, K.S. Prediction and primary prevention of pre-eclampsia. *Best Pract Res Clin Obstet Gynaecol* 25:419–433, 2011.

[19] Hunsberger, M., Rosenberg, K.D., and Donatelle, R.J. Racial/ethnic disparities in gestational diabetes mellitus: Findings from a population-based survey. *Womens Health Issues* 20:323–328, 2010.

[20] Kwak, S.H., Choi, S.H., Jung, H.S., et al. Clinical and genetic risk factors for type 2 diabetes at early or late post partum after gestational diabetes mellitus. *J Clin Endocrin & Metab* 98:E744–E752, 2013.

[21] Food and Nutrition Board, Institute of Medicine. *Dietary Reference Intakes for Energy, Carbohydrates, Fiber, Fat, Protein and Amino Acids.* Washington, DC: National Academies Press, 2002.

[22] Scholtz, S.A., Colombo, J., and Carlson, S.E. Clinical overview of effects of dietary long-chain polyunsaturated fatty acids during the perinatal period. *Nestle Nutr Inst Workshop Ser* 77:145–154, 2013.

[23] Food and Nutrition Board, Institute of Medicine. *Dietary Reference Intakes for Water, Potassium, Sodium, Chloride, and Sulfate.* Washington, DC: National Academies Press, 2004.

[24] Food and Nutrition Board, Institute of Medicine. *Dietary Reference Intakes for Calcium and Vitamin D.* Washington, DC: National Academies Press, 2011.

[25] Berry, R.J., Bailey, L., Mulinare, J., and Bower, C. Fortification of flour with folic acid. *Food Nutr Bull* 31(1 Suppl.):S22–S35, 2010.

[26] De Wals, P., Tiarou, F., Van Allen, M.I., et al. Reduction in neural-tube defects after folic acid fortification in Canada. *N Engl J Med* 357:135–142, 2007.

[27] Fekete, K., Berti, C., Cetin, I., et al. Perinatal folate supply: Relevance in health outcome parameters. *Matern Child Nutr* 6 Suppl 2:23–38, 2010.

[28] Food and Nutrition Board, Institute of Medicine. *Dietary Reference Intakes for Thiamin, Riboflavin, Niacin, Vitamin B-6, Folate, Vitamin B-12, Pantothenic Acid, Biotin, and Choline.* Washington, DC: National Academies Press, 1998.

[29] Pepper, M.R., and Black, M.M. B12 in fetal development. *Semin Cell Dev Biol* 22:619–623, 2011.

[30] Food and Nutrition Board, Institute of Medicine. *Dietary Reference Intakes for Vitamin A, Vitamin K, Arsenic, Boron, Chromium, Copper, Iodine, Iron, Manganese, Molybdenum, Nickel, Silicon, Vanadium, and Zinc.* Washington, DC: National Academies Press, 2001.

[31] Cao, C., and O'Brien, K.O. Pregnancy and iron homeostasis: an update. *Nutr Rev* 71:35–51, 2013.

[32] Chaffee, B.W., and King, J.C. Effect of zinc supplementation on pregnancy and infant outcomes: A systematic review. *Paediatr Perinat Epidemiol* 26 (Suppl. 1):118–137, 2012.

[33] Mills, M.E. Craving more than food: The implications of pica in pregnancy. *Nurs Womens Health* 11:266–273, 2007.

[34] Centers for Disease Control and Prevention. *Birth Defects.* Available online at www.cdc.gov/ncbddd/birthdefects/index.html. Accessed February 25, 2014.

[35] Roseboom, T., de Rooij, S., and Painter, R. The Dutch famine and its long-term consequences for adult health. *Early Hum Dev* 82:485–491, 2006.

[36] Stein, A.D., Zybert, P.A., van de Bor, M., and Lumey, L.H. Intrauterine famine exposure and body proportions at birth: The Dutch Hunger Winter. *Int J Epidemiol* 33:831–836, 2004.

[37] Fall, C.H. Fetal programming and the risk of noncommunicable disease. *Indian J Pediatr* 80 (Suppl. 1):S13–S20, 2013.

[38] Desai, M., Beall, M., and Ross, M.G. Developmental origins of obesity: programmed adipogenesis. *Curr Diab Rep* 13:27–33, 2013.

[39] de Graaf, J.P., Steegers, E.A., and Bonsel, G.J. Inequalities in perinatal and maternal health. *Curr Opin Obstet Gynecol* 25:98–108, 2013.

[40] Casanueva, E., Roselló-Soberón, M.E., and De-Regil, L.M. Adolescents with adequate birth weight newborns diminish energy expenditure and cease growth. *J Nutr* 136:2498–2501, 2006.

[41] National Center for Health Statistics, Centers for Disease Control and Prevention. *Teen Births.* Available online at www.cdc.gov/nchs/fastats/teen-births.htm. Accessed September 3, 2014.

[42] Carolan, M. Maternal age >45 years and maternal and perinatal outcomes: A review of the evidence. *Midwifery* 29:479–489, 2013.

[43] Pediatric and Pregnancy Nutrition Surveillance System, Centers for Disease Control and Prevention. *Maternal Health Indicators.* Available online at www.cdc. gov/pednss/what_is/pnss_health_indicators.htm#Maternal%20Health%20Indicators. Accessed February 26, 2014.

[44] National Down Syndrome Congress. *Down Syndrome Facts.* Available online at http://ndsccenter.org/worpsite/wp-content/uploads/2012/09/Down-Syndrome-Facts.pdf. Accessed February 24, 2014.

[45] American College of Obstetricians and Gynecologists. ACOG Committee Opinion No. 462: Moderate caffeine consumption during pregnancy. *Obstet Gynecol* 116 (2 Pt 1):467–468, 2010.

[46] U.S. Department of Agriculture and U.S. Department of Health and Human Services. *Dietary Guidelines for Americans, 2010,* 7th ed., Washington, DC: U.S. Government Printing Office, 2010.

[47] Mayo Clinic Staff. *Pregnancy nutrition: Foods to avoid during pregnancy.* Mayo Clinic. Available online at http://www.mayoclinic.org/healthy-living/pregnancy-weekby- week/in-depth/pregnancy-nutrition/art-20043844. Accessed March 15, 2014.

[48] Lamont, R.F., Sobel, J., Mazaki-Tovi, S., et al. *Listeriosis* in human pregnancy: A systematic review. *J Perinat Med* 39:227–236, 2011.

[49] U.S. Food and Drug Administration, Center for Food Safety and Nutrition. *Bad Bug Book* (2nd ed.). *Foodborne Pathogenic Microorganisms and Natural Toxins Handbook.* Available online at http://www.fda.gov/food/foodborneillnesscontaminants/causesofillnessbadbugbook/default.htm. Accessed February 18, 2014.

[50] National Toxicology Program. *Toxoplasmosis.* Available online at http://cerhr.niehs.nih.gov/common/toxoplasmosis.html. Accessed February 26, 2014.

[51] Goodlett, C.R., Horn, K.H., and Zhou, F.C. Alcohol teratogenesis: Mechanisms of damage and strategies for intervention. *Exp Biol Med (Maywood)* 230:394–406, 2005.

[52] Riley, E.P., Infante, M.A., and Warren, K.R. Fetal alcohol spectrum disorders: An overview. *Neuropsychol Rev* 21:73–80, 2011.

[53] May, P.A., Gossage, J.P., Kalberg, W.O., et al. Prevalence and epidemiologic characteristics of FASD from various research methods with an emphasis on recent in-school studies. *Devel Disabil Res Rev* 15:176–192, 2009.

[54] Rogers, J.M. Tobacco and pregnancy. *Reprod Toxicol* 28:152–160, 2009.

[55] Clifford, A., Lang, L., and Chen, R. Effects of maternal cigarette smoking during pregnancy on cognitive parameters of children and young adults: A literature review. *Neurotoxicol Teratol* *34*:560–570, 2012.

[56] Xiao, D., Huang, X., Yang, S., and Zhang, L. Direct effects of nicotine on contractility of the uterine artery in pregnancy. *J Pharmacol Exp Ther* *322*:180–185, 2007.

[57] Task Force on sudden infant death syndrome; Moon, R.Y. SIDS and other sleep-related infant deaths: Expansion of recommendations for a safe infant sleeping environment. *Pediatrics* *128*:e1341–e1367, 2011.

[58] Burke, H., Leonardi-Bee, J., Hashim, A, et al. Prenatal and passive smoke exposure and incidence of asthma and wheeze: Systematic review and meta-analysis. *Pediatrics* *129*:735–744, 2012.

[59] Behnke, M., and Smith, V.C.; Committee on Substance Abuse; Committee on Fetus and Newborn. Prenatal substance abuse: Short- and long-term effects on the exposed fetus. *Pediatrics* *131*:e1009–e1024, 2013.

[60] Schempf, A.H. Illicit drug use and neonatal outcomes: A critical review. *Obstet Gynecol Surv* *62*:749–757, 2007.

[61] Fajemirokun-Odudeyi, O., and Lindow, S.W. Obstetric implications of cocaine use in pregnancy: A literature review. *Eur J Obstet Gynecol Reprod Biol* *112*:2–8, 2004.

[62] Innis, S.M. Impact of maternal diet on human milk composition and neurological development of infants. *Am J Clin Nutr* *99*:734S–741S, 2014.

[63] Allen, L.H. B vitamins in breast milk: Relative importance of maternal status and intake, and effects on infant status and function. *Adv Nutr* *3*:362–369, 2012.

[64] Ballard, O., and Morrow, A.L. Human milk composition: nutrients and bioactive factors. *Pediatr Clin North Am* *60*:49–74, 2013.

[65] Centers for Disease Control and Prevention. *Growth Charts: WHO Growth Standards Are Recommended for Use in the U.S. for Infants and Children 0 to 2 Years of Age.* Available online at http://www.cdc.gov/growthcharts/who_charts.htm#The%20WHO%20Growth%20Charts. Accessed March 30, 2014.

[66] Adair, L.S. Long-term consequences of nutrition and growth in early childhood and possible preventive interventions.

Nestle Nutr Inst Workshop Ser 78:111–120, 2014.

[67] Victora, C.G., Adair, L., Fall, C., et al. Maternal and Child Undernutrition Study Group. Maternal and child undernutrition: consequences for adult health and human capital. *Lancet* *371*:340–357, 2008.

[68] Wagner, C.L., and Greer, F.R. American Academy of Pediatrics Section on Breastfeeding, American Academy of Pediatrics Committee on Nutrition. Prevention of rickets and vitamin D deficiency in infants, children, and adolescents. *Pediatrics* *122*:1142–1152, 2008.

[69] American Academy of Pediatrics, policy statement, Committee on Fetus and Newborn. Controversies concerning vitamin K and the newborn. *Pediatrics* *112*:191–192, 2003.

[70] Guesnet, P., and Alessandri, J.M. Docosahexaenoic acid (DHA) and the developing central nervous system (CNS)—Implications for dietary recommendations. *Biochimie* *93*:7–12, 2011.

[71] Kramer, M.S., Aboud, F., Mironova, E., et al. Promotion of Breastfeeding Intervention Trial (PROBIT) Study Group Breastfeeding and child cognitive development: New evidence from a large randomized trial. *Arch Gen Psychiatry* *65*:578–584, 2008.

[72] Tai, E.K., Wang, X.B., and Chen, Z.Y. An update on adding docosahexaenoic acid (DHA) and arachidonic acid (AA) to baby formula. *Food Funct* *4*:1767–1775, 2013.

[73] Lapillonne, A., Groh-Wargo, S., Gonzalez, C.H., and Uauy, R. Lipid needs of preterm infants: Updated recommendations. *J Pediatr* *162* (3 Suppl.):S37–S47, 2013.

[74] Hoffman, D.R., Boettcher, J.A., and Diersen-Schade, D.A. Toward optimizing vision and cognition in term infants by dietary docosahexaenoic and arachidonic acid supplementation: A review of randomized controlled trials. *Prostaglandins, Leukot Essent Fatty Acids* *81*:151–158, 2009.

[75] Birch, E.E., Garfield, S., Castañeda, Y., et al. Visual acuity and cognitive outcomes at 4 years of age in a double-blind, randomized trial of long-chain polyunsaturated fatty acid-supplemented infant formula. *Early Hum Dev* *83*:279–284, 2007.

[76] Qawasmi, A., Landeros-Weisenberger, A., Leckman, J.F., and Bloch, M.H. Meta-analysis of long-chain

polyunsaturated fatty acid supplementation of formula and infant cognition. *Pediatrics* *129*:1141–1149, 2012.

[77] Simmer, K., Patole, S.K., and Rao, S.C. Long-chain polyunsaturated fatty acid supplementation in infants born at term. *Cochrane Database Syst Rev* 7:CD000376, 2011.

[78] Qawasmi, A., Landeros-Weisenberger, A., and Bloch, M.H. Meta-analysis of LCPUFA supplementation of infant formula and visual acuity. *Pediatrics* *131*:e262–e272, 2013.

[79] Gale, C.R., Marriott, L.D., Martyn, C.N., et al. Group for Southampton Women's Survey Study. Breastfeeding, the use of docosahexaenoic acid-fortified formulas in infancy and neuropsychological function in childhood. *Arch Dis Child* *95*:174–179, 2009.

[80] Makrides, M., Smithers, L.G., and Gibson, R.A. Role of long-chain polyunsaturated fatty acids in neurodevelopment and growth. *Nestle Nutr Workshop Ser Pediatr Program* *65*:123–133, 2010.

[81] Section on Breastfeeding. Breastfeeding and the use of human milk. *Pediatrics* *129*:e827–e841, 2012.

[82] Greer, F.R., Sicherer, S.H., and Burks, A.W. Effects of early nutritional interventions on the development of atopic disease in infants and children: The role of maternal dietary restriction, breastfeeding, timing of introduction of complementary foods, and hydrolyzed formulas. *Pediatrics* *121*:183–191, 2008.

[83] Ziegler, E.E. Adverse effects of cow's milk in infants. *Nestle Nutr Workshop Ser Pediatr Program* *60*:185–196, 2007.

[84] American Academy of Pediatrics. Policy Statement: The use and misuse of fruit juice in pediatrics. *Pediatrics* *107*:1210–1213, 2001. Reaffirmed August 2013.

Chapter 12

[1] Institute of Medicine, Food and Nutrition Board. *Dietary Reference Intakes for Energy, Carbohydrate, Fiber, Fat, Protein, and Amino Acids.* Washington, DC: National Academies Press, 2002.

[2] Institute of Medicine, Food and Nutrition Board. *Dietary Reference Intakes for Water, Potassium, Sodium, Chloride, and Sulfate.* Washington, DC: National Academies Press, 2004.

[3] Butte, N.F., Fox, M.K., Briefel, R.R., et al. Nutrient intakes of US infants, toddlers, and preschoolers meet or exceed

dietary reference intakes. *J Am Diet Assoc 110* (12 Suppl.):S27–S37, 2010.

4 Fox, M.K., Condon, E., Briefel, R.R., et al. Food consumption patterns of young preschoolers: Are they starting off on the right path? *J Am Diet Assoc 110* (12 Suppl):S52–S59, 2010.

5 Ogata, B.N., and Hayes, D. Position of the Academy of Nutrition and Dietetics: Nutrition guidance for healthy children ages 2 to 11 years. *J Am Diet Assoc 114*:1257–1276, 2014.

6 Food and Nutrition Board, Institute of Medicine. *Dietary Reference Intakes for Calcium and Vitamin D.* Washington, DC: National Academies Press, 2011.

7 Kumar, J., Muntner, P., Kaskel, F.J., et al. Prevalence and associations of 25-hydroxyvitamin D deficiency in US children: NHANES 2001-2004. *Pediatrics 124*:e362–e370, 2009.

8 Madan, N., Rusia, U., Sikka, M., et al. Developmental and neurophysiologic deficits in iron deficiency in children. *Indian J Pediatr 78*:58–64, 2011.

9 U.S. Department of Agriculture and U.S. Department of Health and Human Services. *Dietary Guidelines for Americans, 2010,* 7th ed. Washington, DC: U.S. Government Printing Office, 2010.

10 American Academy of Pediatrics. The use and misuse of fruit juice in pediatrics. *Pediatrics 107*:1210–1213, 2001.

11 Patrick, H., and Nicklas, T.A. A review of family and social determinants of children's eating patterns and diet quality. *J Am Coll Nutr 24*:83–92, 2005.

12 U.S. Department of Health and Human Services, Centers for Disease Control and Prevention, National Center for Health Statistics. *Growth Charts.* Available online at www.cdc.gov/growthcharts. Accessed March 7, 2014.

13 Rampersaud, G.C., Pereira, M.A., Girard, B.L., et al. Breakfast habits, nutritional status, body weight, and academic performance in children and adolescents. *J Am Diet Assoc 105*: 743–760, 2005.

14 Alaimo, K., Olson, C., and Frongillo, E. Food insufficiency and American school-aged children's cognitive, academic, and psychosocial development. *Pediatrics 108*:44–53, 2001.

15 Adolphus, K., Lawton, C.L., and Dye, L. The effects of breakfast on behavior and academic performance in children and adolescents. *Front Hum Neurosci 7*:425, 2013.

16 Kleinman, R.E., Hall, S., Green, H., et al. Diet, breakfast, and academic performance in children. *Ann Nutr Metab 46* (Suppl. 1):24–30, 2002.

17 Fisk, C.M., Crozier, S.R., Inskip, H.M., et al. Influences on the quality of young children's diets: The importance of maternal food choices. *Br J Nutr 105*:287–296, 2011.

18 U.S. Department of Agriculture, Food and Nutrition Service. *National School Lunch Program.* Available online at http://www.fns.usda.gov/sites/default/files/NSLPFactSheet.pdf. Accessed March 7, 2014.

19 U.S. Department of Agriculture, Food and Nutrition Service. Nutrition standards in the National School Lunch and School Breakfast Programs. Final Rule. *Federal Register 77*(17):4087–4167, January 26, 2012.

20 U.S. Department of Agriculture, Food and Nutrition Service. National School Lunch and School Breakfast Program: Nutrition standards for all foods sold in school as required by the Healthy, Hunger-Free Kids Act of 2010. Interim Final Rule. *Federal Register 78*(125): 39068–39120, June 28, 2013.

21 Hiza, H.A.B., Guenther, P.M., and Rihane, C.I. USDA Center for Nutrition Policy and Promotion. Diet quality of children 2–17 years as measured by the Healthy Eating Index-2010. *Nutrition Insight 52,* July 2013.

22 Centers for Disease Control and Prevention. *Basics about Childhood Obesity.* Available online at www.cdc.gov/obesity/childhood/defining.html. Accessed March 9, 2014.

23 Ogden, C.L. Carroll, M.D., Kit, B.K., and Flegal, K.M. Prevalence of childhood and adult obesity in the United States, 2011–2012. *JAMA 311*:806–814, 2014.

24 American Heart Association. *Cholesterol and Atherosclerosis in Children.* Updated August 7, 2012. Available online at http://www.heart.org/HEARTORG/GettingHealthy/NutritionCenter/Cholesterol-and-Atherosclerosis-in-Children_UCM_305952_Article.jsp. Accessed June 18, 2014.

25 Expert Panel on Integrated Guidelines for Cardiovascular Health and Risk Reduction in Children and Adolescents; National Heart, Lung, and Blood Institute. Expert panel on integrated guidelines for cardiovascular health and risk reduction in children and adolescents:

Summary report. *Pediatrics 128* (Suppl. 5):S213–S256, 2011.

26 Barlow, S.E.; Expert Committee. Expert Committee recommendations regarding the prevention, assessment, and treatment of child and adolescent overweight and obesity: summary report. *Pediatrics 120* (Suppl. 4):S164–S192, 2007.

27 Costa, S.M., Horta, P.M., and dos Santos, L.C. Food advertising and television exposure: Influence on eating behavior and nutritional status of children and adolescents. *Arch Latinoam Nutr 62*:53–59, 2012.

28 *Let's Move! America's Move to Raise a Healthy Generation of Kids. Get Active.* Available online at http://www.lets-move.gov/get-active. Accessed April 8, 2014.

29 Braithwaite, I., Stewart, A.W., Hancox, R.J., et al.; ISAAC Phase Three Study Group. The worldwide association between television viewing and obesity in children and adolescents: Cross sectional study. *PLoS One 8*:e74263, 2013.

30 Batada, A., Seitz, M., Wotan, M., et al. Nine out of ten food advertisements shown during Saturday morning children's television programming are for food high in fat, sodium, or added sugars, or low in nutrients. *J Am Diet Assoc 108*:673–678, 2008.

31 Centers for Disease Control and Prevention. *Attention Deficit/Hyperactivity Disorder. Data and Statistics.* Available online at http://www.cdc.gov/ncbddd/adhd/data.html. Accessed March 9, 2014.

32 Millichap, J.G., and Yee, M.M. The diet factor in attention-deficit/hyperactivity disorder. *Pediatrics 129*:330–337, 2012.

33 Centers for Disease Control and Prevention (CDC). Blood lead levels in children aged 1–5 years—United States, 1999–2010. *MMWR Morb Mortal Wkly Rep 62*:245–248, 2013.

34 Weng, F.L., Shults, J., Leonard, M.B., et al. Risk factors for low serum 25-hydroxyvitamin D concentrations in otherwise healthy children and adolescents. *Am J Clin Nutr 86*:150–158, 2007.

35 Turer, C.B., Lin, H., and Flores, G. Prevalence of vitamin D deficiency among overweight and obese U.S. children. *Pediatrics 131*:e152–e161, 2013.

36 Centers for Disease Control and Prevention (CDC). Iron deficiency—United States, 1999–2000. *MMWR Morb Mortal Wkly Rep 51*:897–899, 2002. Available

Zone (40°–140°)". Available online at http://www.fsis.usda.gov/wps/wcm/connect/8b705ede-f4dc-4b31-a745-836e66eeb0f4/Danger_Zone.pdf?MOD=AJPERES. Accessed April 12, 2014.

22 U.S. Food and Drug Administration. *Pesticide Monitoring Program. 2011 Pesticide Report.* Available online at http://www.fda.gov/Food/FoodborneIllnessContaminants/Pesticides/UCM2006797.htm. Accessed April 5, 2014.

23 U.S. Environmental Protection Agency. *Pesticides: Topical & Chemical Fact Sheets.* Available online at www.epa.gov/pesticides/factsheets/index.htm. Accessed April 5, 2014.

24 U.S. Environmental Protection Agency. *Setting Tolerances for Pesticide Residues in Foods.* Available online at www.epa.gov/pesticides/factsheets/stprf.htm. Accessed April 5, 2014.

25 Organic Trade Association. *2013 Organic Industry Survey.* 2013. Available online at http://insidepenton.com/OTAIndustrySurvey%20Questions.pdf. Accessed September 7, 2014.

26 Crinnion, W.J. Organic foods contain higher levels of certain nutrients, lower levels of pesticides, and may provide health benefits for the consumer. *Altern Med Rev 1*:4–12, 2010.

27 Mukherjee, A., Speh, D., Dyck, E., et al. Preharvest evaluation of coliforms, *Escherichia coli, Salmonella,* and *Escherichia coli* O157:H7 in organic and conventional produce grown by Minnesota farmers. *J Food Prot 67*:894–900, 2004.

28 Dangour, A.D., Lock, K., Hayter, A., et al. Nutrition-related health effects of organic foods: A systematic review. *Am J Clin Nutr 92*:203–210, 2010.

29 Dangour, A.D., Dodhia, S.K., Hayter, A., et al. Nutritional quality of organic foods: A systematic review. *Am J Clin Nutr 90*:680–685, 2009.

30 U.S. Department of Agriculture, Agricultural Marketing Service. *National Organic Program.* Available online at www.ams.usda.gov/AMSv1.0/ams.fetchTemplateData.do?template=TemplateA&navID=NationalOrganicProgram&leftNav=NationalOrganicProgram&page=NOPNationalOrganicProgramHome&acct=AMSPW. Accessed April 5, 2014.

31 U.S. Department of Health and Human Services and U.S. Environmental Protection Agency. *What You Need to Know about Mercury in Fish and Shellfish,* March

2004. Available online at www.fda.gov/Food/ResourcesForYou/Consumers/ucm110591.htm. Accessed September 8, 2014.

32 International Food Information Council. *Fact Sheet: FDA's Approval Process for Food Animal Antibiotics: A Focus on Human Food Safety,* April 2011. Available online at www.foodinsight.org/Resources/Detail.aspx?topic=Fact_Sheet_FDA_s_Approval_Process_for_Food_Animal_Antibiotics. Accessed April 29, 2011.

33 U.S. Food and Drug Administration. *FDA takes significant steps to address antimicrobial resistance,* December 11, 2013. Available online at http://www.fda.gov/AnimalVeterinary/NewsEvents/CVMUpdates/ucm378166.htm. Accessed April 5, 2014.

34 U.S. Food and Drug Administration. *Report on the U.S. Food and Drug Administration's Review of the Safety of Recombinant Bovin Somatotropin.* April 23, 2009. Available online at http://www.fda.gov/animalveterinary/safetyhealth/productsafetyinformation/ucm130321.htm. Accessed April 4, 2014.

35 Riboldi, B.P., Vinhas, A.M., and Moreira, J.D. Risks of dietary acrylamide exposure: A systematic review. *Food Chem 157*: 310–322, 2014.

36 Pedreschi, F., Mariotti, M.S., and Granby, K. Current issues in dietary acrylamide: Formation, mitigation and risk assessment. *J Sci Food Agric 94*:9–20, 2014.

37 U.S. Food and Drug Administration. *U.S. Regulatory Requirements for Irradiating Foods.* May 1999. Available online at http://www.fda.gov/Food/GuidanceRegulation/GuidanceDocumentsRegulatoryInformation/IngredientsAdditivesGRASPackaging/ucm110730.htm. Accessed April 5, 2014.

38 Osterholm, M.T., and Norgan, A.P. The role of irradiation in food safety. *N Engl J Med 350*:1898–1901, 2004.

39 U.S. Department of Health and Human Services. National Institute of Environmental Health Sciences. *Bisphenol A (BPA): Questions and Answers About Bisphenol A.* Available online at http://www.niehs.nih.gov/health/topics/agents/sya-bpa/. Accessed June 24, 2014.

40 Sindelar, J.J., and Milkowski, A.L. Human safety controversies surrounding nitrate and nitrite in the diet. *Nitric Oxide 26*:259–266, 2012.

41 U.S. Food and Drug Administration, International Food Information Center. *Overview of Food Ingredients, Additives, and Colors.* November, 2004; Revised April, 2010. Available online at http://www.fda.gov/Food/IngredientsPackagingLabeling/FoodAdditivesIngredients/ucm094211.htm. Accessed April 7, 2014.

42 U.S. Food and Drug Administration, *Everything Added to Food in the United States (EAFUS),* November, 2011. Available online at http://www.fda.gov/Food/IngredientsPackagingLabeling/FoodAdditivesIngredients/ucm115326.htm. Accessed April 7, 2014.

43 Margawati, E.T. *Transgenic Animals: Their Benefits to Human Welfare.* Available online at www.actionbioscience.org/biotech/margawati.html. Accessed March 21, 2009.

44 Paine, J.A., Shipton, C.A., Chaggar, S., et al. Improving the nutritional value of golden rice through increased pro-vitamin A content. *Nat Biotechnol 23*:482–487, 2005.

45 Sayre, R., Beeching, J.R., Cahoon, E.B., et al. The BioCassava Plus Program: Biofortification of cassava for sub-Saharan Africa. *Annu Rev Plant Biol 62*:251–272, 2011.

46 Gonsalves, D., and Ferreira, S. *Transgenic Papaya: A Case for Managing Risks of Papaya Ringspot Virus in Hawaii.* Available online at www.plantmanagementnetwork.org/pub/php/review/2003/papaya. Accessed April 7, 2014.

47 Smith, N. *Seeds of Opportunity: An Assessment of the Benefits, Safety and Oversight of Plant Genomics and Agricultural Biotechnology.* U.S. House of Representatives report, April 13, 2000. Available online at www.nicksmithconsulting.com/opportunity.pdf. Accessed April 7, 2014.

48 Tang, G., Hu, Y., Yin, S.A., et al. ß-Carotene in Golden Rice is as good as ß-carotene in oil at providing vitamin A to children. *Am J Clin Nutr 96*:658–664, 2012.

49 Nordlee, J.A., Taylor, S. L., Townsend, J. A., et al. Identification of a Brazil-nut allergen in transgenic soybeans. *N Engl J Med 334*:688–692, 1996.

50 Clive, J. Global Status of Commercialized Biotech/GM Crops: 2012. ISAAA Brief No. 44. ISAAA: Ithaca, NY, 2012.

51 U.S. Food and Drug Administration. *Submissions on Bioengineered New Plant Varieties.* Available online at http://www.fda.gov/Food/FoodScienceResearch/

Biotechnology/Submissions/. Accessed September 8, 2014.

Chapter 14

[1] Food and Agriculture Organization of the United Nations. *The State of Food Insecurity in the World 2013, The multiple dimensions of food security.* Available online at www.fao.org/docrep/018/i3434e/i3434e00.htm. Accessed April 2, 2014.

[2] Black, R.E., Victora, C.G., Walker, S.P., et al.; Maternal and Child Nutrition Study Group. Maternal and child undernutrition and overweight in low-income and middle-income countries. *Lancet* 382:427–451, 2013.

[3] World Health Organization. *2008–2013 Action Plan for the Global Strategy for the Prevention and Control of Noncommunicable Diseases.* Available online at whqlibdoc.who.int/publications/2009/9789241597418_eng.pdf?ua=1. Accessed April 4, 2014.

[4] Central Intelligence Agency. Country comparison: Infant mortality rate. *The World Fact Book.* Available online at https://www.cia.gov/library/publications/the-world-factbook/rankorder/2091rank.html. Accessed October 24, 2014.

[5] World Health Organization. *Low Birth Weight: Country, Regional and Global Estimates.* Available online at whqlibdoc.who.int/publications/2004/9280638327.pdf?ua=1. Accessed April 6, 2014.

[6] World Health Organization. *Countdown to 2015 decade report (2000–2010): taking stock of maternal, newborn and child survival.* Available online at http://www.countdown2015mnch.org/documents/2010Report/2010_Report_noprofiles.pdf. Accessed June 25, 2014.

[7] United Nations Children's Fund, World Health Organization, The World Bank, *Joint Child Malnutrition Estimates* (UNICEF/WHO/World Bank). Available online at data.worldbank.org/child-malnutrition. Accessed April 10, 2014.

[8] Fall, C.H. Fetal programming and the risk of noncommunicable disease. *Indian J Pediatr 80* (Suppl. 1):S13–S20, 2013.

[9] World Health Organization. *Obesity and Overweight.* March 2013. Fact sheet no. 311. Available online at www.who.int/mediacentre/factsheets/fs311/en. Accessed June 25, 2014.

[10] Food and Agriculture Organization of the United Nations. *The Nutrition Transition and Obesity.* Available online at www.fao.org/FOCUS/E/obesity/obes2.htm. Accessed April 9, 2014.

[11] Kelly, T., Yang, W., Chen, C.-S., et al. Global burden of obesity in 2005 and projections to 2030. *Int J Obes (Lond) 32*:1431–1437, 2008.

[12] Nikolic, I.A., Stanciole, A.E., and Zaydman, M. Chronic Emergency: Why NCDs Matter. *World Bank Health, Nutrition and Population Discussion Paper,* July, 2011.

[13] Vorster, H. H., Bourne, L. T., Venter, C. S., and Oosthuizen, W. Contribution of nutrition to the health transition in developing countries: A framework for research and intervention. *Nutr Rev* 57:341–349, 1999.

[14] The World Bank. *Poverty Overview.* Available online at www.worldbank.org/en/topic/poverty/overview. Accessed April 10, 2014.

[15] Population Reference Bureau. *2010 World Population Datasheet.* Available online at www.prb.org/pdf13/2013-population-data-sheet_eng.pdf. Accessed April 10, 2014.

[16] Albino, D.K., Bertrand, K.Z., and Bar-Yam, Y. Food for fuel: The price of ethanol. arXiv:1210.6080, October 4, 2012. Available online at necsi.edu/research/social/foodprices/foodforfuel/. Accessed April 18, 2014.

[17] IFAD Policy Report. *Price Volatility in Food and Agricultural Markets: Policy Responses.* Available online at www.ifad.org/operations/food/documents/g20.pdf. Accessed April 10, 2014.

[18] Le Cotty, T., and Dorin, B. A global foresight on food crop needs for livestock. *Animal* 6:1528–1536, 2012.

[19] Steinfeld, H., Gerber, P., Wassenaar, T., et al. Livestock's long shadow: Environmental Issues and Options, 2006. Available online at meteo.lcd.lu/globalwarming/FAO/livestocks_long_shadow.pdf. Accessed April 18, 2014.

[20] World Health Organization. *Preventing and Controlling Micronutrient Deficiencies in Populations Affected by an Emergency.* Available online at www.who.int/nutrition/publications/WHO_WFP_UNICEFstatement.pdf. Accessed April 12, 2014.

[21] Bhutta, Z.A., Salam, R.A., and Das, J.K. Meeting the challenges of micronutrient malnutrition in the developing world. *Br Med Bull 106*:7–17, 2013.

[22] World Health Organization. *Micronutrient Deficiencies: Iodine Deficiency Disorders.* Available online at www.who.int/nutrition/topics/idd/en/index.html. Accessed April 12, 2014.

[23] World Health Organization. *Micronutrient Deficiencies: Iron Deficiency Anemia.* Available online at www.who.int/nutrition/topics/ida/en. Accessed April 12, 2014.

[24] World Health Organization. *Micronutrient Deficiencies: Vitamin A Deficiency.* Available online at www.who.int/nutrition/topics/vad/en. Accessed April 12, 2014.

[25] Coleman-Jensen, A., Nord, M., and Singh, A. Household Food Security in the United States in 2012. *Economic Research Report* No. ERR-155, U.S. Department of Agriculture, Economic Research Service, September 2013. Available online at www.ers.usda.gov/publications/err-economic-research-report/err155.aspx#.U0nxJuZdUqo. Accessed April 12, 2014.

[26] U. S. Census Bureau. *About Poverty 2012 Highlights.* Available online at www.census.gov/hhes/www/poverty/about/overview/index.html. Accessed April 13, 2014.

[27] Centers for Disease Control and Prevention. *A Look inside Food Deserts.* Available online at www.cdc.gov/Features/fooddeserts. Accessed April 13, 2014.

[28] Hampton, T. Food insecurity harms health, well-being of millions in the United States. *JAMA 298*:1851–1853, 2007.

[29] National Vital Statistics Report. Infant Mortality Statistics from the 2010 Period Linked Birth/Infant Death Data Set, December 18, 2013. Available online at www.cdc.gov/nchs/data/nvsr/nvsr62/nvsr62_08.pdf. Accessed April 13, 2014.

[30] U.S. Census Bureau. Table 676: Money income of households—distribution by income level and selected characteristics: 2009. *The 2012 Statistical Abstract.* Available online at www.census.gov/compendia/statab/2012/tables/12s0692.pdf. Accessed April 13, 2014.

[31] U.S. Department of Housing and Urban Development. *The 2013 Annual Homeless Assessment Report to Congress.* January 2013. Available online at www.onecpd.info/resources/documents/ahar-2013-part1.pdf. Accessed April 13, 2014.

Beta-cryptoxanthin (β-cryptoxanthin), 214
Beverages, 111f
    alcoholic, 428f. *See also* Alcohol
    for children and teens, 413f
    for optimizing performance, 351–354
Bicarbonate, 71, 72
Bigorexia, 324t
Bile, 73
Binge drinking, 416, 430
Binge-eating disorder, 318, 318t, 323, 323f
Bioaccumulation, 453
Bioavailability:
    of biotin, 201f
    of minerals, 249
    of vitamins, 190–191, 193
Biochemistry, 19f
Bioelectric impedance, 293f
Biofuels, 157
Biotechnology, 465–469
Biotin, 201, 213t
Birth control, 489f
Birth rate, 487–488
Bisphenol A, 462f
Blackout drinking, 431
Blindness, night, 217
Blood:
    circulation of, 82f
    diluting sodium level in, 350f
    heart disease and lipid level of, 143f
    restoring calcium level of, 263f
    transport of lipids in, 134–136
Blood alcohol levels, 429f
Blood cholesterol, of obese children, 408
Blood clotting, 227f
Blood flow, exercise and, 83f
Blood glucose, 97
    in diabetes, 107f
    managing, 109–110, 110f
    regulation of, 104f
Blood pressure, 241
    and diet, 254f–255f, 256
    high, 142f, 371, 408. *See also*
        Hypertension
    regulation of, 253f
Blood vessels, diabetes complications and,
    109f
BMI (body mass index), 291–293, 292f
BMR (basal metabolic rate), 297
Body:
    balance of water in, 241–242, 241f
    distribution of water in, 240–241, 240f
    electrolyte balance in, 252, 253
    as machine, 58–59
    pregnancy and changes in, 366–371
Body composition, 293, 293f, 334
Body fat:
    health and excess, 291, 291f
    and leptin, 305
    location of, 294f, 295
    subcutaneous, 295
    visceral, 295
Body image, 318, 319

Body mass index (BMI), 291–293, 292f
Body mass index-for-age percentiles, 407f
Body shape, 302–306, 302f, 320
Body size, 261t, 302–306, 320
Body temperature, 244, 244f
Body weight, 288–325. *See also related topics,*
    e.g.: Weight management
    determinants of size/shape and, 302–306
    and eating disorders, 317–325
    and energy balance, 295–301
    and energy expenditure, 345f
    and food choices, 309
    and health, 290–295
    healthy, 39f, 291–295
    ideal, 320
    long-term regulation of, 303–305
    and non-exercise activity thermogenesis,
        306, 306f
Bone, 259–263, 402, 403
Bone mass, 260f, 261
Bone remodeling, 261
Bone resorption, 264
Bottled water, 246
Bottle-feeding technique, 391f
Botulism, 444, 444f, 445
Bovine somatotropin (bST), 457, 457f
Bovine spongiform encephalopathy (BSE),
    447, 449
Bran, 94, 95f
Breakfast, school performance and, 405
Breast milk, 365, 391–395, 492f
    health benefits of feeding, 392–393, 393f
    nutrients in, 392, 392t
    production of, 384–385, 384f
Brush border, 71f
BSE (bovine spongiform encephalopathy),
    447, 449
bST (bovine somatotropin), 457, 457f
Bulimia nervosa, 318, 318t, 322–323, 322f
B vitamins, 206f. *See also specific vitamins*

C

Caffeine, 358, 359, 382
Caffeine toxicity, 358, 359
Calciferol, *see* Vitamin D
Calcitonin, 263
Calcitriol, *see* Vitamin D
Calcium, 263–266, 268t, 269
    adolescents' needs for, 413
    in breast milk vs. formula, 392t
    children's need for, 402
    in food, 264f
    and health/disease, 263–265
    meeting needs for, 265, 266
    pregnant women's need for, 373
Calcium pantothenate, *see* Pantothenic acid
Calcium supplements, 265f
Calories, 4
    balancing, 38–39
    empty, 46, 46f
    kilo-, 8, 11
Campylobacter jejuni, 442, 443f

Cancer, 145, 277, 446f
Canned food, 444f
Capillaries, 71f, 81
Carbohydrates, 92–123
    in breast milk vs. formula, 392t
    choosing foods with, 118–120
    complex, 97, 98
    defined, 8
    Dietary Reference Intakes for, 500t
    digestion and absorption of, 99–103, 99f
    effects of limiting, 106, 106f
    and endurance, 351f
    in food, 9f, 94–95
    functions of, 103–106
    health/disease and intake of, 107–115
    healthy, 117, 118f
    indigestible, 100–102
    meeting dietary needs for, 116–120
    percentage of calories from, 116f
    and physical activity, 347
    recommended intake of, 116–118
    and risk of diabetes, 110
    simple, 97
    structures and sources of, 96f–97f
    types of, 96–98
Carbohydrate loading, 351, 352
Carbohydrate-restricted diets, 313f
Cardiorespiratory endurance, 334
Cardiovascular disease, 140. *See also* Heart
    disease
Cardiovascular system, 62t, 81–84
    blood circulation in, 82f
    blood flow in, 83f
    and delivery of nutrients to liver, 84
    heart and blood vessels in, 82–83
Caries, dental, 111, 280, 411
Carotene, *see* Vitamin A
Carotenoids, 214. *See also* Vitamin A
Cash crops, 491
Cataracts, 424, 424f
Celiac disease, 76–78, 172
Cells:
    getting glucose to, 103–104
    organization in, 60, 60f
Cell differentiation, 216
Cellular respiration, 87, 105f
Cellulose, 97f, 115
Cesarean section, 368
Chemicals, in food, 453–459
Child and Adult Care Food Program, 495t
Childhood obesity, 407–410
Children, 402–411
    beverage choices of, 413f
    dietary supplements for, 230t
    energy and nutrient needs of, 402–403
    health concerns for, 407–411
    healthy eating habits of, 403–407
China, soil selenium in, 276f
Chinese restaurant syndrome, 172, 465
Chloride, 259t
Choice Lists, 47
Cholecalciferol, *see* Vitamin D

Dietary supplements (cont.)
  for fighting hunger, 493
  herbal, 230–233, 231f, 232t
  labels on, 52–54, 53f
  mineral, 230, 230t, 265f, 355, 356, 376, 376f
  need for, 230, 230t
  prenatal, 230t, 376, 376f
  protein, 176f
  vitamin, 230–235, 230t, 355, 376, 376f
  weight-loss, 314–315
Dieters, supplements for, 230t
Diet-induced thermogenesis, 297
Dieting, 308f, 313f
Differentiation, cell, 216
Diffusion, 73
Digestion, 66–85
  and absorption of nutrients, 73
  of carbohydrates, 99–102, 99f
  defined, 64
  and elimination of wastes, 84–85
  in gastrointestinal tract, 66–75
  and health/disease, 75–81
  of lipids, 133–134, 133f
  nutrient delivery after, 81–84
  of proteins, 162f, 163
Digestive system, 64–66. See also Gastrointestinal tract
  bacteria in, 74
  and disease prevention, 75–76
  disorders of, 78–80, 79f
  function of, 63t
  nutrition and changes in, 80
  organs of, 63t, 64
  secretions in, 64, 66
  structure of, 65f
Dihydroxy vitamin D, see Vitamin D
Dipeptides, 160f
Direct food additives, 462
Disaccharides, 96
Dispensable (nonessential) amino acids, 159, 160f
Diuretic, 247
Diverticula, 115
Diverticulitis, 115
Diverticulosis, 115f
DNA, recombinant, 466
Docosahexaenoic acid (DHA), 137f, 390
Down syndrome, 381, 381f
DRIs, see Dietary Reference Intakes
Drug use, in pregnancy, 383–384
Dual-energy X-ray absorptiometry (DXA), 293f
Dutch famine, 380f

E
EARs (Estimated Average Requirements), 34, 35f
Eating disorders, 317–325
  in adolescence, 416

anorexia nervosa, 318, 318t, 321–322, 321f
binge-, 318, 318t, 323, 323f
bulimia nervosa, 318, 318t, 322–323, 322f
causes of, 318–321, 319f
defined, 318
preventing and treating, 324–325
in special groups, 324
types of, 318, 318t
Eating habits:
  of children, 403–407
  in United States, 295–296
Eating patterns, healthy, 37t, 40f–41f, 41–42
Eating recommendations, 44
  for adolescents, 414
  carbohydrate, 120
  for children, 404
  and digestive health, 81
  environmentally friendly, 497
  and exercise, 352–354
  fat and cholesterol, 151
  and food safety, 459
  and healthy diet, 15
  for older adults, 425
  for pregnant women, 378
  protein, 179
  trace mineral, 280
  vitamin, 225
  water and electrolyte, 256
  and weight management, 308
Eclampsia, 371
Economic factors:
  and birth rate, 487, 488
  in food availability with, 491
  for older adults, 424, 427
Edema, 167f, 370
Education:
  and birth rate, 488
  nutrition, 491–492, 496
  and poverty, 485f
EERs, see Estimated Energy Requirements
EER prediction equations, 301t
EFNEP (Expanded Food and Nutrition Education Program), 495t
Eggs, 144, 201f, 440f–441f
Eicosanoids, 138
Eicosapentaenoic acid (EPA), 137f
Electrolytes, 251–259
  balance of, 252, 253
  deficiencies in, 253, 254
  defined, 251
  functions of, 252–253, 252f
  health/disease and intake of, 253–256
  meeting dietary needs for, 256–259
  for pregnant women, 373
  toxicity of, 254
Elements, 8
Elimination of wastes, 84–85, 85f
Embryo, 367
Emergency Food Assistance Program, 495t
Empty calories, 46, 46f

Emulsifiers, 131
Endocrine system, 63t
Endorphins, 331
Endosperm, 94, 95f
Endurance, 334, 351f, 359
Energy:
  from fat, 138–139
  from glucose, 105–106
  and metabolism, 87
  for physical activity, 345–346
  storing and retrieving, 300f
Energy balance, 295–301
  defined, 295
  energy intake and expenditures in, 297–300, 298f–299f
  Estimated Energy Requirements in, 300, 301t
  and storing/retrieving energy, 300f
  in United States, 295–297
Energy drinks, 358
Energy expenditure:
  and body weight, 345f
  in energy balance, 297–300
  and physical activity, 332f, 507f–508f
  TEE equations, 504t
  total, 297
Energy intake:
  and beverages, 111f
  decreasing, 308
  in energy balance, 297–300
  recommendations on, 36, 36f, 501t
Energy needs:
  of adolescents, 413
  of adults, 420
  of children, 402–403, 402f
  of infants, 388, 389f
  and lactation, 385–386, 385f
  and pregnancy, 372, 372f
Energy-yielding nutrients, 8
Enrichment, food, 94
Environment:
  about biotechnology, 468
  and body shape/size, 302–303
  food production and protection of, 488–491
  and food shortages, 481–482
  impact of overfishing on, 482f
Enzymes, 66, 66f
EPA (eicosapentaenoic acid), 137f
Epidemiological studies, 19f
Epidemiology, 20
Epiglottis, 67–68, 67f
Ergocalciferol, see Vitamin D
Ergogenic aids, 355–359
  for building muscle, 356–357
  for enhancing endurance, 359
  for enhancing performance, 357–359
  vitamin and mineral supplements, 355, 356
Escherichia coli, 442–444
Esophagus, 68

Prolactin, 384, 385
Proteases, 72
Proteins, 8, 156–185
    balancing intake and loss of, 173
    breakdown of, 106, 106f
    in breast milk vs. formula, 392t
    choosing foods with, 177–179
    complementary, 177–178
    complete and incomplete dietary, 177
    deficiency in, 170, 171f
    denaturation of, 161, 161f
    Dietary Reference Intakes for, 500t
    digestion and absorption of, 162f, 163
    in food, 9f, 158
    as fuel for exercise, 342
    functions of, 163–168, 167f
    health/disease and intake of, 168–172
    hydrolyzed, 172f
    meeting dietary needs for, 173–182
    and physical activity, 347
    recommended intake of, 174–176, 174f
    structure of, 159–161, 160f
    synthesis of, 163–165, 165f
    in vegetarian diets, 179–182
Protein complementation, 177f, 178
Protein-energy malnutrition (PEM), 170,
    171f
Protein hydrolysates, 172f
Protein quality, 177
Protein supplements, 176f
Prothrombin, 227f
Provitamins, 193
Provitamin A, see Vitamin A
Psychological issues, eating disorders and,
    318, 319
Psychosocial problems, of obese children,
    408
Pteroylglutamic acid, see Folate
PTH (parathyroid hormone), 221
Puberty, 412
Pull-by date, 449t
Pyridoxal phosphate, 201. See also Vitamin B$_6$
Pyridoxamine, see Vitamin B$_6$
Pyridoxine, see Vitamin B$_6$

Q

Qualified health claims, 52
Quality assurance date, 449t

R

Race, as osteoporosis risk factor, 261t
RAEs (retinol activity equivalents), 214
Rancidity, 129
RDAs, see Recommended Dietary Allowances
RDIs (Recommended Dietary Intakes), 506t
Reactive hypoglycemia, 110
Recombinant DNA, 466
Recommended Dietary Allowances (RDAs),
    30, 34, 35f
    for adolescents, 413
    of carbohydrates, 116
    for children, 402, 403

of minerals, 265, 266, 274, 277, 279
    for older adults, 413
    for pregnant women, 372–374
    of protein, 174–176
    of vitamins, 195, 200, 205, 211, 224
Recommended Dietary Intakes (RDIs), 506t
Record-keeping, for HAACP, 441f
Reduced (nutrient content claim), 51t
Reduced-fat diets, 313f
Reduced sodium, 258f
Refined foods, 92–94, 94f
Refined sugar, 95
Regulation:
    of biotechnology, 468
    of blood glucose, 104f
    of blood pressure, 253f
    of body weight, 303–305
    of food additives, 463, 465
    of food intake, 303–304, 304f
    of GM food products, 468–469, 468f
    by proteins, 165
    of protein synthesis, 164
    of stomach activity, 69, 70, 70f
    of water intake, 241–242
    of water loss, 242–243, 243f
Rehydration, 245f
Renewable resources, 481
Reproductive systems, 62t
Resistant starch, 100
Respiration, cellular, 87, 105f
Respiratory system, 62t
Resting heart rate, 334
Resting metabolic rate (RMR), 299f
Restricted diets, supplements and, 230t
Restrictive food intake disorder, 324t
Retailers, 440
Retail stores, 439f
Retinal, see Vitamin A
Retinoic acid, see Vitamin A
Retinoids, 214
Retinol, see Vitamin A
Retinol activity equivalents (RAEs), 214
Retinol-binding protein, 215
Retinyl palmitate, see Vitamin A
Reverse anorexia, 324t
Rhodopsin, 216, 217
Riboflavin, 198–199, 198f, 212t
Rice, golden, 494
Rickets, 221, 221f
RMR (resting metabolic rate), 299f

S

Saccharin, 113t
Saliva, 67
Salivary amylase, 67
Salmonella, 442, 443f
Salt, iodized, 279, 279f, 493f
Satiety, 303, 304f
Saturated fats, 8, 127, 129
Saturated fatty acids, 128f, 129–130
School:
    breakfast and performance in, 405
    meals for children at, 406, 407

School Breakfast Program, 495t
Scientific method, 18f, 19
Scurvy, 211
Secretions, 64, 66, 70f, 71–73
Segmentation, 71
Selective eating disorder, 324t
Selenium, 276–277, 276f, 283t
Self-esteem, 318
Sell-by date, 449t
Semivegetarian diet, 179t
Senior Farmers' Market Program, 495t
Set point, weight, 303
Shakespeare, William, 400–401
Short-term food aid, 487
SIDS (sudden infant death syndrome), 383
Simple carbohydrates, 97
Simple diffusion, 73
Skeletal system, 63t
Skinfold thickness, 293f
Small-for-gestational-age babies, 367
Small intestine, 71–73
    absorption in, 72f, 73, 73f
    digestion in, 72f
    immune function of, 75f
    lipid transport from, 134
    secretions in, 71–73
    structure of, 71f
Smoking:
    by adolescents, 416
    and dietary supplements, 230t
    and heart disease, 143f
    and osteoporosis, 261t
    in pregnancy, 383
Snacks:
    for children, 405–406, 406t
    and exercise, 353
SNAP (Supplemental Nutrition Assistance
    Program), 495t
Social issues, older adults', 424, 427
Sociocultural issues, eating disorders and,
    319–321
Soda, 262
Sodium, 259t
    blood, 350f
    in breast milk vs. formula, 392t
    on food labels, 258f
    iodized salt, 279, 279f, 493f
    in processed foods, 257f
Sodium chloride, 251
Sodium free, 258f
Soluble fiber, 98, 114f
Solutes, 240
Solvent, 243
Special Milk Program, 495t
Special Supplemental Nutrition Program for
    Women, Infants, and Children (WIC),
    380, 495t
Sphincter, 68
Spina bifida, 205f
Spores, bacterial, 444
Sports anemia, 348, 348f
Staphylococcus aureus, 444
Starch, 97, 97f, 98, 100